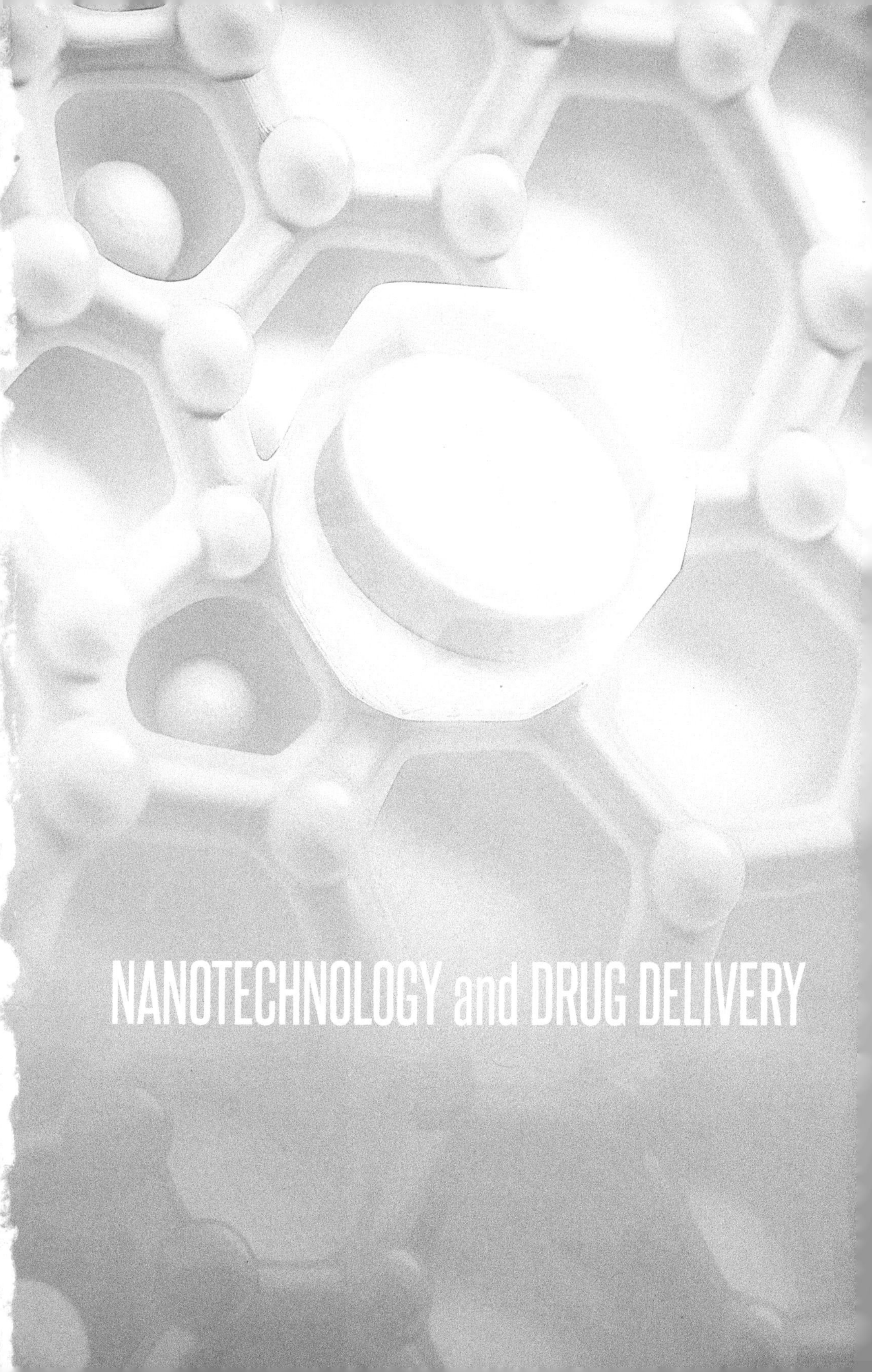

NANOTECHNOLOGY and DRUG DELIVERY

NANOTECHNOLOGY and DRUG DELIVERY

Principles and Applications

edited by

Rakesh K. Sindhu

JENNY STANFORD
PUBLISHING

Published by

Jenny Stanford Publishing Pte. Ltd.
101 Thomson Road
#06-01, United Square
Singapore 307591

Email: editorial@jennystanford.com
Web: www.jennystanford.com

British Library Cataloguing-in-Publication Data
A catalogue record for this book is available from the British Library.

Nanotechnology and Drug Delivery: Principles and Applications

ISBN 978-981-4968-83-6 (Hardcover)
ISBN 978-1-003-43040-7 (eBook)

Contents

Preface

Nanotechnology is playing a new role in creating innovative changes in different life sciences domains, such as biotechnology, drug delivery, agriculture, diagnostics, and allied health sciences.

This book's primary purpose is to serve as a reference textbook on the use of nanotechnology in the design and development of drug delivery systems and to highlight some of this field's most interesting advancements. In order to achieve this, the reader is exposed to several aspects of the principles of drug delivery systems based on nanotechnology as well as their applications. It is also discussed how these systems overcome the problems posed by biological barriers to drug absorption and therapeutic targeting. The book covers the following topics: fundamentals of nanotechnology in drug delivery; nanodrug delivery in therapeutics, including brain targeting, CVS targeting, arthritis, ocular, dermal drug delivery systems, etc.; and regulatory aspects of nanodrug delivery systems. It brings together reviews and unique writings from renowned experts in the interdisciplinary field of nanotechnology in drug delivery. Readers can gain a broad perspective on the new and ongoing potentialities of nanotechnology drug delivery applications based on their thorough and current experience.

I hope that this book will help the reader understand both these tools and the basic science behind them. Each part has been written by one or more well-known experts in the field, and there are a large number of figures and tables to help show the most important points. Many people helped me to finish this book, and I am very grateful to them. I extend my special thanks to the individual chapter contributors and the publisher.

Rakesh K. Sindhu, PhD

Chapter 1

Basics of Nanotechnology and Drug Delivery Systems

Rakesh K. Sindhu,[a] Kailash Rani,[b] Vibha Singh,[b] Yuvraj Singh,[b] Bhavya Hans,[b] M. Arockia Babu,[a] and Anju Goyal[b]

[a]*School of Pharmacy, Sharda University,*
Greater Noida, Gautam Buddha Nagar, Uttar Pradesh 201306, India
[b]*Chitkara College of Pharmacy, Chitkara University, Punjab 140401, India*

rakeshsindhu16@gmail.com

The combination of nanotechnology in medicine, especially medication delivery, is expected to grow substantially. Nanodrug delivery systems are a novel but fast-emerging discipline in which very tiny materials are used as diagnostics or to administer therapeutic drugs to particular targeted locations in a controlled manner. Nanotechnology has several advantages in the treatment of chronic human diseases through the site-specific and target-oriented delivery of precise medications. Interestingly, pharmaceutical scientists are employing nanoparticles to lower medication toxicity and adverse effects. Nanotechnology has the ability to improve the safety profile of medications with high hazardous potential, such as chemotherapeutic cancer treatments and other chronic diseases. As a result, it is a prominent advanced technology for dealing with biology and medicine for therapeutic objectives. In this book chapter, we explore the significance of

Nanotechnology and Drug Delivery: Principles and Applications
Edited by Rakesh K. Sindhu

ISBN 978-981-4968-83-6 (Hardcover), 978-1-003-43040-7 (eBook)
www.jennystanford.com

nanoscience, as well as several nanotechnology platforms employed in other sectors of medicine. In addition, we are looking at the potential applications of nanotechnology in human health.

1.1 Introduction

Nanotechnology is the process of making and employing structures, devices, and systems by changing the size and shape of nanoscale materials. Nanotechnology's innovation is the unique and frequently superior optical, electrical, mechanical, catalytic, and magnetic surface properties of nanostructures, which have fundamentally altered the number of scientific advances. The technique has been implemented in a variety of sectors, including the biomedical field, specifically for diagnostics, therapeutics, bio-imaging, and medication delivery [1]. Particularly nanotechnology-based drug delivery methods have swiftly overcome the challenges of conventional drug delivery systems, including accessibility, drug transport across biological barriers, bioavailability, limited solubility, *in vivo* instability, and undesirable pharmacological effects. According to nanotechnology, it is now possible to create novel pharmaceuticals. Nanotechnology, also known as nanomedicine, has been determined to be the most prevalent and commercially viable technology for improving healthcare procedures [3]. Despite considerable limitations, device businesses, such as pharmaceutical and medical device manufacturers, have been discovered to utilize nanotechnology in the medical industry in certain circumstances, nanotechnology can be utilized to provide drugs with a greater safety profile, such as cancer chemotherapy. Living cells function as virtual devices that participate in many biological processes, including metabolism, energy production, cell-to-cell communication, and nutrient translocation. Considering this, it can be stated that this technology is a strong competitor for usage in biological and medical therapeutic procedures [4].

Nanoscience is the only field that may collaborate with traditional fields, such as molecular chemistry, pharmacological research, healthcare, etc., to discover innovative characteristics in their respective fields [5]. Through the development of a more efficient healthcare system, nanomedicine technologies, and treatment techniques over the past few decades, science and technology have often been well-designed to handle problems in the field of medicine and health sciences (Table 1.1). Common nanoparticles employed as drug delivery vehicles are 100 nm in at least one dimension and consist of biodegradable components including natural or manufactured materials, polymers, lipids, and metals. As per nanotechnology, it is now possible to create novel pharmaceuticals [6].

Table 1.1 Timeline for the development of nanotechnology in medical science [4–7]

Year of innovation	Scientists	Biomedical engineering's advancement of nanotechnology
1857	Michael Faraday	Colloidal ruby gold nanoparticle
1905	Einstein	The size of the sugar molecule or mixture was 1 nm
1931	Max Knoll, Ernest Ruska	Utilized an electron transmission microscope
1953	Francis Crick and James Watson's	Discovery of DNA
1959	Richard Feynman	First nanotechnology presentation on "There's Plenty of Room at the Bottom"
1963	Stephen Papell	The invention of ferrofluids
1974	Norio Taniguchi	Recognized as the origin of the term "nanotechnology"
1977	Richard P. Van Duyne	Introduction of surface-enhanced Raman spectroscopy (SERS)
1981	Eric Drexler	"Molecular engineering" and IBM of scanning rotating microscope
1982	Nadrian Seeman	Development of the concept of DNA nanotechnology
1991	Sumio Iijima	The discovery of carbon nanoparticles
1993	Donald Bethune and Sumio Iijima	Introduced single-wall carbon nanotubes
1996	Chad Mirkin and Robert Letsinger	The exploration of DNA and gold colloids SAM

(*continued*)

Table 1.1 (*continued*)

Year of innovation	Scientists	Biomedical engineering's advancement of nanotechnology
1997	Zyvex	The first nanotechnology firm established
1999	Chad Mirkin	Created Dipped-pen nanolithography (DPN)
2000	Mark Hersam and Joseph Lyding	Feedback-Controlled Lithography (FCL)
2000	United States of America	Announced National nanotechnology effort
2001	Carlo Montemagno	Molecular nanomachines: molecular motor (rotor) utilizing nanoscale silicon devices
2002	Cees Dekker	Carbon nanotubes functionalized with DNA
2004	Royal Society	First report on the implications of nanotechnology
2006	John Paul Rothemund	DNA origami
2007	J. Fraser Stoddart	artificial molecular machines: pH-triggered muscle-like
2008	Martin Chalfie, Osamu Shimomura, and Roger Y. Tsien	The Green Fluorescent Protein (GFP) was awarded the Chemistry Nobel Prize for its discovery and development
2009	Nadrian Seeman	DNA structures fold into 3D rhombohedral crystals
2009	Drug Delivery	Initial use of nanoparticles to target cancerous tissue for drug administration *in vivo*
2016	*In Vivo* study	Analyzing the effects of nanoparticles on living organisms

1.2 Classification of Nanotechnology

Nanoparticles are often classified based on their chemical arrangement, size, state of matter, and shape [1]. Nanoparticles have a particle size range of 10–100 nm, the size of these particles could influence their physical and chemical properties, such as their optical qualities, as in the case of platinum, silver, palladium, and gold. Based on their dimensions, they are classified as 0D or 1D [2], the majority of NPs have characteristic colors which include yellowish-gray (platinum), black (silver), dark black (palladium), and wine red (gold).

The nanoparticle structure comprises three components:

- **Surface layer**: There are several tiny compounds, inorganic compounds, detergents, and macromolecules present.
- **Shell layer:** in this part, the structural component is chemically different.
- **Core:** This is the central portion of the nanoparticle, sometimes known as the nanoparticle (NP) itself [3].

1.3 Nanoparticles Types

It has been discovered that NPs can be employed in a variety of biological and healthcare systems, such as dosage forms, toxic and biological waste detection, as well as CO_2 capture, which have been shown to employ NPs [7] and based on their chemical characteristics, NPs are classified in three categories (Fig. 1.1).

1. Organic-based NPs
2. Inorganic-based NPs
3. Carbon-based NPs

1.3.1 Organic-Based Nanoparticles

Due to their unique properties, nanoparticles are only organic-based due to their unique characteristics, these nanoparticles are biodegradable and non-toxic, requiring a non-covalent interaction for their development and structure. This enables the transition of organic nanoparticles (NPs) into other desired forms such as dendrimers, liposomes, ferritin (polymer), and micelles (Fig. 1.2) related to their hollow cores, some of them are also called nanocapsules and sensitivity to thermal and electromagnetic radiation, also known as heat and light, respectively [8] because of their excellent qualities, they are an ideal material for drug delivery systems with a specific target.

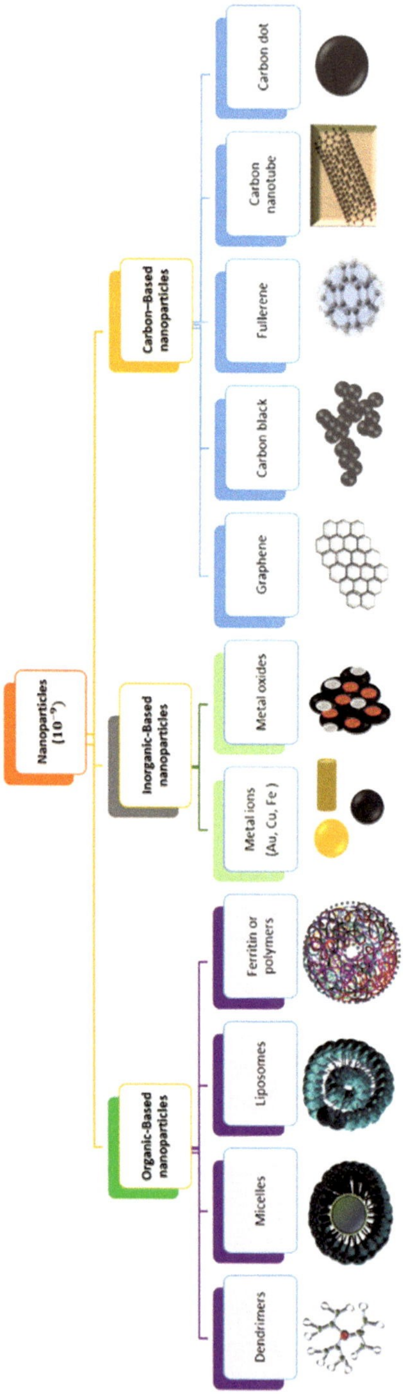

Figure 1.1 Nanoparticles (NPs) are categorized into three groups according to their chemical properties Organic-based, Inorganic-based, and Carbon-based.

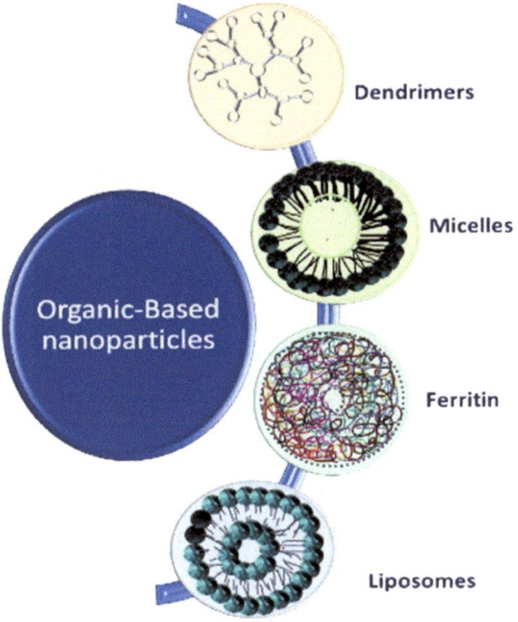

Figure 1.2 Organic-based nanoparticles, dendrimers, micelles, ferritin, and liposomes.

1.3.2 Inorganic-Based Nanoparticles

As the name implies, their structures lack carbon and they consist of inorganic substances such as metal ions (gold, iron, cobalt, zinc, aluminum, cadmium, lead) and metal oxides (Fig. 1.3). Amongst these NPs, many are metallic-primarily based NPs that are created utilizing nanometer-sized metals in two methods known as adverse and constructive [9] in the presence of air (oxygen), metal oxide NPs are generated, which results in the oxidation of metals to create various oxides, such as iron oxide, titanium dioxide, magnetite, silicon dioxide, cerium oxide, etc. On the other hand, certain inorganic NPs are particularly more sensitive to changes in the atmosphere's moisture, and sunlight and the sizes range from 10–100 nm, solid crystalline, and amorphous formations, and circular or tubular geometries, Numerous distinct traits include a high specific surface area ratio, pore, surface charge, and surface density.

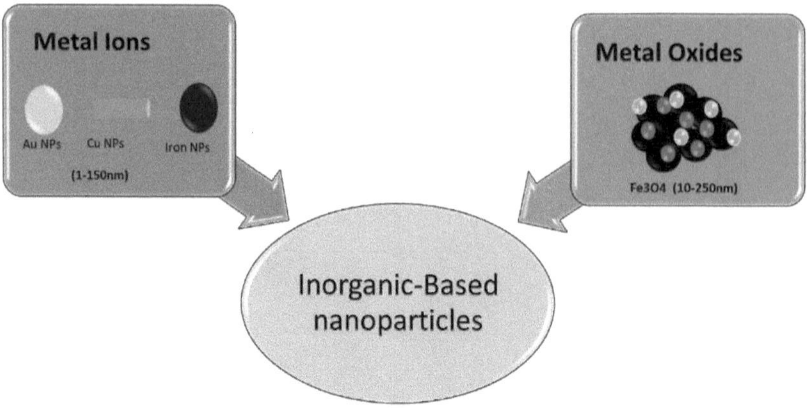

Figure 1.3 Inorganic-based nanoparticles, metal ions (gold, iron, Cu), and metal oxides (Iron oxide).

1.3.3 Carbon-Based Nanoparticles

As their name suggests, they're mostly carbon and the discovery of their unique qualities has led to their use in a wide range of industries, in case mechanical qualities, such as stability, conductivity, and so on, are just a few of their many physical and thermal characteristics [10]. They are classified into various types (Fig. 1.4).

- ***Graphene:*** Graphene is a carbon allotrope that is still being researched. It is used in the manufacture of solar panels, natural LEDs, and the preservation of hydrogen for fuels, supercapacitors, and membranes for gas separation, among others.
- ***Carbon black:*** Its carbon atoms are wound into hollow cylinders, as opposed to the graphene nanofoil, to produce single and multilayered carbon nanotubes of varying lengths that self-align under Van-der-Waals.
- ***Carbon nanotubes:*** Graphene nanofoils are used to create carbon nanofibers in the form of carbon nanotubes coiled into a cup or cone shape. They are employed as scanning electron microscope tips and reinforcement composites in electron emission [11].
- ***Fullerenes (C60) and Carbon dot.***

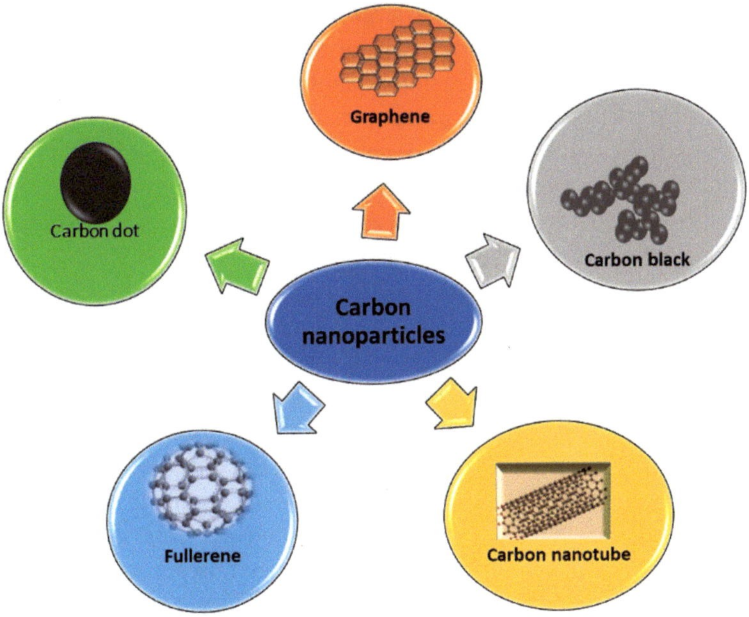

Figure 1.4 Carbon nanoparticles (graphene, carbon black, carbon nanotube, fullerene, and carbon dot.).

1.4 Application

- Contrast agents employed in diagnostic devices
- In the field of Cosmetics research dealing with anti-aging substances
- Used as Catalysts for water purification
- Used as Photovoltaics
- Used to convert methane
- Used in Electronics
- Used as Reinforcement for composites [12]

1.5 Importance of Nanoscale Materials

An essential aspect of nanotechnology for the vast majority of nanoscale constituents is to increase the surface area-to-volume ratio, this enables novel quantum mechanical results due to the "quantum size effect" [13], a large reduction in particle size can change the electrical properties of solids. For instance, due to electron entrapment causing quantum effects, nanoparticles typically exhibit unanticipated visual properties, such as gold nanoparticles, which seem deep red to black when mixed by applying nanoscale design to materials, microscopic and macroscopic features, such as melting temperature, magnetism, and charge capacity [14] can be modified without affecting the chemical ingredients. Theoretically, this should have no effect on the density of the final product, but flow difficulties and the ability of nanoparticles to aggregate create complications. Additionally, the surface action of NPs decreases the initial melting temperature [15], this scale chemistry offers advantages in catalysis due to its high ratio of surface area to volume, and interfacial surface chemistry that is essential for a variety of applications such as catalysis, composites, drug delivery, reactive systems, and energy deposits are excellent applications for nanoscale compounds. However, they are also employed in medicine, and the hue of gold NP varies upon resizing. Introducing green nanotechnology with various features, including enhanced wear resistance and antibacterial qualities even though there are still worries regarding potential health and environmental repercussions [17].

Nanoscale material is also used for material applications, as well as for the design of cleaner industrial processes [14], and the construction of sustainable objects may improve the environment with the unique and novel properties of nanostructured materials, nanotechnology can offer advantages with regard to the construction of catalysts, materials with enhanced strength, and material with reduced environmental impact. In the sectors of catalysis, medicine, solar energy conversion, and water purification [16, 17], these materials can also be employed to provide answers to technical and ecological concerns an important characteristic of molecular structures or biological entities in the body is their orderly nanoscale arrangement. Research and progress in nanotechnology made it possible to introduce tiny objects into living cells [24] through molecular self-assembly, this approach has also made it possible to analyze the micro- and macrostructure of matter. Undoubtedly, this is a highly capable instrument in materials science [18] for instance nanostructured macroscopic systems include enhancing the powder and hardness of nanoparticles and lightweight nanocomposites [14], as well as their compressive characteristics and moldability. Furthermore, such devices may be capable of mechanically changing molecular structures at the nanoscale [19]. In addition, nanosystems can have far greater densities than microstructures and are superior electrical conductors. This could drive the development of new electronic gadgets with more advanced functionality, smaller and faster circuitry, and dramatically decreased energy use. Simultaneously managing nanostructure interactions and their issues [17].

1.6 Design of Nanotechnology

Extensive study has been conducted on the cancer therapeutic uses of colloidal drug delivery systems such as liposomes, micelles, and nanoparticles, and several drug delivery techniques exist compact size, poor drug tolerability, controlled temporal release of the treatment, and alteration of drug pharmacology and physiological distribution. Chemotherapy may fail to treat the disease due to the expansion of cancer cells that develop resistance to anti-cancer medications when resistance develops in cancer cells, p-glycoprotein is able to pump anticancer drugs out of the cell as fast as they pass through the cell's outer membrane. Nanoparticles can be used to carry anticancer medications into cells without activating the p-glycoprotein pump. According to a recent study, new research indicates the effectiveness of paclitaxel-loaded nanoparticles in treating paclitaxel-resistant cancers of the human large intestine and paclitaxel-encapsulated emulsifying wax nanoparticles have also been proven to overcome drug resistance in a human colon glandular cancer cell line that is highly resistant (HCT-15), even though paclitaxel's insolubility difficulties can be solved by conjugating it with albumen, and it has showed biocompatibility with albumin, and other proteins (Abraxane-which is an injectable nanosuspension approved for the treatment of breast cancer). Previously, utilized in paclitaxel formulations, the solvent Chromophore-EL has been associated with acute hypersensitivity responses, and patients should be premedicated with corticosteroids and antihistamines prior to receiving paclitaxel, which should be taken slowly over the course of 2 h and paclitaxel binding to albumin has resulted in the rapid administration of a larger dose of the drug because it is solvent-free, toxicities associated with solvents are also removed. In a clinical investigation, the response rate of Abraxane was discovered to be double that of the medicine Taxol, which contains a solvent.

1.7 Nanomaterial Synthesis

1.7.1 Bottom-Up Approach

1.7.1.1 Arc-discharge

In the arc-discharge synthesis of nanomaterials [20], the discharge of the electrodes produces a fluid that is subsequently utilized to evaporate the electrode matter, and the material selected is dictated by the nanomaterial type required, for instance, graphite electrodes are used to produce carbon nanotubes (CNTs) and produced atomic vaporization will then condense into nanomaterial. CNTs are generated using the arc-discharge process in either gas or liquid-phase systems. certainly, this process was used to make the first CNTs, and it has since been utilized to create an assortment of other nanomaterials, such as silver, silica-coated iron nanoparticles [21], and gold nanoparticles [22].

1.7.1.2 Inert-gas condensation

During inert-gas condensation, metal atoms are evaporated at high temperatures into an inert carrier gas [23] by chilling the gas, a supersaturated vapor is produced, and particles nucleate uniformly across the gas stream as a result. A batch of particles forms and sinter before nucleation and sintering are terminated by further cooling the gas with a stream of gas, the quench gas, or a freezing surface, such as a "cold finger" filled with liquid nitrogen and the particles commonly form agglomerates at this stage, which, under the given conditions, are sufficiently "free" to be separated in a post-processing phase using this process, carbon black, silicon dioxide, and titanium dioxide have been generated [23].

1.7.1.3 Flame synthesis

Flame synthesis is the most common method for generating nanomaterials in commercial quantities [24], the flame synthesis method begins with the vaporization of a precursor in an inert-gas stream [25] before this gas combination is pumped into the flame, it is combined with fuel, and oxidant and nanomaterials are produced in flames, and their properties are dictated by the configuration and composition of the flame. In flame spray pyrolysis, precursors are dissolved in organic solvents that are flammable and then sprayed into a flame using flame synthesis, several nanopowders, including mixed oxides, nano-oxides, fullerenes, and nanotubes, have been created [24, 25].

1.7.1.4 Vapor-phase deposition

The two types of vapor deposition used to generate nanoparticles [26] are chemical vapor deposition (CVD) and physical vapor deposition (PVD) both process deposit components in the gas phase, which combine to form the necessary nanomaterials. Through the method of CVD, a precursor gas is sprayed over a substrate in a furnace, where it reacts chemically with the surfaces to form nanomaterials via deposition of the desired species, and CVD contains chemical interactions between precursors and substrates, as opposed to PVD, which uses just physical techniques to deposit materials without involving chemical processes. PVD and CVD are utilized to produce nanomaterials and deposit a thin coating on a variety of substrates, for instance, CVD is the primary process for creating sapphire crystals using it, and carbon nanotubes (CNTs) were also manufactured commercially [27] and physical structure of the substrate commonly influences the development of nanomaterials to regulate the growth of nanotubes, for instance, the substrate for CNT manufacturing can be composed exclusively of nanoparticles. Vapor-Liquid-Solid (VLS) is a CVD technique that deposits catalytic nanoparticles on the surface of a substrate, condenses the vapor into a liquid, and then solidifies the liquid. It has been used to create numerous types of nanowires, including III-V semiconductor nanowires [26].

1.7.1.5 Colloidal synthesis

Reducing the metal aggregates in dilute solutions is a popular technique for forming colloidal dispersions of metal nanomaterials [28] and the reduction process generates a supersaturated solution of metal atoms, which are then ignited to make nanoparticles, the clustering of these nanoparticles can be prevented by ensuring that the nanomaterial concentration is low or by coating the nanomaterials with a chemical that resists clumping, such as capping agents. In this procedure, Conventionally, chloroauric acid ($HAuCl_4$) is utilized to manufacture gold nanoparticles by slightly overdosing on sodium citrate [29] and sodium citrate transforms the acid's Au^{3+} ions into Au atoms since citrate ions are already present in the solution and can function as stabilizing agents, capping agents are not required for this synthesis. This technique yields a saturated solution of (nearly) spherical gold (Au) nanoparticles, Copper (Cu) nanoparticles can be created using similar methods; in this case, cupric chloride is reduced using hydrazine. However, the surfactant cetrimonium bromide (CTAB) is utilized as a separate capping agent to prevent particle clumping [29] in an endeavor to produce a homogeneous colloidal solution, the experimental conditions must be favorable enough to support diffusion-controlled development and this is made possible by controlling experimental variables such as localized concentration gradients, mixing durations, and temperature gradients. In contrast to reactions happening in equivalent conventional bulk systems, microfluidic reactors can be advantageous for microchannel-based reactions because they permit more precise control of experimental conditions [30, 31].

1.7.2 Synthesis: Top-Down Approach

1.7.2.1 Mechanical milling

Through the use of abrasion, bulk materials are broken down into smaller particles with diminished dimensions [32] and the mechanical milling process demands a great deal of effort and time (or days) to finish among the numerous types of mechanical milling, ball milling is frequently employed for the synthesis of different nanomaterials [33]. A ball mill consists of a revolving chamber partially filled with grinding medium, or balls, and the material to be ground and procedure generates heat, and when paired with mechanical polishing, chemical reactions may occur in different circumstances, this is useful SiO_2 is reduced by carbon in the mill to produce pure silicon nanoparticles and CO_2 during the manufacturing of silicon nanomaterials. For instance, iron oxidation in the presence of water results in the creation of Fe_2O_3 nanoparticles [34], and the size distribution and shape of the particles produced by ball milling are often fairly broad. Therefore, this approach to nanomaterial synthesis is excellent for some applications, such as nanocomposites, where size dispersion is not a concern. However, it is not suited for the synthesis of optical nanoparticles, for which single-mode size distribution and homogeneous shape features are particularly advantageous for optical applications.

1.7.2.2 Laser ablation

It is a technique that utilizes energy that is amplified by nanosecond pulses of laser light [35] to remove and vaporize material from a solid surface in order to create the necessary nanomaterials and this process involves the expulsion of ionized particles into a plume prior to their combination [36], these nanoparticles are capable of being deposited onto the substrate by the plume, and laser ablation is a procedure that can be carried out in the gas, vacuum, or liquid phase such materials are metals, metal oxides, semiconductors, etc.

1.8 Some Key Inventions and Discoveries

In 1985, around 41 years after Feynman's forecast, scientists Binnig, and Rohrer [38] at IBM's Zurich laboratory invented the scanning tunneling microscope (STM), and this was the largest advancement in nanotechnology. Rice paddies A group of IBM scientists using STM to create minute atomic characteristics.

As Feynman predicted [39], one example was the use of xenon atoms to spell "IBM" on a nickel surface. Under extremely controlled conditions, it took almost 24 h to produce the letters "IBM" (including vacuum and liquid He cooling) worth the effort. Moreover, the atoms are not bonded to the surface, they are merely adsorbed and this indicates that they were removed whenever there was a little change in pressure or temperature, to progress in the area of atomic-sized devices, it is necessary to examine this microcosmic ecosystem.

STM enables atomic-resolution imaging of solid surfaces [40] when a sharp tip is affixed to a piezo scanner and delivered to a conductive surface at around 1 nm, a tunneling current begins to flow (1F). In fact, STM can reveal the resolution at the level of individual atoms composing the surface and the creation of STM was followed by a rapid extension of his family of scanning probe microscope (SPM) techniques that are related to STM. In 1986 invention of the atomic force microscope (AFM) was by far the most significant of all the other techniques available at the time [41] and standard AFM is reportedly capable of producing ultra-high resolution line width features with a spatial resolution of 5 nm utilizing the DPN approach. The AFM provides the ability to inspect non-conductive surfaces with its "atomic" chip; van-der-Waals force can be felt, and AFM is comprised of a thin, cantilever-sharp probe tip (radius ~1–10 nm (F)), a piezoelectric 3D scanner, and optics for measuring the cantilever tip's deflection. When a tip touches, taps, or is placed on a surface, both attracting and repulsive surface forces are applied and these forces cause the cantilever to bend and twist. It is continuously measured by deflecting the laser beam that has been reflected. A 3D scanner shifted the specimen in a different design, a given surface area is scanned by moving the cantilever in three dimensions and this instrument has a vertical resolution of 0.01 nm (F), which is on the order of atomic radii, In the first decade of the 20th century, NPs were observed and measured for the first time and these observations were principally attributable to Zsigmondy, who released a book in 1914 after completing extensive research on gold sols and other nanomaterials with sizes <10 nm. In addition, he employed dark-field ultramicroscopy to view particles with sizes far smaller than the wavelengths of visible light and the creation of the scanning tunneling microscope in the 1980s and the discovery of carbon nanotubes and fullerenes marked the beginning of applications. In the 20th century, traditional approaches were established in the fields of interfacial and colloidal research in order to characterize nanobiomaterials widely employed in first-generation passive nanobiomaterials [37], one of the saturated hydrocarbons is the diamonded molecule, which has a fused ring structure similar to a diamond and is extremely valuable in nanotechnology.

1.9 Applications

Diagnosis, prevention, and therapy of numerous diseases have been the primary applications of nanotechnology.

1.9.1 Application in Medicine

Nanotechnology is seen as a promising field of application due to its unique properties that allow it to interact with bodily activities since living cells exist in nanoscale ranges, nanotechnology has a broad use in the field of medicine, and depending on the nature of nanotechnology, and the precision of its distribution, its applicability has increased dramatically. This has enabled numerous nanoscale inventions, including drug delivery, medical imaging at the molecular level, illness diagnosis, and other devices undergoing clinical testing [42, 43]. As it is still a highly competitive field, it is still undergoing development such developments will make it easier for patients to receive improved treatment for cancer, cardiovascular-related, etc. [44]. It has evolved into a centralized platform for assisting and developing several instruments in the fields of biology, medicine, chemistry, etc. Such activities have unlocked previously inaccessible dimensions for therapeutic therapies such as surgery, practice, and the treatment of a variety of ailments [45].

1.9.1.1 Application in drug delivery

There is currently a broad application of interest in nanotechnology for administering various therapeutic substances to their precise sites in order to demonstrate their effectiveness and treat a variety of illnesses (Fig. 1.5) [48], and various new medical discoveries have been made about drug delivery systems, however, there are still many challenges that must be handled before these systems can be used, and administered properly to deliver pharmaceuticals to a specific location, and many researchers are gaining an interest in the utilization of drug delivery systems, making this the main area of study and this enabled the creation of drug targeting techniques that account for the pathophysiological changes that occur during a sick state.

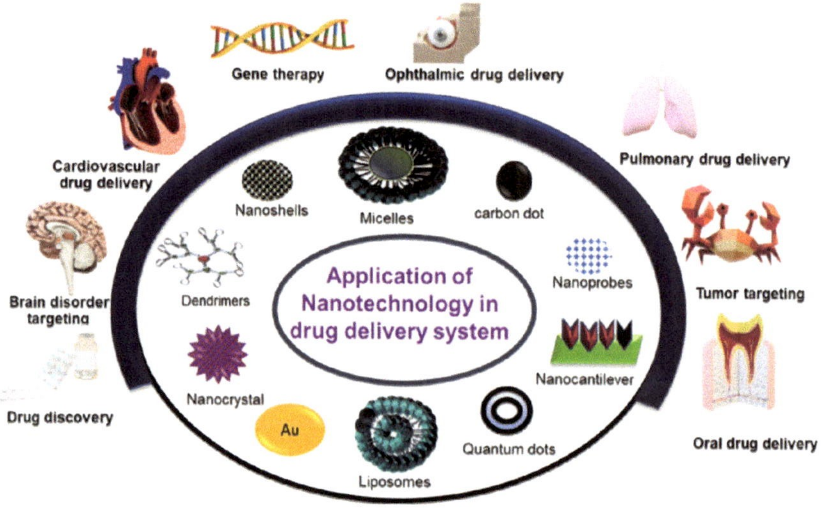

Figure 1.5 Application of nanotechnology in drug delivery system.

1.9.1.2 Nanotechnology in drug development

Drug development relies heavily on the identification of biochemical, biophysical, and drug target features [46] and several sectors are attempting to reduce the price of medicine development despite the increase in competition, the fair market value has risen dramatically, resulting in increased pressure on numerous pharmaceutical industries. This application of nanotechnology to medication research has proven to be both cost-effective and beneficial to work-life balance (Fig. 1.6.), nanoparticles have been demonstrated to drastically reduce toxicity and increase health, due to their excellent bio-physical stability and potential to be produced as controlled-release medications, nanoparticles of solid state have shown to be immensely helpful for the advancement of drug development. Through the utilization of nanoparticles, the formulation of sustained-release medications has become substantially more feasible and several inventions of solid nanoparticles, with or without surface functionality, have been made to date. For instance, aliphatic polyesters such as poly (lactic acid), hydrophilic poly (glycolic acid), and their copolymers poly (lactic acid) and poly (glycolic acid) are aliphatic polyesters (lactide-co-glycolide) maintaining the particle size of NPs throughout their period of action increases the drug's stability.

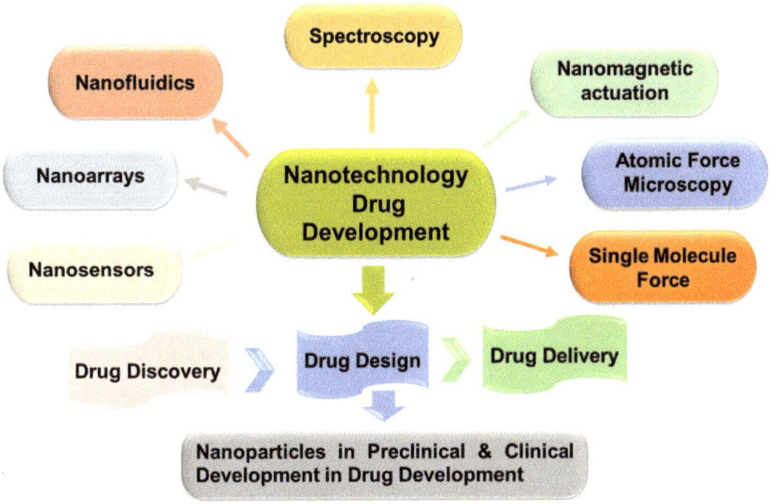

Figure 1.6 Nanotechnology in drug development.

1.9.2 Biological Application

1.9.2.1 Treatment of cancerous diseases

Cancer is the leading cause of death worldwide, and it is a multistage process that is carcinogenic in nature and causes a number of disorders that impact the physiological processes of the cell, such as apoptosis, cell signaling, etc. The utilization of nanotechnology has revitalized conventional cancer treatments. Radiotherapy and chemotherapy are effective treatments used to treat cancer and they continue to experience disadvantages such as severe weakness, hair loss, GIT issues, chemoresistance, etc. [49, 50]. Nanotechnology utilizes genetics, engineering, chemistry, biology, medicine, etc., to create nanoparticles, making it the new frontier for scientific inquiry, development, and multidisciplinary study. It successfully identifies, diagnoses, and treats a variety of cancers by generating biodegradable nanoparticles, the defining characteristic of nanoparticles for medication delivery [51, 52].

Following are the nanomaterials used most frequently in cancer treatment (Fig. 1.7):

(1) Nanocantilevers
(2) Nanoprobes
(3) Nanocrystals
(4) Nanopolymers
(5) Dendrimers
(6) Quantum dots
(7) Nanoshells

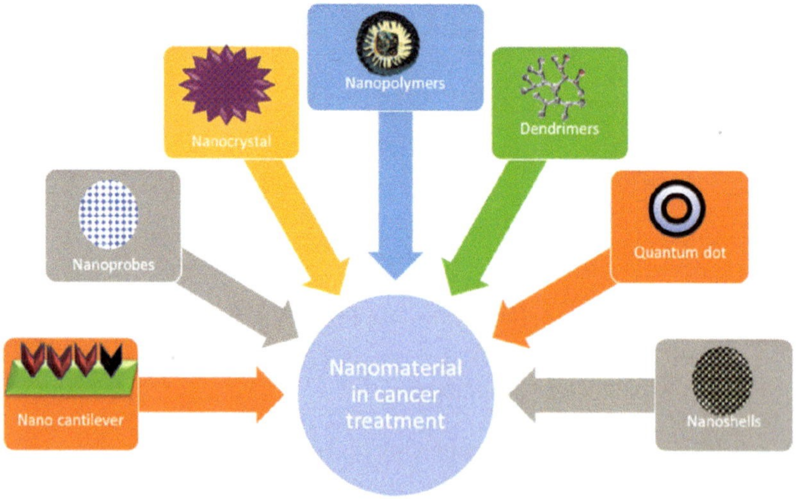

Figure 1.7 Nanomaterial in cancer treatment.

The following are the primary characteristics of nanomaterials used to treat cancer:

1. Tumor detection within the body.
2. Approaching the tumor target without alerting normal cells.

Numerous nanoparticles exist that are very selective and sensitive to cancer cells, but their mechanisms of action vary and these nanoparticles have the following distinctive characteristics:

1. As a result of being coupled to polyvalent ligands, they have a high affinity and accuracy for target cells.
2. They are constructed in a manner that enables their rapid combination for combined cancer therapy.
3. They can inhibit the development of conventional medication resistance.
4. They are designed to provide a wide range of medicinal effects and several investigative qualities.

1.9.2.1.1 MOA of anti-angiogenic and anti-cancer

Anti-angiogenic medications have been discovered to be used interchangeably with chemotherapeutic agents; this has resulted in a significant shift in chemotherapy and this is due to defective condition of tumor blood arteries, which can inhibit the transfer of chemotherapeutic drugs, hence raising drug resistance factors.

For instance, two layers make up their nanoparticles:

It is constructed of PLGA (polylactic-co-glycolic acid) that is attached to PEG and conjugated with doxorubicin.

Combretastatin conjugated with liposomes

- Doxorubicin (an anti-cancer drug) and Combretastatin (anti-angiogenic) in both mouse and human models, it has proven effective against melanoma and lung carcinomas [54] and their nanoparticles have two layers:
  a. Core: PLGA is connected to doxorubicin and attached to PEG.
  b. Liposome-conjugated combretastatin.

This allowed easy absorption of the drug by the tumor on intravenous administration into tumor-mediated mice and positive results were seen as the tumor growth was inhibited.

- Another study showed that upon administration of dual drug-loaded magnetic nanoparticles there was an increase in cell penetration and showed synergistic effects.
- Another study showed the use of double drug delivery through the formation of drugs used for breast cancer which were formulated by encapsulation of hydrophilic and hydrophobic anticancer drugs where HER-2 is the drug target [55].

1.9.2.1.2 Theranostics

Theragnostic is a new field that focuses on the relationship between diagnosis and treatment with its assistance, treatment has become quicker, more effective, and simpler biocompatible nanoparticles are still undergoing investigation to provide effective cancer treatment, noninvasive technology, as well as detection. In recent investigations, scientists have encased SiRNA within tiny gold nanoparticles. Such nanoparticles have been useful for stimulating improved gene silencing and sensory optical imaging [56].

1.9.2.2 Ophthalmic applications

As it would be challenging to maintain enough medication concentrations in the precorneal area, this results in malabsorption in the eye, which is one of the primary complications associated with the topical administration of ophthalmic medications, In comparison to their non-nanotech counterparts, nanoparticles have significantly improved the duration of a drug's effect by extending its half-life by up to 20 min with the introduction of nanoparticle-based ophthalmic medicines, bioavailability has increased, adverse effects have decreased, and intraocular dose levels have increased [55]. The commercially available *Eudragit* polymer was restudied by scientists; rabbits were administered non-steroidal and anti-inflammatory medicines in the eye.

The composition of Eudragit RS and RL is as follows:

1. Poly (ethyl acrylate),
2. Poly (methyl methacrylate),
3. Poly (chloro trimethyl aminoethyl methacrylate).

It was administered in the following way:

1. Drug-polymer combinations were mixed in ethanol and emulsified to generate drug-infused nanoparticles measuring 100 nm.
2. Rabbit eyes had nanoparticles floating in the conjunctival sac.
3. Flurbiprofen and ibuprofen-filled nanoparticles successfully inhibited the post-surgical trauma-induced inflammatory response observed in the rabbit.

This resulted in greater medication concentrations in the ocular region compared to traditional ophthalmic medicines available on the market [56] also known to cause permanent injury and surrounding tissue is cytomegalovirus. Bovine serum albumin (BSA) contains the antiviral drug ganciclovir, which is used to treat CMV (cytomegalovirus) infections, and it is nanoformulated by emulsifying BSA in an aqueous solution during incubation, after which ethanol is added to aid in the production of droplets. Its nanoparticle has an approximate diameter of 280 nm to give this formulation, it is first reconstituted in saline and then administered intravenously [57]. Another study proposed an isotonic solution of HPMC (hydroxyl propyl methylcellulose) with chitosan/hyaluronic acid/sodium tripolyphosphate nanoparticles and ceftazidime as an additional antibiotic, and it was evaluated for efficacy, and shown to possess features such as mucoadhesion, and enhanced contact with ocular mucosa, as well as delayed antibiotic release. This demonstrates that nanoparticles can help prolong a drug's half-life and maintain antibacterial activity, making them appropriate as the first-line drug for ocular drug delivery systems [58]. Dendrimers, another type of nanoformulation, can be utilized as medicine delivery systems for the eyes and these dendrimers are coupled to the substance puerarin and polyamidoamine (PAMAM), which have been found to boost the drug delivery system and therapeutic efficacy when delivered to rabbits in comparison to puerarin eye drops.

1.9.2.3 Application in cardiovascular disease

The primary cause of death for the majority of the population are cardiovascular disorders, which include:

1. Atherosclerosis
2. Myocardial infarction
3. Stroke
4. Hypertension
5. Heart failure

The key method for the prevention and treatment of cardiovascular diseases is early identification, and there are various techniques to diagnose CVDs, which are as follows:

1. X-ray
2. Electrocardiography (ECG)
3. Computed tomography (CT) scan
4. Magnetic resonance imaging (MRI)

Due to the complication of the disease's pathogenesis, early-stage diagnosis is still a difficult issue; hence, the techniques are generally ineffective, despite their continued usefulness. Therefore, procedures that are faster, more reliable, and more exact are required to locate CVDs [59, 60]. The use of nanotechnology and cardiac immunoassay to diagnose and treat early-stage cardiovascular diseases has proven to be more effective than conventional treatments and immunoassays combined with nanotechnology include:

1. Immunoassay for electrochemiluminescence (ECL)
2. Immunofluorescence Assay (IFA)
3. Immunoassay using an enzyme linker (ELISA)

Features of nanotechnology are:

1. Excessive binding cardiac targets
2. Affordable bioavailability
3. Limits non-precise binding sites
4. Allows easy flow across the body
5. Provides better diagnostic accuracy [59]

Fluorescent compounds are a standard option for nanomaterial conjugation, and quantum dots that are fluorescently labeled, and utilized for imaging atherosclerotic plaques are one example.

These nanoparticles have yielded excellent results, as they can be recognized by MRI, which reveals the organization of plaques and thrombi, including macrophagic components, necrotic substances, hemorrhages, etc. Super-paramagnetic nanoparticles are an additional type of material that boosts MRI sensitivity. They contribute to improved signaling [61, 62] using these materials (cross-linked iron oxide nanoparticles), and macrophagic plaques were found in a study [63, 64].

1.9.2.4 Application in respiratory disease

There is limited evidence that nanotechnology-based drug delivery devices can effectively treat respiratory illnesses, Asthma and other anaphylactic disorders are known to cause airway inflammation due to hypersensitivity. This is a result of the patients' decreased interferon (IFN) proliferation when patients deficient in IFN were given chitosan-IFN, a drug-polymer conjugate, their inflamed airways decreased. Thus according to research this therapy boosted the production of IFN by epithelial cells and decreased lung inflammation [65], another work by scientists has demonstrated the use of nanoparticles derived from liposomes as medication delivery devices when supplied to an asthmatic mouse model, the results indicated a decline in inflammation, and this study's primary objective is to inhibit the P-selectin and PSGL 1 receptors on activated endothelial cells in circulation. This demonstrated the least number of contacts between leukocytes and endothelial cells, hence reducing the course of bronchial inflammation [66].

1.9.2.5 Application in CNS disorders

The blood-brain barrier (BBB) has a significant impact on the application of nanotechnology to neurological illnesses, and it surrounds the brain, which is the most intricate organ in the human body. It permits only medications with a high degree of lipophilicity or molecular weight of 400–600 Da or less to be permeable. Furthermore, the presence of BBB is a considerable barrier to the treatment of neurological illnesses due to their high hydrophilicity, many medications used to treat CNS illnesses cannot cross the BBB, preventing them from reaching their intended target. Therefore, treatment choices for neurological illnesses are restricted to prevent this, nanoparticles with conjugated polymer coatings that allow them to penetrate the BBB are utilized, facilitating the early identification and treatment of neurological illnesses, and they can traverse the BBB's tight cell connections, and are encapsulated with ligands to function as site-specific medicines. Majorly, Polymeric nanoparticles are used for example:

1. PIHCA (poly isohexyl cyanoacrylate)
2. Butyl cyanoacrylate
3. PLA (Polylactic acid)
4. PLGA (lactide-co-glycolide), copolymer
5. HSA (Human serum albumin)

Nanoparticles for CNS drug delivery require non-specific binding medications, and surface modifications and BBB transport conjugations such as VEGF, EGF, insulin, albumin, transferrin, lactoferrin, and angiopep-2 will dramatically boost nanoparticle kinetics due to the Lf receptor on the BBB surface. For example, lactoferrin nanoparticle conjugation results in more BBB absorption than non-conjugated nanoparticles. Taxol-carrying NPs may improve brain endothelial cell aggregation in brain cancer when paired with transferrin while doxorubicin is an anti-cancer medication due to the BBB, it's not a good brain tumor treatment when it is encapsulated in a polysorbate-80 nanoparticle, it crossed the BBB. Polysorbate surfactant absorbs surface apolipoprotein B and E the main effect is receptor-mediated brain capillary endocytosis.

Magnetic nanoparticles are also effective at delivering anti-cancer drugs in the presence of a magnetic field, they are first magnetized, and they are utilized successfully because they may be directed to the appropriate places and improve absorption. This aids in minimizing off-target action using cytotoxic medications in conjunction with a magnetic field enabling the drug to be released through the enzymatic process or by altering physiological circumstances, resulting in enhanced absorption at the tumor target sites [67, 68] and multi-functional microbubbles (MBs) containing doxorubicin in combination with MNPs, for instance, blood samples were taken and iron oxide nanoparticles were isolated using RES in one study once iron oxide nanoparticles have penetrated cells, such as macrophages, MRI can detect their presence and this could be a highly efficient method for assessing the composition of the BBB and monitoring macrophage activity in a range of inflammatory illnesses [69]. Ferumoxtran-10, a dextran-coated iron oxide nanoparticle, serves as a stable imaging marker to remove brain tumors during surgery [70]. Ab40 or Ab42 beta-amyloid peptides are utilized to diagnose AD (brain and blood vessel walls) and some of the researchers coupled magnetic nanoparticles (MNPs) with the following substances in a study:

1. Ab1-42 peptide which is used for the identification of amyloid plaque deposition
2. polyethylene glycol which is used for the improvement of brain permeability

Its result was shown through a contrasting MRI where significant imaging capability was seen and the contrasting MRI was done between AD transgenic mice and Wild type mice.

1.9.3 Utilization within Biomedical Engineering

1.9.3.1 Medical types of equipment

1.9.3.1.1 Surgical blades

Since prehistoric times, surgical blades have been utilized due to the transition from traditional instruments to hard-diamond and gold-coated blades, the evolution of surgical blades has gained widespread attention due to their typical low physical adherence to tissues, chemicals, biological membranes, etc., diamonds are utilized as nanocoatings on surgical blades. They are the preferred material given the low coefficient of friction, which reduces the coefficient of penetration force [71], and the blades on the instruments are razor-sharp and extremely thin for making precise cuts because plasma polishing reduces the blade's thickness by 5–25 μm ± 0.5 μm thus, they are ideal for ophthalmic and neurosurgical procedures [72].

1.9.3.1.2 Invasive surgery

After the invention of catheters, low-invasive surgical procedures have been utilized. As a result of the employment of multi-walled carbon nanotubes as filters on the matrix bed (nylon 12), polymer-reinforced catheters comprised of nanotubes are now available *in vivo*, and *in vitro* testing has resulted in the development of better catheters with lower thrombogenicity, maximum fracture toughness, and enhanced mechanical and electrostatic properties [73].

1.9.3.1.3 Optical forceps

There are several types of surgical instruments that feature only one gradient light trap for exploiting nano-sized substances such as viruses and DNA and light is employed to study the dynamics instead of force and tweezers. Consequently, this technique is often characterized as non-invasive [74].

1.9.3.1.4 Tissue engineering

The advancement of tissue engineering has enabled us to replace damaged or destroyed biological tissues [75], and it is believed that this is the primary goal of organ transplants, skin grafts, and bone replacement procedures this section describes tissue engineering.

1.9.3.1.5 Bone tissue engineering

The presence of collagen in bones facilitates their repair and regeneration due to their great compatibility, porous 3D scaffolds with compositions like bone and bio-ceramic are utilized to treat skeletal deformities and massive bone defects [76]. For osteogenesis, these scaffolds employ biomolecular signaling and progenitor cells. According to studies, nanoparticles have been produced that release osteogenic substances *in vitro* to encourage new bone production while preserving the 3D structure [77].

1.9.3.1.6 Nerve tissue engineering

The emergence of nerve tissue engineering, which aids in nerve regeneration and repair, has altered the entire perspective of Neurotherapy, and nerve tissue engineering is incredibly advantageous since it fills the 6 mm gaps between neurons and has a structure very similar to scaffolds [78] utilized nanofibers have a three-dimensional fibrous (3D) structure >1 μm, and it has been discovered that they boost internal cell development and are more tolerant in nature. Electrospinning was utilized by researchers to create Nanofiber PPLA, for instance, the procedure is highly effective and contributes to the formation of polymeric nanofibers, which enhance neural stem adhesion, growth, and differentiation [79].

1.10 The Risk of Nanotechnology

Numerous researchers are interested in nanotechnology, which has diverse applications including medicine, health care, etc. However, with the benefits came dangerous side effects that have garnered considerable attention, and several studies describe the harmful consequences of some nanoparticles as a result of their hazardous features.

1.10.1 Reduced Size of Nanoparticles

Nanoparticle size has both benefits and drawbacks for the human body, on the other hand, they penetrate undesirable cells and tissue to produce pharmacological effects on normal cells, tissues, and so on If this occurs, it becomes nearly impossible to extract these nanoparticles, and doing so may have hazardous effects.

1.10.1.1 Different shapes

Nanoparticles come in a variety of forms. Such a change in form can have hazardous and harmful repercussions on the drug's target, for instance, zinc oxide particles can take the form of rods and spheres, and the latter nanoparticles are less hazardous than rod-shaped nanoparticles that can have harmful effects on the lung epithelium.

1.10.1.2 Motility correlation

Size and mobility are adversely connected as nanoparticles are nanometer-sized, their mobility is high, and high migration speeds allow rapid penetration of cells, tissues, etc. In the cells and tissues, aggregation can have harmful effects.

1.10.1.3 Aggregation

Nanoparticles are stabilized by their aggregation or clustering within cells and tissues and this feature can result in a variety of physiological abnormalities other anomalies are generated by certain nanoparticle features, such as magnetic properties, and strong conductivity [81].

1.11 Limitations of Nanotechnology

Nanomedicine is so new that there isn't much proof that it works yet, and it is still being tested because of this, it is hard to prove that its use is completely safe but we can say for sure that nanoparticles can get into our bodies in many ways and that this is something to worry about it although it is known to have many benefits it still cannot be mentioned as a furnished field. The main reason behind this is due to their decreased particle size which went from being micro-sized to nano-sized.

1. The main limitation of nanoparticles is that there is nothing common between them except for their size, so each particle should be separately tested and judged.
2. Inside our organs, nanoparticles exist in collaboration with the Mononuclear Phagocytic System (MPS) which traps them due to their decreased size, the surface area is significantly accentuated which leads to high chemical reactivity and causing instabilities in their behavior, thereby altering their mechanism of action. This level of chemical reactivity results in the formation of reactive oxygen species (ROS), and ROSs produce oxidative stress, inflammation, and damage to proteins, DNA, and different membranes, all of which have negative consequences.
3. Materials that are non-hazardous in nature at particle size 100 nm turn into hazardous materials when their size becomes 1 nm, and this demonstrates that variations in nanoparticle size result in the development of hazardous compounds.

4. There may be interactions not illustrated that contribute to the creation of dangerous chemicals, therefore, it proves that they are sensitive to the materials present in their environment.

Nanoparticles may reveal undesirable outcomes on administration due to their nano size, they can infiltrate numerous organs, cells, and capillaries, and can even cross the BBB unknown consequences may occur in numerous areas inside the body, including damage to the nucleus, mitochondria, and cellular processes. These systems are designed to reduce undesirable effects, yet they are themselves harmful and there are still numerous difficulties, such as ethical, legal, etc., that must be resolved in order to get support for the administration of nanotechnology, despite its extensive application in future formulations for diseases such as cancer to avert criticism, these difficulties must be addressed, and the public must be made aware of the benefits and risks of nanotechnology.

1.12 Drug Delivery Systems

1.12.1 Drug Delivery

The application and study of drug delivery have expanded significantly, and it enables enhanced methods of administering therapeutically active medicines [48] even though there are several concerns with the medication delivery system that requires public attention, the medical system has deployed numerous drug delivery technologies. Following elements influence the formulation of drug delivery systems:

1. Concentration of the therapeutic agent.
2. Prolonged duration of action
3. Efficacious

Pathophysiological modifications were done to bring this system into effect which may allow easier binding to the target.

It covers a variety of systems that help in controlled drug release, and there are various challenges that pose an issue for the working of such an integrated system. They are as follows:

1. Cross-checking of the intervention context
2. Quantifying the readiness of the system toward a change
3. Cross-checking fidelity and sustainability
4. Cross-check multicomponent interventions and complexes
5. Rationing time in models of delivery systems so that the recommendations can be discussed

Previously utilized techniques, for instance, permit systemic circulation of the drug, resulting in just a tiny amount reaching the tumor target location, this can be remedied by employing tumor-specific drug delivery systems, which will accumulate at the target site without affecting other organs, hence enhancing efficacy while decreasing unwanted effects [82].

Drug delivery has two approaches [83]:

1. Passive drug approach
2. Active drug approach or ligand-based.

For drug targeting and disease-targeting, numerous anticancer medicines have been synthesized as nanoformulations utilizing nanoparticles that facilitate the uptake of poorly soluble medications [84, 85]. Anticancer medicines like paclitaxel [86, 87], doxorubicin [88], 5-fluorouracil [89], and dexamethasone [90], are utilized to produce nanoformulations, for instance, PLGA and polylactic acid (PLA) are used to encapsulate dexamethasone, and dexamethasone, an anticancer medication, has anti-inflammatory and anti-proliferative effects.

Drugs primarily exert their effects by binding to cytoplasmic receptors, which then form drug-receptor complexes and are delivered to the nucleus, where gene expression occurs [90]. The nanoformulations exhibit regulated drug release over a longer period and suppress the proliferation of vascular smooth muscle, and these drug delivery methods are effective due to their tiny size, reduced toxicity, or adverse effects, regulated drug release, and enhanced bioavailability. Certainly, cancers acquire anticancer drug resistance, rendering chemotherapy ineffective, and a protein called p-glycoprotein induces resistance in tumors, causing them to eliminate cancer medications as soon as they cross the cell membrane. Here, nanoformulations can be utilized. According to new research, nanoparticles may be able to deliver anticancer medications to cells without activating the p-glycoprotein pump [87, 91].

1.13 Bio-Polymers

There are various bio-polymeric substances used in medication delivery systems. Following is a discussion of the materials and their qualities.

1.13.1 Chitosan

Chitosan has mucoadhesive characteristics and can influence epithelial tight junctions. Consequently, chitosan-based nano-particles have been widely employed for sustained drug delivery systems in many types of epithelia, such as buccal [94], gut [95], nose [96], eyes [97], and lung [98]. According to a study by Silva et al. [99] for ocular delivery of the antibiotic ceftazidime, an isotonic solution of hydroxyl propyl methylcellulose (HPMC) containing chitosan/sodium tri polyphosphate/hyaluronic acid nanoparticles was produced and assessed by measuring the viscosity of nanoparticles interacting with various mucin mass fractions, rheological synergy parameters were determined in the presence of mucin, chitosan nanoparticles exhibited minimal viscosity. However, nanoparticles are mucoadhesive, resulting in favorable contact with ocular mucosa and long-term release of antibiotics, thereby increasing the drug's lifetime in the eyes with the aid of nanoparticles. Nanoparticles did not affect ARPE-19 and HEK 239T cell lines, and antimicrobial nanoparticles are promising for mucoadhesive ophthalmic medication delivery. Pistone's colleagues [100] made chitosan, alginate, and pectin nanoparticles for oral medicine, and the solubility of nanoparticles in saliva and oral cell lines was used to measure biocompatibility and cytotoxicity following pectin and chitosan, alginate nano-particles are the least stable in artificial saliva after 2 h. and pectin and alginate thereby were cytotoxic, although chitosan was cell-competitive while Zn^{2+} may account for the cytotoxicity (a cross-linker) each formulation has advantages and disadvantages compared to oral delivery and required modification. Carboxymethyl chitosan nanoparticles for intranasal carbamazepine (CBZ) release were developed to overcome the BBB, improving drug delivery to the brain, enhancing therapeutic efficacy, and facilitating systemic distribution. The nanoparticles have a diameter of 218.76±2.41 nm, a drug loading of 35%, and encapsulation efficiency of 80% brain CBZ concentrations were higher than plasma concentrations for 240 min ($P < 0.05$). In a separate investigation, *Jain* [102] analyzed the release profile of 5-fluorouracil (5-FU) from hyaluronic acid-coated chitosan nanoparticles following oral administration, and experiments involving the release of 5-FU exhibited resistance to stomach and small-intestinal excretion in conditions that simulated the gastrocolic transition in the treatment of colon cancer, increased local drug concentrations result in longer exposure durations, hence enhancing anticancer efficacy and reducing systemic toxicity.

1.13.2 Alginate

Alginate is another biopolymer substance that has been utilized for medication delivery, this biopolymer is an anionic mucoadhesive polymer, which sticks to mucus better than cationic polymers and neutral polymers [59, 118]; In order to lower serum glucose levels and increase serum insulin levels in diabetic rats, insulin-loaded alginate nanoparticles containing nicotinamide as a penetrant were developed by Patil and Devarajan [103]. In the presence of nicotinamide, nanoparticles delivered sublingually (5 IU/kg) exhibited high pharmacological availability (>100%) and bioavailability (>80%) using a streptozotocin-induced diabetes mouse model, it was found that NPs can carry insulin through the sublingual route with a pharmacologically higher 20.2% than a 1 IU/kg subcutaneous injection, and there was a potential 24.1% demonstrating the bioavailability of [103]. Haque et al. [104] made alginate nanoparticles that can be used to deliver venlafaxine (VLF) through the nose to treat depression, in fact, the concentration of VLF in the brain was higher when alginate nanoparticles were given through the nose than when VLF was given through the nose or through a vein shows that VLF can enter the brain directly, and we demonstrate the proven delivery superiority of nanoformulations, thus, these nanoparticles have the potential to treat depression. In another instance, Román and colleagues conducted research [105], and the researchers attached the epidermal growth factor to the external surface of alginate microcapsules to target non-small cell lung cancer cells, and carcinogenic cisplatin was also included in the nanoparticles, and the addition of EGF considerably enhanced the specificity of the carrier system, resulting in a higher rate of cell killing (H460 lung cancer line) compared to the medication alone under stomach pH conditions, less than 5% of the AR in the system was released, but rapid and extensive release was seen under conditions of gut pH. Hence, the carrier demonstrated the ability to preserve molecules released from the gastrointestinal tract following oral delivery. Costa et al. [107] designed chitosan-coated alginate nanoparticles to improve the ocular epithelial penetration of daptomycin and produce an antibacterial effect using an eye epithelial cell culture paradigm, the permeability was evaluated *in vitro*, the antibacterial efficacy of nano-encapsulated daptomycin against pathogens associated with bacterial endophthalmitis seemed promising. According to ocular permeability investigations, a 4 h treatment with 9–12% HCE and ARPE-19 cells was permeable to total daptomycin enclosed within chitosan-alginate nanoparticles such investigations imply that this method improved the retention of drugs in the ocular epithelium.

1.13.3 Xanthan Gum

Xanthan gum (XG) is a high-molecular-weight heteropoly-saccharide produced by Xanthomonas campestris, and this polyanionic polysaccharide possesses outstanding bioadhesive properties, Xanthan gum, which is non-toxic and non-irritating, can be used as a cosmetic ingredient [108]. The violation of xanthan gum has increased the buccal mucosa's adherence as compared to indigenous xanthan gum, additionally, the xanthan gum thiolate absorbs more saliva than the oral mucosa-drying tannic acid. Therefore, this technique will be an effective method for lowering salivary flow in people with sialorrhea, and angiogenesis is a crucial aspect of soft tissue regeneration. Huang et al. [110] developed injectable hydrogels consisting of aldehyde-modified xanthan, and carboxymethyl-modified chitosan that contained a potent angiogenic agent (anti-vascular endothelial growth factor, VEGF) to enhance abdominal wall restoration, and hydrogel is more effective in the digestive tract and wound tissues. Hydrogel VEGF stimulated angiogenesis and repaired the abdominal wall in a recent study, Menzel et al. [111] sought to identify new excipients for usage as nasal release systems, Cys-MNA was linked with xanthan gum, the primary polymer in the resultant conjugation, characteristics such as the quantity of the associated binder, mucoadhesive qualities, and stability against degradation was evaluated each gram of polymer underwent ligation with 252.5220.54 mol of the binder compared to thiolated xanthan, the grafted polymer has 1.7 times the mucoadhesion. Moreover, nasal epithelial cell ciliary beating was reduced and only reversed when the polymer was removed.

1.13.4 Cellulose

Cellulose and its derivatives are commonly utilized in drug delivery systems to improve solubility and gelation and control drug release [112]. Elseoud et al. [113] investigated repaglinide's oral release (an anti-hyperglycemic mic), and RPG nanoparticles are chitosan and cellulose nanocrystal hybrid nanoparticles. Nanocrystals made of oxidized cellulose and chitosan hybrid had an RPG mean diameter of 251–310 nm. Their sustained release is owing to the presence of hydrogen bonds between the cellulose nanocrystals and the drug, and the nanoparticles synthesized with oxidized cellulose nanocrystals had a reduced release behavior than those manufactured with native cellulose nanocrystals. In a study conducted by Hansen and colleagues [115] four cellulose derivatives were identified, including:

- Methylcellulose
- Hydroxypropyl methylcellulose
- Sodium carboxymethylcellulose
- Cationic hydroxyethyl cellulose

They are mostly utilized for medication delivery to the nasal mucosa and the combination of these cellulose analogs including an extra-active ingredient was also evaluated, the prototype medicine for this approach was acyclovir. Moreover, the ciliary beat frequency (CBF) and nasal tissue infusion were assessed to determine the suitability of these polymers for nasal release applications when cellulose derivatives and polymer graft copolymers were mixed, thermally induced viscosity improved. Additionally, when acyclovir was coupled with cationic hydroxyethyl cellulose, nasal mucosal penetration was enhanced analysis of CBF demonstrated that none of the natural polymers had harmful impacts on the nasal mucosa's tissues and cells.

1.13.5 Liposomes

Alec Bangham developed liposomes during the 1960s, In the pharmaceutical and cosmetic industries, liposomes are utilized for the delivery of numerous compounds, and they are one of the most studied vehicle systems for drug delivery, and liposomes are a prevalent formulation technique for improving medication delivery, and they are spherical vesicles consisting of phospholipids and steroids with a typical size range of 50–450 nm [116]. Their membrane features resemble those of cell membranes, and they are regarded as superior drug delivery vehicles because they enhance drug absorption into the plasma stream [116]. In addition, it has been demonstrated to stabilize therapeutic molecules, enhance biodistribution, compatibility with hydrophilic and hydrophobic medicines, biocompatibility, and biodegradability. The following four types of liposomes are distinguished.

(1) Conventional liposomes: They consist of a lipid bilayer capable of forming either anionic, cationic, or neutral cholesterol or phospholipids surrounding an aqueous core element. In this case, both the lipid bilayer and the aqueous space can be filled with hydrophobic and hydrophilic materials, respectively.

(2) PEGylated types: The liposome surface incorporates polyethylene glycol (PEG) to provide steric balance.

(3) ligand-targeted type: The liposome surface incorporates polyethylene glycol (PEG) to provide steric balance.

(4) Type of theranostic liposomes: It consists of nanoparticles in addition to targeting, imaging, and therapeutic characteristics [117].

The following is an example of a method for synthesizing liposomes among these include thin-layer hydration, mechanical agitation, solvent evaporation, solvent infusion, and surfactant solubilization [118]. Notably, the drugs enclosed within liposomes are inaccessible until they are released to maximize the bioavailability of medications inside the therapeutic window at the ideal rate and duration, it is essential that they accumulate at certain sites liposomes can be loaded with drugs both actively (drug trapping following liposome synthesis) and passively (synthesis of liposomes with drug entrapment) [119] in aqueous core of liposomes, hydrophilic medications like ampicillin and its 5-fluoro-deoxyuridine are typically found; thus, the drug/lipid ratio is irrelevant for encapsulation. However, hydrophobic ones were discovered in the acyl hydrocarbon chains of liposomes, including amphotericin B and indomethacin indicating that acyl chain composition influences their entanglement [120]. Mechanically, solvent dispersion, and surfactant removal techniques are all examples of passive loading strategies [119]. RES (Reticuloendothelial System), Opsonization, and Immunogenic Drug Delivery Formulations, to overcome these difficulties. However, properties like enhanced permeability and the EPR (retention impact) can be used to the drug's advantage as they circulate through the bloodstream, liposomes meet opsonins, high-density lipoproteins (HDL), and low-density lipoproteins (LDL) after they enter the body. Opsonins (including immunoglobulins and fibronectin) assist RES in identifying and eliminating liposomes. HDL and LDL interact with liposomes to destabilize them and liposomes tend to concentrate in organs like the liver and spleen. This is advantageous because high concentrations of liposomes are beneficial for treating pathogenic disorders, whereas the clearance of lipophilic liposomes is delayed in malignancies drugs can result in drug use as stated at the outset, various forms of liposomes have been generated as a result. Dymov et al. [121] described a continuous synthesis, functionalization, and purification of liposomes using flow systems, and the study includes sub-300 nm vesicles in a lab-on-a-chip, which are candidates to produce expensive medications and protein encapsulation [121]. The production cost of medicine impacts whether it can be commercialized.

1.13.6 Polymeric Micelles

Micelles are nanostructures of amphiphilic block copolymers that self-assemble in an aqueous solution to form core-shell structures, and the hydrophobic core can be loaded with hydrophobic medicines (camptothecin, docetaxel, paclitaxel, etc.), while the hydrophilic shell makes the entire system water soluble and stabilizes the hydrophobic core. Polymeric micelles are often narrowly dispersed to avoid rapid renal elimination and accumulate in tumor tissue through EPR effects. Moreover, their polymeric coating inhibits nonspecific interactions with biological components, and the inner core structure of these nanostructures allows for the inclusion of hydrophobic medicines, resulting in increased stability and bioavailability [123, 122]. There are two methods for creating polymeric micelles:

(1) Direct polymer dissolving using a solvent, followed by a dialysis process.

(2) Addition of a solvent causes one block to precipitate [123, 124].

Micelle production is influenced by variables such as the amphiphilic molecule's hydrophobic chain length, concentration, solvent system, and temperature [125]. When amphipathic molecules reach a minimum concentration known as the critical micelle concentration (CMC) [124], micelle production commences amphipathic molecules are tiny and arise independently at low quantities [124]. In general, three methods are utilized to load medicines into polymeric micelles: (1) direct dissolution, (2) solvent evaporation, and (3) dialysis. In direct dissolution, the copolymer and active ingredient self-assemble in an aqueous media to generate micelle-containing active ingredients in the solvent evaporation method, a volatile organic solvent is used to dissolve the copolymer and the drug of interest, and in the dialysis method, both the drug in solution and the copolymer in the organic solvent are inserted into the dialysis bag, the substance is dialyzed, then bind to form micelles [126]. Different methods of action, such as boosting permeability and stimulating retention effects, are proven using distinct polymeric micelles to target pharmaceuticals. Complexation of target-specific ligand molecules to the surface of micelles; or by combining monoclonal antibodies against micellar coronas [127] according to reports, polymeric micelles can be used for both anticancer drug administration [124] and ocular medication delivery [128].

1.13.7 Dendrimers

Dendrimers are monodispersed, highly branching, well-defined 3Dl structures due to their spherical form and the ease with which their surfaces can be functionalized in a regulated manner, these structures are attractive drug targets [129, 130]. Dendrimers can be synthesized in two different ways, the first is an alternative path in which the dendrimer is generated from its core and subsequently grows outward, whereas the second is a convergent route beginning from the dendrimer's exterior [130, 131] according to their functionalization units, dendrimers are categorized as PAMAM, PPI, liquid crystal, core-shell, chiral, peptide, glycodendrimer, and PAMAMOS. PAMAM is extensively explored for oral medication delivery due to its water solubility and ability to be bridged to promote transmission via paracellular and epithelial routes [132] due to the presence of amine groups, dendrimers have restricted therapeutic applicability. These groups are positively charged or cationic and poisonous, hence dendrimers are typically altered to decrease or remove this issue, and the processes for drug loading onto dendrimers are simple encapsulation, electrostatic interactions, and covalent binding [133].

Dendrimers essentially release drugs in two distinct ways, alterations towards the environment's physical conditions, which covers temperature and pH, and impact in medication effects [133] for transdermal, oral, ocular, respiratory, and selective drug administration, dendrimers have been synthesized [134]. Jain et al [135] "As a model, they presented folic acid-conjugated poly-L-lysine dendrimers (doxorubicin hydrochloride) for pH-dependent drug release, target selectivity, anti-angiogenic and anti-neoplastic properties as a potential cancer prevention medication carrier". Those individuals were administered doxorubicin-folic acid after 24 h, compared to free doxorubicin, coupled poly-L-lysine dendrimers elevated the doxorubicin level in tumors by 121.5%. Similarly, Kaur et al. [136] exhibited delayed release, enhanced cellular uptake, and low cytotoxicity against the MCF-7 cell line MTX -FAPPI) must also be mentioned compared to free methotrexate, it is selectively taken up by cancer cells (MTX).

1.13.8 Inorganic Nanoparticles

Inorganic nanoparticles consist of nanoparticles of silver, gold, iron oxide, and silica, and they are not the subject of as many studies as other nanoparticle varieties covered in this section, even though they have certain outstanding applications. However, only a few nanoparticles have been approved for their respective clinical applications, while the majority are still undergoing clinical trials. Metal nanoparticles, such as silver and gold, possess certain properties, such as SPR (surface Plasmon resonance). Liposomes, dendrimers, and micelles do not possess such features, they have demonstrated numerous benefits, including biocompatibility and surface functionalization adaptability studies of drug delivery-related activity do not reveal whether the drug exists in particulate or ionized form, or if they are associated with its toxicity.

Two methods have been suggested:

1. paracellular transport
2. transcytosis

However, there are limited data on their *in vivo* transport and absorption process [137] by methods of ionic or covalent bonding and physical absorption, gold nanoparticles (Au NPs) can be employed in conjugated forms with pharmaceuticals, and their release and distribution can be regulated by biological cues or light activation [138]. Silver nanoparticles are believed to exhibit antimicrobial activity, but in the case of drug delivery, only a few studies have been conducted, such as Prusty and Swain's [139] synthesis of an interlinked and spongy polyacrylamide/dextran nanohydrogels hybrid system with covalently connected silver nanoparticles for the release of ornidazole, leading to a 98.5% *in vitro* release [139]. Additionally, another study found that nanoparticles of iron oxide were generated using laser pyrolysis and coated with Violamycine B1 and anthracycline antibiotics using commercial formulations, researchers compared the cytotoxicity, and anti-proliferation properties of iron oxide nanoparticles against MCF-7 cells [140].

1.13.9 Nanocrystals

Drug particles with a diameter of 1000 nm are called nanocrystals in order to soften the suspension of the nanocrystals in the liquid rim media, surfactants are frequently used in nanosuspension. In this scenario, the dispersion medium is predominantly water or non-aqueous solution including liquid polyethylene glycols and oils [141, 142]. Unique characteristics of nanocrystals allow them to overcome hurdles such as improved saturation solubility, higher dissolving rate, and improved surface/cell membrane adherence. The nanocrystal production method can be separated into top-down and bottom-up ways; Top-down procedures include sonocrystallization, precipitation, high-gravity controlled precipitation techniques, multi-inlet vortex mixing techniques, and restricted liquid-jet precipitation techniques [141]. However, the use of organic solvents and their subsequent cleanup make this procedure quite costly. In the bottom-up method, grinding and high-pressure homogenization occur at the same time [141]. Milling, high-pressure homogenization, and precipitation are the most often employed techniques for producing nanocrystals improved solubility, suspension velocity, and intestinal wall adhesion are among the mechanisms by which nanocrystals facilitate medication absorption [141]. Ni et al. [142] to carry hydrophobic medicines via the lung, nanocrystals of cinaciguate are encased in chitosan microparticles utilizing the swelling, and mucoadhesive capabilities of the polymer, nanoparticles for continuous medication release were created, and they discovered that inhalation efficacy may be demonstrated during illness settings; however, additional research is required to demonstrate this system's greater potential [142].

1.13.10 Metallic Nanoparticles

Metallic nanoparticles have seen an increase in use in a variety of medicinal applications in recent years, including:

- bioimaging
- biosensors
- sustained drug delivery
- hyperthermia
- photoablation therapy [143]

Furthermore, there are various modifications and functionalization of these nanoparticles consisting of specific functional groups that permit them to bind to antibodies, drugs, and other ligands, hence making these systems more promising in biomedical applications [144]. Although the most substantially studied metallic nanoparticles are gold, silver, iron, and copper, interest has been exploited regarding other kinds of metallic nanoparticles, such as zinc oxide, titanium oxide, platinum, selenium, gadolinium, palladium, cerium dioxide, etc. [144].

1.13.10.1 Mechanism

As a result of the development of nanomedicine and the improvement of drug discovery and drug delivery systems, a variety of therapeutic procedures and ancient clinical diagnostic methods have been investigated in order to increase drug specificity and diagnostic precision, for instance, new routes of medication delivery are being investigated, with an emphasis on assuring their focused action in particular places, Consequently, overall cytotoxicity will be reduced, and overall bioavailability will rise within the body, and this method has resulted in the development of novel lead medications that are based on biological targets using drug design as a promising component. For this industry to grow and expand, experimental techniques for categorizing and purifying proteins, peptides, and biological targets must be created. furthermore, there are a few studies and reviews on this subject that emphasize the necessity of investigating alternate drug release mechanisms and the rational design of various molecules. Moreover, natural compounds might provide plausible and intriguing answers to drug design issues and serve as a source of inspiration for drug development with the needed chemical features. Additionally, medication delivery technologies have gained prominence in recent years. Such systems are frequently constructed in a straightforward manner and can encourage the controlled release of active components in the body. As an exception, Chen et al. studied "the medicinal benefits of these systems and gave a vivid overview of how nanocarriers are used for imaging and sensory applications". In addition, Pelaz et al. studied the new opportunities and problems facing the industry while providing an up-to-date description of the many applications of nanocarriers to nanomedicine, and it's interesting to note that each of these drug delivery methods has unique chemical, physical, and morphological characteristics. Additionally, these methods should attract different medicinal polarities through chemical interactions (such as covalent and H-bonds) as well as physical interactions (e.g., electrostatic and van der Waals interactions). Mattos et al. discovered biogenic oxide nanoparticles grafted with *Azadirachta indica* bark extract had a worse discharge profile than biogenic silica nanoparticles loaded with the extract. Consequently, these characteristics influence the interaction of nanocarriers with biological systems, also because of the active ingredient's release mechanism within the organism. In addition, Sethi et al. constructed a cross-linkable lipoid shell (CLS) containing docetaxel and wortmannin as the initial pharmaceuticals used to control the drug release kinetics; they then analyzed its release profile, which was discovered to be influenced by both *in vivo* and *in vitro* conditions. Other factors, such as the composition of nanocarriers (e.g., organic, inorganic, and hybrid materials) and the type of medicines connected with them (e.g., core-shell system or matrix system), are required for understanding their drug delivery profile. Several investigations are undertaken regarding unlocking mechanisms of medication in nanocarriers. Kamaly et al. offered a comprehensive overview of controlled-release systems, with an emphasis on studies pertaining to dominating drug release from chemical compound nanocarriers. However, there are numerous nanocarriers with different drug release profiles, strategies are being developed to improve the specificity of the nanostructures to target areas of the organism and to decrease their immunogenicity by coating or chemically functionalizing them with a variety of substances, such as polymers, natural polysaccharides, antibodies, cell membrane, and turnable surfactants, peptides, etc. In cases where drugs do not show interaction and affinity with a specific target or do not cross the BBB or even the blood–body fluid boundary, these ligand-modified nanocarriers are used to tolerate the semipermeable membrane and enable programmable drug delivery in a very specific environment, for instance, mucopolysaccharide (a carbohydrate found in the animal matrix) has been used as a ligand-appended in several nanocarriers, demonstrating promising results to enhance antitumor action against the skin cancer stem-like cells, carcinoma cells, pneumonic glandular cancer cells, and to facilitate intravitreal drug delivery for retinal cistron medical care and to reduce the immunogenicity of the shaped super-molecule corona. In addition, few studies are conducted to evaluate the interaction of ligands attached to nanocarriers with cell membranes, and their absorption process is unknown. Therefore, it has been demonstrated that the uptake of nanoparticles by cells occurs via somatic cell or non-phagocytic pathways (e.g., clathrin-mediated endocytosis, caveolae-mediated endocytosis, and others), whereas it has been difficult to standardize the mechanism of action/interaction of those systems within the cells due to the specific physicochemical characteristics of each delivery system. In a review, Islamin and Khosrowshahi identified the endocytosis pathways responsible for the cellular uptake of carbohydrate nanoparticles containing active chemicals in contrast, stimuli-responsive nanocarriers have demonstrated the ability to regulate the release profile of a drug (as a triggered release) by exploiting external factors such as ultrasound, heat, magnetism, light, pH, and ionic strength, which can improve targeting and permit greater titration control, for example, super-paramagnetic iron compound nanoparticles are coupled to chemical compound nanocarriers or lipids in order to induce a controlled-release system when an external magnetic field is applied. moreover, Ulbrich et al. explored the impact of covalently or noncovalently attached drugs for cancer treatment and reviewed current advancements in drug delivery methods, focusing specifically on the concept of chemical and magnetic nanoparticles. Thereby further, Au/Fe_3O_4 polymer nanoparticles were synthesized for use in NIR-triggered chemo photothermal treatment, Therefore, hybrid nanocarriers are currently among the most promising technologies for nanomedicine, since they provide a combination of features from many systems in a single system, thereby enhancing the performance of materials for therapeutic and diagnostic purposes (i.e., theranostic systems). Despite this, little is known about the actual mechanisms of action and toxicity of drug delivery systems, which presents an opportunity for new research. additionally, the number of studies specializing in the manufacture of nanocarriers using plant extracts and microorganisms to promote ecologically friendly chemical processes has expanded.

1.14 Future of Nanomedicine

Nanomedicine science is currently one of the most alluring study fields, and there is extensive work in this subject over the past two decades has resulted in the issuance of 1500 patents and the completion of dozens of clinical investigations [145]. Cancer looks to be a prime example of a disease whose diagnosis and treatment benefit from non-medical technologies, as stated in several sections above. Nanomedicine and nanotechnology provide precise doses of medications to afflicted cells, such as cancer/tumor cells, without interfering with normal cellular physiology without a doubt, the use of drug delivery systems will continue to increase in the future and the research and development landscape of the coming decades, the nanoparticles presented in this release are measured in nanometers and submicrons (100 nm and above). More research will be undertaken on materials with improved drug loading, and release capabilities, and this review also highlights major advancements in the diagnostic use of metal-based nanoparticles. In the coming years, the diagnostic and therapeutic use of these metals, such as gold and silver, may contribute to the extension of nanomedicine's applications. Gold nanoparticles, which appear to be well absorbed by soft tumor tissue, and radiation (IFR)-based heat for targeted ablation of tumors have sparked significant interest in this area increases your susceptibility to therapy even in cancer treatment/diagnosis, the impact of nanomedicine and nanodrug delivery systems on healthcare systems is quite limited despite the widespread recognition of their future potential. As a result, the topic is a new scientific discipline in which just 20 years of genuine research have been conducted on the subject and many fundamentally significant qualities remain undiscovered. Fundamental markers of sick tissue, such as fundamental potential biomarkers that allow for precise targeting without causing disruption of cellular activities, this is an important area for future research eventually, as our molecular understanding of disease expands, nanomedicine applications will develop, or the finding of markers corresponding to the intracellular size of nanoparticles will open new routes.

Understanding the molecular markers of diseases will therefore result in future improvements in nanomedicine applications utilizing well-known nanoprobes and nanotheranostics tools, additional study beyond what is mentioned in this review paper will be essential for larger applications of nanomedicine, and the concept of controlled release of specific medications to impacted areas, methods for assessing these events, pharmacological effects at the tissue/cellular level, and mathematical models for predicting the future have yet to be refined, and multiple research in the field of nanomedicine has concentrated on biomaterials and formulation research, and biological applications are likely in their infancy animal experiments and inter-disciplinary investigations that require a substantial amount of time yield valuable data with potential uses in drug therapy and diagnostic research. Smarter, multicenter approaches to nanomedicine and nanodrug delivery technologies have a promising future as the global drive toward more precise medications and diagnostics grows. A simplified view of the creation of nanorobots that work in tissue diagnostic and repair mechanisms with total external control has sparked considerable interest. This is not yet a reality, but it is futuristic research that humanity may be able to accomplish in the near future. However, in addition to its benefits, nanomedicine has the potential to help both individuals and the environment. Therefore, it is necessary to conduct a thorough analysis of the potential acute or chronic harmful effects of novel nanomaterials on humans and the environment as nanomedicine grows in popularity, its affordability will make it yet another scientific field requiring additional study as described in the preceding section, the regulation of nanomedicine evolves in tandem with improvements in nanomedicine applications.

1.15 Conclusion

This study examines recent breakthroughs in nanotherapeutics, including improvements in medication administration and diagnostic methods, nanorobots, and nano-sensors that can diagnose, deliver to targets accurately, and activate live system materials. Nanotechnology improved drug solubility, absorption, bioavailability, and controlled-release nanomedicine design entails significant levels of uncertainty, and identifying pharmacologically active compounds from natural sources, thus it's not desired nanotechnology enhances bioactive substance efficiency. Application of nanotechnology when: Curcumin, Resveratrol, Curcumin, Quercetin, Ellagic acid, Berberine, etc. Utilizing nanocarriers formulated with gold, silver, cadmium sulfide, and titanium dioxide, polymeric nanoparticles, solid lipid nanoparticles, crystal nanoparticles, liposomes, micelles, superparamagnetic iron oxide nanoparticles, and dendrimers have significantly increased the efficacy of these natural products due to their biodegradable, biocompatible, readily available, renewable, and low toxicity. Identifying polysaccharides and proteins as natural biopolymers and making them more stable by cross-linking are cutting-edge research disciplines. Nanocapsules and Nanospheres are two types of polymeric nanoparticles that can be created via solvent evaporation, emulsion polymerization, and surfactant-free emulsion. Polymerization is another approach that has been utilized extensively in recent years, cancer has served as a disease model for the integration of therapy and diagnosis, often known as theranostic exceptional examples have been encapsulated, including oleic acid-coated iron oxide nanoparticles, which are currently benign and used for diagnostic applications via near-infrared, photodynamic detection of colorectal cancer through the use of alginate and folic acid-based chitosan nanoparticles, utilization of cathepsin B in the form of fluorogenic peptide probes conjugated to glycol chitosan nanoparticles, and The number of nanotechnology-based goods and clinical trials authorized by the FDA has grown during the 1990s. It frequently combines synthetic polymer particles, liposome formulations, micellar nanoparticles, protein nanoparticles, and nanocrystals with other drugs. Nanomedicine has already transformed the discovery and administration of pharmaceuticals in biological systems, even though it will be the subject of important future advancements, including regulatory frameworks for nanomedications and safety/toxicity assessments as a result of breakthroughs in nanomedicine, it is now possible to diagnose disorders and integrate diagnosis with treatment.

References

1. I Khan, K Saeed, I. Khan, Nanoparticles: properties, applications, and toxicities. *Arab J Chem* 2019; 12(7): 908–931.
2. D Chenthamara, et al., Therapeutic efficacy of nanoparticles and routes of administration. *Biomater Res* 2019; 23(1): 20.
3. H Heinz, et al., Nanoparticle decoration with surfactants: molecular interactions, assembly, and applications. *Surf Sci Rep* 2017; 72(1): 1–58.
4. SB Ghaffari, et al., Functionalization of ZnO nanoparticles by 3-mercaptopropionic acid for aqueous curcumin delivery: synthesis, characterization, and anticancer assessment. *Mater Sci Eng C Mater Biol Appl* 2017; 79: 465–472.
5. JE Lee, et al., Multifunctional mesoporous silica nanocomposite nanoparticles for theranostic applications. *Accounts Chem Res* 2011; 44(10): 893–902.
6. M Mansha, et al., Synthesis, characterization and visible-light-driven photoelectrochemical hydrogen evolution reaction of carbazole-containing conjugated polymers. *Int J Hydrogen Energy* 2017; 42(16): 10952–10961.
7. H Ullah, et al., Sonochemical-driven ultrafast facile synthesis of SnO_2 nanoparticles: growth mechanism structural electrical and hydrogen gas sensing properties. *Ultrason Sonochem* 2017; 34: 484–490.
8. Y Xin, et al., Recent progress on nanoparticle-based drug delivery systems for cancer therapy. *Canc Biol Med* 2017; 14(3): 228–241.
9. A Heuer-Jungemann, et al., The role of ligands in the chemical synthesis and applications of inorganic nanoparticles. *Chem Rev* 2019; 119(8): 4819–4880.

10. A Kaushik, in: Akash Deep, Sandeep Kumar, eds, *Advances in Nanosensors for Biological and Environmental Analysis*: Book Review, Elsevier, 2019, ISBN 978-0-12-817456-2, p. 101.
11. Y Zhu, DK James, JM Tour, New routes to graphene, graphene oxide and their related applications. *Adv Mater* 2012; 24(36): 4924–4955.
12. E Ghavaminezhad, M Mahnama, N Zolfaghari, The effects of van der Waals interactions on the vibrational behavior of single-walled carbon nanotubes using the hammer impact test: a molecular dynamics study. *Phys Chem Chem Phys* 2020; 22(22): 12613–12623.
13. DM Dabbs, IA Aksay, Self-assembled ceramics produced by complex-fluid templation. *Ann Rev Phys Chem* 2000; 51(1): 601–622.
14. T Kaehler, Nanotechnology: basic concepts and definitions. *Clin Chem* 1994; 40(9): 1797–1799.
15. M Ghorbanpour, M Khanuja, A Varma, eds, *Nanoscience and Plant-Soil Systems*. Springer, Technology & Engineering, Soil Biology; 2017.
16. B Bhushan, ed, *Springer Handbook of Nanotechnology*. Technology & Engineering, Springer Science & Business Media; 2010.
17. Y Li, NH Lee, DS Hwang, JS Song, EG Lee, SJ Kim, Synthesis and characterization of nano titanania powder with high photoactivity for gas-phase photo-oxidation of benzene from $TiOCl_2$ aqueous solution at low temperatures. *Langmuir* 2004; 20(25): 10838–10844.
18. Y Xue, GA Mansoori, Self-assembly of diamondoid molecules and derivatives (MD simulations and DFT calculations). *Int J Mol Sci* 2010; 11: 288–303.
19. B Wang, P Král,, Thanopoulos I. Docking of chiral molecules on twisted and helical nanotubes: nanomechanical control of catalysis. *Nano Lett* 2006; 6(9): 1918–1921.
20. JA Kent, *Handbook of Industrial Chemistry and Biotechnology*, 12th ed, Vol. 1. New York: Springer; 2012.
21. The Project on Emerging Nanotechnologies. 2014. Consumer products inventory. Available at: http://www.nanotechproject.org/cpi/. Accessed.
22. MC Roco, CA Mirkin, MC Hersam, Nanotechnology research directions for societal needs in 2020: Summary of international study. *J Nanoparticle Res* 2011; 13(3): 897–919.
23. G Oberdorster, E Oberdorster, J Oberdorster, Nanotoxicology: an emerging discipline evolving from studies of ultrafine particles. *Environ Health Perspect* 2005; 113(7): 823–839.

24. Y Ju-Nam, JR Lead, Manufactured nanoparticles: an overview of their chemistry, interactions and potential environmental implications. *Sci Total Environ* 2008; 400(1–3): 396–414.

25. YM Li, GA Somorjai, Nanoscale advances in catalysis and energy applications. *Nano Lett* 2010; 10(7): 2289–2295.

26. Y Yu, P Zhang, L Guo, Z Chen, Q Wu, Y Ding, W Zheng, Y Cao, The design of TiO_2 nanostructures (nanoparticle, nanotube, and nanosheet) and their photocatalytic activity. *J Phys Chem C* 2014; 118(24): 12727–12733.

27. E Petryayeva, WR Algar, IL Medintz, Quantum dots in bioanalysis: a review of applications across various platforms for fluorescence spectroscopy and imaging. *Appl Spectrosc* 2013; 67(3): 215–252.

28. CHM Chuang, PR Brown, V Bulovic, MG Bawendi, Improved performance and stability in quantum dot solar cells through band alignment engineering. *Nat Mater* 2014; 13(8): 796–801.

29. RE Messersmith, GJ Nusz, SM Reed, Using the localised surface Plasmon resonance of gold nanoparticles to monitor lipid membrane assembly and protein binding. *J Phys Chem C* 2013; 117(50): 26725–26733.

30. G Lövestam, H Rauscher, G Roebben, BS Klüttgen, N Gibson, J-P Putaud, H Stamm, Considerations on a definition of nanomaterial for regulatory purposes. *Eur Commission Joint Res Centre*; 2010.

31. ISO. ISO/TS 27687:2008 Nanotechnologies – Terminology and Definitions for Nano-Objects – Nanoparticle, Nanofibre and Nanoplate. ISO; 2008.

32. JM Green, Peer reviewed: a practical guide to analytical method validation. *Anal Chem* 1996; 68(9): 305A–309A.

33. SA Bell, A beginner's guide to uncertainty of measurement, in Measurement Good Practice Guide. National Physical Laboratory; 2001.

34. J Wüthrich, M Weber, ISO/IEC 17025. Double Accreditation Brings a New Class of CRMs. Switzerland: Sigma-Aldrich Marketing Communications Europe; 2008. p 4.

35. ISO. Available at http://www.iso.org/iso/home/standards.htm. accessed 2015 Nov 19.

36. British Standards Institute. BS 0: 2011 A Standard for Standards–Principles of Standardization. British Standards Institute.

37. K Subramani, W Ahmed, JK Hartsfield, eds, *Nanobiomaterials in Clinical Dentistry*. Elsevier Inc.; 2012.

38. G Binnig, H Rohrer, Scanning tunnelling microscope. *Sci Am* 1985; 253: 50–56.
39. DM Eigler, EK Schweizer, Positioning single atoms with a scanning tunnelling microscope. *Nature* 1990; 344: 524–526.
40. MF Crommie, CP Lutz, DM Eigler, Confinement of electrons to quantum corrals on a metal surface. *Science* 1993; 262: 218–220.
41. G Binnig, CF Quate, C Gerber, Atomic force microscope. *Phys Rev Lett* 1986; 56: 930–933.
42. B Pelaz, et al., Diverse applications of nanomedicine. *ACS Nano* 2017; 11(3): 2313–2381.
43. S Chen, et al., Nanomaterials in medicine and pharmaceuticals: nanoscale materials developed with less toxicity and more efficacy. *Eur J Nanomed* 2013; 5(2): 61.
44. M Chandarana, A Curtis, C Hoskins, The use of nanotechnology in cardiovascular disease. *Appl Nanosci* 2018; 8(7): 1607–1619.
45. M Mozafari, Nanotechnology in wound care: one step closer to the clinic. *Mol Ther J Am Soc Gene Ther* 2018; 26(9): 2085–2086.
46. S Bayda, et al., The history of nanoscience and nanotechnology: from chemical-physical applications to nanomedicine. *Molecules* 2019; 25(1): 112.
47. D Bobo, et al., Nanoparticle-based medicines: a review of FDA-approved materials and clinical trials to date. *Pharm Res (NY)* 2016; 33(10): 2373–2387.
48. MA Obeid, et al., Delivering natural products and biotherapeutics to improve drug efficacy. *Ther Deliv* 2017; 8(11): 947–956.
49. S Russi, et al., Adapting and surviving: intra and extra-cellular remodelling in drug-resistant gastric cancer cells. *Int J Mol Sci* 2019; 20(15): 3736.
50. HK Verma, Exosomes facilitate chemoresistance in gastric cancer: future challenges and openings. *Precis Radiat Oncol* 2019; 3(4): 163–164.
51. J Larocque, DJ Bharali, SA Mousa, Cancer detection and treatment: the role of nanomedicines. *Mol Biotechnol* 2009; 42(3): 358–366.
52. JK Patra, et al., Nano based drug delivery systems: recent developments and future prospects. *J Nanobiotechnol* 2018; 16(1): 1–33.
53. R Misra, S Acharya, SK Sahoo, Cancer nanotechnology: application of nanotechnology in cancer therapy. *Drug Discov Today* 2010; 15(19–20): 842–850.

54. S Sengupta, et al., Temporal targeting of tumour cells and neovasculature with a nanoscale delivery system. *Nature* 2005; 436(7050): 568–572.

55. A Singh, et al., Composite polymeric magnetic nanoparticles for co-delivery of hydrophobic and hydrophilic anticancer drugs and MRI imaging for cancer therapy. *ACS Appl Mater Interfaces* 2011; 3(3): 842–856.

56. MS Shim, et al., Combined multimodal optical imaging and targeted gene silencing using stimuli-transforming nanotheranostics. *J Am Chem Soc* 2010; 132(24): 8316–8324.

57. M Merodio, et al., Ocular disposition and tolerance of ganciclovir-loaded albumin nanoparticles after intravitreal injection in rats. *Biomaterials* 2002; 23(7): 1587–1594.

58. MM Silva, et al., Chitosan nanoparticles as a mucoadhesive drug delivery system for ocular administration. *Mar Drugs* 2017; 15(12): 370.

59. C Shi, et al., Nanoscale technologies in highly sensitive diagnosis of cardiovascular diseases. *Front Bioeng Biotechnol* 2020; 8(June): 1–18.

60. Y Deng, et al., Application of the nano-drug delivery system in treatment of cardiovascular diseases. *Front Bioeng Biotechnol* 2020; 7(January): 1–18.

61. IY Chen, JC Wu, Cardiovascular molecular imaging: focus on clinical translation. *Circulation* 2011; 123(4): 425–443.

62. FA Jaffer, P Libby, R Weissleder, Molecular imaging of cardiovascular disease. *Circulation* 2007; 116(9): 1052–1061.

63. E Aikawa, et al., Osteogenesis associated with inflammation in early-stage atherosclerosis evaluated by molecular imaging *in vivo*. *Circulation* 2007; 116(24): 2841–2850.

64. A Saraste, SG Nekolla, M Schwaiger, Cardiovascular molecular imaging: an overview. *Cardiovasc Res* 2009; 83(4): 643–652.

65. M Kumar, et al., Chitosan IFN-gamma-pDNA nanoparticle (CIN) therapy for allergic asthma. *Genet Vaccine Ther* 2003; 1(1): 3.

66. AE John, et al., Discovery of a potent nanoparticle P-selectin antagonist with anti-inflammatory effects in allergic airway disease. *Faseb J* 2003; 17(15): 2296–2298.

67. M Saeedi, et al., Applications of nanotechnology in drug delivery to the central nervous system. *Biomed Pharmacother* 2019; 111(December 2018): 666–675.

68. F Dilnawaz, SK Sahoo, Therapeutic approaches of magnetic nanoparticles for the central nervous system. *Drug Discov Today* 2015; 20(10): 1256–1264.
69. Z Fan, D Chen, CX Deng, Improving ultrasound gene transfection efficiency by controlling ultrasound excitation of microbubbles. *J Control Release* 2013; 170(3): 401–413.
70. KK Jain, Role of nanotechnology in developing new therapies for diseases of the nervous system. *Nanomedicine* 2006; 1(1): 9–12.
71. MF Yanik, et al., Neurosurgery: functional regeneration after laser axotomy. *Nature* 2004; 432(7019): 822.
72. ED Kirson, Y Yaari, A novel technique for micro-dissection of neuronal processes. *J Neurosci Methods* 2000; 98(2): 119–122.
73. T Kubik, K Bogunia-Kubik, M Sugisaka, Nanotechnology on duty in medical applications. *Curr Pharmaceut Biotechnol* 2005; 6(1): 17–33.
74. S Shrivastava, D Dash, Applying nanotechnology to human health: revolution in biomedical sciences. *J Nanotechnol* 2009; 2009: 184702.
75. K Ma, et al., Electrospun nanofiber scaffolds for rapid and rich capture of bone marrow-derived hematopoietic stem cells. *Biomaterials* 2008; 29(13): 2096–2103.
76. A Chaubey, et al., Surface patterning: tool to modulate stem cell differentiation in an adipose system. *J Biomed Mater Res B Appl Biomater* 2008; 84(1): 70–78.
77. S Ber, G Torun Kose, V Hasirci, Bone tissue engineering on patterned collagen films: an *in vitro* study. *Biomaterials* 2005; 26(14): 1977–1986.
78. H Kenar, et al., Chemical and topographical modification of PHBV surface to promote osteoblast alignment and confinement. *J Biomed Mater Res* 2008; 85(4): 1001–1010.
79. A Khademhosseini, et al., Microfluidic patterning for fabrication of contractile cardiac organoids. *Biomed Microdevices* 2007; 9(2): 149–157.
80. S Bayda, et al., The history of nanoscience and nanotechnology: from chemicalphysical applications to nanomedicine. *Molecules* 2019; 25(1): 112. doi: 10.3390/molecules25010112.
81. B Issa, et al., Magnetic nanoparticles: surface effects and properties related to biomedicine applications. *Int J Mol Sci* 2013; 14(11): 21266–21305.

82. N Bertrand, J-C Leroux, The journey of a drug-carrier in the body: an anatomo physiological perspective. *J Control Release* 2012; 161(2): 152–163.

83. RH Prabhu, VB Patravale, MD Joshi, Polymeric nanoparticles for targeted treatment in oncology: current insights. *Int J Nanomed* 2015; 10: 1001.

84. T Lian, RJ Ho, Trends and developments in liposome drug delivery systems. *J Pharm Sci* 2001; 90: 667–680.

85. OC Farokhzad, J Cheng, BA Teply, et al., Targeted nanoparticle-aptamer bioconjugates for cancer chemotherapy *in vivo*. *Proc Natl Acad Sci U S A* 2006; 103: 6315–6320.

86. KG Janoria, S Gunda, SH Boddu, et al., Novel approaches to retinal drug delivery. *Expert Opin Drug Deliv* 2007; 4: 371–388.

87. R Langer, Implantable controlled-release systems. *Pharmacol Ther* 1983; 21: 35–51.

88. RS Langer, NA Peppas, Present and future applications of biomaterials in controlled drug delivery systems. *Biomaterials* 1981; 2: 201–214.

89. R Langer, J Folkman, Polymers for the sustained release of proteins and other macromolecules. *Nature* 1976; 263: 797–800.

90. R Langer, Drug delivery and targeting. *Nature* 1998; 392S: 5–10.

91. R Chess, Economics of drug delivery. *Pharm Res* 1998; 15: 172–174.

92. MK Swamy, UR Sinniah, Patchouli (PogostemoncablinBenth.): botany, agrotechnology and biotechnological aspects. *Ind Crops Prod* 2016; 87: 161–176.

93. K McNamara, SA Tofail, Nanosystems: the use of nanoalloys, metallic, bimetallic, and magnetic nanoparticles in biomedical applications. *Phys Chem Chem Phys* 2015; 17: 27981–27995.

94. A Portero, C Remuñán-López, M Criado, M Alonso, Reacetylated chitosan microspheres for controlled delivery of antimicrobial agents to the gastric mucosa. *J Microencapsul* 2002; 19: 797–809.

95. P Artursson, T Lindmark, SS Davis, L Illum EffectEffect of chitosan on the permeability of monolayers of intestinal epithelial cells (Caco-2). *Pharm Res* 1994; 11: 1358–1361.

96. R Fernández-Urrusuno, P Calvo, C Remuñán-López, JL Vila-Jato, MJ Alonso, Enhancement of nasal absorption of insulin using chitosan nano-particles. *Pharm Res* 1999; 16: 1576–1581.

97. AM De Campos, A Sánchez, MJ Alonso, Chitosan nanoparticles: a new vehicle for the improvement of the delivery of drugs to the ocular surface. Application to cyclosporin A. *Int J Pharm* 2001; 224: 159–168.

98. S Al-Qadi, A Grenha, D Carrión-Recio, B Seijo, C Remuñán-López, Micro-encapsulated chitosan nanoparticles for pulmonary protein delivery: *in vivo* evaluation of insulin-loaded formulations. *J Control Release* 2012; 157: 383–390.

99. MM Silva, R Calado, J Marto, A Bettencourt, AJ Almeida, L Gonçalves, Chitosan Nanoparticles as a mucoadhesive drug delivery system for ocular administration. *Mar Drugs* 2017; 15: 370.

100. S Pistone, FM Goycoolea, A Young, G Smistad, M Hiorth, Formulation of polysaccharide-based nanoparticles for local administration into the oral cavity. *Eur J Pharm Sci* 2017; 96: 381–389.

101. S Liu, S Yang, PC Ho, Intranasal administration of carbamazepine-loaded carboxymethyl chitosan nanoparticles for drug delivery to the brain. *Asian J Pharm Sci* 2018; 13: 72–81.

102. A Jain, SK Jain, Optimization of chitosan nanoparticles for colon tumours using experimental design methodology. *Artif Cells Nanomed Biotechnol* 2016; 44: 1917–1926.

103. NH Patil, PV Devarajan, Insulin-loaded alginic acid nanoparticles for sublingual delivery. *Drug Deliv* 2016; 23: 429–436.

104. S Haque, S Md, JK Sahni, J Ali, S Baboota, Development and evaluation of brain targeted intranasal alginate nanoparticles for treatment of depression. *J Psychiatr Res* 2014; 48: 1–12.

105. JV Román, MA Galán, EMM del Valle, Preparation and preliminary evaluation of alginate crosslinked microcapsules as potential drug delivery system (DDS) for human lung cancer therapy. *Biomed Phys Eng Expr* 2016; 2: 035015.

106. G Garrait, E Beyssac, M Subirade, Development of a novel drug delivery system: chitosan nanoparticles entrapped in alginate microparticles. *J Microencapsul* 2014; 31: 363–372.

107. J Costa, N Silva, B Sarmento, M Pintado, Potential chitosan-coated alginate nanoparticles for ocular delivery of daptomycin. *Eur J Clin Microbiol Infect Dis* 2015; 34: 1255–1262.

108. S Goswami, S Naik, Natural gums and its pharmaceutical application. *J Sci Innovative Res* 2014; 3: 112–121.

109. F Lafeur, M Michalek, Modified xanthan gum for buccal delivery—a promising approach in treating sialorrhea. *Int J Biol Macromol* 2017; 102: 1250–1256.

110. J Huang, Y Deng, J Ren, G Chen, G Wang, F Wang, X Wu, Novel in situ forming hydrogel based on xanthan and chitosan re-gelifying in liquids for local drug delivery. *CarbohydrPolym* 2018; 186: 54–63.

111. C Menzel, M Jelkmann, F Lafeur, A Bernkop-Schnürch, Nasal drug delivery: design of a novel mucoadhesive and in situ gelling polymer. *Int J Pharm* 2017; 517: 196–202.

112. B Sun, M Zhang, J Shen, Z He, P Fatehi, Y Ni, Applications of cellulose-based materials in sustained drug delivery systems. *Curr Med Chem* 2017. https://doi.org/10.2174/0929867324666170705143308.

113. WSA Elseoud, ML Hassan, MW Sabaa, M Basha, EA Hassan, SM Fadel, Chitosan nanoparticles/cellulose nanocrystals nanocomposites as a carrier system for the controlled release of repaglinide. *Int J Biol Macro Mol* 2018; 111: 604–613.

114. T Agarwal, SGH Narayana, K Pal, K Pramanik, S Giri, I Banerjee, Calcium alginate-carboxymethyl cellulose beads for colon-targeted drug delivery. *Int J Biol Macromol* 2015; 75: 409–417.

115. K Hansen, G Kim, KG Desai, H Patel, KF Olsen, J Curtis-Fisk, E Tocce, S Jordan, SP Schwendeman, Feasibility investigation of cellulose polymers for mucoadhesive nasal drug delivery applications. *Mol Pharm* 2015; 12: 2732–2741.

116. G Bozzuto, A Molinari, Liposomes as nanomedical devices. *Int J Nanomed* 2015; 10: 975.

117. L Sercombe, T Veerati, F Moheimani, SY Wu, AK Sood, S Hua, Advances and challenges of liposome assisted drug delivery. *Front Pharm* 2015; 6: 286.

118. NG Kotla, B Chandrasekar, P Rooney, G Sivaraman, A Larrañaga, KV Krishna, A Pandit, Y Rochev, Biomimetic lipid-based nanosystems for enhanced dermal delivery of drugs and bioactive agents. *ACS Biomater Sci Eng* 2017; 3: 1262–1272.

119. A Akbarzadeh, R Rezaei-Sadabady, S Davaran, SW Joo, N Zarghami, Y Hanifehpour, M Samiei, M Kouhi, K Nejati-Koshki, Liposome: classifca-tion, preparation, and applications. *Nanoscale Res Lett* 2013; 8: 102.

120. A Mohan, S Narayanan, S Sethuraman, UM Krishnan, Novel resveratrol and 5-fluorouracil co encapsulated in PEGylated nanoliposomes improve chemotherapeutic efficacy of combination against head and neck squamous cell carcinoma. *BioMed Res Int* 2014; 2014: 424239.

121. N Dimov, E Kastner, M Hussain, Y Perrie, N Szita, Formation and purifca-tion of tailored liposomes for drug delivery using a module-based micro continuous-flow system. *Sci Rep* 2017; 7: 12045.

122. K Miyata, RJ Christie, K Kataoka, Polymeric micelles for nano-scale drug delivery. *React FunctPolym.* 2011; 71: 227–234.

123. W Xu, P Ling, T Zhang, Polymeric micelles, a promising drug delivery system to enhance bioavailability of poorly water-soluble drugs. *J Drug Deliv* 2013; 2013: 340315.

124. SS Kulthe, YM Choudhari, NN Inamdar, V Mourya, Polymeric micelles: authoritative aspects for drug delivery. *Design Monomers Polym* 2012; 15: 465–521.

125. PV Devarajan, S Jain, *Targeted Drug Delivery: Concepts and Design*. Berlin: Springer; 2016.

126. V Mourya, N Inamdar, R Nawale, S Kulthe, Polymeric micelles: general considerations and their applications. *Ind J Pharm Educ Res* 2011; 45: 128–138.

127. RR Wakaskar, Polymeric micelles for drug delivery. *Int J Drug Dev Res* 2017; 9: 1–2.

128. A Mandal, R Bisht, ID Rupenthal, AK Mitra, Polymeric micelles for ocular drug delivery: from structural frameworks to recent preclinical studies. *J Control Release* 2017; 248: 96–116.

129. P Kesharwani, L Xie, S Banerjee, G Mao, S Padhye, FH Sarkar, AK Iyer, Hyaluronic acid-conjugated polyamidoamine dendrimers for targeted delivery of 3,4-difluorobenzylamine curcumin to CD44 overexpressing pancreatic cancer cells. *Coll Surf B* 2015; 136: 413–423.

130. K Madaan, S Kumar, N Poonia, V Lather, D Pandita, Dendrimers in drug delivery and targeting: drug-dendrimer interactions and toxicity issues. *J Pharm Bioallied Sci* 2014; 6: 139.

131. Y Cheng, Z Xu, M Ma, T Xu, Dendrimers as drug carriers: applications in different routes of drug administration. *J Pharm Sci* 2008; 97: 123–143.

132. B Noriega-Luna, LA Godínez, FJ Rodríguez, A Rodríguez, G Larrea, C Sosa Ferreira, R Mercado-Curiel, J Manríquez, E Bustos, Applications of dendrimers in drug delivery agents, diagnosis, therapy, and detection. *J Nanomater* 2014; 2014: 39.

133. S Tripathy, M Das, Dendrimers and their applications as novel drug delivery carriers. *J Appl Pharm Sci* 2013; 3: 142–149.

134. P Kesharwani, K Jain, NK Jain, Dendrimer as nanocarrier for drug delivery. *ProgrPolym Sci* 2014; 39: 268–307.

135. K Jain, U Gupta, NK Jain, Dendronized nanoconjugates of lysine and folate for treatment of cancer. *Eur J Pharm Biopharm* 2014; 87: 500–509.

136. A Kaur, K Jain, NK Mehra, N Jain, Development and characterization of surface engineered PPI dendrimers for targeted drug delivery. *Artif Cells Nanomed Biotechnol* 2017; 45: 414–425.

137. S-J Choi, JK Lee, J Jeong, J-H Choy, Toxicity evaluation of inorganic nanoparticles: considerations and challenges. *Mol Cell Toxicol* 2013; 9: 205–210.

138. F-Y Kong, J-W Zhang, R-F Li, Z-X Wang, W-J Wang, W Wang, Unique roles of gold nanoparticles in drug delivery, targeting and imaging applications. *Molecules* 2017; 22: 1445.

139. K Prusty, SK Swain, Nano silver decorated polyacrylamide/dextran nanohydrogels hybrid composites for drug delivery applications. *Mater Sci Eng* 2018; 85: 130–141.

140. A Marcu, S Pop, F Dumitrache, M Mocanu, C Niculite, M Gherghiceanu, C Lungu, C Fleaca, R Ianchis, A Barbut, Magnetic iron oxide nanoparticles as drug delivery system in breast cancer. *Appl Surf Sci* 2013; 281: 60–65.

141. VB JunyaPrasert, B Morakul, Nanocrystals for enhancement of oral bioavailability of poorly water-soluble drugs. *Asian J Pharm Sci* 2015; 10: 13–23.

142. R Ni, J Zhao, Q Liu, Z Liang, U Muenster, S Mao, Nanocrystals embedded in chitosan-based respirable swellable microparticles as dry powder for sustained pulmonary drug delivery. *Eur J Pharm Sci* 2017; 99: 137–146.

143. K McNamara, SA Tofail, Nanoparticles in biomedical applications. *Adv Phys* 2017; 2: 54–88.

144. J Kudr, Y Haddad, L Richtera, Z Heger, M Cernak, V Adam, O Zitka, Magnetic nanoparticles: from design and synthesis to real world applications. *Nanomaterials* 2017; 7: 243.

145. A Pandit, DI Zeugolis, Twenty-five years of nano-bio-materials: have we revolutionised healthcare? *Fut Med* 2016; 11(9): 985–987.

Chapter 2

Regulatory Barriers to the Marketing Authorization of Nanodrug Delivery System

Simran,[a,*] Bharathi Kannan,[a,*] Amruta Nandagawale,[a,*] Praveena Karnati,[a] Ramesh Joga,[a] Chetan Dushantrao Sabanis,[a] Parul Grover,[b] Rakesh K. Sindhu,[c] and Sandeep Kumar[a]

[a]*Department of Regulatory Affairs,*
National Institute of Pharmaceutical Education and Research,
Hyderabad, Balanagar, Hyderabad 500037, Telangana, India
[b]*KIET School of Pharmacy, KIET Group of Institutions,*
Delhi-NCR, Ghaziabad 201206, Uttar Pradesh, India
[c]*School of Pharmacy, Sharda University, Greater Noida,*
Uttar Pradesh 201310, India

sandeepkumar.ra@niperhyd.ac.in, katariatniper@gmail.com

Nanotechnology is an emerging field due to its prominent effect on unmet medical needs like cancer treatment. Along with advantages, lots of risks are also associated with this technology. Nowadays, due to comparatively high risk over benefits, this technology is limited to only severe diseases. Many pharma giants filed investigational new drug applications for nanoformulation. However, only few get marketed because according to regulatory

*These authors contributed equally.

Nanotechnology and Drug Delivery: Principles and Applications
Edited by Rakesh K. Sindhu

ISBN 978-981-4968-83-6 (Hardcover), 978-1-003-43040-7 (eBook)
www.jennystanford.com

bodies safety is the prior requirement. Benefits should overcome the risk for the approval of any drug whether it is normal or nanoformulations. In the case of nanoformulation, most of the drugs reach clinical trials after a successful preclinical trial. But jammed in clinical trials due to the insufficiency of risk-benefits data. Some countries consider nanomaterials as hazardous chemicals and regulate them accordingly. However, there is an urge to frame common applicable preclinical toxicity studies to minimize clinical trial failure.

2.1 Introduction

The emerging and highly explored science in the last two decades is nanoscience which is the study of materials, which have at least one dimension of the particle size in the nanometer range. It was observed that the size of the material controlled to the subatomic level resulted in unique properties and drastic alterations in its properties (physicochemical, biological, mechanical, optical, electronic so on and so forth). These novel or altered properties are further explored to the extent of nearly all the research applications to produce improved products. Apart from having its application in diverse fields (e.g., electronic industry, environment treatment technologies), it showed a great impact on the pharmaceutical field. The demand for nanotechnology has been augmented over 10 years. For example, the submission of applications like New Drug Application (NDA), Abbreviated New Drug Application (ANDA), and Investigational New Drug (IND) towards drug products containing nanomaterials has increased as depicted in Fig. 2.1. Along with the demands, advancements like carbon-based nanoparticles, metal nanoparticles, polymeric nanoparticles, and lipid-based nanoparticles were also established [1]. This unique technology finds different properties of the material at this scale of size which was not observed in bulk size. Such unique properties of materials are found to overcome many limitations of conventional pharmaceuticals and older formulations of drug delivery systems, for instance by increasing the efficacy and reducing the toxicity.

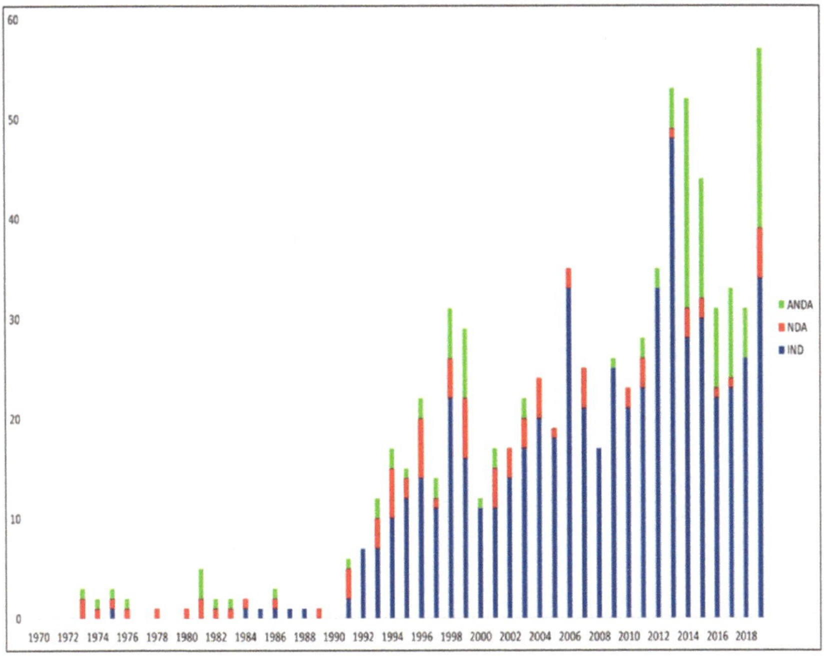

Figure 2.1 Nanotechnology-Over a Decade of Progress and Innovation "A Report by the US Food and Drug Administration" issued on July 2020. The figure has been taken from the USFDA website 2020 [2].

The efficacy was enhanced mostly due to the comparatively smaller size than the normal formulations. Stringent regulations regarding nanoformulations can be considered the root cause of these limitations. Nowadays several studies are going on the nanoformulations; however, only a few medicines can reach the market by going through the regulatory requirements [3]. According to the United States-food and drug administration (USFDA) this unique nanotechnology covers the size range between 1 to 100 nm [4]. Any technology that involves these kinds of size particles is considered nanotechnology [5]. In 2011 European Commission (EC) provided a definition that includes any manufactured or natural preparations involving 1–100 nm particles either in unbound or aggregated states and the threshold of distribution is 50% or in random cases can be considered as 1 to 50%. Moreover, the EC took the initiative to define the term nanoparticles but this definition is only to determine whether a formulation has nanoparticles or not [6, 7]. Nanotechnology is a broad spectrum of technology covering various health branches like biologicals, medical devices, and drugs. Many researchers have been attracted to this technology because it overcomes many conventional drug barriers like absorption, distribution, dose reductions, and permeability. Nowadays every researcher works on nanotechnology but not every formulation reaches the market. Because for regulatory bodies safety is the priority even more than efficacy and many safety risks are associated with this technology. This chapter gives a deep insight regarding nanotechnology along with various regulations associated with nanotechnology and the barrier faced by the formulator to market nanoformulations.

2.2 Criteria for the Selection of Nanoparticles in the Formulation

Before proceeding to the nanoformulations many criteria should be followed by the scientist while selecting the nanoparticles to avoid toxicity and regulatory hurdles in the marketing of nanoformulation. Although the selection of raw material or drug discovery is not a part of regulatory approval still if some criteria are followed by the formulator regarding safety and efficacy, will ultimately help to get the regulatory approval in later stages. Various criteria for the selection of nanoparticles have been given below [3, 7]:

1. Nanoformulation should be controlled and slow release instead of immediate release.
2. Nanoformulation should have the capability to bind the selected target to show efficacy.
3. Stable physicochemical properties lead to better penetration through the membrane barrier.
4. Considerations should be taken while selecting nanoparticles like non-immunogenicity, biocompatibility, and biodegradability.
5. Avoid the use of the organic and toxic substances as a solvent while preparing a formulation.

6. Raw materials used in the preparations should be cheap, safe, and easily available. Although price does not affect the regulatory approval decision but decreases competition with other marketed approved drugs for the same indication.
7. Stability is another parameter that should be fulfilled by the formulations while storage.

2.3 The Need for Nanomedicine Regulation

Previously nanoformulations were considered the same as the other conventional drugs. But later the nanomedicines were found to have general toxicity along with genotoxicity and mutagenicity. Due to its smaller size, it can easily cross the blood-brain barrier [8] and directly interact with cellular physiology and produce toxicity [9]. Most of the recorded cases are on free radical accumulation [1]. Till now many studies have been done on nanotechnologies. In the area of health, this technology demonstrated the potential in various lab-scale experiments and has been explored in almost all applications of pharmaceutical sciences. However, the irony is that most of the nanoformulations failed in clinical trials; Sinerem is an example. Sinerem was developed by Guerbet for the purpose of the diagnosis of pelvic cancer. This product includes ultra-small iron oxide which is super-paramagnetic. The product's unique technology and sensitivity make it able to reach the clinical trial. However, in the phase III clinical trial, this diagnostic device got revoked by the company itself. The reason behind the self-revocation was that the company was unable to submit the additional data asked by the Committee for Medicinal Product for Human Use (CHMP) while processing the application. When the European regulatory body asks for additional data regarding the risk-benefit ratio. This case emphasized the need for new methods for the analysis of nanomaterials so that these formulations do not show failure in clinical trials.

Nanoformulations are different from conventional formulations. Their toxicity profile and high absorption and permeability make them different from the conventional drug so their regulatory approval criteria should also be different because not every shoe size is meant for every foot. Similarly, different formulations need different regulations. After back-to-back case studies awakened the regulatory bodies to prepare separate guidelines regarding nanotechnology. As discussed in the introduction, nanotechnology is involved in pharmaceuticals, medical devices, and biological as well. All products have their own regulatory guidelines for regulatory approval. The nano regulations should also vary on the type of the product for example nanobiologicals and nanodevices. Moreover, these different guidelines for different pathways are important but still will extend the complexity for the stakeholder. To resolve the issue of the regulation regarding nanotechnology, a community like the Environment Protection Act (EPA), European Medicines Agency (EMA), and many small communities joined hands and prepared regulatory science framework nano(bio) material-based medical products and devices named as REFINE project. Its objectives were decided in 2019 and provided regulatory suggestions and guidelines for devices, biologicals, and pharmaceuticals that involve nanotechnology. This project provides new methods for testing and validation of the products involved in nanotechnology. These products involved both regulatory bodies and stakeholders to develop a new method for testing of toxicology of the products and work on regulatory sciences. As discussed in the introduction only a few nanopreparations reach the market because of the regulatory barrier. The REFINE project objective is to assist the formulator to overcome the regulatory barrier through its regulatory science tool [10–12].

2.4 REFINE Project

In 2017, the European Technology platform initiated a REFINE project for the regulatory framework of nanomedicines to provide the required data to the regulatory body in a suitable manner with respect to the safety profile of the drug product as well as medical devices [13, 14]. Formulators found many issues to standardize their formulations. However, some products are combinations of biological nanoparticles. Then the formulators become confused about which pathway will be suitable for their product. In these kinds of cases, REFINE plays a key role in regulatory approval by using regulatory sciences. REFINE is the result of collaborations of various communities like EC and other small communities. It consists of various stakeholders of science, regulatory, and technology along with the end-user. The team of experts develops methods for testing and validations. Apply regulatory science to reduce the chances of product failure in clinical trials. This project is only applicable to biomaterials and nanomedicines [15, 16]. The organizations and regulations of the REFINE project have been given in Fig. 2.2.

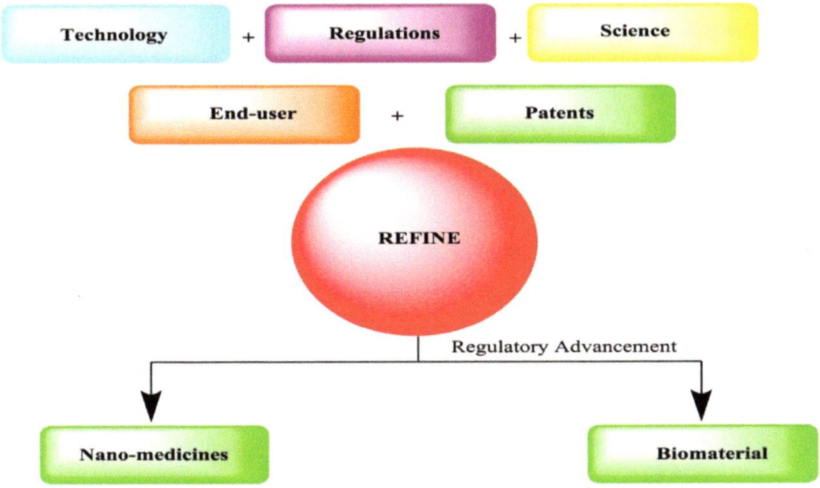

Figure 2.2 REFINE project stakeholders and regulated products.

2.5 Regulatory Challenges of Nanomedicines

Many regulatory challenges have been faced by the inventor to get approval for marketing their product in respective countries. Meanwhile, every country has their own regulatory bodies and regulations, and due to variations in regulations, it will be difficult to impose the same nanomedicine regulations on every country. Nano guidelines and their challenges in various countries have been discussed in further sections.

2.5.1 European Union (EU) Guidelines

According to EU legislation, the substance covered under the nanomaterial is considered chemical. In the EU all chemicals which can harm humans, as well as the environment, are regulated by European Chemicals Agency (ECHA) and have to go through the Registration, Evaluation, Authorisation and Restriction of Chemicals (REACH) registration and Classification, Labelling, and Packaging (CLP). The consideration of nanomaterials as chemicals somehow clears the path for nanomedicines in Europe [17]. The REACH was developed by the EU to protect humans and the environment from exposure to harmful chemicals. Although the nanomaterials are different from other hazardous chemicals because all tests for chemicals do not apply to nanomaterials. The issue has been acknowledged by REACH and in response to that, its developed requirements which are specially meant for the nanomaterials which include additional dissolution in water or other media to be performed in addition to solubility data, and dispersion stability data in different media can be a replacement for n-octanol/water partition coefficient. According to Annexure VI of REACH guidelines, if any treatment and surface functionalization have been done on nanomaterial then the proper description and IUPAC name along with the CAS number is required for each agent used. REACH also mention specific surface area by mass and volume or both are required. The shape of nanomaterial is also associated with toxicity. So, morphological characterization, shape and aspect ratio are mentioned as the special requirements in the case of nanomaterial [18]. Likewise, nanomaterials should be classified according to its hazards capacity and labeled according to the CLP guidelines provided by ECHA. After the clarification from REACH and CLP, the product went through the marketing authorization procedure likewise other pharmaceutical products [19, 20]. The process of marketing authorizations showing the role of above mention agency and guidelines for nanomedicines has been given in Fig. 2.3.

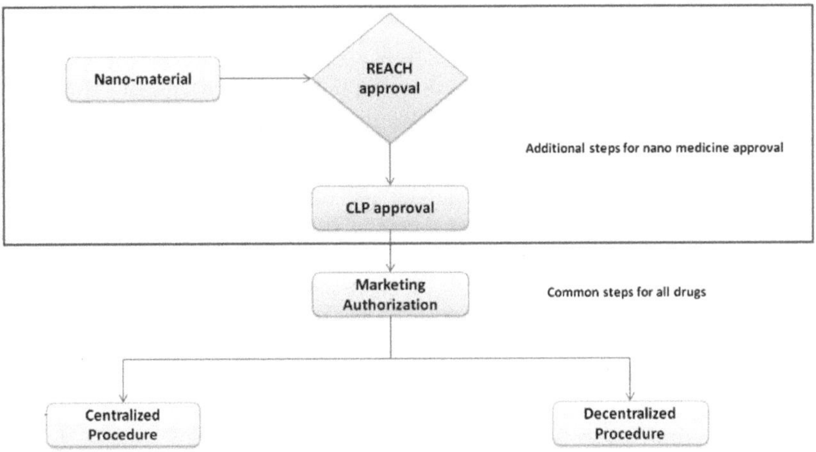

Figure 2.3 Process of marketing authorizations for nanomedicines. (REACH-Registration, Evaluation, Authorisation and Restriction of Chemicals, CLP—Classification, Labelling and Packaging).

In the approval process in the EU, there is no major difference. Medicinal products can be approved within 210 days of the procedure or can be shortened by 150 days based on the public health interest [21].

2.5.2 United States Guidelines

In 2000, USFDA created the National Nanotechnology Initiative (NNI) to minimize the hurdles associated with the development of nanoformulation. Then in 2006, Nanotechnology Task Force (NTF) was developed by the relevant authority [22]. According to the NTF report 2007, a bulk of products associated with the nanomaterial were applied for approval in the US [23]. This gradual increase in the applications of pharmaceutical products including nanomaterials increases the concern of the regulatory bodies with regard to nanomaterials. This forces the agency to develop separate guidelines regarding nanomedicines to ensure that only safe and effective products reach the US population. The basic challenge was that nanomaterials are not limited to drugs they are also implied in the devices and biologicals as well. The USFDA has different departments for different health products which has been described in (Fig. 2.4). To resolve that issue the US-FDA established different requirements of nano guidelines with respect to their categories [24].

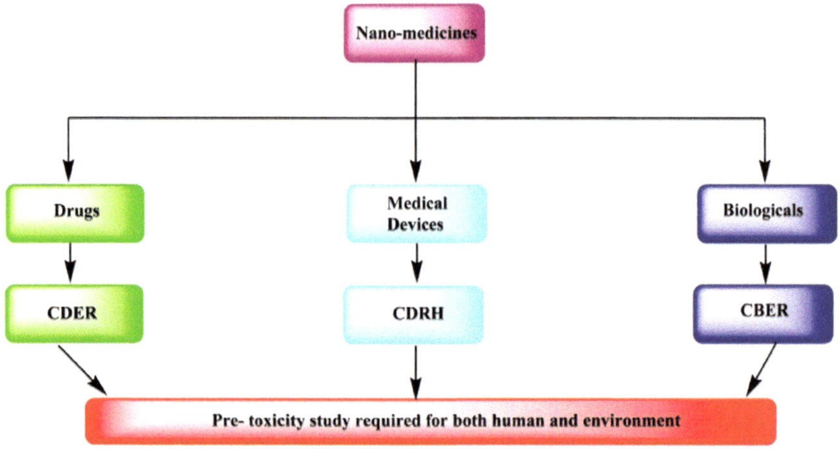

Figure 2.4 Different regulators for approval in USFDA.

2.5.2.1 The process to get approval for nanomedicines in the US market

As discussed in Fig. 2.4, different regulators and approval pathways will vary from product to product. However general approval processes have been given in Fig. 2.5. According to US legislation, if the product comes under the category of nanomedicines, then the product should go through all the toxicity studies in the preclinical stages. Likewise, the EU and the US also considered nanomaterials as hazardous chemicals that can harm humans as well as the environment. That means any nanoformulation whether it is a pre-approved drug, has to go through all preclinical and clinical trials to ensure the safety and efficacy of the drug. The main drawback of the formulator is that the USFDA has not provided any authentic definition of nanomaterial. Moreover, the scientist-recommended range of up to 100 is accepted by the USFDA.

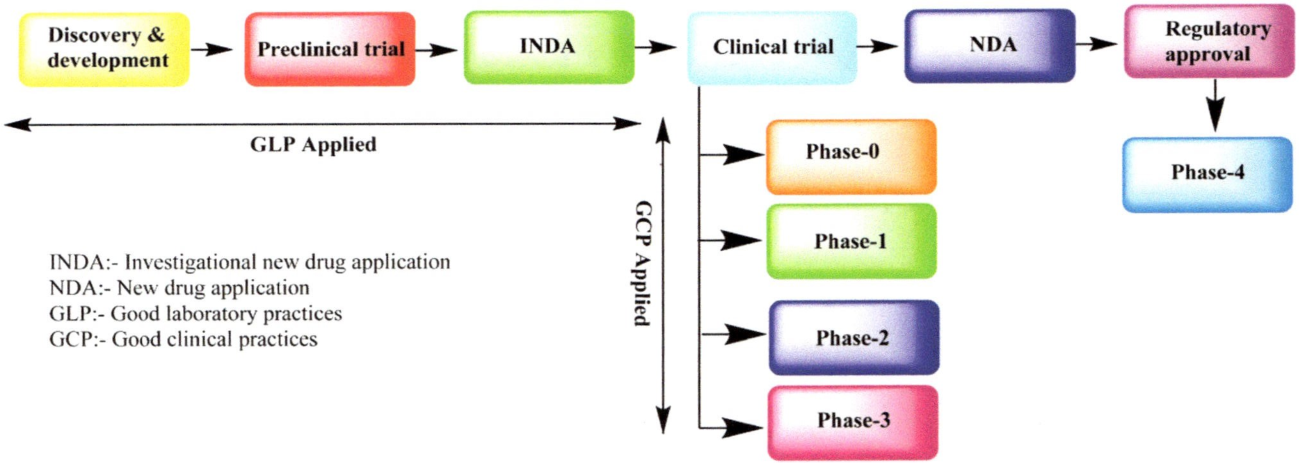

Figure 2.5 General drug approval process.

2.5.2.2 Guidance for formulators regarding the application of nanomedicines

If the applicant wants to market their drug including the nanomaterial, they have to follow 505(b)(2) which is for the new drug, and in the case of generic the applicant should go for 505(J) [23]. However if the application is for the devices, then it will depend on the class of the medical device in the case of high-risk medical devices the applicant should follow the Pre-marketing approval which needs clinical data. Likewise, 510(k) is for medium-risk medical devices. Generally, devices containing nanomaterial do not come under the low-risk devices which need only notification [25]. In the case of biologics 351(k) same applies [25, 26].

2.5.3 Indian Guidelines

As per the Guidelines for Evaluation of Nanopharmaceuticals released in October 2019, a nanopharmaceutical has been suggested as any drug formulation or pharmaceutical preparation having nanomaterials, i.e., material of particle size 1–100 nm in one or more dimensions, also including those materials of up to 1000 nm size which has its property (chemical, physical and biological) attributed to its size with the intention of internal use or external application on humans for therapeutics, diagnostics, and health benefits [27].

2.5.3.1 Evolution of regulations regarding nanopharmaceuticals in India

In 2006, the Indian government empower the Department of Pharmaceuticals to carry out the project of framing the regulation for nanomedicine to the National Institute of Pharmaceutical Education and Research (NIPER) Mohali then after a few years in 2012, it was handed over to NIPER Kolkata that it will be answerable for nanotoxicology assessment and regulations of nanodrugs and devices [28]. In the year 2007, As a part of the government's National Nanotechnology strategy plan, the National Center for Nano-Structured Materials was created and it was handled by the

Council for Scientific and Industrial Research (CSIR). Then CSIR launched the project Nano-SHE, i.e., Nanomaterials: Application and Impact on Safety, Health, and Environment for toxicological evaluation of nanostructured materials [29]. In the same year 2007, the Department of Science and Technology (DST) working group was formed for the regulation of nanotechnology it launches a mission on Nanoscience and Technology (NanoMission) [30]. DST's Nano-mission program announced establishing a Framework Roadmap for National Regulatory Authorities in the field of nanotechnology. Nano-mission has also developed a draft guideline and best practices for the safe handling of nanomaterials in 2019 [31].

2.5.3.2 Draft guidelines issued in 2019

Nanomaterials are generally tiny particles that can perforate into the cell very quickly and it is likely to have a greater impact. Their special characteristic properties and features make the drug utilization wider. As a result of this perforation, it can cause harmful effects on human health and surrounding also. For this reason, various studies are currently going around the world to assess the toxicity because the works of literature based on nanomaterials are insufficient. The Centre for Knowledge Management of Nanoscience and Technology (CKMNT) & International Advanced Research Centre for Powder Metallurgy & New Materials (ARCI) had stepped up to make the guideline regarding good handling practices on nanomaterials in their respective working areas. They proposed that scientists who are working or going to work on nanomaterials should follow the guidelines like equipment for personal protection, work practices, etc., to reduce hazardous exposure. A framework for nanomaterial regulation done by the European Union called REACH will be followed and adopted efficiently wherever required.

Indian guidelines regarding nanoformulation are still in their budding stage. Regulatory bodies in collaboration with technical and science experts are working hard to establish proper guidelines concerning the pharmaceuticals associated with nanoformulations. Plenty of time is needed to build ideal regulations. However, the work on nano regulations is going on, and to minimize the risk, in 2019 India provided draft guidelines associated with nanomedicines. These guidelines provided basic handling methods given in (Fig. 2.6) to avoid safety risks associated with nanoformulations.

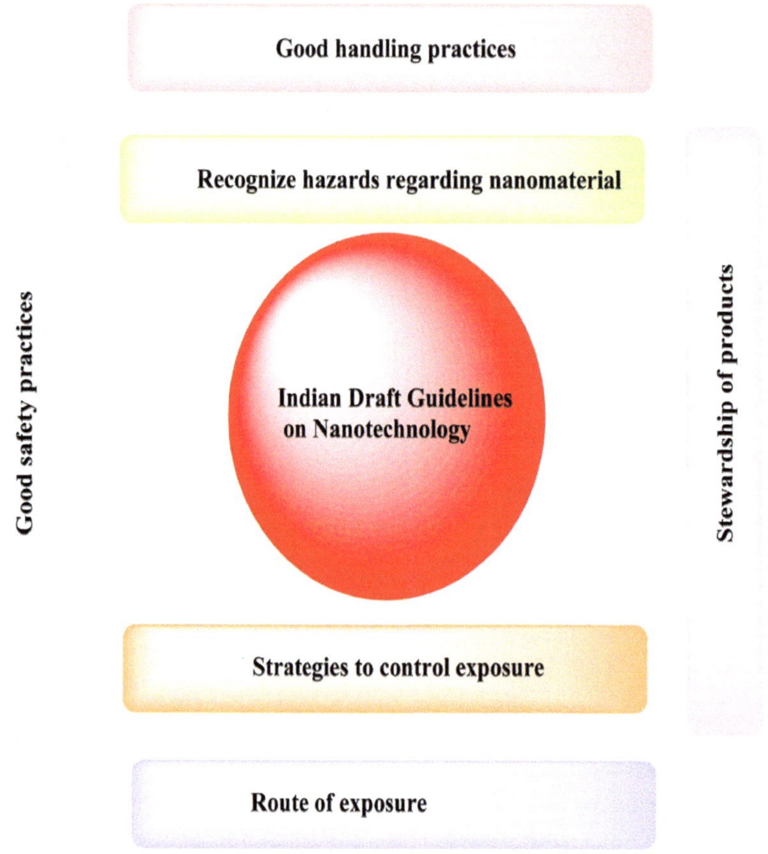

Figure 2.6 Methods of handling of nanomaterial according to Indian draft guidelines [31].

2.5.3.2.1 Recognizing hazards

Identification is the prior step to avoid hazards. There are various categories through which the identification of hazards has been done. Surface charge is an important parameter to recognize the severity of the hazards like cationic charge is more cytotoxic and neutral charge is least cytotoxic. Accumulation of free radical produce toxicity, through surface chemistry it can be identified. Different shapes of nanomaterials are associated with different kinds of toxicity; for example, fibrous nanomaterials produce lung toxicity. Solubility plays a key role to identify hazards; for example, low-solubility nanomaterials have a higher ability to develop cancer and oxidative stress compared with high-solubility ones. If the flash point of nanomaterial is below 200°F, then it will be characterized aa s fire hazard. The value of flash point will vary with types of materials; for example, in the case of flammable liquid, the value should not exceed 100°F. Meanwhile, in the case of combustible liquids, the value is ≥100°F. Toxic Hazard helps in deciding the safety preventive measures with Threshold Limit Values (TLV) or Permissible Exposure Limits (PEL) should have a value less than 50 parts per million and will be handled with care mostly in the fume hood. Explosion Hazard can be identified by calculating with minimum ignition energy and minimum exposable dust concentration.

2.5.3.2.2 Route of exposure

Nanomaterials can penetrate the body through various routes like inhalation, dermal absorption, and ingestion. It is important to understand all the possible routes through which nanomaterials can enter the human body to avoid further risks. Safety precautions should be carried out according to the exposure route. For example, N95 mask should be used while dealing with powder form of nanomaterial because in powder form there are high chances of inhalation as compared to suspension. Likewise in the case of the dermal route, safety measures like, gloves, lab coats are used while handling nanoformulations to minimize the exposure.

2.5.3.2.3 Strategies to control exposure

(A) Control of Engineered Particles

Appropriate measures should be taken before unveiling nanoparticles. These techniques are:

1. Revealing the source of generation

2. Filters are used to catch airborne particles. For example- High-Efficiency Particulate Air (HEPA) filter
3. Nanomaterials from the reactors are collected by appropriate containers such as airlocks and sealed containers

(B) Control of Administration

It consists of various other additional procedure techniques such as training, housekeeping, work practice, health check-ups, keeping records of work done, supervision of workstations, and storage. Various considerations should be taken care of while imparting training to personnel:

(1) Proper understanding of nanoparticles
(2) Standard operating procedure knowledge
(3) Maintaining equipment associated with nanomaterials
(4) Handling of waste materials and their labeling
(5) Regular checking of the health status of employees
(6) Understanding the impact on the atmosphere

2.5.3.2.3.1 *Supervisions of workstations*

Regular supervision is important in the case of nanomaterials. Through supervision concentration of nanomaterials at the workplace can be detected by using various methods like, condensation particle counters.

2.5.3.2.3.2 *Storage*

Storage of nanoparticles should be taken under special precautions to protect the product as well as the personnel.

2.5.3.2.3.3 *Waste disposal*

In sealed containers, we are able to pour milligrams of nanoparticles that should be correctly labeled and should be disposed of in front of responsible authorities. If it is more than a milligram then disposal will be based on the solubility of the chemicals. If the solubility is less, it is considered as chemical waste, it can be metals or metal oxides, etc., on the other hand, if the solubility is more, based on the toxicity class its disposal is carried out.

2.5.3.2.4 Nanomaterials handling and production

(1) Transportation and storage are done in containers which is shatter resistant, along with defined labeling
(2) Dry powders quantification and weighting have to be done in closed areas
(3) Multiple processing steps are used to produce nanoparticles at a greater concentration. In this step, staff can be exposed to nanomaterials so the generation of nanomaterials will be done under sufficient operating controls
(4) Caution must be taken to avoid any interruption of the enclosed chambers, and cleaning should be carried out on a wet stage or in the liquid medium so that spreading can be avoided
(5) Working stations should be monitored on a regular basis to avoid the exposure of nanomaterials to staff
(6) Waste disposal should be done by the production department with reduced risk to humans and the atmosphere

2.5.3.2.5 Safety practices

In this transportation, buddy system, outburst safety, controlling access, and dry materials are discussed. When a staff is working lonely in his labs, he should make friends in his nearby labs so that they will notice us in and out the time of the labs, especially when you are doing highly hazardous operations this is called a buddy system.

2.5.3.2.5.1 *Outburst safety*

Nanomaterials are oxidizable in powder form so that when it becomes in contact with water, they will show pyrophoric activities so outburst can happen. When these outburst materials activities are done in labs anti-static shoes and mates are highly preferred. Tests for pyrophoricity should be done on small quantities of nanomaterial.

2.5.3.2.5.2 *Dry materials*

A walk-off mat should be placed in the exit area. While cleaning the materials which are collected should be disposed of properly. Nanomaterials in HEPA vacuum are labeled separately as "For Use with Nanomaterials Only."

2.5.3.2.6 Product supervision

This product will be delivered to the customers with supporting information such as a material safety data sheet, a sheet of information about the product, operating manuals, and a sheet of specifications [31].

2.5.3.3 Required information for the evaluation of nanomaterials

Nanopharmaceuticals are classified based on functions and their nature and the current status of marketing approval of nanomaterial and active pharmaceutical ingredient forms of the drug.

Nanomaterial is classified based on their:

1. Degradation characteristics
2. Nature of Nanomaterials
3. Ingredient in Nanoform

2.5.3.3.1 Based on their degradation characteristics, it is further classified into biodegradable and non-biodegradable

2.5.3.3.1.1 *Biodegradable*

These materials are breakdown or decompose naturally, so it is often used in drug delivery as vehicles. For example, proteins, lipids, etc.

2.5.3.3.1.2 *Non-biodegradable*

These materials do not decompose naturally, so they are infrequently used in pharmaceuticals. But often used in cosmetics. For example, gold, platinum, silver, etc. Non-biodegradables are stored in the body over a period of time which is the biggest disadvantage while using them.

2.5.3.3.2 Based on the nanomaterial's nature, they are further classified into organic and inorganic materials

2.5.3.3.2.1 *Organic nanomaterials*

A drug which has carbon molecules in its structure will fall under this category which is primarily focused on reduction in toxicity and improved bioavailability at the site. For example, polymers, liposomes, and proteins.

2.5.3.3.2.2 *Inorganic nanomaterials*

It generally contains an inorganic portion. Based on the combination, size and others there are various adjustable properties. It generally has higher stability than organic nanomaterials. It has several benefits over organic nanomaterials and it is very easy to prepare.

2.5.3.3.2.3 *Multi-component nanomaterials*

Made up of more than two diverse materials so, this makes the drug for fulfilling several functions along with its physico-chemical properties. For example, magnetic liposomes. Although the stability of the nanomaterials remains challenging.

2.5.3.3.3 Based on the ingredient used in the nanoform

2.5.3.3.3.1 *Nanocarriers loaded with API*

These are transporters used along with the drug. Due to their small size, they can easily release the drug at a particular site or a convenient site within the body. Examples are liposomal amphotericin B, etc.

2.5.3.3.4 Based on drug approval status along with nanomaterial in other countries

The need for data may vary according to the drug approval status along with its nanomaterials. The Central Drug Standard Control Organization (CDSCO) evaluates all nanopharmaceutical formulations as new drugs based on four categories:

1st Category: Here the drug and nanocarrier are new to the market and not yet approved in any other country. Therefore, it will be considered as an IND application. The requirements for the application data have been given in the second schedule of New Drug Clinical Trials (NDCT) Rules, 2019.

2nd Category: The New Molecular Entity (NME) is not yet approved but the carrier is utilized already in nanopharmaceuticals. This will also be treated as an IND application. The requirement for data is given in the second schedule of NDCT Rules, 2019. Relaxation for this category is safety studies on nanocarrier molecules.

3rd Category: The NME is approved in other countries but the carrier molecule is not approved or regulated in any other countries. In this formulation, the data for the IND application is given in the second schedule of NDCT Rules. But sufficient data on the safety of the final formulation should be reported to the regulatory body at the time of submission.

4th Category: In this category, both the drug and carrier molecule are approved as the particular formulation is still to be approved in India. This type of application is considered as abbreviated or bridging studies as per the second schedule of NDCT Rules, 2019.

2.5.3.3.5 Evaluation of nanopharmaceuticals with respect to the second schedule of the NDCT Rules, 2019

The guidelines and general requirements for the manufacture or import of a new drug or to undertake a clinical trial with consideration to nanopharmaceuticals have been outlined in the second schedule of New Drug and Clinical Trails along with their chemical and pharmaceutical information, non-clinical and clinical data concerning a nanotechnology-based pharmaceutical product. Although the complexity of these products varies case-by-case, products should be taken on for evaluating their quality, safety, and efficacy. The impact of waste disposal of these nanomaterials and their effect on the environment should also be discussed. India accepts USFDA guidelines for liposomal formulations.

2.5.3.3.6 Testing for the stability of nanopharmaceutical formulations

Based on the methods given in the 5th clause of the second schedule (i.e., stability testing of new drugs) of NDCT Rules, 2019 and International Conference on Harmonization Q1 Guidelines. In specified storage conditions, the drug should be tested from time to time to confirm its stability when the drug is loaded with a carrier molecule. So, attention should be given to the effectiveness, size, and stability of formulation and carrier along with its degradation products. Stability studies have been conducted on marketing packs along with the parameters that are particular to nanomaterial-based formulations e.g. size & size distribution and drug loading by suitable methods. These parameters should be measured at suitable time intervals. For example, if we use PEG for surface coating the thickness of PEG will be quantified by appropriate analytical methods. The characterization should be done for the nanomaterial system as well.

2.5.3.3.7 Data on animal pharmacology

Data should be based on the toxicity of active pharmaceutical ingredients as well as the drug's intended use and also the delivery system which influences the drug release. For this purpose, the guidelines are established in animal pharmacology (i.e., 3rd clause) of the second schedule of NDCT Rules, 2019. However, evaluating the nanopharmaceutical drug effectiveness, the response of the product should be noted in preclinical testing. Evaluation of the properties should result in the increase of therapeutic effectiveness, drug accumulation at the site of release. For example, in cancer studies, data should be collected with respect to accumulation in the tumor cells or biodistribution, circulation, and bioavailability. In the case of nanopharmaceuticals with brain targeting action, some special studies have to be performed with appropriate drug concentration in a different location in the brain when compared to other studies.

2.5.3.3.8 Data on animal toxicology

Data generated in the area of toxicological studies for nanopharmaceuticals should follow the guidelines based on the administered route which is given in animal toxicology studies (i.e., clause 2) of the second schedule of NDCT Rules, 2019. The most preferred animal models are rodent and non-rodent species. Commonly rats and dogs are preferred in both sexes.

2.5.3.3.9 Information required for evaluation of nanopharmaceuticals

Data which are generally submitted to the regulatory authority along with the clinical trials and manufacture of nanopharmaceuticals for marketing in India will be the same as those requirements mentioned in NDCT Rules, 2019 [27].

2.6 Roles of Intellectual Property (Patent) in Regulatory Approval

A patent is an exclusive right provided to the inventor that nobody can use his invention without permission. On the other hand, regulatory approval is the method by which an inventor can launch their drug into the market. The regulatory approval is not limited to the patented product. The non-patented drugs can also get regulatory approval through the pathways like repurposing and generic drugs. In the case of nanodrug delivery systems, bulk formulations got patents. However, out of them, only a few reaches the market (a few are listed in Table 2.1) which means patents do not assure that the innovation got marketing approval or not. The differences between a patent and regulatory approval have been given in Table 2.2.

2.7 Comparison of Various Countries' Regulations with Regard to Nanotechnology

Regulations regarding nano varied from country to country. The US has separate guidelines for devices, drugs and biologicals which includes nanomaterial. Meanwhile, the EU considers all nanomaterials in the range of 1 to 100 nm as harmful chemicals and regulated by a separate body named ECHA. In ECHA, the nanomaterial should go through REACH and CLP approval. In India, the guidelines regarding nanomaterials are still in the development stage. Till now only draft guidelines regarding the careful handling of nanomaterials have been given. However, REACH is accepted in India for nanomaterials. The comparison and challenges associated with nano in various countries have been described in Table 2.3.

Table 2.1 List of globally marketed nanomedicines approved by the FDA and the EMA

Type	Trade name	Company	Date of approval	Active ingredients	Indication
Nanocrystals	Emend®	Merck & Co. Inc.	FDA (2003)	aprepitant	antiemetic drug
	Ivemend®	Merck & Co. Inc.	FDA, EMA (2008)	fosaprepitant dimeglumine (prodrug of aprepitant)	antiemetic drug
	Ostim®	Osartis GmbH & Co	FDA (2004)	calcium hydroxyapatite	bone-grafting material
	Rapamune®	Wyeth Pharmaceuticals Inc. (a subsidiary of Pfizer Inc.)	EMA(2001), FDA (2010)	sirolimus (rapamycin)	prevents rejection of kidney transplants (immunosuppressant)
	Vitoss®	Orthovita Inc	FDA (2003)	β-tricalcium phosphate	bone-grafting material
	Ritalin LX®	Novartis	FDA (2002)	methylphenidate	attention deficit hyperactivity disorder (ADHD) in children
	Avinza®	Pfizer Pharmaceuticals	FDA (2002)	morphine sulfate	psychostimulant
	Focalin XR®	Novartis	FDA (2008)	dexmethylphenidate HCl	ADHD in children
	Invega®	Janssen Pharmaceuticals	FDA (2009)	paliperidone	schizophrenia
	Invega Sustenna®	Janssen Pharmaceuticals	FDA (2009)	paliperidone Palmitate	schizophrenia
	Megace ES®	Par Pharmaceuticals	FDA (2005)	megestrol acetate	Anti-anorexic
	NanOss®	RTI Surgical	FDA (2005)	hydroxyapatite	bone substitute

(Continued)

Table 2.1 (*Continued*)

Type	Trade name	Company	Date of approval	Active ingredients	Indication
	EquivaBone®	Zimmer Biomet	FDA (2009)	hydroxyapatite	bone substitute
	OsSatura®	IsotisOrthobiologics Inc	FDA (2003)	hydroxyapatite	bone substitute
	Epaxal®	Crucell Berna Biotech	EMA (1993)	inactivated hepatitis A virus vaccine	prevents hepatitis A infection
	Zanaflex®	Acorda	FDA (2002)	tizanidine HCl	muscle relaxant
	Ryanodex®	Eagle pharm	FDA (2014)	dantrolene sodium	malignant hyperthermia
	TriCor®	Abbott Laboratories	FDA (2004)	fenofibrate	antihyperlipidemic
Lipid-based nanoparticles	Doxil®	Johnson & Johnson	FDA (1995), EMA (1996)	doxorubicin (adriamycin)	metastatic ovarian cancer, HIV-associated Kaposi's sarcoma
	Lipodox®	Sun Pharma Global FZE	FDA (2013)	doxorubicin hydrochloride	metastatic ovarian cancer, HIV-associated KS
	DaunoXome®	Galen Ltd.	FDA, EMA (1996)	daunorubicin	cancers and HIV-associated KS
	Onivyde®	Merrimack Pharmaceuticals	FDA (2015)	irinotecan	metastatic pancreatic cancer
	DepoCyt®	Pacira Pharmaceuticals	EMA (2002), FDA (2007)	cytarabine	lymphomatous meningitis
	Myocet®	Teva Pharmaceutical Industries Ltd.	EMA (2000)	doxorubicin hydrochloride	breast cancer

Type	Trade name	Company	Date of approval	Active ingredients	Indication
	Mepact®	Takeda France SAS	EMA (2009)	mifamurtide	osteogenic sarcoma
	Marqibo®	Talon Therapeutics	FDA (2012)	vincristine	Philadelphia chromosome-negative chronic myelogenous leukemia in adult patients
	Onpattro®	Alnylam	FDA & EMA (2018)	Patisiran	hereditary transthyretin (TTR) mediated amyloidosis
	AmBisome®	NeXstar Pharmaceuticals	EMA (1990), FDA (1997)	Amphotericin B	antifungal drug
	Abelcet®	Defiante Farmaceutica	FDA (1995)	amphotericin B	antifungal drug
	DepoDur®	Skyepharma	FDA (2004), EMA (2006)	liposomal morphine sulfate	postoperative analgesia
	Curosurf®	Chiesi	FDA (1999)	liposomal morphine sulfate	respiratory distress syndrome (RDS)
	Inflexal®	Crucell Berna Biotech	EMA (1997)	inactivated influenza virus vaccine	prevents influenza infection
	Moderna COVID-19 Vaccine	ModernaTX Inc.	FDA (2020)	mRNA vaccine	prevents COVID-19 infection

(Continued)

Table 2.1 *(Continued)*

Type	Trade name	Company	Date of approval	Active ingredients	Indication
	Visudyne®	QLT Phototherapeutics	FDA & EMA (2000)	photosensitizer (PS), benzoporphyrin	choroidal neovascularization caused by wet age-related macular degeneration
Polymer-based nanoparticles	Cimzia®	UCB	FDA (2008), EMA (2009)	IgG Fab' fragment that specifically recognizes and binds to TNF-α	rheumatoid arthritis, Crohn's disease, psoriatic arthritis, and ankylosing spondylitis
	Apealea®	Oasmia Pharmaceutical AB	EMA (2018)	paclitaxel	ovarian cancer, peritoneal cancer, fallopian tube cancer
	Neulasta®	Amgen, Inc	FDA (2002)	filgrastim	febrile neutropenia, consequent infections arising due to lack of neutrophils
	Oncaspar®	Enzon Pharmaceuticals Inc.	FDA (1994), EMA (2016)	L-asparaginase	Acute lymphoblastic leukemia, chronic myelogenous leukemia
	General-PM®	Lupin Ltd.	FDA (2007)	paclitaxel	breast cancer
	Diprivan®	Fresenius Kabi	FDA (1989), EMA (2001)	propofol	(Sedative-hypnotic agent) used in surgery to induce relaxation before and during general anesthesia
	Somavert	Pfizer Pharmaceuticals	EMA (2002), FDA (2003)	Analog of human growth hormone acts as an antagonist of GH receptors	acromegaly

Type	Trade name	Company	Date of approval	Active ingredients	Indication
	Macugen®	Pfizer Pharmaceuticals	FDA (2004)	pegaptanib sodium	choroidal neovascularization caused by wet age-related macular degeneration
	Mircera®	Vifor	EMA (2007), FDA (2018)	epoetin β (EPO) (EPO is a genetically recombinant form of erythropoietin)	anemia
	PegIntron®	Merck & Co. Inc	EMA (2000), FDA (2001)	alpha interferon (INF) molecule	hepatitis C
	Krystexxa®	Savient Pharmaceuticals	FDA (2010)	pegloticase is a recombinant porcine like uricase	refractory chronic gout
	Plegridy®	Biogene	FDA (2014)	recombinant IFN-β	relapsing-remitting multiple sclerosis (RRMS) in adult patients
	Adynovate®	Baxalta US Inc	FDA (2015)	coagulation factor VIII	hemophilia A
	Copaxone®/ FOGA	Teva Pharmaceutical Industries Ltd.	FDA (1996), EMA (2016)	glatiramer acetate	multiple sclerosis (MS)
	Eligard®	Tolmar Pharmaceuticals Inc.	FDA (2002)	leuprolide acetate	prostate cancer
	Renagel®	Sanofi	FDA (2000)	sevelamer carbonate	hyperphosphatemia is caused by chronic kidney disease (CKD)

(*Continued*)

Table 2.1 (*Continued*)

Type	Trade name	Company	Date of approval	Active ingredients	Indication
	Renagel®/ Renvela®	Genzyme	EMA (2007)	sevelamer HCL	hyperphosphatemia caused by CKD
	Rebinyn®	NovoNordisk	FDA (2017)	Recombinant DNA-derived coagulation FIX	hemophilia B
	Estrasorb™	Novavax, Inc.	FDA (2003)	estradiol (17β-estradiol) hemihydrate	moderate vasomotor symptoms due to menopause
	Zilretta®	Flexion Therapeutics	FDA (2017)	triamcinolone acetonide	knee osteoarthritis
Dendrimer-based nanoparticles	VivaGel® BV	Starpharma	FDA (2015)	stormier sodium	anti-infective for the prevention of recurrent bacterial vaginosis (BV)
Protein-based nanoparticles	Abraxane®	Celgene Pharmaceutical Co. Ltd.	FDA (2005, 2012, 2013), EMA (2008)	paclitaxel	approved by the FDA for the treatment of metastatic breast cancer, lung cancer, and metastatic pancreatic adenocarcinoma
	Ontak®	Eisai	FDA (1999)	diphtheria toxin	leukemia, T-cell lymphoma
Inorganic nanoparticles	Feraheme™	AMAG Pharmaceuticals	FDA (2009)	ferumoxytol	anemia
	Venofer®	Luitpold Pharma	FDA (2000)	iron sucrose	iron deficiency in CKD
	Dexferrum®	American Regent	FDA (1996)	iron dextran	iron deficiency in CKD

Type	Trade name	Company	Date of approval	Active ingredients	Indication
	Ferinject®	Vifor	FDA, EMA (2013)	iron carboxymaltose colloid	Iron-deficient anemia
	Ferrlecit®	Sanofi-Aventis	FDA (1999), EMA (2013)	sodium ferric gluconate	iron deficiency in CKD
	Hensify®	Nanobiotix	EMA (2019)	hafnium oxide nanoparticles	locally advanced squamous cell carcinoma
	Infed®	Actavis Pharma	FDA (1992)	iron dextran	iron deficiency in CKD
	Feridex®/ Endorem	AMAG Pharma	FDA (1996) Disc.* 2008	SPION-dex	imaging agent

Table 2.2 Difference between patent and regulatory approval

Patent	Regulatory approval
Only new and innovative products got patent	Not limited to new, like generic also got approval
Patent given by the patent office or respective country	Approval was given by the regulatory authority of the respective country
The patent will not give any approval to drug products for marketing until and unless the drug fulfills all preclinical and clinical requirements of the respective regulatory body	The regulatory body provides approval for a drug to get marketed

Table 2.3 Comparison of various country regulations with respect to nanotechnology

Country	Regulatory body	Definition	Approval pathway	Regulation of nanomedicine	Regulator	Challenges for industry	Refs
Europe	European Medicine Agency (EMA)	It defines nanomaterial as a natural, incident or manufactured material containing particles in an unbound state or as an aggregate or as an agglomerate and where, for 50% or more of the particles in the number size distribution, one or more external dimensions is in the size range 1–100 nm.	Centralized procedure	REACH REFINE project	European Commission	There will be always a regulatory hurdle whenever any device and biological is incorporated with nano. Reach hasn't differentiated between the drug devices and biologicals that include nano. It will provide the same testing method for all. REFINE project somehow resolves the problem but still, method development takes time.	[16, 32]
USA	United States Food and	USFDA itself doesn't recommend any proper definition,	505(b2)-CDER 505(J)-CDER	Separate guidelines for	Medical Devices-CDRH	USFDA provided the requirement for all nano-incorporated drugs, devices, and biologicals separately. However,	[26, 33]

Country	Regulatory body	Definition	Approval pathway	Regulation of nanomedicine	Regulator	Challenges for industry	Refs
	Drug Administration	according to scientists' consideration the nanomaterial with a size range of 1 to 100 nm.	510(K)-CDRH 351(K)-CBER	each type of product	Biologics-CBER Drugs-CDER	the agency hasn't provided any proper method for evaluation of safety regarding nanoformulations.	
INDIA	Central Drug Standard Control Organization (CDSCO)	The nanomaterial is generally defined as material having a particle size in the range of 1 to 100 nm in at least one dimension. However, if a material exhibits physical, chemical, or biological phenomena or activities that are attributable to its dimension beyond the nanoscale range of up to 1000 nm, the material should also be considered a nanomaterial.	Form 44	Nano-mission follows REACH as well as OECD guidelines	Drug Controller General of India(DCGI)	Still no proper guidelines for medical devices, biologics including nano.	[27, 31]

Note: This table is taken from open source of NCBI as per creative common attribute license [3].

2.8 Conclusion

Nanotechnology is the future of the pharmaceutical industry. Regulatory bodies put their maximum efforts to establish proper guidelines for the nanomedicines. USFDA still does not have any definition for nanomaterials. However, scientist-generated definitions are acceptable by the regulatory body. Meanwhile, USFDA provides product-specific guidelines for nanomaterials along with stringent requirements regarding safety. Europe required CLP and REACH certifications along with the marketing authorization application. Till now India has only draft guidelines associated with the careful handling of nanomaterial. REACH guidelines related to nanomaterial is also acceptable in India. Still, there is a massive difference between the applications and approval regarding nanomaterials. The REFINE project is a great initiative to resolve those regulatory barriers by providing product-specific methods to ensure that the product does not fail in clinical trials. However, this project is limited to only a few countries. There is a need for collaboration between industry and regulatory bodies to establish suitable methods to resolve regulatory issues associated with nanomedicine approval.

References

1. Foulkes R, Man E, Thind J, Yeung S, Joy A, Hoskins C. (2020). The regulation of nanomaterials and nanomedicines for clinical application: Current and future perspectives, *Biomaterials Science*. 8(17), 4653–64.
2. USFDA. Nanotechnology-Over a Decade of Progress and Innovation 2020 [cited 2022 5 June]. Available from: https://www.fda.gov/media/140395/download.
3. Halwani AA. (2022). Development of Pharmaceutical Nanomedicines: From the Bench to the Market, Pharmaceutics. 14(1), 106.
4. USFDA. Guidance for Industry Considering Whether an FDA-Regulated Product Involves the Application of Nanotechnology 2014 [cited 2022 1 June]. Available from: https://www.fda.gov/regulatory-information/search-fda-guidance-documents/considering-whether-fda-regulated-product-involves-application-nanotechnology.

5. USFDA. Drug Products, Including Biological Products, that Contain Nanomaterials – Guidance for Industry 2022 [cited 2022 4 June]. Available from: https://www.fda.gov/regulatory-information/search-fda-guidance-documents/drug-products-including-biological-products-contain-nanomaterials-guidance-industry.
6. Soares S, Sousa J, Pais A, Vitorino C. (2018). Nanomedicine: principles, properties, and regulatory issues, *Frontiers in Chemistry*. 6, 360.
7. Majuru S, Oyewumi MO. (2009). Nanotechnology in drug development and life cycle management. In *Nanotechnology in Drug Delivery*: Springer, pp. 597–619.
8. Saraiva C, Praça C, Ferreira R, Santos T, Ferreira L, Bernardino L. (2016). Nanoparticle-mediated brain drug delivery: overcoming blood–brain barrier to treat neurodegenerative diseases, *Journal of Controlled Release*. 235, 34–47.
9. Soenen SJ, Rivera-Gil P, Montenegro J-M, Parak WJ, De Smedt SC, Braeckmans K. (2011). Cellular toxicity of inorganic nanoparticles: common aspects and guidelines for improved nanotoxicity evaluation, *Nano Today*. 6(5), 446–65.
10. EMA. Questions and Answers on the withdrawal of marketing application for Sinerem 2008 [cited 2022 18 May]. Available from: https://www.ema.europa.eu/en/documents/medicine-qa/questions-answers-withdrawal-marketing-application-sinerem_en.pdf.
11. EMA. Guerbet withdraws its marketing authorisation application for Sinerem 2007 [cited 2022 18 MAY]. Available from: https://www.ema.europa.eu/en/documents/press-release/guerbet-withdraws-its-marketing-authorisation-application-sinerem_en.pdf.
12. EMA. Withdrawal assessment Report for Sinerem 2008 [cited 2022 18 May]. Available from: https://www.ema.europa.eu/en/documents/withdrawal-report/withdrawal-assessment-report-sinerem_en.pdf.
13. Platform ET. REFINE Project 2022 [cited 2022 10 June]. Available from: https://etp-nanomedicine.eu/about-nanomedicine/european-nanomedicine-projects/.
14. European Commission. Regulatory Science Framework for Nano(bio) material-based Medical Products and Devices 2022 [cited 2022 10 June]. Available from: https://cordis.europa.eu/project/id/761104.
15. REFINE. About Refine Framework 2022 [cited 2022 29 May]. Available from: http://refine-nanomed.eu/about/.

16. REFINE. Regulatory Science Framework for Nano(bio)material-based Medical Products and Devices 2022 [cited 2022 29 May]. Available from: http://refine-nanomed.eu/.
17. EUON. EUON Regulations 2022 [cited 2022 30 May]. Available from: https://euon.echa.europa.eu/regulation.
18. ECHA. REGULATION (EC) No 1907/2006 OF THE EUROPEAN PARLIAMENT AND OF THE COUNCIL of 18 December 2006 [cited 2022 15 June]. Available from: https://eur-lex.europa.eu/legal-content/en/TXT/HTML/?uri=CELEX:02006R1907-20220301.
19. European Commission. REGULATION (EC) No 1272/2008 OF THE EUROPEAN PARLIAMENT AND OF THE COUNCIL 2008 [cited 2022 29 May]. Available from: http://publications.europa.eu/resource/cellar/e3f31046-b274-11eb-8aca-01aa75ed71a1.0013.02/DOC_1.
20. ECHA. CLP Legislation 2008 [cited 2022 15 June]. Available from: https://echa.europa.eu/regulations/clp/legislation.
21. Hafner A, Lovrić J, Lakoš GP, Pepić I. (2014). Nanotherapeutics in the EU: an overview on current state and future directions, *International Journal of Nanomedicine*. 9, 1005.
22. USFDA. Nanotechnology Task Force 2021 [cited 2022 7 June]. Available from: https://www.fda.gov/science-research/nanotechnology-programs-fda/nanotechnology-task-force.
23. USFDA. Center for Drug Evaluation and Research Nanotechnology Programs 2018 [cited 2022 25 May]. Available from: https://www.fda.gov/science-research/nanotechnology-programs-fda/center-drug-evaluation-and-research-nanotechnology-programs.
24. USFDA. Nanotechnology Guidance Documents 2018 [cited 2022 1 June]. Available from: https://www.fda.gov/science-research/nanotechnology-programs-fda/nanotechnology-guidance-documents.
25. USFDA. Center for Devices and Radiological Health Nanotechnology Programs 2018 [cited 2022 21 May]. Available from: https://www.fda.gov/science-research/nanotechnology-programs-fda/center-devices-and-radiological-health-nanotechnology-programs.
26. USFDA. Drug Products, Including Biological Products, that Contain Nanomaterials Guidance for Industry 2022 [cited 2022 30 May]. Available from: https://www.fda.gov/media/157812/download.
27. CDSCO. Guidelines for Evaluation of Nanopharmaceuticals in India 2019 [cited 2022 2 JUNE]. Available from: https://dbtindia.

gov.in/sites/default/files/uploadfiles/Guidelines%20For%20 Evaluation%20of%20Nanopharmaceuticals%20in%20India.pdf.

28. Kaur G, Malhotra R. (2021). Artificial intelligence and nanomedicine: legal and ethical challenges in India.
29. DST. CSIR Nano-tech 2022 [cited 2022 5 JUNE]. Available from: https://www.csirnano.co.za/about-us/.
30. DST. Mission on Nano Science and Technology (Nano Mission) 2022 [cited 2022 24 May]. Available from: https://dst.gov.in/scientific-programmes/mission-nano-science-and-technology-nano-mission.
31. DST. Guidelines and Best Practices for Safe Handling of Nanomaterials in Research Laboratories and Industries 2022 [cited 2022 28 May]. Available from: https://dst.gov.in/sites/default/files/Draft-Guidelines%20.pdf.
32. Medicine EAfAtS. The Nanomedicine Regulatory Coalition 2022 [cited 2022 10 June]. Available from: https://eunanomedicinescoalition.eu/.
33. USFDA. cosmetic nanotechnology 2022 [cited 2022 22 May]. Available from: https://www.fda.gov/cosmetics/cosmetics-science-research/cosmetics-nanotechnology.

Multiple Choice Questions (MCQ)

1. For which category of medicinal products are 510(K) approvals needed?
   a. Drug product
   b. Food and Cosmetic
   c. Medical Devices
   d. Veterinary Medicines
2. Generally nanoparticle size range is ________________.
   a. 0.001 to 0.1 micrometer
   b. 0.1 to 1 micrometer
   c. 0.001 to 2 micrometers
   d. 0.01 to 2 micrometers
3. Expand the term REACH.
   a. Registration, Evaluation, Authorization and Restriction of chemicals

   b. Registration, Examination, Authorization and Restriction of chemicals
   c. Restriction, Evaluation, Authorization and Registration of chemicals
   d. Regulation, Examination, Audits and Report of Chemicals

4. What type of application do we have to submit to the regulatory body while selecting generic formulations?
   a. 505 (b1) application
   b. 505 (j) application
   c. 505 (k) application
   d. None of the above

5. To which country is the Nano-mission program related?
   a. Europe
   b. United States
   c. India
   d. Australia

6. Expand the term CDER.
   a. Center for Dosing, Evaluation and Regulation
   b. Center for Drug Evaluation and Research
   c. Current Drug Exporting Regulations
   d. None of above

7. Which procedure is followed by Europe for the evaluation of nanomedicines?
   a. Centralized Procedure
   b. Decentralized Procedure
   c. National Competent Authority
   d. Mutual Recognition Procedure

8. If both the drug and the nanocarrier are not previously approved in other countries then in which category will they fall for the marketing authorization application as per Indian regulation?
   a. 1st Category
   b. 2nd Category
   c. 3rd Category
   d. 4th Category

9. Basic criteria for a grant of patent
   a. Novelty and Non-obviousness
   b. Inventive step
   c. Industrial Application
   d. All the above

10. Regulatory Body of United States
    a. MHRA
    b. CDSCO
    c. FDA
    d. CBER

11. Which of the following is the odd one out?
    a. Nanoformulation have the capability to bind the selected target to show good efficacy
    b. Due to stable physicochemical properties, it can penetrate the membrane barrier
    c. Nanoformulation are mostly formulated as immediate release
    d. Organic substance can be avoided in formulation

12. Device that failed in submission of clinical trial data in Europe
    a. Sinerem
    b. Vitossa
    c. Ontak
    d. Infed

13. What is CLP?
    a. Classification, labelling and preparation
    b. Categorization, labelling and packaging
    c. Classification, labelling and packaging
    d. Categorization, labelling and preparation

14. CDSCO stands for
    a. Central drug standard control operation
    b. Central drug standard control organization
    c. Center for drug standardization and control and organization

d. Center for drug standardization and control and operation

15. Which is the form required for the drug approval in India?
    a. Form 22
    b. Form 44
    c. Form 22
    d. Form 41
16. When did the European Technology platform initiate the REFINE project?
    a. 2015
    b. 2010
    c. 2000
    d. 2017
17. What is ECHA?
    a. European control agency
    b. European chemical agency
    c. European chemical administration
    d. European chemical authorization
18. What is the temperature criteria for the fire hazard of flash point for chemical?
    a. Should be below 200°F
    b. Should be above 200°F
    c. At 200°F
    d. At 100°F
19. Which type of nanomedicine is Onivyde?
    a. Nanocrystal
    b. Lipid-based nanoparticle
    c. Polymer-based nanoparticle
    d. Protein-based nanoparticle
20. Find the odd one out:
    a. Renagel
    b. Rebinyen
    c. Zilretta
    d. Abraxane

21. Example of dendrimer-based nanoparticles
    a. Venofer
    b. Infed
    c. Vivagel
    d. Somavert

22. Which clause of second schedule of NDCT indicates stability testing of a new drug?
    a. Fourth
    b. Fifth
    c. Seventh
    d. Tenth

23. Guidelines for the evaluation of nanopharmaceuticals were given in
    a. 2020
    b. 2019
    c. 2018
    d. 2017

24. Permissible exposure limits for a toxic hazard should be
    a. Less than 20 ppm
    b. Less than 50 ppm
    c. Less than 70 ppm
    d. Less than 100 ppm

25. Liposomal amphotericin B is an example of
    a. Nanocarriers loaded with API
    b. Nanocarrier only
    c. Nanocarrier without API
    d. None of the above
    e.

Answer Key

1.	(c)	**2.**	(a)	**3.**	(a)	**4.**	(b)	**5.**	(c)	**6.**	(b)	**7.**	(a)
8.	(a)	**9.**	(d)	**10.**	(c)	**11.**	(c)	**12.**	(a)	**13.**	(c)	**14.**	(b)
15.	(b)	**16.**	(d)	**17.**	(b)	**18.**	(a)	**19.**	(b)	**20.**	(d)	**21.**	(c)
22.	(b)	**23.**	(b)	**24.**	(b)	**25.**	(a)						

Short-Answer Questions

1. What are the ideal properties of nanoparticles delivery systems?
2. What is the definition of nanoparticles according to the EMA?
3. List some of the nanomedicines that are marketed globally.
4. What is the REFINE project and what is the main aim of the project regarding nanoparticles?
5. Define REACH.
6. What are differences between patent and regulatory approval?
7. What are the four categories for drug approval of nanopharmaceuticals according to CDSCO?
8. What are the criteria to be considered while choosing the nanoparticles for formulation?
9. Who are the regulators for the different types of products in USFDA?
10. Which schedule mainly focuses on nanomedicines requirement in India?

Long-Answer Questions

1. What are the major challenges faced in the regulation of nanomedicine?
2. Write a note on regulatory guidelines of nanomedicine in the EMA.
3. Discuss in detail the REFINE project.
4. Write a note on USFDA regulatory guidelines for nano-medicines.
5. Establish the comparison between USFDA and EMA guide-lines with respect to nanomedicines.

Chapter 3

Nanodrug Delivery System for Brain Targeting

Adeola Tawakalitu Kola-Mustapha,[a] Olufunke Dorothy Akin-Ajani,[b] Oluwakorede Joshua Adedeji,[a] and Oluwatoyin Adepeju Odeku[b]

[a]*Department of Pharmaceutics & Industrial Pharmacy, Faculty of Pharmaceutical Sciences, University of Ilorin, Ilorin, Nigeria*
[b]*Department of Pharmaceutics & Industrial Pharmacy, Faculty of Pharmacy, University of Ibadan, Ibadan, Nigeria*

pejuodeku@yahoo.com

Conventional drugs face limitations crossing into the brain allowing for only ideal drug candidates. These candidates should possess properties such as high lipophilicity, moderate molecular weight, charge, etc. This leaves out many other drugs and prevents entry into the brain. The brain protects itself via several barriers that limit drug entry and reduce effectiveness. These barriers include the blood-brain barrier, the blood-cerebrospinal fluid barrier, and the arachnoid barrier. These barriers reduce the efficacy of drugs in the therapy of brain-related diseases. This has necessitated the development of novel strategies such as nanodrug delivery systems, to target drugs to the brain for effective therapies. Nanodrug delivery systems such as liposomes, carbon dots, viral vectors, polymeric micelles, etc., are increasingly being tested in preclinical models and clinical trials in the management of

Nanotechnology and Drug Delivery: Principles and Applications
Edited by Rakesh K. Sindhu

ISBN 978-981-4968-83-6 (Hardcover), 978-1-003-43040-7 (eBook)
www.jennystanford.com

brain-related diseases. So far, some successes have been recorded for diseases such as Parkinson's disease, Alzheimer's disease, Huntington's Disease, Multiple Sclerosis, etc., While nanodrug systems show promise in future applications, some limitations affect the use in clinical settings. This chapter highlights the current advances in nanodrug delivery systems and their benefits in brain targeting to enhance clinical outcomes.

3.1 Introduction

Targeted drug delivery systems have received increasing attention in the past several decades to achieve better therapeutic outcomes and reduced side effects [1]. There are numerous examples of targeted drug delivery systems undergoing clinical trials; however, clinical translation of targeted drug delivery systems is relatively slow [2]. Major efforts have been made to identify high-affinity ligands and identify nanodrug delivery system strategies, particularly for enhanced brain targeting [3–5].

Nanodrug delivery systems (NDDS) are drug delivery systems for the delivery of medications in nano sizes (1 billionth of a meter) to specific organs. These systems are encapsulated in vesicles or polymer matrices with one or more medicinal compounds [1, 2]. They provide a means of administering medications to improve drug delivery and efficacy at the targeted organ [6]. They are also used to improve drug stability and water solubility, prolong cycle time, boost target cell or tissue absorption rate, and limit enzyme degradation, hence improving drug safety and effectiveness [7–9]. They have unique properties which make them suitable for targeting drugs to specific organs such as the brain where drug uptake could present some challenges.

3.2 Physiological Barriers of the Brain to Drugs

The brain is one of the most important organs in the human body and no harm must come to it [10]. The blood-brain barrier (BBB)—a highly selective, partially permeable barrier between the brain and the rest of the body is one of the most important defense systems of the brain [11]. The blood-brain barrier has a very strict regulation of solutes, ions and molecules that it permits into the central nervous system (CNS) and brain. This is a result of the tight junctions formed by densely packed endothelial cells and a complex efflux transporter system which actively removes molecules from the brain and the cerebrospinal fluid transporting them back into the systemic circulation [11–13]. the BBB's highly selective nature has posed a big challenge for scientists to treat CNS or brain disorders or diseases, as many of the drugs that need to reach the brain to be effective are unable to do so [14].

For decades, drug delivery to the brain in the treatment of CNS disorders has been faced with the problem of poor drug targeting. Irrespective of the development of active drugs in the therapy of diseases, efficacy may still be limited due to low drug delivery across the BBB. Endothelial cells are an integral part of the BBB structure and they are encompassed by pericytes with tight junctions in between. They utilize a high amount of ATP to maintain the structure of the barrier. Endothelial cells regulate the permeability of substances from the circulatory vasculature into the neuronal system [15]. The blood is separated from the brain parenchyma by endothelial cells that line the capillaries in the brain. The brain capillaries' endothelium monolayer serves as a vital interface for the exchange of nutrients, gases, and metabolites between blood and brain, as well as a barrier for neurotoxic plasma components and xenobiotics [16, 17]. Astrocytes enable strong attachment of endothelial cells and maintain strong tight junctions. It is the most common cellular component type in the brain and is involved in several functions such as gliotransmitter release, dopamine metabolism, glutamate uptake, etc. [17]. Pericytes are found between endothelial cells and astrocytes and very essential in maintaining homeostasis. It also enables angiogenesis and the increase of endothelial cells [17]. Besides all cellular components, the non-cellular component (the basement membrane), is a composite of four proteins, all of which help in the support and anchoring of cells. Collagen IV is essential for the maintenance of the Basement membrane, but not for its formation. The role of laminin is not well known, but nidogen, the third protein, stabilizes the network between the two former proteins. Perlecan is large in size but invaluable in embryogenesis [18]. All components of the basement membrane work to protect the brain from the entry of exogenous compounds and regulate the movement of blood solutes across the barrier.

The BBB is not the only physiological barrier that limits brain drug delivery, another barrier is the blood-cerebrospinal fluid (CSF) barrier [19]. The choroid plexus regulates the flow of drugs via the blood to the CSF. Drug transfer via the choroid plexus and the BBB occurs via unrelated pharmacokinetics. The choroid plexus is not as tight as the BBB in limiting the entry of substances owing to the difference in the cells forming the barrier. At an inverse proportion to the drug's rate, the molecules penetrate the CSF [20]. While the drug enters the CSF much more easily than the BBB, it exits rather quickly. A drug injected into the CSF compartment travels quickly from the brain to the bloodstream like "a slow intravenous infusion". Almost all drugs enter into the CSF irrespective of the ability to cross BBB. There is minimal entry into the brain parenchyma and drugs rapidly exit into the blood.

The arachnoid barrier, which also limits the entry of drugs from the circulatory system into the brain, may be considered a part of the blood-CSF barrier. The arachnoid barrier cells form one of the three layers of the meninges covering the CNS. The meninges are made up of an outermost dura layer (adjacent to the skull) and two innermost layers (leptomeninges), which include the arachnoid mater [21]. The subarachnoid space accounts for more than 80% of the cerebrospinal fluid space thereby playing a major role in the level of drugs transported into the CSF [22]. The spinal cord and blood-spinal cord barrier are rate-limiting factors in the entry of drugs into the other part of the CNS. This barrier regulates the entry of endogenous and exogenous substances into the spinal environment [23].

These physiological barriers limit the entry of drugs for brain targeting and necessitate the use of novel methods such as nanodrug delivery systems in the treatment of central nervous disorders.

3.3 Strategies for Effective Brain Targeting

Currently, several strategies are effective for brain drug delivery. While some are invasive, others are not invasive. The reasons for this special delivery system for the brain stem from the unique nature of the organ and the number of barrier systems in place to protect this delicate organ. The strategies that have been used are discussed in the following section.

3.3.1 Exosomes

Studies have shown exosomes to be of advantage as a useful delivery system for drugs to the brain [24, 25]. Exosomes are vesicles secreted from cells; in this case, endothelial cells are used to produce exosomes which are then used in brain targeting. Exosomes work as vesicles for the drug which can easily cross the BBB [24]. When compared to nanoparticulate drug delivery systems like liposomes and polymeric nanoparticles, using exosomes as drug delivery vehicles have several advantages [26]. Exosomes are intracellular vesicles for the natural transport of substances outside the cell, thus, can be adapted for drug delivery. Despite the potential advantages of exosomes, some issues limit its clinical applications; choice of donor cell for exosome (because exosomes can vary in composition depending on the source), further toxicity studies, etc. [24].

3.3.2 Blood Permeability Enhancers

Some compounds can enable the transport of drugs to the brain by temporarily opening the BBB. These molecules, known as permeability enhancers, are effective in overcoming the BBB and provide efficient drug targeting. In a study by Liang et al., a new glioma-targeting approach based on enhancer-modified albumin nanoparticles was created to safely and efficiently deliver medications to glioma areas in the brain [27]. Breitkreuz et al. [28] also utilized a new compound, M01, to effect a transient increase in BBB permeability resulting in improved delivery of paclitaxel to the mouse brain leading to reduced orthotopic glioblastoma growth [28].

In recent years, ultrasound has become well known for enhancing the entry of medications across the BBB [24]. Ultrasound can improve medication administration to the brain by improving distribution via a BBB that is already impaired, such as in tumors and by disrupting the BBB in normal brain tissue [29]. When used together with microbubbles in the brain, ultrasound can increase BBB permeability and enable drugs to easily cross the barrier. Microbubbles are micro-sized vesicles with rigidity maintained by lipids and polymers. The outer layer (shell) can be attached to different moieties, whether in diagnostic (imaging agents) or therapeutic agents (drugs) [30]. The mechanical index magnitude can affect the properties of the microbubble. It can cause to oscillate (sonoporation) or implode (sono-permeabilization). The oscillating activity (cavitation) can help open up membranes and blood vasculature [30]. Both components (ultrasound and microbubbles) affect the extent of permeability. This technique has been applied in the therapy of different diseases [30].

3.3.3 Chemical Modification

Chemical modifications such as prodrug formation involve the modification of the drug structure for it to cross the BBB, then it is metabolized to the original drug in the CNS. The use of prodrugs has been applied in the delivery of dopamine to the brain. Due to its polar nature, hydrophilic dopamine cannot cross the BBB, hence, it is administered as L-dopa which enters the CNS and is converted to dopamine [31]. The use of prodrugs is also seen in the delivery of azidothymidine to the brain via the simple formation of the ester prodrug [32, 33]. Another study utilized a prodrug ester in the transfer of ketoprofen across the BBB [34]. The formation of dimers as a prodrug has also been applied in the CNS delivery of anti-HIV drugs like abacavir [32]. The necessity for a drug to be hydrophobic enough to cross the BBB underlies the basis for the formation of prodrug forms which are often non-polar enough to cross the barrier [24]. Yue et al. (2018) experimented with the use of a dual-targeting prodrug in the delivery of Ibuprofen to the CNS [35]. Several prodrugs are currently utilizing the L-type amino acid transporter 1 (LAT-1) which is found in the BBB. LAT1 belongs to a larger family of L-transporters that help to transfer some amino acids across membranes into cells in the body [36]. The ability of LAT1 to detect specific amino acids and physiological hormones as important endogenous substrates and several medications as exogenous substrates determine its impact on human metabolism [36].

3.3.4 Transport Systems

The use of transport systems also represents another mode of drug delivery to the brain. These transport systems are endogenous structures that physiologically transport endogenous molecules across cell membranes. It is thus exploited in the delivery of drugs as well by modifying the structures of the drugs to resemble endogenous molecules recognized by the transporters. Examples of transporters used to mediate drug transfer across the BBB include the above-mentioned LAT1, glucose transporter type 1 (GLUT 1), monocarboxylic acid transporter type 1 (MCT1), equilibrative nucleoside transporter type 1 (ENT 1), and cationic amino acid transporter 1 (CAT1) [37]. It is also possible for two or more modes of drug delivery to be combined as seen in the delivery of L-dopa in the treatment of parkinsonism which combines a prodrug to resemble an L-amino acid which is then taken up by LAT1 (prodrug + transport system) [31].

3.3.5 Direct Administration

Another method of bypassing the BBB is the direct administration of the drug into the brain. This may either be intracerebral or intracerebroventricular. The intracerebral route involves the administration of the drug through microinjection guide sleeves that are implanted stereotaxically to enable the targeted entry of the drug to a specific part of the brain [38]. The latter requires the administration of the drug via the ventricles of the brain [38]. Unlike the other systems, these methods are invasive and require special care. Intracerebroventricular administration has long been utilized for several CNS diseases such as refractory pain, infection in the brain and brain tumors [39]. The same route can be applied whether, in the treatment of meningitis, where antimicrobials are administered intracerebroventricularly, or in chemotherapy, treatment of CNS lymphoma. Some existing strategies in brain drug delivery are presented in Table 3.1.

Table 3.1 Strategies in brain drug delivery

S/N	Delivery system	Uses	Refs
1.	Direct administration (Intracerebroventricular or Intracerebral)	Administration of anti-epileptic drugs	[40]
2.	Prodrug	Administration of dopamine	[31]
3.	Prodrug	Treatment of HIV infection in the brain	[33]
4.	Prodrug transport systems (LAT1)	Administration of ketoprofen, an anti-inflammatory drug	[34]
5.	Transport system (MCT1)	Brain cancers	[41]
6.	Viral Vector delivery	Gene therapy	[42]
7.	BBB disruption (Ultrasound)	Delivery of irinotecan to the brain in an animal model	[43]
8.	Polymeric micelles	Treatment of premature ejaculation using dapoxetine	[44]
9.	Solid Lipid Nanoparticles	Administration of clozapine, an antipsychotic	[45]

3.4 Characteristics of an Ideal Drug Candidate for Effective Brain Targeting

Effective brain targeting requires that drugs should possess essential characteristics. Typically, this would depend on the intended mode of transport across the BBB (exosomal delivery, transporter-mediated, viral-vectored, etc.). These characteristics would enhance adequate exposure and optimal drug delivery. Due to the nature of the BBB, an essential characteristic is its high lipophilicity, which determines the membrane transport and action binding ability [46]. Moreover, it is a parameter that determines the ability of drugs to bind to active sites and is very important for pharmacokinetics - absorption, distribution, metabolism, excretion; pharmacodynamics and toxicity properties [46]. It is measured in terms of the partition coefficient (Log *P*), which is a measure of the distribution of the drug in the organic phase (unionized) ratio to the amount in the aqueous phase (ionized). Drugs with high lipophilicity can enter the CNS via solubilization into the lipid layer of the endothelial cells or diffusion. For an ideal drug candidate, the Log *P* value ranges between 1.5 and 2.7 [47].

Only when a drug's molecular weight is less than or substantially equal to 400–600 Da can its lipophilicity be used as a measure of BBB transit [48]. The molecular weight of an ideal drug for brain targeting entering the brain compartment via passive diffusion requires a molecular weight <400 Da or between 400–600 Da. The rate of diffusion across membranes relies on the molecule's ability. The larger the molecular weight, the more the number of hydrogen bond donor molecules and acceptor moieties and the lesser the lipophilicity and thus, the ability to diffuse across the blood-brain barrier [49]. Ideal drug candidates for brain drug delivery require high lipophilicity, small molecular weight and a low number of hydrogen bonds (<8) [50].

The charge is another essential requirement for crossing the BBB. The cell membrane of the BBB is negatively charged and the use of an equally negatively charged compound may create a form of repulsion and limit diffusion. Polymers, cationic lipids, albumin, and nanoparticles are examples of positively charged materials that can interact with the negatively charged cell membrane and internalize via adsorptive endocytosis [51]. Carrier-mediated drug delivery requires essential properties such as the high affinity of the drug for the cell transporter [52]. Transporters recognize endogenous molecules, hence the need to enable drugs to acquire similar properties to enhance affinity. In some cases, the formation of a prodrug is necessitated. An ideal drug candidate should be able to revert to its active state on entering the brain compartment and retain activity. For nanomedicines, properly understanding the pharmacokinetics, toxicity, and distribution properties of drugs and conjugates is essential in enhancing the clinical application of medicines for brain drug targeting [53]. The key characteristics of ideal drug candidates for brain targeting are shown in Fig. 3.1.

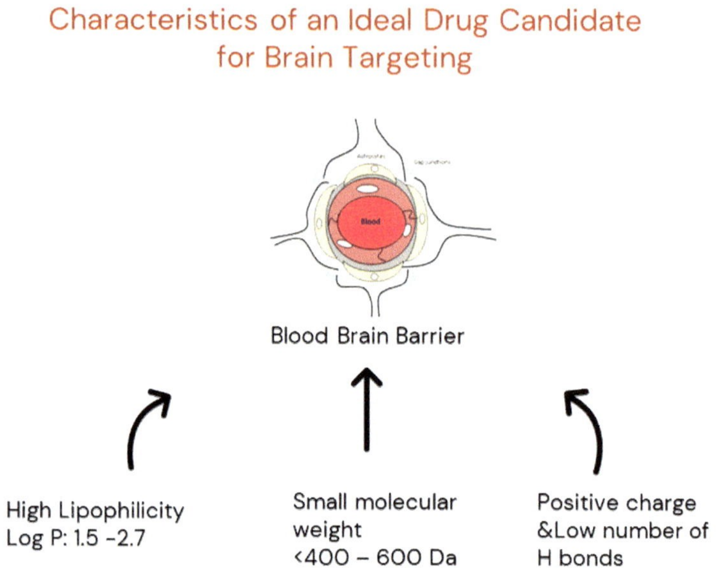

Figure 3.1 Key characteristics of ideal drug candidates for brain targeting [53].

3.5 Nanodrug Delivery System Strategies for Enhanced Brain Targeting

Different strategies have been employed for the formulation of nanodrug delivery systems to enhance drug delivery to the brain. These strategies include the following:

3.5.1 Micelles

Micelles are uni-layered amphiphilic nanocarriers that allow the controlled release of encapsulated drugs [10, 54, 55] They are characterized by their unique spherical shape, with the hydrophobic part(s) set apart from the hydrophilic part(s), which leads to the formation of an inner hydrophobic core surrounded by external hydrophilic terminals [11]. Their stability in physiological environments is a result of their amphiphilic nature, which results in long circulation times, providing them with sufficient time to reach the target tissue [56].

Despite the long systemic circulation, they have poor cellular binding and uptake [57]. Due to their amphiphilic nature, both lipophilic and hydrophilic drugs can be loaded into micellar DDSs. However, micellar drug delivery systems possess low drug loading capacities compared to other systems. In a study by Yin et al., doxorubicin-loaded poly(lactic-glycolic) acidlysoGM1 micelles was developed with an encapsulation efficiency of about 61%. These micelles easily crossed the BBB and accumulate inside the brain parenchyma of mice and zebrafish used in the *in vivo* studies through micropinocytosis and lysosomal pathways [10, 55].

Amphiphilic block copolymers generate nano-sized encapsulating structures known as polymeric micelles. The formation of micelles is based on the ability of these block copolymers to aggregate/coalesce into a larger spherical vesicle when present in an aqueous solvent [58]. Micelles can vary based on the forming polymers. While some of these polymers are largely hydrophobic, others are more hydrophilic. Polyethylene oxide, for example, contains hydrophilic blocks while poly propylene oxide contains hydrophobic blocks. A combination of these two creates a highly useful polymeric micelle in the solubilization of drugs [59]. Polymeric micelles are particularly well suited for drug administration because of their inherent and adjustable characteristics [60]. They are commonly characterized by a hydrophilic, water-loving coating known as the 'corona' with an inner lipophilic or hydrophobic 'core' [61] due to the amphiphilic nature of forming copolymers. Polymeric micelles provide useful advantages due to their unique properties of solubility, low toxicity, compatibility with biological systems, structure, arrangement, etc., hence their diverse use in various treatment applications [62]. They are also uniquely target-specific. The interesting nature of the micelle enables it to protect the coated drug from degradation, and enhance its solubility, particularly for poorly soluble drugs [62]. In the treatment of brain diseases, micelles are useful in the delivery of anti-cancer drugs. Polyethylene glycol (PEG micelles) help deliver drugs such as doxorubicin and camptothecin, which were found to be effective in the treatment of glioblastoma. Its applications are not limited only to brain drug targeting, but to other organs as well due to its target specificity and bioavailability. An advanced application of micelles in drug delivery is the ultrasound micelle drug delivery, which is a form of augmentation that utilizes ultrasound waves in stimulating the release of drugs from the micelles [58]. Interestingly, this modification involves the use of ultrasound which is comprised of waves that are transmitted through the skin without any need for invasive procedures or surgery, and rupture or stimulate the release of drug-containing micelles in specific locations of the body, minimizing avoidable side effects [58].

3.5.2 Liposomes

Liposomal drug delivery is a major means of overcoming restrictions of BBB transport. It has been shown that liposome surface modifications can improve the circulation time in blood, the therapeutic index, and the bioavailability, as well as change the drug distribution to the brain [63]. Liposomes are composed of phospholipids and cholesterol formed into small spherical-shaped vesicles consisting of one or more phospholipid bilayers that can hold various therapeutic molecules including drugs, vaccines, nucleic acids, and proteins [10]. In general, the components of the liposomes make them biologically inert, non-immunogenic, and biodegradable, with low inherent toxicity [64]. Liposomes can be used as carriers for biologically active compounds and have been widely used as a drug delivery system (DDS) to improve drug efficacy and eliminate drug-related toxicity or unwanted effects [65–67]. Even though liposomes have lipophilic characteristics, they are very large and cannot simply diffuse across cell membranes or between BBB cells [68]. Instead, liposomes cross the BBB via transport systems, such as adsorptive-mediated transcytosis (AMT), receptor-mediated transcytosis (RMT), and carrier-mediated transcytosis (CMTs) [69, 70] To efficiently cross the BBB, instead of using conventional liposomes, further surface modification is possible. This includes cationic liposomes, specifically targeted liposomes and long-circulating liposomes; to which immunoliposomes belong (see Table 3.2). Liposome-based strategies can be classified as physiological since the liposome adds physiological interactions to that of the drug on its own, whereby it influences drug distribution characteristics [63].

Table 3.2 Types of liposomes [63]

Liposome type	Description
Conventional liposome	Entraps hydrophilic compounds such as small molecules or biological-based compounds in the liposome's core and lipophilic compounds in the phospholipid bilayer membrane Compounds are stabilized thus avoiding early degradation in the systemic circulation
Non-specific targeted liposome	
Cationic liposome	Increases drug transport across the BBB by maximizing liposome-endothelial tissue retention while lipid surface can facilitate adsorption of polyanions, such as DNA and RNA
Anionic liposome	Monocyte can bind to anionic liposome and facilitates drug transport across the BBB via the mononuclear cell migration pathway
Cationic PEGylated liposome	Enhances the brain uptake by increasing plasma concentration and tissue retention
Specifically targeted liposome	Polyethylene glycol (PEG) acts as a shield to protect liposomes from plasma protein binding or RES uptake. Thus, it increases plasma concentration. However, PEGylation is only able to prolong liposome circulation without improving BBB penetration
Long-circulating liposome	Achieved by conjugating liposome or PEGylated liposome to single functional ligand or multiple ligands to facilitate a specific binding to the BBB surface receptors or carrier proteins Targeted delivery leverages the delivery efficiency of liposomes to the brain, and improves the therapeutic index by increasing target site drug accumulation while decreasing peripheral toxicity. This opens a possibility for reducing dose or dosing frequency Targeted ligands can be antibodies, cell-penetrating peptides, or endogenous molecules, e.g., transferrin, GSH, ApoE, and lactoferrin

3.5.2.1 Immunoliposomes

Immunoliposomes; antibody-directed liposomes have been recognized as a promising tool for the site-specific delivery of drugs and diagnostic agents [71]. However, the *in vivo* use of classical immunoliposomes is hampered by the very rapid clearance of immunoliposomes from the circulation by the reticuloendothelial system [72]. This obstacle can be avoided if gangliosides or PEG-derivatized lipids are inserted within the bilayer of the conventional liposomes, as these modifications will prolong considerably the liposome half-life in circulation [71, 73, 74]. In a study by Huwyler et al., [71] immunoliposomes were used to target an encapsulated drug, daunomycin, to the rat brain *in vivo*. This was achieved using vector-mediated drug delivery systems, which have been previously used for peptides or peptide nucleic acids [75] to apply small molecule drug delivery to the brain. Thus, micromolar drug concentrations in the brain were achieved using BBB drug delivery vectors with increased carrying capacity by logarithmic orders. As micromolar concentrations of many small drug molecules in the brain are required for pharmacological activity. This was possible with the use of PEG-conjugated immunoliposomes and monoclonal antibodies that target the brain and BBB receptors [71].

3.5.3 Dendrimers

Dendrimers are highly branched spherical polymers that are now used as drug delivery systems due to the ease with which they can be produced and modified compared to other nanotechnology-based drug delivery systems and their size. Dendrimers are sometimes referred to as "starburst" polymers as a result of their branching. They are made up of three main, distinct components; an initiator core, to which interior layers (i.e., generations) of repeating subunits (dendrons) are radially linked, and the terminals, where the functionalization (such as the linking of bioconjugates such as proteins or antibodies onto the dendrimer surface), as well as drug loading, takes place [76–79].

One of the most studied classes of dendrimers used in the delivery of therapeutics to the brain are the polyamidoamine dendrimers, which have an ethylenediamine ($C_2H_4(NH_2)_2$) core, amide (RC(=O)NR0R00) branches (where R, R0 and R00 are organic groups or hydrogen atoms) forming the walls of cavities and amino ($-NH_2$), hydroxyl (–OH), or carboxylic acid (–COOH) functional groups as terminals [80, 81]. These dendrimers are small, highly stable, highly water-soluble, and functional groups can easily be attached to them, making them very suitable for the delivery of therapeutics [82]. The amino-terminated variants of polyamidoamine dendrimers are the most popular in pharmaceutical research owing to their ease of bioconjugation using a variety of protein and/or peptide ligands [11]. Through the use of chemical linkages or encapsulation, drugs can be conjugated to the amino terminals of polyamidoamine dendrimers [80]. Drug delivery systems based on Dendrimers can use any among the transport system at the BBB to travel across it due to the significant variation in size and other physical characteristics of dendrimers [81].

3.5.4 Polymeric Nanoparticles

Polymeric nanoparticles are solid, colloidal particles formed by polymers in which drugs can be dissolved, adsorbed, or encapsulated [83, 84]. They have gone forward to be one of the most successful candidates for drug delivery systems owing to their ability to undergo surface modification (e.g., PEGylation), nanosizing, bioactivity, controlled and sustained drug release, nontoxicity, bioavailability, biocompatibility, reticuloendothelial clearance bypass, and the encompassing of various active molecules including drugs, oligonucleotides, and peptides [10, 85]. Similarly to other solid nanoparticulate drug delivery systems, polymeric nanoparticles can be used for the active or passive targeting of drugs to different tissues as a result of their high functional ability, exhibiting a broad range of physicochemical and biochemical characteristics [77]. The different types of polymeric nanoparticulate drug carrier systems are discussed below:

3.5.4.1 PLGA nanoparticles

Currently, attention is being paid to PLGA nanoparticles as potential nanocarriers of drugs across the BBB owing to their high biocompatibility, biodegradability and functional ability [86, 87]. This is because the hydrolysis products of PLGA; lactic acid (LA) and glycolic acid (GA) in aqueous environments are easily metabolized and eliminated from the body through the Krebs cycle

[87]. PLGA nanoparticles on their own do not have a sufficiently long half-life after IV administration however, this can be significantly prolonged by using the polymer's highly modifiable end-group [87, 88]. PLGA has a poor uptake by cells due to its negative surface charge thus, it does not readily cross the BBB. These problems can be solved through the use of crosslinkers, surface adsorption and end-group modifications [87, 89].

Barbara et al. [90] showed that PLGA nanoparticles loaded with curcumin and decorated with the glycopeptide "g7" significantly reduced b-amyloid aggregation, which is a significant indicator of Alzheimer's disease [90] while Wang et al. [91] showed increased accumulation of trimethylated chitosan conjugated PLGA nanoparticles (TMC-PLGA NPs) in the periventricular region of the cortex and the third ventricle of the brain with negligible cytotoxicity using an *in vivo* model. The researchers believe adsorptive-mediated transcytosis to be responsible for TMC-PLGA NPs' ability to cross the BBB [91].

3.5.4.2 PEG nanoparticles

PEG like PLGA has low toxicity levels in the body, is biocompatible, though not biodegradable, is easily eliminated from the body by the kidneys, and is a highly modifiable polymer for drug delivery [92]. Thus, PEG is a commonly used polymer in several pharmaceutical applications, including nanomedicine [86]. Covalently linking PEG onto another molecule (i.e., polymer, NP, drug, protein, antibody, etc.), is known as PEGylation. It is a common technique used for the conferring of function on several nanoparticulate drug carriers. An example of such an FDA approved drug is doxorubicin (used in the treatment of ovarian cancer, breast cancer, multiple myeloma and Kaposi's sarcoma) sold under the brand name DOXIL® (in the US) by Tibotec Therapeutics—a division of Ortho Biotech Products in New Jersey, USA [93, 94].

3.5.4.3 Copolymer nanoparticles

Copolymers are polymers made from more than one single type of monomer. The surface modification to PLGA NPs by PEGylation of drug-loaded PLGA nanoparticles (PEG-PLGA NPs) for brain drug delivery is an effective technique as the nanoparticles possess noticeably improved BBB permeating properties [86, 95]. Jeong et al. [96] first synthesized the triblock copolymer PLGA–PEG–PLGA (PEP), which has exhibited a considerable increase in the delivery of encapsulated drugs to the brain in a study conducted by Chen et al. [97].

3.5.5 Nanoemulsion

These are nano-sized (<200 nm) heterogeneous dispersions of water-in-oil or oil-in-water stabilized using a suitable emulsifier [98, 99]. They are appropriate for the delivery of both the hydrophilic and lipophilic drugs and their permeation through the BBB via receptor-mediated transcytosis (RMT) is facilitated by surface functionalization with suitable ligands. Nanoemulsions are commonly made of vegetable or animal oils, e.g., peanut oil, flaxseed oil, sunflower oil, hemp oil, wheat germ oil, fish oil, egg phosphatidylcholine, etc., making them highly compatible with biological membranes. Stability issues, however, limit its application [100].

Recent studies have shown the use of nanoemulsions for direct nose-to-brain delivery of drugs as well as drug delivery through the parenteral route [101]. Ling Tan et al. [102] used parenteral nanoemulsion for brain targeting of carbamazepine to treat seizures and evaluated its pharmacokinetic efficiency. The study revealed a higher pharmacokinetic profile and lower side effects of the drug when delivered as nanoemulsion than when delivered as the free drug solution [102]. In another study, Abdou et al. [103] assessed the brain targeting efficiency of encapsulated zolmitriptan; an anti-migraine agent nanoemulsion as a mucoadhesive and delivered it via the intranasal route. They found that the mucoadhesive intranasal nanoemulsion significantly enhanced the drug permeability, AUC and bio-availability in the brain [103].

3.5.6 Viral Vectors

Viruses are known to replicate by attacking their host to introduce their genetic material into the host cell [11]. This genetic material is composed of instructions to produce more viruses. Thus, viruses end up taking over the host cell completely to fulfil their own needs with eventual taking over of more host cells [104, 105]. The genetic material that guides the replication of viruses can be substituted with instructions that would be beneficial for the host, such as instructions to attack, poison and destroy cancerous cells. In essence, viral vectors can be used to deliver specific genes to treat or prevent diseases through gene therapy [106, 107]. In addition to gene therapy, viral vectors have recently been used as drug carriers, in which the drugs are encapsulated or infused with a vector that can be functionalized for targeted delivery [11]. Viral vectors compared to other drug delivery systems in gene transduction to the brain have about 80% transfection efficiency and long-term expression of transgenes within the non-dividing cells [10]. Lentivirus, herpes simplex virus (HSV), adenovirus (AdV) and adeno-associated virus (AAV) are examples of the viral vectors that have been used to achieve drug delivery into the brain [10]. Viral vectors as drug delivery systems, however, still have issues linked to the high cost of production and their safety, as the administration of viruses carries a certain level of risk [24, 108, 109].

3.5.7 Carbon Nanotubes

Carbon nanotubes (CNTs) are nanoscaled cylinders of graphene sheets, which have become a promising nanocarrier system for therapeutic agents in many brain-specific therapies [10]. The potential activity of CNTs is due to their ability to undergo surface functionalization easily with specific chemical compounds, which leads to the variation in their physical and biological properties [101, 110]. Polymer-coated carbon nanodots and chemically functionalized multiwalled carbon nanotubes (MWCNTs) can easily bypass the BBB and also form an interface with neurons based on several *in vitro* and *in vivo* models experiments. Thus resulting in enhanced uptake of CNTs at the site of a tumor [101, 110]. The limitations associated with CNTs include toxicity, high cost of production, no control over CNT length and chirality, batch-to-batch variation, and polydispersity in CNT type.

3.5.8 Carbon Dots (CDs)

These are a new class of zero-dimensional carbonaceous nanomaterials. Compared to traditional inorganic quantum dots or noble metal nanoclusters, CDs display improved properties thus, making them promising luminescent nanocarriers and probes [10]. One of the most fascinating characteristics of CDs is their fully color-tunable fluorescent from the blue to the near-infrared regions and the ease of surface modification for targeted delivery. CDs are mostly used in the biomedical field due to their physical and optical properties that include feasible fluorescence, adjustable stability, and water solubility. These have made them powerful tools for use in chemo- or biosensing based on their tunable luminescence properties. The synthesis of CDs is cost-effective. While CDs have good biocompatibility and low toxicity, their limitations include photobleaching, instability, particle-particle aggregation, creation of a nonhomogeneous mixture, inability to be stored for very long, and size-induced toxicity; sizes <5 nm showed more toxic effects than sizes >10 nm [111].

3.5.9 Carbon Nano-Onions (CNOs)

These onion-like carbonaceous zero-dimensional nanostructures are synthesized by thermal annealing of nanodiamonds at very high temperatures and pressure in an inert atmosphere [112, 113]. They are composed of an average of six to eight graphitic shells with sizes ranging between 5 to 6 nm and the distance between two graphitic layers being 0.335 nm. They appear to be suitable candidates for biomedical applications due to their unique electronic and structural features, which include a broad absorption band, a large surface area to volume ratio, the ability to reversibly accept multiple electrons, biocompatibility, and thermal stability [114]. Limitations to their use include poor dispersibility of CNOs in aqueous solution due to their hydrophobic nature resulting in bioaccumulation and hence the toxicity of these nanocarriers, batch-to-batch variation due to the method of synthesis, and difficulty to easily bypass the BBB due to their high molecular weight, which could lead to disruption of the integrity of the

BBB [114]. As a result of the poor solubility of CNOs, surface functionalization is carried out to avoid aggregation in organic and inorganic solvents due to intermolecular interactions such as van der Waals forces between the original nanostructures.

3.6 Mechanisms of Nanodrug Release

Nanodrug delivery systems are considered not only for the ability to convey drugs to the target site but also for the ability to release the drugs. There are a variety of mechanisms of drug release from different nanodrug delivery systems. Ensuring that polymers or composite materials or any form of nanocoating are easily degradable in the active site is essential for activity. Maintaining favorable release kinetics is highly paramount for overall drug efficacy. For liposomes, drugs are released after the dissolution of the lipid layers [115]. This occurs when the cellular membrane lipids fuse with the lipophilic layers of the liposome, releasing drug contents [116]. Polymeric micelles release drugs via a diffusion mechanism of the drug and the rate at which the polymer is depolymerized [117]. Common mechanisms that underlie the different nanocarrier systems include diffusion, disintegration, dissolution, stimuli-controlled release and chemical interaction [118]. The stimuli-controlled release mechanism is observed in ultrasound micelle drug delivery. In this mechanism, an ultrasound device is used to stimulate the rupture of polymeric micelles in target tissues. This form of controlled release utilizes pressure waves. Other types of stimuli include temperature, pH gradient, etc., some of which are internal stimuli. This way, enhanced target specificity is achieved via the external or internally stimulated drug release mechanism [58]. The diffusion mechanism is usually observed in polymeric-encapsulated drugs in which drug dissolution first occurs within the capsule before it diffuses across the polymer nanocapsule into the target site [118]. For drugs with matrix-type nano-enclosure, there is no polymeric barrier hence the initial fast release of drugs is observed [118].

Some types of dendrimers release drugs via a degradation mechanism by which the polymers are degraded enzymatically or hydrolytically *in vivo* at the target site. Polymers such as polylactic acid (PLA) are bulk degraded, while in cases, where water entry into the matrix occurs much slower than the rate of degradation, surface erosion is typically observed [118]. In some cases, special drug release mechanisms are employed via surface changes. This is observed in liposomes adapted into pH-sensitive liposomes to trigger release in the acidic or basic medium of tissue [119] or with magnetic resonance imaging [120]. For polymeric micelles, the rate of drug release can be determined by the hydrophobicity and molecular weight of copolymers [118]. Some polymers show responses to heat and ultrasound as well.

3.7 Applications of Nanodrug Delivery Systems in Brain-Related Disorders

Nanodrug delivery systems are increasingly applied in the treatment of brain-related disorders, enhancing outcomes and improving the quality of life. There is a wide range of brain-related disorders affecting different parts of the brain resulting in different signs and symptoms. Examples of these include Parkinson's disease, Alzheimer's disease, Amyotrophic lateral sclerosis/multiple sclerosis, Huntington's disease, frontotemporal dementia, prion diseases, and; brain tumors, epilepsy, stroke, HIV encephalopathy, etc.

3.7.1 Parkinson's Disease

Parkinson's disease is a neurodegenerative disease evident by the following symptoms: tremors, rigidity, akinesia and postural instability resulting from the loss of dopaminergic neurons in the nigrostriatal region [121]. While it is inheritable, studies have shown that it may be caused by a combination of genetic and environmental factors. Commonly used drugs in the management of Parkinson's include dopamine agonists such as ropinirole, pramipexole; levodopa, and monoamine oxidase-B inhibitors such as rasagiline, and selegiline. While these treatments have been effective in improving symptoms, novel nano delivery systems help with new treatments and modifying disease therapies. In preclinical studies, the use of liposomes in loading dopamine into the brain has been tested [122]. For sustained release, polymeric nanoparticles have also been tested for other drugs such as ropinirole, apomorphine, selegiline, etc. [123]. Polyethylene glycol attached to nanoparticles can be used to increase retention time and reduce the clearance of these drugs [123].

Nanoparticles in Parkinson's disease have useful advantages not only in increasing retention time but also in cell targeting, triggered release, anti-aggregation, etc. For instance, phenylboronic acid can be used to modify nanoparticles for the triggered release of apomorphine [123, 124]. This helps to prevent unwanted side effects by enabling release only in selective environments. Nanoparticles may sometimes have useful therapeutic effects, such as gold nanoparticles, which have shown protective effects in clinical trials for patients with Parkinson's [123, 125].

3.7.2 Alzheimer's Disease

Alzheimer's disease (AD) is a progressive disease in which the brain cells undergo atrophy and die. This leads to symptoms such as loss of memory, difficulty performing tasks, and inability to cater for oneself, then eventually leads to death. It is characterized by the presence of abnormal protein build-up in the brain and it is accountable for the majority of dementia around the world. In preclinical models, polymeric nanoparticles coupled with poly ethylene glycol have been tested in the management of AD [126]. A study was undertaken in which memantine was loaded into biodegradable polymeric NPs generated by the double emulsion process to improve the efficacy of memantine against AD. Targeting the AD brain with memantine-loaded NPs can reduce Aβ plaques and AD-related inflammation significantly [127]. Zinc-loaded polymeric nanoparticles tested in animal models in the management of AD showed sustained effect and target specificity [126]. Nanogels containing deferoxamine have also been found useful in the management of Alzheimer's disease [128].

3.7.3 Huntington's Disease

Huntington's disease (HD) is a rare disease in which the brain's nerve cells continue to degenerate and this usually affects cognition, functional abilities, and locomotion, and may also cause psychiatric disorders. Symptoms usually appear in middle age after a person has had children, however, the disease can appear during any period between childhood and senescence [129]. Huntington is found in all human and mammalian cells, with the largest quantities found in the brain and testes; modest amounts can also be found in the liver, heart, and lungs [130]. The function of the wild-type protein, as well as the pathophysiology of Huntington's disease, are yet unknown. Common drugs used to control the jerking include tetrabenazine and deutetrabenazine. In the management of Huntington's disease, intranasal administration of chitosan nanoparticles loaded with siRNA was found effective in lowering Huntington's disease gene expression [131]. To replenish selenium levels associated with HD, selenium nanoparticles were also tested in preclinical models to regulate cognitive decline [132].

3.7.4 Brain Tumors

Brain tumors and cancers are a group of related disorders characterized by the abnormal proliferation of cells without regulated apoptosis. Brain cancers are more complicated because of difficulty inaccessibility, hence the need for novel systems such as nanodrug delivery systems. A wide variety of nanosystems have been tested for selectivity, ability to cross BBB, enhance retention time, etc. Based on evidence that nanoparticles can accumulate in tissue sites with tumors, they can be used to treat intracranial tumors [133]. Polymeric nanoparticles made from polymers such as poly (D,L-lactide-co-glycolide) are approved for use in clinical applications. The hydrophobic shell of polymeric micelles also serves as a useful means of encapsulating anti-cancer drugs such as platinum [134]. Nanoliposomes are also useful in enhancing the cytotoxicity of anti-cancer drugs in tumors such as glioblastoma [134].

3.7.5 HIV Encephalopathy

HIV encephalopathy is an HIV complication which occurs when the virus reaches the CNS resulting in mental symptoms and disorders. The emergence of nanomedicine may be used to manage this disease through nano-ARTs. A variety of nanoparticles have been tested and these include gold nanoparticles, silver nanoparticles, etc. The inhibition of CCR5 by TAK-779, an effective agent by conjugation of gold nanoparticles with a fragment is an example [135]. Silver nanoparticles were also found to be effective against the virus *in vitro* [135].

3.8 Nanodrug Delivery Systems at the Clinical Trials Stage

Nanodrugs have been tested in various animal models under preclinical settings. Now, they are increasingly being tested in humans at different phases of clinical trials. Some of the nanodrug delivery systems at the clinical trials stage are shown in Table 3.3.

Despite the great advantages of nanodrug delivery systems, nanoneurotherapeutics still possess certain limitations that hamper their full implementation in clinical settings. One limitation is that as the size of the particles reduces to the nanoscale, certain physicochemical properties changes, which may result in unintended effects.

Table 3.3 Nanodrug delivery systems at the clinical trials stage

Nanodrugs	Disease/condition	Phase of clinical trials	Year
AGuIX nanoparticles with radiotherapy plus concomitant temozolomide	Glioblastoma	Phase I/II	[136]
Novel nanosensor array	Multiple Sclerosis	Diagnostic	[137]
NA-NOSE artificial olfactory system	Multiple Sclerosis	Diagnostic	[138]
Nano-sized gadolinium particles	Brain tumor	Phase I	[139]

Nanoparticles have larger surface areas and hence tend to become sticky with each other. The increased surface area of nanoparticles as a result of their smaller size causes an increase in chemical reactivity, which may impact how these nano-sized particles will react under different conditions and in the presence of cell membranes [140]. This may lead to the production of reactive species that may cause oxidative damage and cause toxicity. In addition, unpredicted effects may occur when they cross other membranes and barriers besides the blood-brain barrier. Nanoparticles may also cause damage to the lungs, although unclear [140]. Gold nanorods have been reported to be cytotoxic due to the formulation.

Another major factor that may hinder the progress in the use of nanomedicines is ethical concerns. Risk assessment, risk management, and risk communication in clinical trials are currently the most important ethical challenges in nanomedicine. To win and sustain public support, it is critical to educate members of society on the benefits and risks of nanomedicine [141].

3.9 Future Research Direction/Development

Nanotherapeutics hold unlimited potential in the management and treatment of diseases, especially for CNS disorders such as Alzheimer's disease, Parkinson's, mania, depression, schizophrenia, brain tumors, cancer, etc. The field is dynamic and rapidly evolving with researchers all over the world inventing and discovering new liposomes, nanoparticles, extracellular vesicles, and medical devices to improve drug delivery to the brain [142]. Future research points in the direction of fully elucidating the unique properties of nanomedicines and the influence of nanosize on the behavior of molecules. Numerous *in vitro* models would be required to ascertain this to suggest the direction for regulatory understanding. Evaluation of compounds on a nanoscale and their impact on biological processes points the arrow for new research.

Many more developments will likely spring up in the nanodrug delivery system for brain drug targeting in the coming years. Overcoming significant challenges in some systems like exosomes, for example, could be alleviated with artificial exosomes that do not precipitate host immune reactions in the patients. Achieving precision in cell targeting could provide a gainful step in transformative systems in brain drug delivery. Nano-based drugs are yet to be fully implemented in clinical settings suggesting the need for more studies [142, 143]. While the permeation of the BBB is the priority for nanosystems, protection from neurotoxicity is important. More data is needed on the toxicity profile of nanodrug delivery systems to ensure safety and suitability [142].

Nanomedicine is indeed exciting and provides a unique way of solving formulation and delivery problems. Brain drug targeting is much more desirable since it eliminates the need for invasive delivery processes. In the future, more research may also be directed towards personalized treatments-pharmacogenomics. Pharmacogenomics ignores a 'one-size-fits-all' approach, studies the individual response to drugs based on expressed genes, and provides care to the patient uniquely. With a unique combination of a nano approach in this field, particularly in cancer treatment where it has achieved significant results, enhanced decisions can be made in enabling optimal outcomes [144].

It is conceivable that nanodrug delivery systems will be largely optimized across the management of an array of brain diseases following increased profile studies, characterization, and pharmacokinetic analyses. Increasing industrial acceptability and reducing manufacturing costs are largely key to facilitating availability and use, and application in clinical settings.

3.10 Conclusion

The applications of nanomedicine in brain targeting are immense and extremely useful in the treatment of brain diseases. Whether glioblastoma, multiple sclerosis, Parkinson's, Alzheimer's or any other disease, existing drugs can be modified to improve delivery, enhance retention and reduce clearance, and new drugs can be formulated in nano delivery systems to improve therapeutic outcomes. Future research may further help eliminate limitations and improve their application in clinical settings.

References

1. Li C, Wang J, Wang Y, Gao H, Wei G, Huang Y, et al. Recent progress in drug delivery. *Acta Pharmaceutica Sinica B*. 2019; 9(6): 1145–62.

2. Zhang Z, Guan J, Jiang Z, Yang Y, Liu J, Hua W, et al. Brain-targeted drug delivery by manipulating protein corona functions. *Nature Communications.* 2019; 10(1), 3561.
3. Hwang SR, Kim K. Nano-enabled delivery systems across the blood-brain barrier. *Archives of Pharmacal Research.* 2014; 37(1): 24–30.
4. Zhao Z, Ukidve A, Kim J, Mitragotri SJC. Targeting strategies for tissue-specific drug delivery. *Cell.* 2020; 181(1), 151–67.
5. Wang J, Zhou T, Liu Y, Chen S, Yu Z. Application of nanoparticles in the treatment of lung cancer with emphasis on receptors. *Frontiers in Pharmacology.* 2021; 12: 781425.
6. Babu A, Templeton AK, Munshi A, Ramesh RJAP. Nanodrug delivery systems: a promising technology for detection, diagnosis, and treatment of cancer. *AAPS PharmSciTech.* 2014; 15(3): 709–21.
7. Cho K, Wang X, Nie S, Shin DMJCcr. Therapeutic nanoparticles for drug delivery in cancer. *Clinical Cancer Research.* 2008;14(5): 1310–6.
8. Quan X-Q, Kang L, Yin X-Z, Jin Z-H, Gao Z-GJCCL. Synthesis of PEGylated hyaluronic acid for loading dichloro (1,2-diaminocyclohexane) platinum (II)(DACHPt) in nanoparticles for cancer treatment. *Chinese Chemical Letters.* 2015; 26(6): 695–9.
9. Gupta P, Garcia E, Sarkar A, Kapoor S, Rafiq K, Chand HS, et al. Nanoparticle based treatment for cardiovascular diseases. *Cardiovascular & Hematological Disorders Drug Targets.* 2019; 19(1): 33–44.
10. Ahlawat J, Guillama Barroso G, Masoudi Asil S, Alvarado M, Armendariz I, Bernal J, et al. Nanocarriers as potential drug delivery candidates for overcoming the blood-brain barrier: challenges and possibilities. *ACS Omega.* 2020; 5(22): 12583–95.
11. Ayub A, Wettig S. An overview of nanotechnologies for drug delivery to the brain. *Pharmaceutics.* 2022; 14(2): 224.
12. Kusuhara H, Sugiyama YJDdt. Efflux transport systems for drugs at the blood–brain barrier and blood–cerebrospinal fluid barrier (Part 1). *Drug Discovery Today.* 2001; 6(3): 150–6.
13. Abbott NJ, Patabendige AA, Dolman DE, Yusof SR, Begley DJ. Structure and function of the blood–brain barrier. *Neurobiology of Disease.* 2010; 37(1): 13–25.
14. Jones AR, Shusta EVJ Pr. Blood–brain barrier transport of therapeutics via receptor-mediation. *Pharmaceutical Research.* 2007; 24(9): 1759–71.

15. Bernardo-Castro S, Sousa JA, Brás A, Cecília C, Rodrigues B, Almendra L, et al. Pathophysiology of blood–brain-barrier permeability throughout the different stages of ischemic stroke and its implication on hemorrhagic transformation and recovery. *Frontiers in Neurology.* 2020: 11, 594672.

16. Helms HC, Abbott NJ, Burek M, Cecchelli R, Couraud P-O, Deli MA, et al. *In vitro* models of the blood–brain barrier: an overview of commonly used brain endothelial cell culture models and guidelines for their use. *Journal of Cerebral Blood Flow and Metabolism.* 2016; 36(5): 862–90.

17. Cabezas R, Ávila M, Gonzalez J, El-Bachá RS, Báez E, García-Segura LM, et al. Astrocytic modulation of blood–brain-barrier: perspectives on Parkinson's disease. *Frontiers in Cellular Neuroscience.* 2014; 8: 211.

18. Xu L, Nirwane A, Yao YJS, neurology v. Basement membrane and blood–brain barrier. *Stroke and Vascular Neurology.* 2019; 4(2): 78–82

19. Islam Y, Leach AG, Smith J, Pluchino S, Coxon CR, Sivakumaran M, et al. Physiological and pathological factors affecting drug delivery to the brain by nanoparticles. *Advanced Science.* 2021; 8(11): 2002085.

20. Pardridge WMJF, CNS Bot. Drug transport in brain via the cerebrospinal fluid. *Fluids and Barriers of the CNS.* 2011; 8(1): 7.

21. Yasuda K, Cline C, Vogel P, Onciu M, Fatima S, Sorrentino BP, et al. Drug transporters on arachnoid barrier cells contribute to the blood–cerebrospinal fluid barrier. *Drug Metabolism and Disposition.* 2013; 41(4): 923–31.

22. Huttunen KM, Terasaki T, Urtti A, Montaser AB, Uchida YJPr. Pharmacoproteomics of brain barrier transporters and substrate design for the brain targeted drug delivery. *Pharmaceutical Research,* 2022: 39(7): 1363–92.

23. Jin L-Y, Li J, Wang K-F, Xia W-W, Zhu Z-Q, Wang C-R, et al. Blood–spinal cord barrier in spinal cord injury: a review. *Journal of Neurotrauma.* 2021; 38(9): 1203–24.

24. Dong X. Current strategies for brain drug delivery. *Theranostics.* 2018; 8(6): 1481–93.

25. Haqqani AS, Delaney CE, Tremblay T-L, Sodja C, Sandhu JK, Stanimirovic DB. Method for isolation and molecular characterization of extracellular microvesicles released from brain endothelial cells. *Fluids and Barriers of the CNS* 2013; 10(1): 4.

26. Ha D, Yang N, Nadithe V. Exosomes as therapeutic drug carriers and delivery vehicles across biological membranes: current perspectives and future challenges. *Acta Pharmaceutica Sinica. B*, 2016; 6(4): 287–96.
27. Liang J, Gao C, Zhu Y, Ling C, Wang Q, Huang Y, et al. Natural brain penetration enhancer-modified albumin nanoparticles for glioma targeting delivery. *ACS Applied Materials & Interfaces* 2018; 10(36): 30201–13.
28. Breitkreuz-Korff O, Tscheik C, Del Vecchio G, Dithmer S, Walther W, Orthmann A, et al. M01 as a novel drug enhancer for specifically targeting the blood-brain barrier. *Journal of Controlled Release*. 2021; 338: 137–48.
29. O'Reilly MA, Hynynen K. Ultrasound enhanced drug delivery to the brain and central nervous system. *International Journal of Hyperthermia*. 2012; 28(4): 386–96.
30. Dasgupta A, Liu M, Ojha T, Storm G, Kiessling F, Lammers T. Ultrasound-mediated drug delivery to the brain: principles, progress and prospects. *Drug Discovery Today: Technologies*. 2016; 20: 41–8.
31. Rautio J, Laine K, Gynther M, Savolainen J. Prodrug approaches for CNS delivery. *AAPS Journal*. 2008; 10(1): 92–102.
32. Zeiadeh I, Najjar A, Karaman R. Strategies for enhancing the permeation of CNS-active drugs through the blood-brain barrier: a review. *Molecules*. 2018; 23(6): 1289.
33. Dalpiaz A, Paganetto G, Pavan B, Fogagnolo M, Medici A, Beggiato S, et al. Zidovudine and ursodeoxycholic acid conjugation: design of a new prodrug potentially able to bypass the active efflux transport systems of the central nervous system. *Molecular Pharmaceutics*. 2012; 9(4): 957–68.
34. Gynther M, Laine K, Ropponen J, Leppänen J, Mannila A, Nevalainen T, et al. Large neutral amino acid transporter enables brain drug delivery via prodrugs. *Journal of Medicinal Chemistry*. 2008; 51(4): 932–6.
35. Yue Q, Peng Y, Zhao Y, Lu R, Fu Q, Chen Y, et al. Dual-targeting for brain-specific drug delivery: synthesis and biological evaluation. *Drug Delivery*. 2018; 25(1): 426–34.
36. Zhang J, Xu Y, Li D, Fu L, Zhang X, Bao Y, et al. Review of the correlation of LAT1 with diseases: mechanism and treatment. *Frontiers in Chemistry*. 2020; 8: 564809.
37. Bellettato CM, Scarpa M. Possible strategies to cross the blood–brain barrier. *Italian Journal of Pediatrics*. 2018; 44(Suppl 2): 131.

38. Haley T, McCormick WG chemotherapy. Pharmacological effects produced by intracerebral injection of drugs in the conscious mouse. *British Journal of Pharmacology and Chemotherapy.* 1957; 12(1): 12–5.

39. Cook AM, Mieure KD, Owen RD, Pesaturo AB, Hatton J. Intracerebroventricular administration of drugs. *Pharmacotherapy.* 2009; 29(7): 832–45.

40. Barcia JA, Gallego JM. Intraventricular and intracerebral delivery of anti-epileptic drugs in the kindling model. *Neurotherapeutics.* 2009; 6(2): 337–43.

41. Sun Y, Sun J, He Z, Wang G, Wang Y, Zhao D, et al. Monocarboxylate transporter 1 in brain diseases and cancers. *Current Drug Metabolism.* 2019; 20(11): 855–66.

42. Fu H, McCarty DM. Crossing the blood–brain-barrier with viral vectors. *Current Opinion in Virology.* 2016; 21: 87–92.

43. McDannold N, Zhang Y, Supko JG, Power C, Sun T, Vykhodtseva N, et al. Blood-brain barrier disruption and delivery of irinotecan in a rat model using a clinical transcranial MRI-guided focused ultrasound system. *Scientific Reports.* 2020; 10: 8766.

44. Abourehab MA, Ahmed OA, Balata GF, Almalki WH. Self-assembled biodegradable polymeric micelles to improve dapoxetine delivery across the blood–brain barrier. *International Journal of Nanomedicine.* 2018; 13: 3679–87.

45. Manjunath K, Venkateswarlu V. Pharmacokinetics, tissue distribution and bioavailability of clozapine solid lipid nanoparticles after intravenous and intraduodenal administration. *Journal of Controlled Release.* 2005; 107(2): 215–28.

46. Lawther BK, Kumar S, Krovvidi H. Blood–brain barrier. *JCEiA, Critical Care, Pain.* 2011; 11(4): 128–32.

47. Constantinescu T, Lungu CN, Lung IJM. Lipophilicity as a central component of drug-like properties of chalchones and flavonoid derivatives. *Molecules.* 2019; 24(8): 1505.

48. Pajouhesh H, Lenz GR. Medicinal chemical properties of successful central nervous system drugs. *NeuroRx.* 2005; 2(4): 541–53.

49. Banks WA, Greig NH. Small molecules as central nervous system therapeutics: old challenges, new directions, and a philosophic divide. *Future Medicinal Chemistry.* 2019; 11(6): 489–93.

50. Pardridge WM. Drug transport across the blood–brain barrier. *Journal of Cerebral Blood Flow and Metabolism.* 2012; 32(11): 1959–72.

51. Warren KE. Beyond the blood: brain barrier: the importance of central nervous system (CNS) pharmacokinetics for the treatment of CNS tumors, including diffuse intrinsic pontine glioma. *Frontiers in Oncology*. 2018; 8: 239.

52. Pulgar VM. Transcytosis to cross the blood brain barrier, new advancements and challenges. *Frontiers in Neuroscience*. 2019: 12: 1019.

53. Abioye AO, Tangyie Chi G, Kola-Mustapha AT, Ruparelia K, Beresford K, Arroo R. Polymer-drug nanoconjugate–an innovative nanomedicine: challenges and recent advancements in rational formulation design for effective delivery of poorly soluble drugs. *Pharmaceutical Nanotechnology*. 2016; 4(1): 38–79.

54. Shiraishi K, Wang Z, Kokuryo D, Aoki I, Yokoyama M. A polymeric micelle magnetic resonance imaging (MRI) contrast agent reveals blood–brain barrier (BBB) permeability for macromolecules in cerebral ischemia-reperfusion injury. *Journal of Controlled Release*. 2017; 253: 165–71.

55. Yin Y, Wang J, Yang M, Du R, Pontrelli G, McGinty S, et al. Penetration of the blood–brain barrier and the anti-tumour effect of a novel PLGA-lysoGM1/DOX micelle drug delivery system. *Nanoscale*. 2020; 12(5): 2946–60.

56. Zhang Y, Huang Y, Li S. Polymeric micelles: nanocarriers for cancer-targeted drug delivery. *AAPS PharmSciTech*. 2014; 15(4): 862–71.

57. Owen SC, Chan DP, Shoichet MS. Polymeric micelle stability. *Nano Today*. 2012; 7(1): 53–65.

58. Husseini GA, Pitt WG. Micelles and nanoparticles for ultrasonic drug and gene delivery. *Advanced Drug Delivery Reviews*. 2008; 60(10): 1137–52.

59. Chiappetta DA, Sosnik A. Poly (ethylene oxide)–poly (propylene oxide) block copolymer micelles as drug delivery agents: improved hydrosolubility, stability and bioavailability of drugs. *European Journal of Pharmaceutics and Biopharmaceutics*. 2007; 66(3): 303–17.

60. Croy S, Kwon G. Polymeric micelles for drug delivery. *Current Pharmaceutical Design*. 2006; 12(36): 4669–84.

61. Galetti M, Rossi S, Caffarra C, Gerboles AG, Miragoli M. Innovation in nanomedicine and engineered nanomaterials for therapeutic purposes. In *Exposure to Engineered Nanomaterials in the Environment*. 2019; Elsevier, pp. 235–62.

62. Yadav HK, Almokdad AA, Sumia I, Debe MS. Polymer-based nanomaterials for drug-delivery carriers. In *Nanocarriers for Drug Delivery*. 2019; Elsevier, pp. 531–56.

63. Juhairiyah F, de Lange ECM. Understanding drug delivery to the brain using liposome-based strategies: studies that provide mechanistic insights are essential. *AAPS Journal*. 2021; 23(6): 114.

64. Akbarzadeh A, Rezaei-Sadabady R, Davaran S, Joo SW, Zarghami N, Hanifehpour Y, et al. Liposome: classification, preparation, and applications. *Nanoscale Research Letters*. 2013; 8(1): 102.

65. Wu S, Li G, Li X, Lin C, Yu D, Luan S, et al. Transport of glial cell line-derived neurotrophic factor into liposomes across the blood-brain barrier: *in vitro* and *in vivo* studies. *International Journal of Molecular Sciences*, 2014; 15(3): 3612–23.

66. Gao J, Wang Z, Liu H, Wang L, Huang G. Liposome encapsulated of temozolomide for the treatment of glioma tumor: preparation, characterization and evaluation. *Drug Discoveries & Therapeutics*. 2015; 9(3): 205–12.

67. So P-W, Ekonomou A, Galley K, Brody L, Sahuri-Arisoylu M, Rattray I, et al. Intraperitoneal delivery of acetate-encapsulated liposomal nanoparticles for neuroprotection of the penumbra in a rat model of ischemic stroke. *International Journal of Nanomedicine*. 2019; 14: 1979–91.

68. Pardridge WM. Transport of small molecules through the blood-brain barrier: biology and methodology. *Advanced Drug Delivery Reviews*. 1995; 15(1–3): 5–36.

69. Torchilin VP. Recent advances with liposomes as pharmaceutical carriers. *Drug Discovey*. 2005; 4(2): 145–60.

70. Lai F, Fadda AM, Sinico C. Liposomes for brain delivery. *Expert Opinion on Drug Delivery*. 2013; 10(7): 1003–22.

71. Huwyler J, Wu D, Pardridge WM. Brain drug delivery of small molecules using immunoliposomes. *Proceedings of the National Academy of Sciences of the United States of America*, 1996; 93(24): 14164–9.

72. Gupta R, Gupta J, Pathak A. Immunoliposomes: a targeted drug delivery system for cancer therapeutics and vaccination. *Current Pharmaceutical Biotechnology*. 2023; 24(3): 366–390.

73. Molnar D, Linders J, Mayer C, Schubert R. Insertion stability of poly(ethylene glycol)-cholesteryl-based lipid anchors in liposome membranes. *European Journal of Pharmaceutics and Biopharmaceutics*. 2016; 103: 51–61.

74. Dolor A, Kierstead P, Dai Z, Szoka FC. Sterol-modified PEG lipids: alteration of the bilayer anchoring moiety has an unexpected effect on liposome circulation. *Chemical Communications.* 2018; 54(84): 11949–52.

75. Pardridge WM. Vector-mediated drug delivery to the brain. *Advanced Drug Delivery Reviews.* 1999; 36(2–3): 299–321.

76. Tomalia DA, Baker H, Dewald J, Hall M, Kallos G, Martin S, et al. A new class of polymers: starburst-dendritic macromolecules. *Polymer Journal.* 1985; 17(1): 117–32.

77. Sahoo SK, Labhasetwar V. Nanotech approaches to drug delivery and imaging. *Drug Discovery Today.* 2003; 8(24): 1112–20.

78. Abbasi E, Aval SF, Akbarzadeh A, Milani M, Nasrabadi HT, Joo SW, et al. Dendrimers: synthesis, applications, and properties. *Nanoscale Research Letters.* 2014; 9: 247.

79. Madaan K, Kumar S, Poonia N, Lather V, Pandita D. Dendrimers in drug delivery and targeting: drug-dendrimer interactions and toxicity issues. *Journal of Pharmacy and Bioallied Sciences.* 2014; 6(3): 139–50.

80. Mekuria SL, Debele TA, Tsai H-C. PAMAM dendrimer based targeted nano-carrier for bio-imaging and therapeutic agents. *RSC Advances.* 2016; 6: 63761–72.

81. Zhu Y, Liu C, Pang Z. Dendrimer-based drug delivery systems for brain targeting. *Biomolecules.* 2019; 9(12): 790.

82. Florendo M, Figacz A, Srinageshwar B, Sharma A, Swanson D, Dunbar GL, et al. Use of polyamidoamine dendrimers in brain diseases. *Molecules.* 2018; 23(9): 2238.

83. Gulati M, Chopra DS, Singh SK, Saluja V, Pathak P, Bansal P. Patents on brain permeable nanoparticles. *Recent Patents on CNS Drug Discovery.* 2013; 8(3): 220–34.

84. Patil V, Patel A. Biodegradable nanoparticles: a recent approach and applications. *Current Drug Targets.* 2020; 21(16): 1722–32.

85. Ahlawat J, Henriquez G, Narayan M. Enhancing the delivery of chemotherapeutics: role of biodegradable polymeric nanoparticles. *Molecules.* 2018; 23(9): 2157.

86. Kumari A, Yadav SK, Yadav SC, biointerfaces sB. Biodegradable polymeric nanoparticles based drug delivery systems. *Colloids and Surfaces. B, Biointerfaces* 2010; 75(1): 1–18.

87. Danhier F, Ansorena E, Silva JM, Coco R, Le Breton A, Préat V. PLGA-based nanoparticles: an overview of biomedical applications. *Journal of Controlled Release.* 2012; 161(2): 505–22.

88. Makadia HK, Siegel SJ. Poly lactic-co-glycolic acid (PLGA) as biodegradable controlled drug delivery carrier. *Polymers.* 2011; 3(3): 1377–97.

89. Tosi G, Bortot B, Ruozi B, Dolcetta D, Vandelli MA, Forni F, et al. Potential use of polymeric nanoparticles for drug delivery across the blood–brain barrier. *Current Medicinal Chemistry.* 2013; 20(17): 2212–25.

90. Barbara R, Belletti D, Pederzoli F, Masoni M, Keller J, Ballestrazzi A, et al. Novel Curcumin loaded nanoparticles engineered for blood-brain barrier crossing and able to disrupt Abeta aggregates. *International Journal of Pharmaceutics.* 2017; 526(1–2): 413–24.

91. Wang ZH, Wang ZY, Sun CS, Wang CY, Jiang TY, Wang SL. Trimethylated chitosan-conjugated PLGA nanoparticles for the delivery of drugs to the brain. *Biomaterials.* 2010; 31(5): 908–15.

92. Calzoni E, Cesaretti A, Polchi A, Di Michele A, Tancini B, Emiliani C. Biocompatible polymer nanoparticles for drug delivery applications in cancer and neurodegenerative disorder therapies. *Journal of Functional Biomaterials.* 2019; 10(1): 4.

93. Gabizon AA. Pegylated liposomal doxorubicin: metamorphosis of an old drug into a new form of chemotherapy. *Cancer Investigation* 2001; 19(4): 424–36.

94. Green AE, Rose PG. Pegylated liposomal doxorubicin in ovarian cancer. *International Journal of Nanomedicine.* 2006; 1(3): 229.

95. Hu K, Shi Y, Jiang W, Han J, Huang S, Jiang X. Lactoferrin conjugated PEG-PLGA nanoparticles for brain delivery: preparation, characterization and efficacy in Parkinson's disease. *International Journal of Pharmaceutics.* 2011; 415(1–2): 273–83.

96. Jeong B, Bae YH, Kim SW. Thermoreversible gelation of PEG–PLGA–PEG triblock copolymer aqueous solutions. *Macromolecules.* 1999; 32(21): 7064–9.

97. Chen Y-C, Hsieh W-Y, Lee W-F, Zeng D-T. Effects of surface modification of PLGA-PEG-PLGA nanoparticles on loperamide delivery efficiency across the blood–brain barrier. *Journal of Biomaterials Applications.* 2013; 27(7): 909–22.

98. Ganta S, Amiji MJ. Coadministration of paclitaxel and curcumin in nanoemulsion formulations to overcome multidrug resistance in tumor cells. *Molecular Pharmaceutics.* 2009; 6(3): 928–39.

99. Ganta S, Deshpande D, Korde A, Amiji M. A review of multifunctional nanoemulsion systems to overcome oral and CNS drug delivery barriers. *Molecular Membrane Biology.* 2010; 27(7): 260–73.

100. Li X, Tsibouklis J, Weng T, Zhang B, Yin G, Feng G, et al. Nano carriers for drug transport across the blood–brain barrier. *Journal of Drug Targeting.* 2017; 25(1): 17–28.

101. Alexander A, Agrawal M, Uddin A, Siddique S, Shehata AM, Shaker MA, et al. Recent expansions of novel strategies towards the drug targeting into the brain. *International Journal of Nanomedicine.* 2019; 14: 5895–909.

102. Ling Tan S, Stanslas J, Basri M, Karjiban RA A, P Kirby B, Sani D, et al. Nanoemulsion-based parenteral drug delivery system of carbamazepine: preparation, characterization, stability evaluation and blood-brain pharmacokinetics. *Current Drug Delivery.* 2015; 12(6): 795–804.

103. Abdou EM, Kandil SM, El Miniawy HMFE. Brain targeting efficiency of antimigrain drug loaded mucoadhesive intranasal nanoemulsion. *International Journal of Pharmaceutics.* 2017; 529(1–2): 667–77.

104. Lodish H, Berk A, Zipursky S, Matsudaira P, Baltimore D, Darnell J. Viruses: structure, function, and uses. In *Molecular Cell Biology*, 4th Edition, Freeman and Company, New York. 2000.

105. Tong S, Revill P. Overview of hepatitis B viral replication and genetic variability. *Journal of Hepatology.* 2016; 64(1): S4–S16.

106. Robbins PD, Tahara H, Ghivizzani SC. Viral vectors for gene therapy. *Trends in Biotechnology.* 1998; 16(1): 35–40.

107. Gonçalves GAR, Paiva RMA. Gene therapy: advances, challenges and perspectives. *Einstein.* 2017; 15 (3): 369–75.

108. Thomas CE, Ehrhardt A, Kay MA. Progress and problems with the use of viral vectors for gene therapy. *Nature Reviews.* 2003; 4(5): 346–58.

109. Lockney D, Franzen S, Lommel S. Viruses as nanomaterials for drug delivery. *Methods in Molecular Biology.* 2011; 726: 207–21.

110. Ma X, Zhong L, Guo H, Wang Y, Gong N, Wang Y, et al. Multiwalled carbon nanotubes induced hypotension by regulating the central nervous system. *Advanced Functional Materials.* 2018; 28(11): 1705479.

111. Yao K, Lv X, Zheng G, Chen Z, Jiang Y, Zhu X, et al. Effects of carbon quantum dots on aquatic environments: comparison of toxicity to organisms at different trophic levels. *Environmental Science and Technology.* 2018; 52(24): 14445–51.

112. Mykhailiv O, Lapinski A, Molina-Ontoria A, Regulska E, Echegoyen L, Dubis AT, et al. Influence of the synthetic conditions on the structural and electrochemical properties of carbon nano-onions. *Chemphyschem.* 2015; 16(10): 2182–91.

113. Berman D, Narayanan B, Cherukara MJ, Sankaranarayanan S, Erdemir A, Zinovev A, et al. Operando tribochemical formation of onion-like-carbon leads to macroscale superlubricity. *Nature Communications.* 2018; 9: 1164.

114. Plonska-Brzezinska ME. Carbon nano-onions: a review of recent progress in synthesis and applications. *ChemNanoMat.* 2019; 5(5): 568–80.

115. Hashmi MP, Koester TM. Applications of synthetically produced materials in clinical medicine. In *Reference Module in Materials Science and Materials Engineering*, Elsevier. 2018.

116. Yadav D, Sandeep K, Pandey D, Dutta RK. Liposomes for drug delivery. *Journal of Biotechnology and Biomaterials.* 2017; 7(4): 276.

117. Wang Z, Deng X, Ding J, Zhou W, Zheng X, Tang G. Mechanisms of drug release in pH-sensitive micelles for tumour targeted drug delivery system: a review. *International Journal of Pharmaceutics.* 2018; 535(1–2): 253–60.

118. Lee JH, Yeo Y. Controlled drug release from pharmaceutical nanocarriers. *Chemical Engineering Science.* 2015; 125: 75–84.

119. Yuba E, Harada A, Sakanishi Y, Watarai S, Kono K. A liposome-based antigen delivery system using pH-sensitive fusogenic polymers for cancer immunotherapy. *Biomaterials.* 2013; 34(12): 3042–52.

120. Torres E, Mainini F, Napolitano R, Fedeli F, Cavalli R, Aime S, et al. Improved paramagnetic liposomes for MRI visualization of pH triggered release. *Journal of Controlled Release.* 2011; 154(2): 196–202.

121. Paul A, Yadav KS, Parkinson's disease: current drug therapy and unraveling the prospects of nanoparticles. *Journal of Drug Delivery Science and Technology.* 2020; 58: 101790.

122. During MJ, Freese A, Deutch AY, Kibat PG, Sabel BA, Langer R, et al. Biochemical and behavioral recovery in a rodent model of Parkinson's disease following stereotactic implantation of dopamine-containing liposomes. *Experimental Neurology.* 1992; 115(2): 193–9.

123. Jo S, Sun I-C, Ahn C-H, Lee S, Kim K. Recent trend of ultrasound-mediated nanoparticle delivery for brain imaging and treatment. *ACS Applied Materials & Interfaces.* 2023; 15(1), 120–37.

124. Tan JPK, Voo ZX, Lim S, Venkataraman S, Ng KM, Gao S, et al. Effective encapsulation of apomorphine into biodegradable polymeric nanoparticles through a reversible chemical bond for

delivery across the blood–brain barrier. *Nanomedicine: Nanotechnology, Biology, and Medicine.* 2019; 17: 236–45.

125. Gao G, Chen R, He M, Li J, Li J, et al. Gold nanoclusters for Parkinson's disease treatment. *Biomaterials.* 2019; 194: 36–46.

126. Khan NH, Mir M, Ngowi EE, Zafar U, Khakwani MMAK, Khattak S, et al. Nanomedicine: a Promising way to manage Alzheimer's disease. *Frontiers in Bioengineering and Biotechnology.* 2021; 9: 630055.

127. Sánchez-López E, Ettcheto M, Egea MA, Espina M, Cano A, Calpena AC, et al. Memantine loaded PLGA PEGylated nanoparticles for Alzheimer's disease: *in vitro* and *in vivo* characterization. *Journal of Nanobiotechnology.* 2018; 16(1): 32.

128. Ashrafi H, Azadi A, Mohammadi-Samani S, Hamidi M. New candidate delivery system for Alzheimer's disease: deferoxamine nanogels. *Biointerface Research in Applied Chemistry.* 2020; 10(6): 7106–19.

129. Walker FO. Huntington's disease. *Seminars in Neurology.* 2007; 27(2): 143–50.

130. DiFiglia M, Sapp E, Chase K, Schwarz C, Meloni A, Young C, et al. Huntingtin is a cytoplasmic protein associated with vesicles in human and rat brain neurons. *Neuron.* 1995; 14(5): 1075–81.

131. Sava V, Fihurka O, Khvorova A, Sanchez-Ramos J. Enriched chitosan nanoparticles loaded with siRNA are effective in lowering Huntington's disease gene expression following intranasal administration. *Nanomedicine: Nanotechnology, Biology, and Medicine.* 2020; 24: 102119.

132. Cong W, Bai R, Li Y-F, Wang L, Chen C. Selenium nanoparticles as an efficient nanomedicine for the therapy of Huntington's disease. *ACS Applied Materials and Interfaces* 2019; 11(38): 34725–35.

133. Fisusi FA, Schätzlein AG, Uchegbu IF. Nanomedicines in the treatment of brain tumors. *Nanomedicine.* 2018. 13(6): 579–83.

134. Kumar LA, Pattnaik G, Satapathy BS, Swapna S, Mohanty D, Targeting to brain tumor: nanocarrier-based drug delivery platforms, opportunities, and challenges. *Journal of Pharmacy and Bioallied Sciences.* 2021; 13(2): 172–7.

135. Nowacek A, Gendelman HE. NanoART, neuroAIDS and CNS drug delivery. *Nanomedicine.* 2009; 4(5): 557–74.

136. NCT04881032. Clinical Trials. AGuIX Nanoparticles With Radiotherapy Plus Concomitant Temozolomide in the Treatment of Newly Diagnosed Glioblastoma (NANO-GBM) https://www.

clinicaltrials.gov/ct2/show/NCT04881032?term=nano&cond=Glioblastoma&draw=2&rank=1 2021 (accessed 17 May 2022).

137. NCT04074629. Novel Nanosensor Array for Detection of Volatile Biomarkers From Skin in Multiple Sclerosis (Nano-Skin-MS) https://www.clinicaltrials.gov/ct2/show/NCT04074629?term=nano&cond=Multiple+Sclerosis&draw=2&rank=1 2022 (accessed 17 May 2022).

138. NCT01465087. Nanotechnology for Detection of Multiple Sclerosis Compared to Autoimmune and Neurological Diseases by Exhaled Samples https://www.clinicaltrials.gov/ct2/show/NCT01465087?term=nano&cond=Multiple+Sclerosis&draw=2&rank=4 ClinicalTrials.gov 2016 (accessed 17 May 2022).

139. NCT02820454. Radiosensitization of Multiple Brain Metastases Using AGuIX Gadolinium Based Nanoparticles (NANO-RAD) https://www.clinicaltrials.gov/ct2/show/NCT02820454?term=nano&cond=Brain+Tumor&draw=2&rank=1 ClinicalTrials.gov 2019 (Accessed 17 May 2022).

140. Shubhika K. Nanotechnology and medicine-The upside and the downside. *International Journal of Drug Development and Research.* 2013; 5(4): 1–10.

141. Kazemi A, Majidinia M, Jamali AA,. The question of ethics in nanomedicine. *Journal of Clinical Research and Bioethics.* 2014; 5(4): 1000193.

142. Masserini M. Nanoparticles for brain drug delivery. *International Scholarly Research Notices.* 2013; 2013: Article ID 238428.

143. Lundy DJ, Nguyễn H, Hsieh PC. Emerging nano-carrier strategies for brain tumor drug delivery and considerations for clinical translation. *Journal of Pharmaceutics.* 2021; 13(8): 1193.

144. Chawla R, Rani V, Mishra M, Kumar K. Integrated role of nanotechnology and pharmacogenetics in diagnosis and treatment of diseases. *Pharmacogenetics.* IntechOpen; 2021.

Multiple Choice Questions

1. Which one of the following is a nanodrug delivery system?

   A. Tablets
   B. Capsules
   C. Liposomes
   D. Syrups

2. ___________ are spherical colloidal structures that possess an outer lipid bilayer.

   A. Liposomes
   B. Dendrimers
   C. Micelles
   D. Capsules

3. The surface of Liposomes can be modified with ________ to increase retention time in circulation.

   A. Ethylenediamine
   B. Poly ethylene glycol
   C. Poly propylene glycol
   D. Micelles

4. _________ is a dynamic structure that regulates the entry of substances into the brain and exit out of, and is key to maintaining its homeostasis.

   A. Cell membrane
   B. Blood-Brain Barrier
   C. Skull
   D. Blood

5. One of the following is not part of the blood-brain barrier?

   A. Endothelial cells
   B. Astrocytes
   C. Pericytes
   D. None of the above

6. One of the following is not a major protein found in the basement membrane of the blood–brain barrier

   A. Laminin
   B. Perlecan
   C. Keratin
   D. Nidogen

7. How many layers of meninges cover the central nervous system?

   A. 1
   B. 2
   C. 3
   D. 4

8. Prodrug formation belongs to what type of strategy for brain drug targeting?
   A. Chemical modification
   B. BBB permeability enhancer
   C. Transport systems
   D. Direct administration
9. Drugs with high lipophilicity are able to cross the blood-brain barrier via:
   A. Disintegration
   B. Erosion
   C. Solubilization
   D. pH-gradient transfer
10. Amphilic block Copolymers constitute ______________
    A. Liposomes
    B. Micelles
    C. Opsonins
    D. Vectors
11. Polymeric micelles are characterized by an inner lipophilic ______________ and an outer hydrophilic ______________ respectively.
    A. Core, corona
    B. Corona, core
    C. Polymer, block
    D. None of the above
12. Coupling antibodies to surfaces of liposomes result in the formation of ______________
    A. Micelles
    B. Dendrimers
    C. Immunoliposomes
    D. Exosomes
13. Three different layers make up dendrimers and they include core, corona and ______________
    A. Middle layer
    B. Branching layer

C. Outer layer
D. Inner layer

14. ______________ contains minuscule droplet sizes.

A. Liposomes
B. Micelles
C. Nanoemulsion
D. Viral vectors

15. Which one of the following is not used as a viral vector?

A. Adenovirus
B. Adeno-associated virus
C. Herpes virus
D. Ebola virus

16. Which one of the following is fluorescent in nature?

A. Carbon dots
B. Carbon nanotubes
C. Liposomes
D. Micelles

17. Common mechanisms that underlie the release of drugs from different nanocarrier systems include:

A. Diffusion
B. Stimuli-controlled release
C. Chemical Interaction
D. All of the above

18. Nanodrug delivery systems (NDDS) are tested in the treatment of all but one of the following brain diseases:

A. Parkinson's disease
B. Alzheimer's disease
C. Duodenal ulcer
D. Huntington's disease

19. ________ is attached to nanoparticles to enhance retention time and reduce clearance of drugs

A. Micelles
B. Poly ethylene glycol
C. Poly lactic acid
D. Liposomes

20. ____________ can be used to modify nanoparticles for triggered release of apomorphine
    A. Ethanol
    B. Poly ethylene glycol
    C. Phenylboronic acid
    D. Benzoic acid

21. Curcumin in the management of Alzheimer's Disease is faced with the following issues:
    A. Low bioavailability
    B. Poor stability
    C. All of the above
    D. None of the above

22. Huntingtin is found in all mammalian cells with the largest quantities found in:
    A. Brain
    B. Testes
    C. All of the above
    D. None of the above

23. Polymeric nanoparticles made from ________ polymer are approved for use in clinical applications
    A. Poly ethylene glycol
    B. Poly (D,L-lactide-co-glycolide)
    C. Polyacrylamide
    D. Poly propylamide

24. Which one of the following minerals were tested as nanoparticles in Huntington's?
    A. Calcium
    B. Magnesium
    C. Nickel
    D. Selenium

25. ____________ and ____________ nanoparticles have been tested in the management of HIV encephalopathy
    A. Gold and silver
    B. Selenium and zinc

C. Iron and gold
D. Selenium and silver

26. Nano-sized gadolinium particles were tested in the treatment of brain tumors in ____________ of clinical trials.
    A. Phase I
    B. Phase II
    C. Phase III
    D. Phase IV

27. AGuIX nanoparticles with radiotherapy plus concomitant Temozolomide were tested in clinical trials in the management of ________________
    A. Alzheimer's disease
    B. Huntington's disease
    C. Glioblastoma
    D. Multiple sclerosis

28. Which one of the following is not a limitation of nanoneurotherapeutics?
    A. Ethical concerns
    B. Toxicity
    C. Tissue selectivity
    D. Lung damage

29. Which one of the following is not an advantage of nanodrug delivery systems?
    A. Tissue selectivity
    B. Increased drug concentration in the brain
    C. Increased efficacy
    D. Increased deposition in vital organs

30. Production of reactive oxygen species may cause __________.
    A. Enhanced treatment outcomes
    B. Oxidative damage
    C. Tissue selectivity
    D. Reduced clearance

Answer Key

1.	C	**2.**	A	**3.**	B	**4.**	B	**5.**	D	**6.**	C
7.	C	**8.**	A	**9.**	C	**10.**	B	**11.**	A	**12.**	C
13.	B	**14.**	C	**15.**	D	**16.**	A	**17.**	D	**18.**	C
19.	B	**20.**	C	**21.**	C	**22.**	C	**23.**	B	**24.**	D
25.	A	**26.**	A	**27.**	C	**28.**	C	**29.**	D	**30.**	B

Short-Answer Questions

1. The use of prodrug is also seen in the delivery of Azidothymidine to the brain via the simple formation of the ____________ prodrug.
2. The blood is separated from the brain parenchyma by ________ that line the capillaries in the brain.
3. ____________, ____________ and ____________ barriers limit drug entry into the brain.
4. The oscillating activity of ultrasound devices that can help open up membranes and blood vasculature is known as ____________.
5. Dendrimers release drugs via degradation mechanism by which the polymers are degraded by ____________ or ____________.
6. Common mechanisms that underlie the release of drugs from different nanocarrier systems include ________, ________, ________, ____________and ______.
7. Curcumin, however beneficial, is faced with the problem of ____________ and ____________.
8. The increasing surface area of nanoparticles leads to a rise in ____________.

Answers

1. Ester
2. Endothelial cells
3. Blood-brain barrier, blood-cerebrospinal fluid barrier and arachnoid barrier

4. Cavitation
5. Enzymatic activity, hydrolysis
6. Diffusion, disintegration, dissolution, stimuli-controlled release, and chemical interaction
7. Low bioavailability, stability issues
8. Chemical reactivity

Long-Answer Questions

1. Briefly describe the role of liposomes as a nanodrug delivery system in enhancing drug delivery to the brain.
2. Explain the difference between micelles and dendrimers.
3. How does chemical modification increase drug delivery to the brain?
4. Explain the various characteristics of ideal drug candidates for brain targeting.
5. Elucidate the various advantages of nanomedicine in brain targeting as compared to conventional drug administration.

Chapter 4

Reconnoitring the Beneficial Role of Nanodrug Delivery System in Treating Cardiovascular Disorders

Ankita Sood,[a] Suman Baishnab,[a] Damanpreet K. Lang,[a] Ashok Kumar,[b] and Rakesh K. Sindhu[c]

[a]*Chitkara College of Pharmacy, Chitkara University, Punjab, India*
[b]*Department of Cardiology, Sadbhawan Hospital, Fatehabad, Haryana, India*
[c]*School of Pharmacy, Sharda University, Greater Noida, Uttar Pradesh, India*

rakeshsindhu16@gmail.com

Cardiovascular disorders inflict a consequential danger to human health and well-being and are regarded as a preeminent cause of morbidity and mortality worldwide. Numerous conventional formulations or drug delivery systems are available in the market for treating cardiovascular disorders, but they are still inadequate due to various inferior pharmaceutical and pharmacological properties exhibited by them such as decreased water solubility and biological activity, drug resistance and non-targeting actions. With the expansion of nanotechnology, nanodrug delivery systems (NDDSs) such as liposomes, metal nanomaterials and dendritic macromolecules provide a novel drug delivery mechanism for treating disorders associated with

Nanotechnology and Drug Delivery: Principles and Applications
Edited by Rakesh K. Sindhu

ISBN 978-981-4968-83-6 (Hardcover), 978-1-003-43040-7 (eBook)
www.jennystanford.com

the cardiovascular system and, hence, display significant benefits in addressing the issues. Nanoparticles and nanocarriers have garnered considerable attention in the field of cardiology because of various characteristics such as enhanced target selectivity, and sensitivity followed by both active and passive targeting towards cardiac organs and tissues. Moreover, NDDS could act as a noteworthy and promising approach for treating cardiovascular disease patients by providing effective treatment, enhanced prognosis, and fewer non-target tissue side effects. This review will highlight the particulars of the prospective alternatives to the current inadequate and conventional therapies available in the market as well as the promising future of nanotechnology in cardiovascular treatment and the challenges associated with their use.

4.1 Introduction

Cardiovascular diseases are considered to be a major public health concern worldwide, with the increased incidence of morbidity and mortality among all the other diseases. Due to such a dire situation, finding suitable medications to treat these disorders has surged to the top of the priority list [1]. There are numerous challenges faced in treating cardiovascular disorders, including, failure to identify gaps in diagnosis and management, failure in identifying risk factors, inability to identify and meet individual needs, failure to diagnose these disorders, failure to access first-line treatment approaches and lastly inability to recognize and use advanced treatment options and supportive care [2]. Overcoming these obstacles will result in the technological innovations, novel diagnostic procedures, and the utilization of modern technologies to aid in the management and therapy of CVDs [3]. With the technological advances in the field of nanoscience and the astounding functioning of nanomaterials, nanotechnology has surfaced as a promising approach for overcoming the limitations of existing cardiovascular disease treatment [4]. Nanodrug delivery systems or NDDSs are nanomaterials with a dimension of 1–100 nm that can enhance the stability of drugs, improve water solubility, lengthen cycle periods, augment target cell or tissue absorption rates, and restrict enzyme degradation, hence enhancing medicine safety and effectiveness [5]. NDDSs are available in various formulations and can be delivered through a variety of routes including inhalation, oral route, and parenteral route such as intravenous injection, all of which have an enhanced bioavailability [6]. Prolonged circulating nanoparticles in the blood can increase drug retention in the bloodstream, resulting in higher nanoparticle extravasation from arteries and drug accumulation in other compromised organs possessing leaky microvasculature [7]. The targeted nanoparticles can be specifically permeated into the intended tissue after being armed with a homing device, resulting in much reduced adverse effects [8]. Because of the increased accumulation in diseased regions via passive and active targeted pathways, nanoscaled drug delivery systems can enhance pharmacokinetic and pharmacodynamic features. Nanoparticles could also be surface coated using a variety of targeted, imaging, diagnostic, and therapeutic agents due to their large surface area to volume ratio [9]. For instance, various homing elements, including monoclonal antibodies and their components such as Fv, scFv and Fab, peptides, aptamers, and low molecular weight molecules that recognize a tissue ligand, are bound to the nanoparticle surface chemically in targeted drug delivery approach [10].

Numerous inorganic, organic, lipidic, and polymeric materials are used in formulating NDDSs [11]. The structural and physicochemical characteristics of nanoparticles including size, shape, stability surface charge, and perturbations of the surface have been proven to affect their performances both *in vitro* and *in vivo* [12]. Moreover, enhanced surface-to-volume ratios make it easier to design multifunctional nanosystems [13]. Apparently, nanoparticle shape and surface charge can influence their penetration across blood-tissue and blood-brain barriers, cellular uptake and organ distribution [7]. Nanoparticles can be broadly classified on the basis of morphological and physiochemical characteristics as demonstrated in Fig. 4.1.

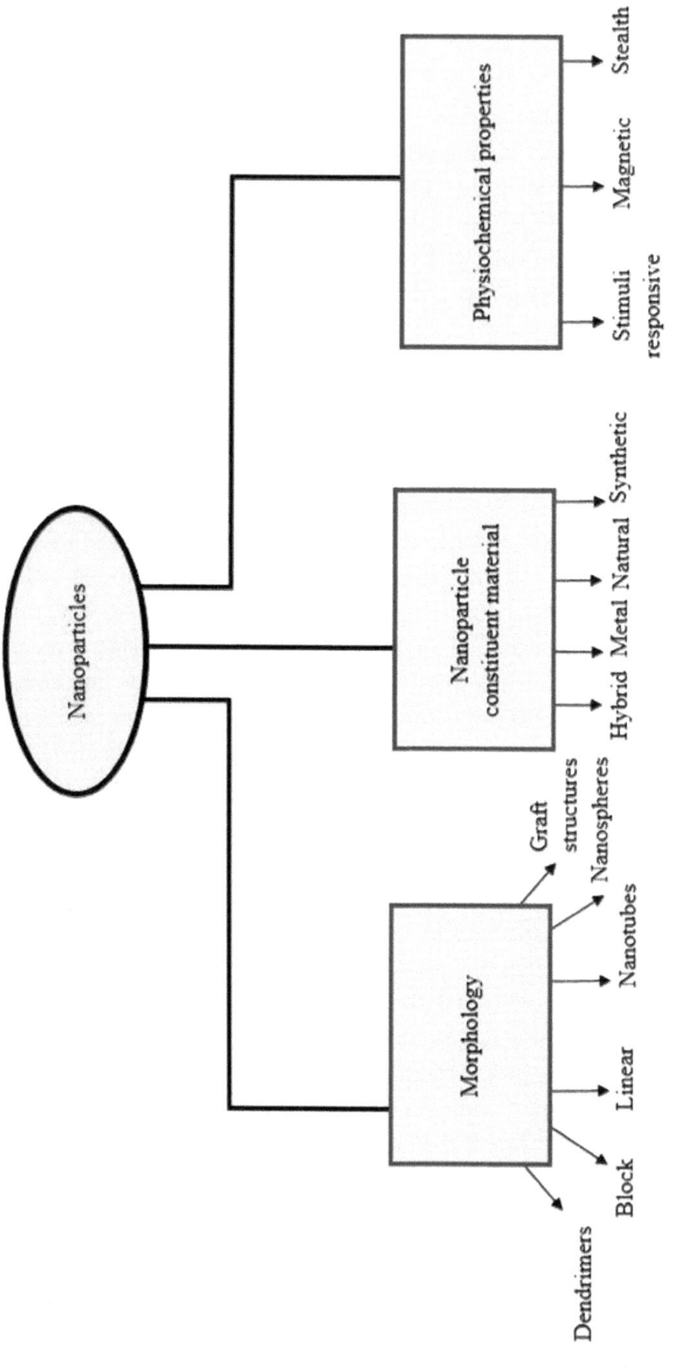

Figure 4.1 Broad classification of the nanoparticles.

4.2 Various Cardiovascular Diseases and Their Mechanisms

Atherosclerosis: Atherosclerosis, which occurs as a result of hyperlipidemia and oxidation of lipids, is considered to be the prominent cause of illness and death worldwide. It can be defined as a disease involving vascular intima that can affect any part of the vascular system, from the aorta to the coronary arteries, and is described by the formation of intimal plaques [14]. The term atherosclerosis is derived from the words of Greek origin 'gruel' or 'porridge,' referring to the lipid substance found in the center of an atherosclerotic plaque or atheroma [15]. The risk factors for the disease comprise smoking cigarettes, drinking alcohol, obesity, hypertension, sedentary lifestyle, hypercholesterolemia, family history, age and diabetes mellitus. The clinical manifestations include stroke, vascular dementia, acute coronary syndrome, aortic aneurysm, stable angina, renovascular hypertension, and acute mesenteric ischemia [16, 17]. Every year, around 610,000 individuals living in the United States succumb to cardiovascular disorders. This equates to one out of every four deaths. Coronary heart disease is regarded as the major reason for mortality in the Western world, taking away the lives of more than 370,000 people each year. Annually, over 735,000 American individuals are prone to heart attack. Notably, around 525,000 people suffer from an initial attack, whereas 210,000 individuals are prone to a recurring attack. Approximately, 75% of acute myocardial infarction cases can be attributed to plaque rupture, with the maximum likelihood of rupture occurring in men over the age of 45 years, while the risk increases in women after the age of 50 [18]. Various factors including oxidative stress, imbalance in lipid metabolism, misconducted immune response, genetic predisposition and inflammation are involved in the pathophysiology of atherosclerosis [19]. The process begins with the formation of fatty streaks due to migration of low-density lipoprotein cholesterol (LDL-c) into the vasculature wall further causing endothelial dysfunction [20]. Furthermore, LDL-c gets trapped in the arterial walls and undergoes the lipid peroxidation process to convert into oxidized LDL via the release of reactive oxygen species and the free radicals. In addition, the oxidized LDL triggers the endothelial cells to release inflammatory cytokines and chemokines and causes up-regulation of vascular cell adhesion molecule-1 (VCAM-1), intercellular adhesion molecule-1 (ICAM-1), interleukin-8 (IL-8), monocyte chemoattractant protein-1 and selectins [21]. This leads to the monocyte adhesion to endothelial cells, thereby further causing migration to subendothelial space [22]. Under the influence of macrophage-colony stimulating factor, monocytes procure the characteristics of macrophage and express numerous scavenger receptors such as CD36, CD68, A and B1, which bind Ox-LDL, anionic phospholipids and native lipoproteins [23, 24]. Moreover, the macrophages induce the release of IL-6, IL-1 β and tumor necrosis factor-α (TNF-α), which further lead to atherosclerotic lesion progression [25]. Apparently, the growth and expansion of atherosclerotic plaque is promoted by smooth muscle cell proliferation, their growth as well as migration towards tunica intima and chemoattraction of platelets towards the plaque [26]. The current treatment strategies for atherosclerosis comprise surgical procedures such as angioplasty and bypass grafting, whereas pharmacological therapy comprises statins (inhibitors of 3-hydroxy-3-methylglutaryl coenzyme A (HMG-CoA) reductase) such as pravastatin, proprotein convertase subtilisin/kexin type 9 (PCSK9) inhibitors such as alirocumab and evolocumab, immunosuppressant comprising of methotrexate and rapamycin [27].

Hypertension: Recurrently increased blood pressure in the systemic arteries is known as systemic arterial hypertension. The elevated blood pressure is the most common chronic risk factor for various cardiovascular diseases such as heart failure, myocardial infarction, coronary heart disease, stroke, chronic kidney disease, atrial fibrillation, and peripheral artery disease, and remains the foremost cause of death and mortality globally [28]. Approximately 1.28 billion individuals in the age group of 30–79 years are affected by this ailment, with the majority of them living in low and middle-income nations [29]. Poor dietary habits such as excessive salt intake, more consumption of a diet rich in saturated fats, decreased fruit and vegetable intake, lack of exercise, smoking and alcohol consumption, and obesity are etiological factors for hypertension, which are also modifiable.

Any past family history of hypertension, age above 65 years, and comorbidities including diabetes mellitus or renal problems are considered as non-modifiable risk factors [30]. A decline in renal pressure natriuresis, feedback system involving increased blood pressure and concomitant elevation in water and salt elimination are together implicated in the pathophysiology of hypertension. Moreover, pressure natriuresis can be caused by poor renal function, inappropriate hormone activation that controls the excretion of water and salt in the renin-angiotensin-aldosterone system, or excessive sympathetic nervous system stimulation [31]. The combination of cardiac output and systemic vascular resistance can be considered as defining factors for blood pressure. Patients with arterial hypertension might have an increase in cardiac output, raised systemic vascular resistance, or both. In younger patients, cardiac output is typically increased, whereas in older patients, enhanced systemic vascular resistance and sustained vasculature stiffness have a significant effect. An increased vascular tone can be caused by the activation of the α-adrenoceptor and the secretion of peptides such as angiotensin or endothelin [32]. The current treatment strategies for hypertension comprise diuretics (thiazide, loop, potassium sparing), calcium channel blockers, ACE inhibitors, Angiotensin receptor blockers, vasodilators (arteriolar or venous), β receptor and α receptor antagonists [33]. But, all of these antihypertensive medications have significant shortcomings, such as a low plasma half-life, poor bioavailability, and adverse effects such as angioedema, reflex tachycardia, upper respiratory tract abstraction, extreme hypotension. The nanoemulsions decrease blood pressure substantially, have an extended maintenance period, and could also yield approximately three times the dosage reduction when compared to the traditional dose [34].

Pulmonary Hypertension: A resting mean pulmonary arterial pressure of 25 mm Hg or higher is considered as pulmonary hypertension. The disease has a very poor prognosis and survival rate is also very less [35]. Pulmonary arterial hypertension is described by pulmonary arterial remodeling of the precapillary pulmonary arteries, as well as excessive vascular cell proliferation. Although the specific etiology is uncertain, there is growing evidence that inflammation might play a major role [36]. This disease is characterized by increased levels of pro-inflammatory cytokines and chemokines such as IL-6, IL-1β, IL-10, ICAM-1, VCAM-1 and TNF-α, which furthermore recruit various immune cells like macrophages and neutrophils [37]. The current treatment strategies focus on suppressing proliferative or vasoconstriction pathways and increasing anti-proliferative pathways to restore normal pulmonary artery pressure. The common vasodilators used for treating the condition comprise type 5 phosphodiesterase inhibitors, antagonists of Prostaglandin I and Endothelin receptor. These vasodilators possess efficacy, but only limited and with greater systemic side effects [34]. Figure 4.2 gives a pictorial representation of pulmonary hypertension classification according to the updated World Symposium on Pulmonary Hypertension.

Ischemic Heart Disease and Myocardial Infarction: Ischemic heart disease is a comprehensive term that refers to a group of closely related disorders induced by myocardial ischemia, which is defined as an unbalance amongst cardiac circulatory system perfusion, myocardial oxygen, and nutrient intake. Ischemic heart disease is the leading factor of mortality in the U.S and other developed countries, claiming the lives of seven million people every year [38]. It is indeed caused primarily by thrombotic occlusion of a high-risk coronary artery, which leads to myocardial infarction or cardiovascular mortality. There is narrowing of blood vessels supplying to the myocardium which can be due to constriction or atherosclerosis leading to death of heart muscles which is termed myocardium infarction. Continuous pain can help confirm a diagnosis of myocardial infarction, but confirmation requires QRS abnormalities on an electrocardiograph (ECG), along with ST segment T changes and a rise in blood biomarkers produced from the damaged heart [39]. (The QRS complex represents the spread of a stimulus through the ventricles.) A multidisciplinary treatment strategy incorporates all these concerns in each patient. Use of angiotensin-converting enzyme inhibition, aspirin, and efficient cholesterol reduction are three widely used approaches that have been shown to minimize mortality and morbidity in these patients. Beta-blockers have been proven to lower mortality in people who have previously experienced myocardial infarction. Other treatment strategies, including nitrates, calcium channel blockers, ranolazine, and beta-blockers have indeed been proven to improve angina, ischemia, and exercise performance [40].

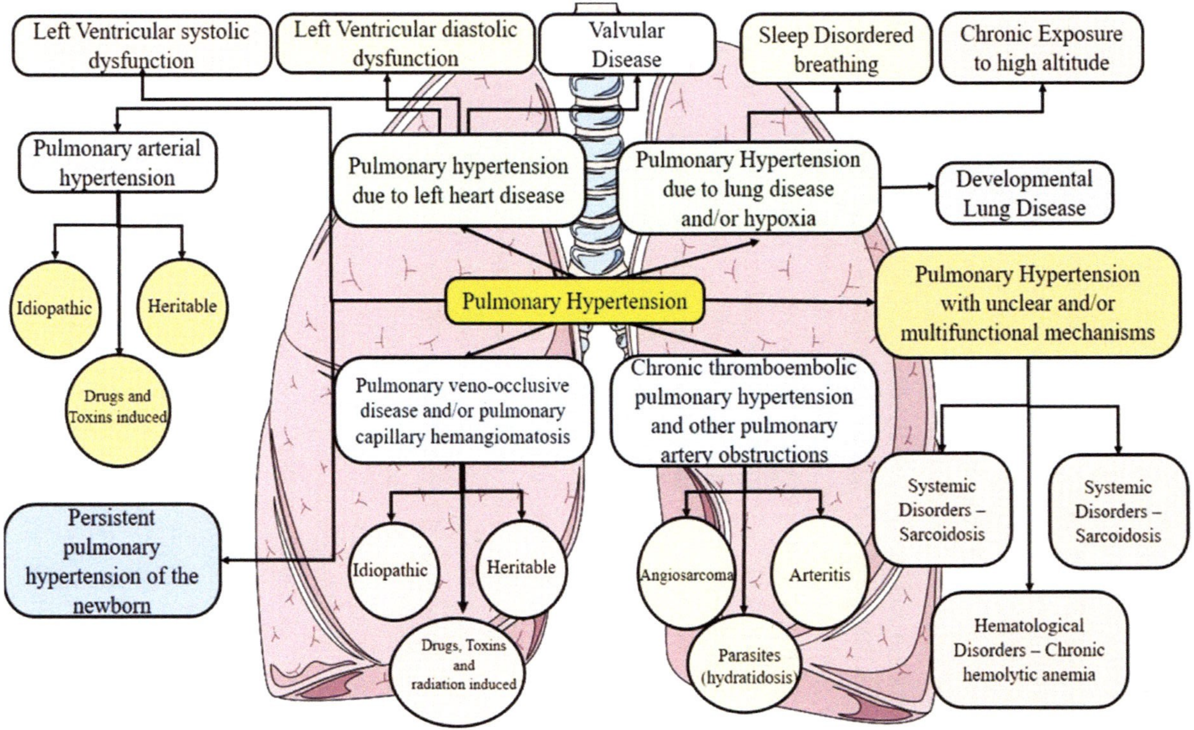

Figure 4.2 Pulmonary hypertension classification (in accordance with World Symposium on Pulmonary Hypertension).

Stroke and Thrombosis: The majority of strokes are thromboembolic in origin. If a cerebral blood artery becomes clogged, the tissues around it become hypoxic, glucose-, and hypo-perfused deficient. That section of brain tissue eventually dies. Ischemic stroke can also be caused by minor and big arterial thromboembolism with identified cardiac or vascular causes. Systemic hypoperfusion or venous thrombosis can also induce it. The brain tissue injured by hypoperfusion is not uniformly affected; however, the intensity spectrum reflects the affected subject's collateral circulation [41]. The Willis circle can be used to provide collateral flow, although it is usually just partial, and the obstruction occurs largely downstream, limiting compensating flow. As a result, the center of the infarct zone is severely hypoperfused and suffers from acute necrotic cell mortality, while the rest of the region is partially damaged and has a higher rate of apoptotic cell death. Mitochondrial adenosine triphosphate (ATP) production is impaired whenever the ischemia cascade is activated. This has various molecular and cellular implications, including inflammation or vascular changes. Cellular hypoxic ischemia finally results in membrane ion pump dysfunction, potassium ion loss, as well as increased gain of sodium, calcium, and chloride ions, and production of cytotoxic edema [42, 43]. The platelet cascade and coagulation cascade both initiate the process known as thrombogenesis. The synthesis of fibrin from its own inactive state forms fibrinogen, via thrombin cleavage is of special importance. Thrombin also stimulates glycoprotein IIb/IIIa on platelets in an indirect manner, therefore it is implicated in both cascades. Active glycoprotein IIb/IIIa subsequently binds fibrin, causing the attached platelets to release secondary messengers, including a burst of thrombin, speeding up the formation of the thrombus [44]. Furthermore, all thrombi have limited space amongst their building elements, rendering them very dense. This makes thrombi more difficult to break down and restricts therapeutic penetration, emphasizing the need for new treatment techniques [45].

4.3 Nanodrug Delivery Systems as an Emerging Therapeutic Option for Treating Cardiovascular System (CVS) Disorders

Potential Role of NDDSs in Treating Atherosclerosis: Nanoparticles can be used to treat atherosclerosis by improving drug solubility, lowering drug dosages, minimizing cytotoxicity, enhancing targeted drug delivery at particular concentrations, and combining diagnostic and therapeutic procedures to develop an effective theranostics [46]. The targets for drug therapy comprise macrophage aggregation, protease expression, enhanced platelet endothelial cell adhesion molecules and increased vascular permeability [47]. The medication could be targeted towards the plaques using a nanodrug carrier to efficiently enhance the plasma half-life of the drug, enhance the lesion concentration, and limit adverse effects [27]. The therapy techniques of these carriers include controlling lipoprotein levels, decreasing inflammation, blocking neovascularization and minimizing coagulation [48]. Matoba et al. have demonstrated using an experimental mouse model of plaque rupture that the phagocytic cells, monocytes and neutrophils in the circulation and aortas assimilated FITC-loaded poly lactic-co-glycolic acid (PLGA) nanoparticles 2 h after injection using flow cytometric analysis. In the aortic arch, FITC-NP developed in atherosclerotic lesions. Moreover, FITC-NP delivery towards monocytes was accompanied by its transmission to aortic macrophages 2–7 days post injection, implying that PLGA nanoparticles are delivered directly to blood monocytes, which then further move towards the atheromatous aorta [49]. It has been revealed that in rabbits that underwent iliac artery stenting, liposomal preparations of the bisphosphonate alendronate reduced neointimal development and thereafter inhibited circulating monocytes. In clinical testing, liposomal alendronate was proven to be safer for infusion during percutaneous coronary intervention [46]. Some reports have revealed the beneficial role of surface-modified copper sulfide nanoparticles in aiming towards transient receptor potential vanilloid-1 and preventing the accumulation of lipids in the arteries.

Hyperlipidemia is a known risk factor for causing atherosclerosis. The cytotoxic medication paclitaxel was demonstrated to accelerate atherosclerosis stagnation in a cholesterol-rich nanoemulsion and, when evaluated *in vivo*, it exhibited a 65% decrease in the volume of the atheroma with reduced toxicity [50]. It has been demonstrated that encapsulated prednisolone phosphate amid PEGylated 3,5-dipentadecyloxybenzamidine hydrochloride liposomes significantly reduced in-stent neointimal development in atherosclerotic rabbits. The addition of glycosaminoglycans (GAGs) to these liposomes caused their binding to chondroitin sulfate proteoglycans. Moreover, these findings also revealed that the synthesized liposomes have fewer systezmic adverse effects [51]. In another experimental study, VCAM-1-directed target sensitive liposomes (TSL) carrying Teijin (chemokine receptor 2 antagonist) were created to target the early inflammation process by eliminating monocyte adhesion and transmigration, which are frequently involved processes in atherosclerosis. The dioleoylphosphatidylethanolamine (DOPE) and dihydroxyphenylalanine (DOPA) mixture was used to make PEG-stabilized TSLs, and a synthesized phospholipid anchor, namely Mal-PEG-DSPE was attached to the liposome surface to pair with VCAM-1 binding peptide. Various characteristics including release patterns, size, and serum stability of the manufactured targeted liposomes were all measured. The binding affinity with the target was used to verify its functionality. TSL binding efficiency was measured using activated endothelial cells in a competitive binding assay employing flow cytometry. The results revealed significant selective binding of targeted liposomes to cell surface [52]. Table 4.1 demonstrates the various nanocarriers used as diagnostic and therapeutic agents in treating atherosclerosis.

Potential Role of NDDSs in Treating Hypertension and Pulmonary Hypertension: Nanotechnology is being used to enhance the therapeutic management of hypertension. Gold and silica nanoparticles have been produced to improve the bioavailability of nitric oxide (NO) to dysfunctional vasculature [61]. In addition, cerium dioxide nanoparticles having antioxidant capacity have been shown to reduce both antioxidant levels and microvascular impairment when evaluated *in vivo* [62].

Table 4.1 Nanoparticle-mediated drug delivery system in targeting atherosclerosis

S. No.	Type of nanocarrier	Target	Ligand being used	Role and action	Refs
1.	Liposome	Anti-ICAM1 antibody	ICAM1	Imaging (CT scan and MRI)	[53]
2.	Polymer-based nanocarriers	Peptide γ3 of human fibrinogen	ICAM1	Drug delivery to the target site	[54]
3.	Poly (dl-lactide-co-glycolide-b-ethylene glycol-b-dl-lactide-co-glycolide) (PLGA-PEG-PLGA)	cLABL Peptide	ICAM1	Targeted drug delivery (in vitro)	[55]
4.	Liposome	SAINT-O-Somes (Antibodies)	E-Selectin and VCAM1	Drug delivery	[56]
5.	Micelles	CREKA peptide	Plasma proteins (clotted)	Drug delivery to the target site	[57]
6.	Paramagnetic nanoparticles	Antagonists of Peptidomimetic vitronectin	Alpha-v beta-3 integrin	Drug delivery to the target site	[58]
7.	Nanoparticles	Poly (dl-lactide-co-glycolide-b-ethylene glycol-b-dl-lactide-co-glycolide) (PLGA-PEG-polymer)	Collagen IV	Drug delivery	[59]
8.	Dendrimeric nanoparticles	Macrophages	Mannose	Attenuation of plaque burden	[60]

Table 4.2 represents the FDA-approved antihypertensive agents used along with nanoparticles *in vivo*. Although there are no medically authorized nanoformulations for treating pulmonary hypertension, preclinical studies are underway to see if they may be used to treat the condition. The NF-κB polymeric nanoformulation is one such example. There is a build-up in the amount of NF-κB in the presence of pulmonary hypertension lesions. Targeting the NF-κB receptors using a polymeric nanoparticle-NF-κB antagonist combination forestalled the disease and increased the life expectancy of such patients [63]. Incorporation of statins such as HMG-CoA reductase inhibitors to polymeric nanoparticles has been proven to be beneficial in attenuating inflammation and decreasing lipid levels and might be useful in treating pulmonary hypertension [64]. Encapsulation of polylactide-glycolide (PLGA) nanoparticles with beraprost in a rat model revealed that beraprost nanoparticles reduced right ventricular pressure and hypertrophy after a single treatment. The rate of survival of the monocrotaline (MCT) rat model was dramatically improved by Beraprost-nanoparticles. After their administration, no inflammatory cell infiltration, bleeding, or fibrosis was identified in the heart, kidney, liver and spleen [65]. In another experimental model of rats, a single intratracheal injection of imatinib-incorporated nanoparticles prevented MCT-induced pulmonary hypertension. On human pulmonary hypertension-pulmonary artery smooth muscle cells, imatinib-incorporated nanoparticles demonstrated a long-lasting antiproliferative impact [66]. In MCT-induced pulmonary hypertensive rats, Gupta et al. found that the administration of liposomal fasudil via intratracheal route lowered mPAP and that lasted for around 3 h, implying that liposomal pharmaceutical preparations caused pulmonary selective vasodilation [67]. Strikingly, in another experimental study performed on Sugen5416/hypoxia rat models by Kanaya et al., the beneficial role of nanospheres of ONO1301 (prostacyclin agonist) was demonstrated. The treatment of ONO1301 nanospheres resulted in decreased IL-6, 1L-1β, transforming growth factor-β levels, lowered the number of proliferating cell nuclear antigen-positive smooth muscle cells, resulted in a higher right ventricle/left ventricle pressure ratio and hence ameliorated pulmonary arterial hypertension [68]. Table 4.3 describes nanocarriers experimentally tested in pulmonary hypertensive rat models.

Table 4.2 Nanoparticle-mediated drug delivery system in targeting hyper-tension

S. No.	Type of nanocarrier	Medication	Animal model	Reference
1.	Niosomes	Lacidipine	Hypertensive rats	[34]
2	Poly (D,L-lactide)	Aliskiren	Hypertensive rats (Male)	[34]
3	Polymeric nanoparticle	Ramipril, felodipine,	Male Wistar rats	[69]
4.	Liposome	Valsartan	Hypertensive rats	[34]
5	Chitosan and polyethylene glycol	Nitric oxide, nitrite	—	[34]
6.	Chitosan polymer	Captopril, valsartan amlodipine	—	[34]
7.	Solid Lipid nanoparticle	Nisoldipine, Isradipine	Male Wistar rats	[69]
8.	Nanostructured Lipid Carrier	Lacidipine	Male Wistar albino rats	[69]
9.	Nanoemulsion	Ramipril	Male Wistar albino rats	[69]
10.	Liposome encapsulation	superoxide dismutase	Rats	[70]
11.	Proliposome	Lercanidipine	Rats	[70]
12.	PLGA	Felodipine	Rats	[70]
13.	Magnetic Poly (D,L-lactide)	Aliskiren	Hypertensive rats	[70]

Table 4.3 Nanodrug delivery system in targeting pulmonary hypertension

S. No.	Type of nanocarrier	Medication	Animal model	Refs
1.	Nanostructured lipid carriers	Sildenafil	Rat (A549 cells)	[34]
2.	Liposome	Cerivastatin	Rat	[34]
3.	Polymeric nanoparticles	Nitric oxide	Hepatic stellate cells	[34]
4.	Poly (D,L-lactide-co-glycolide) nanoparticles	Sildenafil	—	[34]
5.	PLGA polymer	Pitavastatin	Monocrotaline (MCT)-induced rat model	[71]
6.	PEG-PLGA polymer	NF-kB decoy	MCT-induced rat model	[71]
7.	PLGA polymer	Imatinib	MCT-induced rat model	[71]
8.	Liposome	Fasudil	MCT-induced rat model	[71]

Potential Role of NDDSs in Treating Ischemic Heart Disease and Myocardial Infarction: In the infarcted heart, lipid nanoparticles are considered as an effective drug delivery system. This drug delivery system has been widely used for delivery of imaging diagnostic substances, proteins, peptides, and low molecular therapeutic agents. A study conducted by Paulis and co-workers considered micelles as a promising system to deliver cardioprotective drugs in the acute stage of myocardial infarction and even in infarcted heart of patients that are in chronic myocardial infarction stage [72, 73]. Liposomes, on the other hand, are better at delivering pro-angiogenic medicines to the infarcted microvessels. Dendrimers have enhanced binding capability and effective binding with antibodies and certain ligands. Nanomaterials are nano-sized vesicles that can operate as a controlled release delivery mechanism for therapeutic substances and improve myocardial restoration in ischemic heart disease. A study conducted by Xue et al. reported the reduction in infarct size and showed apoptosis of cardiomyocytes when microRNA-1 inhibitor was encapsulated inside dendrimer in an acute myocardial ischemia mouse model [74]. Another study conducted by Katsuki et al. showed that the positive impact of polymeric nanoparticles encapsulated in a statin matrix in the treatment of myocardial ischemia reperfusion injury, rupturing or destabilization of plaque and remodeling of ventricles after an acute myocardial infarction episode [64]. Copper contains antioxidant, anti-inflammatory, and cardioprotective properties. Sharma et al. administered the infarcted rat with a small dosage of copper nanoparticles and found that it reduced inflammatory cytokines and oxidative stress and induced apoptosis via pathways like phosphorylate GSK-3 kinase. Gold nanoparticles injected intravenously at a dosage of 400 μg/kg/day for 14 days may indeed ameliorate myocardial damage following myocardial infarction event in rats by decreasing endothelial nitric oxide synthase immune reactivity, Bcl-2, and collagen fibers. In the rat acute myocardial infarction model, intramyocardial administration of a nanodrug delivery system composed of graphene oxide packed with the vascular endothelial growth factor-165 gene results in a considerable reduction in infarct size reduction and augmentation capillary density [75]. Overall large percentage of *in vivo* investigations have revealed that nanoparticle approaches have a high potential for enhancing the performance and tissue repair of the infarcted heart. However, decorating these nanoparticle systems with cardioactive molecules or non-invasive physical signals can increase the recruitment and distribution of these nanoparticles, as well as their therapeutic benefits, to the target tissues. Various types of nanodrug delivery systems that have been tested in myocardial infarction are discussed in Table 4.4.

Potential Role of NDDSs in Treating Stroke and Thrombosis: To guarantee optimal patient care, stroke damage is very dynamic and complicated, necessitating accurate treatment and diagnosis using modern technologies. In this area, nanotechnology and its derivatives are showing promising outcomes. To identify macrophages inside atherosclerotic plaques, gold nanoparticles have been utilized as a contrast media in intravascular photoacoustic imaging. Intravascular photoacoustic imaging is indeed an invasive method that scans atherosclerotic tissues using ultrasonography through a catheter [83]. To avoid the negative implications of delivering large gold nanoparticles, MRI-guided targeted ultrasonography is employed using thiolated polyethylene glycol (PEG)-coated gold nanoparticles 50 nm total diameter. These gold nanoparticles have an improved kinetic profile and can pass the blood-brain barrier, as well as better solubility and stability [84]. Several liposomal systems have indeed been described for the management of ischemic stroke. Liposomal compositions for ischemic stroke have shown promising outcomes in animal testing, as seen by decreases in infarct volume and brain edema, as well as advances in behavioral outcomes. Surface modification using PEG across the lipid layer slowed opsonization and increased liposome lifespan. Stimuli-responsive liposomes were also produced, allowing therapeutic drugs for stroke to be delivered in a controlled fashion [85, 86]. When injected further into cisterna magna of rats having ischemic stroke, iron-tagged neural progenitor cells migrated to the ischemic area and stimulated angiogenesis [87]. Nanofibers have also been proven to nourish transported stem cells, allowing them to multiply and thrive, leading to glial migration and neurite sprouting [88].

A variety of theranostic nanoparticles carrying different imaging moieties and medicines have been created for the detection, mitigation, and management of thrombosis. A study conducted by Groult et al. utilized iron oxide nanoparticles for delivering anti-coagulant agent Heparin and the same system was utilized by McCarthy et al. for delivery of tissue plasminogen activator in a retrospective treatment study [89, 90]. Silica-based ceramic vehicles have now been employed in stroke medication delivery. It has been demonstrated that tissue plasminogen activator coupled to silica-coated magnetic nanoparticles accumulates at the thrombus location. Huang et al. described an activated platelet-sensitive nanocarrier effective for causing preferential thrombolysis by active targeting and regulated release of tissue plasminogen activator to blood clots [91]. Various types of nanodrug delivery systems that have been tested in thrombosis are discussed in Table 4.5.

Table 4.4 Nanoparticle-mediated drug delivery system in targeting myocardial infarction

Type of nanodrug delivery system	Loaded agent	Outcome	Refs
Graphene Oxide Gold Nanosheets	Chitosan-Graphene-Gold Scaffold	Improvement in cardiac contractility and restoration of ventricular functionality	[76]
Graphene Oxide Complex	IL-4 pDNA	Mitigation of fibrosis, attenuation of inflammation and enhancement of heart functionality	[77]
PEG-PLGA	Liraglutide	Reduction in size of the infarct, progression in angiogenesis, improvement in cardiac functionality and prevention of cardiomyocyte apoptosis	[78]
PLGA	IGF1	Reduction in size of the infarct prevents apoptosis of cardiomyocytes	[79]
Micelles	Nitroxyl radical	Reduction in size of the infarct and apoptosis of myocardium	[80]
Lipid	siRNA CRMP2	Reduction in heart failure rate after post myocardium infarction event	[81]
PLGA	Pitavastatin	Reduction in apoptosis of cardiomyocytes	[82]

Table 4.5 Nanoparticle-mediated drug delivery system in targeting thrombosis

Type of nanoparticle	Therapeutic agent	Refs
Aspirin-polymer	Aspirin	[92]
Polymersome	HBA	[93]
PFC nanodroplet	PPACK	[94]
Erythrocyte microvesicle	Tissue plasminogen activator	[95]
PLGA polymersome	rtPA	[96]
PLGA shell-coated nanodroplets	Microbubble	[97]
Carbon dot	Urokinase	[98]

4.4 Conclusion and Future Perspectives

Cardiovascular ailments and their related health comorbidity are certainly a major cause of deaths globally. Even though some of the ailments are treatable, healthcare experts continue to be concerned about coronary artery diseases due to the rapid lifestyle changes in humans. For the prevention and treatment of cardiovascular disorders, there are several cardioprotective medications accessible, and newer therapeutic strategies such as natural products and traditional Chinese medicine are gaining popularity in the medical system. These techniques and substances are favored over synthetic medications since they have fewer negative effects. However, because these drugs have not been validated by scientific investigations, they have often struggled to reach inpatient practice. The conventional treatment approaches are associated with a greater risk of adverse effects including thrombosis, abnormal immune system activation and toxicity. As a result, nanodrug delivery systems are being used as an alternate medium to deliver medications to damaged cardiac tissue in an efficient and appropriate manner. Similarly, nanoparticles offer a wide range of applications in the detection and imaging of cardiovascular disorders, allowing for quick diagnostic approaches and real-time monitoring while the treatment is going on. Numerous cardiovascular nanoformulations have been studied *in vitro* and *in vivo* in clinical studies, but their clinical adaptation is still being worked on. Furthermore, as the utility of nanomaterials expands, so does the vulnerability to nanoparticles in clinical settings. As a result, nanomaterials will have additional ways of engaging with vasculature and systemic components, which will further impose significant repercussions on the overall well-being of the human. There is limited research information on biological outcomes to evaluate the association between nanoparticle physiochemical properties such as size, shape, surface structure and cardiovascular system toxicity. As a result, more intensive research approaches are required for evaluating these harmful effects and pathways of ordinary nanomaterial exposure, so that experts can use nanomaterials in a better way to prevent, mitigate, or decrease the incidence of potential health risks.

Table 4.6 Demonstration of ongoing clinical trials for various nanoformulations and devices in treating cardiovascular disorders [99]

Identifier	Title of the study	Study details	Condition	Intervention	Phase
NCT00428662	Evaluating new Nanotechnology Based drug-eluting Stent for opening of narrowed arteries of the heart	Interventional, Non-Randomized	Coronary Stenosis	Device: drug-eluting nonpolymeric nanoporous stent	Not applicable
NCT04616872	Treating patients having atherosclerotic disease using methotrexate-associated to LDL Like nanoparticles	Interventional, Randomized	Coronary Artery Disease (CAD), Atherosclerosis, , Inflammation	Drug: Methotrexate-LDE and Placebo-LDE	Phase 2 Phase 3
NCT01270139	Plasmonic Nanophotothermal Therapy of Atherosclerosis (NANOM-FIM)	Interventional (Clinical Trial), Randomized	Stable Angina Heart Failure Atherosclerosis Multivessel CAD	Procedure: Nanoparticle, iron-bearing nanoparticles transplantation Device: Stenting	Not applicable
NCT03659864	Eicosanoids in the Cardiovascular Actions of Inhaled Nanoparticles (ECOARM)	Interventional (Clinical Trial), Randomized	Blood Biomarkers Vasodilation Blood Clotting Lung Function Healthy Volunteers	Other: diesel exhaust particulate Other: carbon nanoparticles Other: small graphene oxide Other: ultrasmall graphene oxide Other: filtered air	Not applicable

(*continued*)

Table 4.6 (*continued*)

Identifier	Title of the study	Study details	Condition	Intervention	Phase
NCT04148833	Treating Patients having Atherosclerotic Disease with Paclitaxel-associated to LDL Like Nanoparticles (PAC-MAN)	Interventional (Clinical Trial), Randomized	CAD Atherosclerosis Inflammation	Drug: LDE-Paclitaxel and LDE-Placebo	Phase 2 Phase 3
NCT02467673	Nanoparticulate Versus Micronized Steroids Delivery for Transdermal Hormone Replacement Therapy	Interventional, Randomized	Menopause	Drug: Micronized estradiol + progesterone and Nanoparticulate estradiol + progesterone	Phase 2
NCT01925027	Efficacy and Safety of Nano + Polymer-free Sirolimus-Eluting Stent: An Optical Coherent Tomography Study	Interventional (Clinical Trial)	CAD	Device: Nano+ DES	Phase 4
NCT01435031	EXPERT CTO: Evaluation of the XIENCE PRIME™ LL and XIENCE Nano™ Everolimus Eluting Coronary Stent Coronary Stents, Performance, and Technique in Chronic Total Occlusions (EXPERT CTO)	Interventional (Clinical Trial)	CAD Chronic Total Occlusion (CTO)	Device: CTO Treatment Device	Not applicable

In addition, more *in vivo* approaches and clinical trial studies are needed to fully understand the impact of nanoparticles on the human body system and cardiac cells. Prospective nanocarrier designs and improvements will necessitate further research. Various nanoformulations and nanodevices are being investigated under clinical trials for treating cardiovascular diseases such as atherosclerosis, angina and heart failure as depicted in Table 4.6.

References

1. Roth, G. A., Mensah, G. A., Johnson, C. O., Addolorato, G., Ammirati, E., Baddour, L. M., ... and GBD-NHLBI-JACC Global Burden of Cardio-vascular Diseases Writing Group. (2020). Global burden of cardiovascular diseases and risk factors, 1990–2019: update from the GBD 2019 study. *J. Am. Coll. Cardiol.*, 76(25), 2982–3021.
2. McClellan, M., Brown, N., Califf, R. M., and Warner, J. J. (2019). Call to action: urgent challenges in cardiovascular disease: a presidential advisory from the American Heart Association. *Circulation*, 139(9), e44–e54.
3. Thompson, S. C., Nedkoff, L., Katzenellenbogen, J., Hussain, M. A., and Sanfilippo, F. (2019). Challenges in managing acute cardiovascular diseases and follow up care in rural areas: a narrative review. *Int. J. Environ. Res. Public Health*, 16(24), 5126.
4. Li, T., Liang, W., Xiao, X., and Qian, Y. (2018). Nanotechnology, an alternative with promising prospects and advantages for the treatment of cardiovascular diseases. *Int. J. Nanomed.*, 13, 7349.
5. De Jong , W. H., and Borm, P. J. (2008). Drug delivery and nanoparticles: applications and hazards. *Int. J. Nanomed.*, 3(2), 133–149.
6. Gelperina, S., Kisich, K., Iseman, M. D., and Heifets, L. (2005). The potential advantages of nanoparticle drug delivery systems in chemotherapy of tuberculosis. *Am. J. Respir. Crit. Care Med.*, 172(12), 1487–1490.
7. Blanco, E., Shen, H., and Ferrari, M. (2015). Principles of nanoparticle design for overcoming biological barriers to drug delivery. *Nat. Biotechnol.*, 33(9), 941–951.
8. Shi, J., Votruba, A. R., Farokhzad, O. C., and Langer, R. (2010). Nanotechnology in drug delivery and tissue engineering: from discovery to applications. *Nano Lett.* 10(9), 3223–3230.
9. Ud Din, F., Aman, W., Ullah, I., Qureshi, O. S., Mustapha, O., Shafique, S., and Zeb, A. (2017). Effective use of nanocarriers as drug delivery

systems for the treatment of selected tumors. *Int. J. Nanomed.*, 12, 7291.

10. Puri, A., Loomis, K., Smith, B., Lee, J. H., Yavlovich, A., Heldman, E., and Blumenthal, R. (2009). Lipid-based nanoparticles as pharmaceutical drug carriers: from concepts to clinic. *Crit. Rev. Ther. Drug Carrier Syst.*, 26(6).
11. Liechty, W. B., Kryscio, D. R., Slaughter, B. V., and Peppas, N. A. (2010). Polymers for drug delivery systems. *Annu. Rev. Chem. Biomol. Eng.*, 1, 149–173.
12. Gatoo, M. A., Naseem, S., Arfat, M. Y., Mahmood Dar, A., Qasim, K., and Zubair, S. (2014). Physicochemical properties of nanomaterials: implication in associated toxic manifestations. *BioMed Res. Int.*, 2014. Article ID: 498420.
13. Khan, I., Saeed, K., and Khan, I. (2019). Nanoparticles: properties, applications and toxicities. *Arab. J. Chem.*, 12(7), 908–931.
14. Rafieian-Kopaei, M., Setorki, M., Doudi, M., Baradaran, A., and Nasri, H. (2014). Atherosclerosis: process, indicators, risk factors and new hopes. *Int. J. Prev. Med.*, 5(8), 927.
15. Li, J. J., and Fang, C. H. (2004). Atheroscleritis is a more rational term for the pathological entity currently known as atherosclerosis. *Med. Hypotheses.*, 63(1), 100–102.
16. Libby, P. (2002). Atherosclerosis: the new view. *Sci. Am.*, 286(5), 46–55.
17. Herrington, W., Lacey, B., Sherliker, P., Armitage, J., and Lewington, S. (2016). Epidemiology of atherosclerosis and the potential to reduce the global burden of atherothrombotic disease. *Circ. Res.*, 118(4), 535–546.
18. Pahwa, R., and Jialal, I. (2021). Atherosclerosis. (Updated 2021 Sep 28). In: StatPearls (Internet). Treasure Island (FL): StatPearls Publishing; 2022 Jan. Available from: https://www.ncbi.nlm.nih.gov/books/NBK507799/.
19. Alfarisi, H. A. H., Mohamed, Z. B. H., and Ibrahim, M. B. (2020). Basic pathogenic mechanisms of atherosclerosis. *Egypt. J. Basic Appl. Sci.*, 7(1), 116–125.
20. Bergheanu, S. C., Bodde, M. C., and Jukema, J. W. (2017). Pathophysiology and treatment of atherosclerosis. *Neth. Heart J.*, 25(4), 231–242.
21. Sakakura, K., Nakano, M., Otsuka, F., Ladich, E., Kolodgie, F. D., and Virmani, R. (2013). Pathophysiology of atherosclerosis plaque progression. *Heart Lung Circ.*, 22(6), 399–411.

22. Čejková, S., Králová-Lesná, I., and Poledne, R. (2016). Monocyte adhesion to the endothelium is an initial stage of atherosclerosis development. *Cor et Vasa*, 58(4), e419–e425.
23. Shaposhnik, Z., Wang, X., and Lusis, A. J. (2010). Arterial colony stimulating factor-1 influences atherosclerotic lesions by regulating monocyte migration and apoptosis (S). *J Lipid Res.*, 51(7), 1962–1970.
24. Moore, K. J., and Freeman, M. W. (2006). Scavenger receptors in atherosclerosis: beyond lipid uptake. *Arterioscler. Thromb. Vasc. Biol.*, 26(8), 1702–1711.
25. Xu, H., Jiang, J., Chen, W., Li, W., and Chen, Z. (2019). Vascular macrophages in atherosclerosis. *J. Immunol. Res.*, 2019.
26. Bennett, M. R., Sinha, S., and Owens, G. K. (2016). Vascular smooth muscle cells in atherosclerosis. *Circ. Res.*, 118(4), 692–702.
27. Nasr, S. H., and Huang, X. (2021). Nanotechnology for targeted therapy of atherosclerosis. *Front. Pharmacol.* 12.
28. Oparil, S., Acelajado, M. C., Bakris, G. L., Berlowitz, D. R., Cífková, R., Dominiczak, A. F., Grassi, G., Jordan, J., Poulter, N. R., Rodgers, A., and Whelton, P. K. (2018). Hypertension. *Nat. Rev. Dis. Primers*, 4, 18014.
29. World Health Organization. Hypertension. https://www.who.int/news-room/fact-sheets/detail/hypertension (accessed on 1 May 2022).
30. Singh, S., Shankar, R., and Singh, G. P. (2017). Prevalence and associated risk factors of hypertension: a cross-sectional study in Urban Varanasi. *Int. J. Hypertens.*, 2017, 5491838.
31. Harrison, D. G., Coffman, T. M., and Wilcox, C. S. (2021). Pathophysiology of hypertension: the mosaic theory and beyond. *Circ. Res.*, 128(7), 847–863.
32. Foëx, P., and Sear, J. W. (2004). Hypertension: pathophysiology and treatment. *Continuing Ed. Anaesth. Crit. Care Pain*, 4(3), 71–75.
33. Gupta, R., and Guptha, S. (2010). Strategies for initial management of hypertension. *Indian J. Med. Res.*, 132(5), 531–542.
34. Deng, Y., Zhang, X., Shen, H., He, Q., Wu, Z., Liao, W., and Yuan, M. (2020). Application of the nano-drug delivery system in treatment of cardiovascular diseases *Front. Bioeng. Biotechnol.*, 489.
35. Thenappan, T., Ormiston, M. L., Ryan, J. J., and Archer, S. L. (2018). Pulmonary arterial hypertension: pathogenesis and clinical management. *BMJ (Clinical research ed.)*, 360, j5492.

36. Price, L. C., Wort, S. J., Perros, F., Dorfmüller, P., Huertas, A., Montani, D., and Humbert, M. (2012). Inflammation in pulmonary arterial hypertension. *Chest*, 141(1), 210–221.

37. Groth, A., Vrugt, B., Brock, M., Speich, R., Ulrich, S., and Huber, L. C. (2014). Inflammatory cytokines in pulmonary hypertension. *Respir. Res.*, 15(1), 1–10.

38. Pu, J., Mintz, G. S., Biro, S., Lee, J. B., Sum, S. T., Madden, S. P., ... and Maehara, A. (2014). Insights into echo-attenuated plaques, echolucent plaques, and plaques with spotty calcification: novel findings from comparisons among intravascular ultrasound, near-infrared spectroscopy, and pathological histology in 2,294 human coronary artery segments. *J. Am. Col. Cardiol.*, 63(21), 2220–2233.

39. Tejtel, S. K. S., Munoz, F. M., Al-Ammouri, I., Savorgnan, F., Guggilla, R. K., Khuri-Bulos, N., ... and Engler, R. J. (2022). Myocarditis and pericarditis: case definition and guidelines for data collection, analysis, and presentation of immunization safety data. *Vaccine*, 40(10):1499–1511.

40. Manolis, A. J., Boden, W. E., Collins, P., Dechend, R., Kallistratos, M. S., Poulimenos, L. E., ... and Rosano, G. (2021). State of the art approach to managing angina and ischemia: tailoring treatment to the evidence. *Eur. J. Intern. Med.*, 92, 40–47.

41. Campbell, B. C., De Silva, D. A., Macleod, M. R., Coutts, S. B., Schwamm, L. H., Davis, S. M., and Donnan, G. A. (2019). Ischaemic stroke. *Nat. Rev. Dis. Primers*, 5(1), 1–22.

42. Rocha, M., and Jovin, T. G. (2017). Fast versus slow progressors of infarct growth in large vessel occlusion stroke: clinical and research implications. *Stroke*, 48(9), 2621–2627.

43. Fukuda, A. M., and Badaut, J. (2012). Aquaporin 4: a player in cerebral edema and neuroinflammation. *J. Neuroinflammation*, 9(1), 1–9.

44. Mackman, N., Bergmeier, W., Stouffer, G. A., and Weitz, J. I. (2020). Therapeutic strategies for thrombosis: new targets and approaches. *Nat. Rev. Drug Discov.*, 19(5), 333–352.

45. Chernysh, I. N., Nagaswami, C., Kosolapova, S., Peshkova, A. D., Cuker, A., Cines, D. B., ... and Weisel, J. W. (2020). The distinctive structure and composition of arterial and venous thrombi and pulmonary emboli. *Sci. Rep.*, 10(1), 1–12.

46. Pala, R., Anju, V. T., Dyavaiah, M., Busi, S., and Nauli, S. M. (2020). Nanoparticle-mediated drug delivery for the treatment of cardiovascular diseases. *Int. J. Nanomed.*, 15, 3741.

47. Simone, E., Ding, B. S., and Muzykantov, V. (2009). Targeted delivery of therapeutics to endothelium. *Cell Tissue Res.*, 335(1), 283–300.

48. Manners, N., Priya, V., Mehata, A. K., Rawat, M., Mohan, S., Makeen, H. A., ... and Muthu, M. S. (2022). Theranostic nanomedicines for the treatment of cardiovascular and related diseases: current strategies and future perspectives. *Pharmaceuticals*, 15(4), 441.

49. Matoba, T., Koga, J. I., Nakano, K., Egashira, K., and Tsutsui, H. (2017). Nanoparticle-mediated drug delivery system for atherosclerotic cardiovascular disease. *J. Cardiol.*, 70(3), 206–211.

50. Mohamed, N. A., Marei, I., Crovella, S., and Abou-Saleh, H. (2022). Recent developments in nanomaterials-based drug delivery and upgrading treatment of cardiovascular diseases. *Int. J. Mol. Sci.*, 23(3), 1404.

51. Joner, M., Morimoto, K., Kasukawa, H., Steigerwald, K., Merl, S., Nakazawa, G. ... and Virmani, R. (2008). Site-specific targeting of nanoparticle prednisolone reduces in-stent restenosis in a rabbit model of established atheroma. *Arterioscler. Thromb. Vasc. Biol.*, 28(11), 1960–1966.

52. Calin, M., Stan, D., Schlesinger, M., Simion, V., Deleanu, M., Constantinescu, C. A., ... and Simionescu, M. (2015). VCAM-1 directed target-sensitive liposomes carrying CCR2 antagonists bind to activated endothelium and reduce adhesion and transmigration of monocytes. *Eur. J. Pharm. Biopharm.*, 89, 18–29.

53. Danila, D., Partha, R., Elrod, D. B., Lackey, M., Casscells, S. W., and Conyers, J. L. (2009). Antibody-labeled liposomes for CT imaging of atherosclerotic plaques: *in vitro* investigation of an anti-ICAM antibody-labeled liposome containing iohexol for molecular imaging of atherosclerotic plaques via computed tomography. *Tex. Heart Inst. J.*, 36(5), 393.

54. Garnacho, C., Serrano, D., and Muro, S. (2012). A fibrinogen-derived peptide provides intercellular adhesion molecule-1-specific targeting and intraendothelial transport of polymer nanocarriers in human cell cultures and mice. *J. Pharmacol. Exp. Ther.*, 340(3), 638–647.

55. Zhang, N., Chittasupho, C., Duangrat, C., Siahaan, T. J., and Berkland, C. (2008). PLGA nanoparticle–peptide conjugate effectively targets intercellular cell-adhesion molecule-1. *Bioconjug. Chem.*, 19(1), 145–152.

56. Kowalski, P. S., Lintermans, L. L., Morselt, H. W., Leus, N. G., Ruiters, M. H., Molema, G., and Kamps, J. A. (2013). Anti-VCAM-1 and anti-E-selectin SAINT-O-Somes for selective delivery of siRNA into inflammation-activated primary endothelial cells. *Mol. Pharm.*, 10(8), 3033–3044.

57. Peters, D., Kastantin, M., Kotamraju, V. R., Karmali, P. P., Gujraty, K., Tirrell, M., and Ruoslahti, E. (2009). Targeting atherosclerosis by using modular, multifunctional micelles. *Proc. Natl. Acad. Sci.*, 106(24), 9815–9819.

58. Winter, P. M., Neubauer, A. M., Caruthers, S. D., Harris, T. D., Robertson, J. D., Williams, T. A., ... and Lanza, G. M. (2006). Endothelial αvβ3 integrin–targeted fumagillin nanoparticles inhibit angiogenesis in atherosclerosis. *Arterioscler. Thromb. Vasc. Biol.*, 26(9), 2103–2109.

59. Roată, C. E., Iacob, Ş., Morăraşu, Ş., Livadaru, C., Tudorancea, I., Luncă, S., and Dimofte, M. G. (2021). Collagen-binding nanoparticles: a scoping review of methods and outcomes. *Crystals*, 11(11), 1396.

60. He, H., Yuan, Q., Bie, J., Wallace, R. L., Yannie, P. J., Wang, J., ... and Ghosh, S. (2018). Development of mannose functionalized dendrimeric nanoparticles for targeted delivery to macrophages: use of this platform to modulate atherosclerosis. *Transl. Res.*, 193, 13–30.

61. Das, A., Mukherjee, P., Singla, S. K., Guturu, P., Frost, M. C., Mukhopadhyay, D., and Patra, C. R. (2010). Fabrication and characterization of an inorganic gold and silica nanoparticle mediated drug delivery system for nitric oxide. *Nanotechnology*, 21(30), 305102.

62. Minarchick, V. C., Stapleton, P. A., Sabolsky, E. M., and Nurkiewicz, T. R. (2015). Cerium dioxide nanoparticle exposure improves microvascular dysfunction and reduces oxidative stress in spontaneously hypertensive rats. *Front. Physiol.*, 6, 339.

63. Kimura, S., Egashira, K., Chen, L., Nakano, K., Iwata, E., Miyagawa, M. ... and Sunagawa, K. (2009). Nanoparticle-mediated delivery of nuclear factor κB decoy into lungs ameliorates monocrotaline-induced pulmonary arterial hypertension. *Hypertension*, 53(5), 877–883.

64. Katsuki, S., Matoba, T., Koga, J. I., Nakano, K., and Egashira, K. (2017). Anti-inflammatory nanomedicine for cardiovascular disease. *Front. Cardiovasc. Med.*, 4, 87.

65. Ishihara, T., Hayashi, E., Yamamoto, S., Kobayashi, C., Tamura, Y., Sawazaki, R., and Mizushima, T. (2015). Encapsulation of beraprost sodium in nanoparticles: analysis of sustained release properties,

targeting abilities and pharmacological activities in animal models of pulmonary arterial hypertension. *J. Control. Release,* 197, 97–104.

66. Akagi, S., Nakamura, K., Miura, D., Saito, Y., Matsubara, H., Ogawa, A., and Ito, H. (2015). Delivery of imatinib-incorporated nanoparticles into lungs suppresses the development of monocrotaline-induced pulmonary arterial hypertension. *Int. Heart J.*, 56(3):354–359.
67. Gupta, V., Gupta, N., Shaik, I. H., Mehvar, R., McMurtry, I. F., Oka, M., and Ahsan, F. (2013). Liposomal fasudil, a rho-kinase inhibitor, for prolonged pulmonary preferential vasodilation in pulmonary arterial hypertension. *J. Control. Release,* 167(2), 189–199.
68. Kanaya, T., Miyagawa, S., Kawamura, T., Sakai, Y., Masada, K., Nawa, N. ... and Sawa, Y. (2021). Innovative therapeutic strategy using prostaglandin I2 agonist (ONO1301) combined with nano drug delivery system for pulmonary arterial hypertension. *Sci. Rep.*, 11(1), 1–11.
69. Alam, T., Khan, S., Gaba, B., Haider, M. F., Baboota, S., and Ali, J. (2017). Nanocarriers as treatment modalities for hypertension. *Drug Deliv.*, 24(1), 358–369.
70. Fancher, I. S., Rubinstein, I., and Levitan, I. (2019). Potential strategies to reduce blood pressure in treatment-resistant hypertension using food and drug administration–approved nanodrug delivery platforms. *Hypertension*, 73(2), 250–257.
71. Nakamura, K., Matsubara, H., Akagi, S., Sarashina, T., Ejiri, K., Kawakita, N., Yoshida, M., Miyoshi, T., Watanabe, A., Nishii, N., and Ito, H. (2017). Nanoparticle-mediated drug delivery system for pulmonary arterial hypertension. *J. Clin. Med.*, 6(5), 48.
72. Cheraghi, M., Negahdari, B., Daraee, H., and Eatemadi, A. (2017). Heart targeted nanoliposomal/nanoparticles drug delivery: an updated review. *Biomed. Pharmacoth.*, 86, 316–323.
73. Paulis, L. E., Geelen, T., Kuhlmann, M. T., Coolen, B. F., Schäfers, M., Nicolay, K., and Strijkers, G. J. (2012). Distribution of lipid-based nanoparticles to infarcted myocardium with potential application for MRI-monitored drug delivery. *J. Controlled Release,* 162(2), 276–285.
74. Xue, X., Shi, X., Dong, H., You, S., Cao, H., Wang, K., ... and Li, Y. (2018). Delivery of microRNA-1 inhibitor by dendrimer-based nanovector: an early targeting therapy for myocardial infarction in mice. *Nanomed. Nanotechnol. Biol. Med.*, 14(2), 619–631.

75. Paul, A., Hasan, A., Kindi, H. A., Gaharwar, A. K., Rao, V. T., Nikkhah, M., Shin, S. R., Krafft, D., Dokmeci, M. R., Shum-Tim, D., Khademhosseini, A. (2014). Injectable graphene oxide/hydrogel-based angiogenic gene delivery system for vasculogenesis and cardiac repair. *ACS Nano*, 8(8), 8050–62.

76. Saravanan, S., Sareen, N., Abu-El-Rub, E., Ashour, H., Sequiera, G. L., Ammar, H. I., ... and Dhingra, S. (2018). Graphene oxide-gold nanosheets containing chitosan scaffold improves ventricular contractility and function after implantation into infarcted heart. *Sci. Rep.*, 8(1), 1–13.

77. Han, J., Kim, Y. S., Lim, M. Y., Kim, H. Y., Kong, S., Kang, M., ... and Kim, B. S. (2018). Dual roles of graphene oxide to attenuate inflammation and elicit timely polarization of macrophage phenotypes for cardiac repair. *ACS Nano*, 12(2), 1959–1977.

78. Qi, Q., Lu, L., Li, H., Yuan, Z., Chen, G., Lin, M., ... and Zhao, Q. (2017). Spatiotemporal delivery of nanoformulated liraglutide for cardiac regeneration after myocardial infarction. *Int. J. Nanomed.*, 12, 4835.

79. Herrán, E., Pérez-González, R., Igartua, M., Pedraz, J. L., Carro, E., and Hernández, R. M. (2013). VEGF-releasing biodegradable nanospheres administered by craniotomy: a novel therapeutic approach in the APP/Ps1 mouse model of Alzheimer's disease. *J. Controlled Release*, 170(1), 111–119.

80. Asanuma, H., Sanada, S., Yoshitomi, T., Sasaki, H., Takahama, H., Ihara, M., ... and Kitakaze, M. (2017). Novel synthesized radical-containing nanoparticles limit infarct size following ischemia and reperfusion in canine hearts. *Cardiovas. Drugs Ther.*, 31(5), 501–510.

81. Zhou, J., Yang, X., Liu, W., Wang, C., Shen, Y., Zhang, F., ... and Wang, C. (2018). Injectable OPF/graphene oxide hydrogels provide mechanical support and enhance cell electrical signaling after implantation into myocardial infarct. *Theranostics*, 8(12), 3317.

82. Mao, Y., Koga, J. I., Tokutome, M., Matoba, T., Ikeda, G., Nakano, K., and Egashira, K. (2017). Nanoparticle-mediated delivery of pitavastatin to monocytes/macrophages inhibits left ventricular remodeling after acute myocardial infarction by inhibiting monocyte-mediated inflammation. *Int. Heart J.*, 58(4), 615–623.

83. Etame, A. B., Diaz, R. J., O'Reilly, M. A., Smith, C. A., Mainprize, T. G., Hynynen, K., and Rutka, J. T. (2012). Enhanced delivery of gold nanoparticles with therapeutic potential into the brain using MRI-guided focused ultrasound. *Nanomed. Nanotechnol. Biol. Med.*, 8(7), 1133–1142.

84. Xi, G., Keep, R. F., and Hoff, J. T. (2006). Mechanisms of brain injury after intracerebral haemorrhage. *Lancet Neurol.*, 5(1), 53–63.

85. Kang, X., Chen, H., Li, S., Jie, L., Hu, J., Wang, X., ... and Du, Y. (2018). Magnesium lithospermate B loaded PEGylated solid lipid nanoparticles for improved oral bioavailability. *Colloids Surf. B Biointerfaces*, 161, 597–605.

86. Zarhri, Z., Houmad, M., Ziat, Y., El Rhazouani, O., Slassi, A., Benyoussef, A., and El Kenz, A. (2016). Ab initio study of magnetism behavior in TiO_2 semiconductor with structural defects. *J. Magn. Magn. Mater.*, 406, 212–216.

87. Sarmah, D., Saraf, J., Kaur, H., Pravalika, K., Tekade, R. K., Borah, A., ... and Bhattacharya, P. (2017). Stroke management: an emerging role of nanotechnology. *Micromachines*, 8(9), 262.

88. Mahairaki, V., Lim, S. H., Christopherson, G. T., Xu, L., Nasonkin, I., Yu, C., ... and Koliatsos, V. E. (2011). Nanofiber matrices promote the neuronal differentiation of human embryonic stem cell-derived neural precursors *in vitro*. *Tissue Eng. Part A*, 17(5–6), 855–863.

89. Groult, H., Poupard, N., Herranz, F., Conforto, E., Bridiau, N., Sannier, F., ... and Maugard, T. (2017). Family of bioactive heparin-coated iron oxide nanoparticles with positive contrast in magnetic resonance imaging for specific biomedical applications. *Biomacromolecules*, 18(10), 3156–3167.

90. McCarthy, J. R., Sazonova, I. Y., Erdem, S. S., Hara, T., Thompson, B. D., Patel, P., ... and Jaffer, F. A. (2012). Multifunctional nanoagent for thrombus-targeted fibrinolytic therapy. *Nanomedicine*, 7(7), 1017–1028.

91. Huang, Y., Yu, L., Ren, J., Gu, B., Longstaff, C., Hughes, A. D., ... and Chen, R. (2019). An activated-platelet-sensitive nanocarrier enables targeted delivery of tissue plasminogen activator for effective thrombolytic therapy. *J. Controlled Release*, 300, 1–12.

92. Lee, J., Jeong, L., Jung, E., Ko, C., Seon, S., Noh, J., and Lee, D. (2019). Thrombus targeting aspirin particles for near infrared imaging and on-demand therapy of thrombotic vascular diseases. *J. Controlled Release*, 304, 164–172.

93. Kang, C., Gwon, S., Song, C., Kang, P. M., Park, S. C., Jeon, J., ... and Lee, D. (2017). Fibrin-targeted and H_2O_2-responsive nanoparticles as a theranostics for thrombosed vessels. *ACS Nano*, 11(6), 6194–6203.

94. Myerson, J., He, L., Lanza, G., Tollefsen, D., and Wickline, S. (2011). Thrombin-inhibiting perfluorocarbon nanoparticles provide a novel

strategy for the treatment and magnetic resonance imaging of acute thrombosis. *J. Thromb. Haemostasis*, 9(7), 1292–1300.

95. Vankayala, R., Corber, S. R., Mac, J. T., Rao, M. P., Shafie, M., and Anvari, B. (2018). Erythrocyte-derived nanoparticles as a theranostic agent for near-infrared fluorescence imaging and thrombolysis of blood clots. *Macromol. Biosci.*, 18(4), 1700379.

96. Zhou, J., Guo, D., Zhang, Y., Wu, W., Ran, H., and Wang, Z. (2014). Construction and evaluation of Fe_3O_4-based PLGA nanoparticles carrying rtPA used in the detection of thrombosis and in targeted thrombolysis. *ACS Appl. Mater. Interfaces*, 6(8), 5566–5576.

97. Xu, J., Zhou, J., Zhong, Y., Zhang, Y., Liu, J., Chen, Y., ... and Guo, D. (2017). Phase transition nanoparticles as multimodality contrast agents for the detection of thrombi and for targeting thrombolysis: *in vitro* and *in vivo* experiments. *ACS Appl. Mater. Interfaces*, 9(49), 42525–42535.

98. Niu, Y., Tan, H., Li, X., Zhao, L., Xie, Z., Zhang, Y., ... and Qu, X. (2020). Protein–carbon dot nanohybrid-based early blood–brain barrier damage theranostics. *ACS Appl. Mater. Interfaces*, 12(3), 3445–3452.

99. Clinicaltrials.gov https://www.clinicaltrials.gov/ (accessed on 1 May 2022).

Chapter 5

Smart Targeted Novel Nanocarriers-Based Treatment of Arthritis

Rakesh K. Sindhu,[a] Shuchi Goyal,[b] Divya Thirumal,[b] Kailash Rani,[b] Ashok Kumar Gupta,[a] M. Arockia Babu,[c] and Sandeep Kumar[d]

[a]*School of Pharmacy, Sharda University, Greater Noida, Gautam Buddha Nagar, Uttar Pradesh, India*
[b]*Chitkara College of Pharmacy, Chitkara University, Punjab, India*
[c]*Institute of Pharmaceutical Sciences, GLA University, Mathura 281406, Uttar Pradesh, India*
[d]*Department of Regulatory Affairs, National Institute of Pharmaceutical Education and Research, Hyderabad, Balanagar, Hyderabad, Telangana, India*

rakeshsindhu16@gmail.com

An acute or persistent joint infection is known as arthritis, and it may cause a huge variety of symptoms, along with pain, stiffness, a decrease in the variety of motion, and joint abnormalities. The kinds of arthritis, i.e., rheumatoid arthritis (RA) and osteoarthritis had been mentioned in this article. In RA patients, infection was caused by means of pro-inflammatory cytokines like IL-1, IL-6, IL-8, and IL-10. Nonsteroidal anti-inflammatory medications (NSAIDs), corticosteroids, disease-modifying antirheumatic drugs (DMARDs), and a few biological agents are the most popular RA remedies. However, not one of the remedies available is capable

Nanotechnology and Drug Delivery: Principles and Applications
Edited by Rakesh K. Sindhu

ISBN 978-981-4968-83-6 (Hardcover), 978-1-003-43040-7 (eBook)
www.jennystanford.com

of attaining the final purpose for treating, i.e., drug-free remission. Microemulsions, microspheres, micelles, liposomes, microballoons, co-crystals, nanoemulsions, dendrimers, microsponges, and different strategies had been employed for intrasynovial medicine administration. Because of their size and chemical composition, liposomes have been demonstrated to be specifically effective for maintaining the drugs in the synovial cavity. In contrast to present drugs, novel nanotherapeutic strategies have proven greater selective targeting, extended half-life, subtle bioavailability, and decreased systemic toxicity with the use of nanomaterials and sensible nanomedicines.

5.1 Introduction to Arthritis

The term "disease of joints" in Greek is the origin of the word "arthritis." Arthritis is defined as an acute or chronic inflammation of joints which is often accompanied by pain and structural damage. Numerous symptoms such as pain, stiffness, reduced movement, and joint abnormalities can be attributed to arthritis. The kind of arthritis can be identified through history and physical examination. Apart from this, laboratory and imaging tests may also be necessary to confirm the diagnosis. More than 100 different forms of arthritis have been identified among which osteoarthritis is the most prevalent. Osteoarthritis is a non-inflammatory type of arthritis. There are numerous circumstances which can lead to the development of inflammatory arthritis. These may be caused through autoimmune processes (psoriatic arthritis, RA, ankylosing spondylitis, etc.), inflammation caused by crystal deposition (gout, alkaline calcium phosphate disease, pseudogout). Other autoimmune connective tissue diseases such as Sjoergen's syndrome, myositis, and celiac disease may also be associated with inflammatory arthritis [1].

Depending on the kind of arthritis, many causes can be identified. The main contributing causes of osteoarthritis are advanced aging, joint damage, female sex and obesity. A few genetic variables have been identified, including mutations in genes that produce collagen types II, IV, V and VI [2]. On the other hand, RA is an inflammatory autoimmune disease. Smoking and other environmental variables interact to cause the immune system's activation and dysfunction, which in turn causes inflammation in RA [3–4].

On imaging, more than one third of the population in America has arthritis, and this percentage will inevitably rise as the average population age rises. 19–30% of adults of osteoarthritis, 27% of adults are suffering from hip osteoarthritis [5–7]. One percent of Caucasians have RA, with females (lifetime risk of 3.6%) more typically affected than males (lifetime risk of 1.7%). The condition often manifests in early adulthood, with the prevalence of disease up to 5% in women over 65 years of age [8].

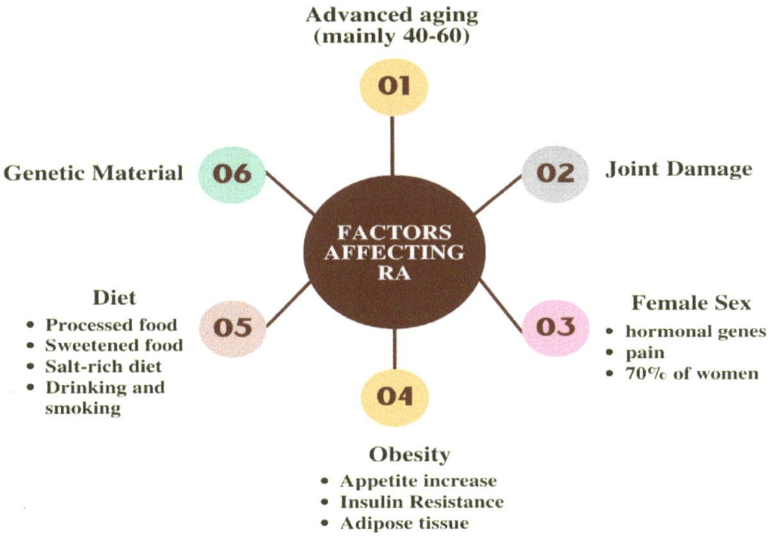

Figure 5.1 Various factors affecting RA.

A degenerative cascade of gradual cartilage loss results in bone deterioration is the hallmark of osteoarthritis. Subchondral cysts, osteophytes and the thickening of the subchondral plate are the necessary characteristic features. Joint collagen is degraded as a result of the induction of proteolytic enzymes like matrix metallo-proteinases, serine proteases and cysteine proteinases by IL-6, interferon-induced protein 10, monokines and macrophages chemotactic protein [9]. The thickness of the cartilaginous matrix is decreased and subsequently destroyed by the calcification of the articular cartilage around it. Additionally, when chondrocyte function declines with age, osteoarthritic degeneration susceptibility increases. RA often has more severe symptoms than that of osteoarthritis. An autoimmune reaction to an environmental stimulus results in the systemic and persistent inflammatory condition known as RA. Endothelial cell activation and synoviocyte hyperplasia precede cartilage and, ultimately, bone destruction. Following the abnormal generation of inflammatory mediators, the disease develops [10]. Various factors affecting RA as shown in Fig. 5.1.

5.2 Nanotechnology for RA Therapy

Nanotechnology deals with the exploitation of nuclear-level issues to produce newer novel nanomaterials, which has increased in recent years, due to its capacity to manufacture sophisticated nanomaterials, items, and procedures chosen at the nanoscale. Because of nanotechnology's ability to create complex nanoscale materials, products, and processes, there has been an interest in using concerns at the nuclear level to create new nanomaterials that have seen growth in recent years [11–12]. This technique has progressively expanded the potential uses of nanoparticles in cosmetics during the past few years. In order to improve their solubility and change their physical characteristics, liposomal technologies have been used. These technologies have produced hydrophilic vesicles with phosphatidylcholine membranes [13].

(a) Nanotechnology-based gene therapy: Synovial cytokines are important in the pathophysiology of RA, and they also serve as the basis for the current RA treatment approaches, which include monoclonal antibodies against IL-6 and IL-1β because of their damaging effects on articular cartilage and bone. Despite their success, there are still a number of restrictions on how these biologics can be used [14–15]. A promising therapeutic strategy for many human diseases is gene therapy, in which nucleic acids are introduced into cells to silence, suppress, or abrogate the aberrant expression of proteins. In RA, gene therapy shows promise for a local, joint-specific, targeted approach to suppress pro-inflammatory cytokine expression or overexpress pro-inflammatory cytokines. Arthritis medications provide long-lasting anti-inflammatory benefits while avoiding systemic side effects.

A constantly expanding field includes the exploration for the appropriate non-viral, nanotechnology-based vectors for gene therapy that have many benefits such as low immunogenicity, infection threat and no insertional mutagenesis. Numerous of these nanotechnological methods have already received in-depth reviews elsewhere [16–19]. As per different studies conducted in pre-clinical animal models, non-viral delivery techniques for gene therapy appears to be promising. The difficulty though, will be managing the possibility of off-target side effects while overcoming the silencing effect's transient nature.

(b) Nanotechnology-based antiangiogenic approaches: Angiogenesis is the formation of new blood vessels from pre-existing vessels. It is one of the initial histological signs of RA and is typically observed in inflammatory regions. Angiogenic blood vessels help leukocytes be recruited to the region of inflammation and provide nourishment for the RA synovium [20]. The synovium produces numerous important pro-angiogenic molecules, which include growth factors, cytokines, chemokines, adhesion molecules and proteases. In addition, there are a variety of endogenous antiangiogenic substances such as angiostatin, theombospordin, IL-4, endostatin, IL-3, etc. It is widely acknowledged that a new vessel development and inflammation are sustained in RA due to an imbalance between antiangiogenic and pro-angiogenic agents [21]. Many of the current RA medications have an indirect impact on angiogenesis through altering cytokines and growth factors. For example, combined treatment using MTX and GCs modifies the amount of VEGF and FGF produced by RA patients' serum and cultured cells [22]. Recent years have seen the emergence of nanosystems designed specially to prevent pro-angiogenic mediators or pathways. Recent research has demonstrated the antiangiogenic capabilities of nanogold particles. Although VEGF is a key player in angiogenesis and its suppression is a topic of active research for the treatment of cancer, direct targeting of this pathway from a nanotechnology perspective has not yet been fully developed for treating RA. Integrin $\alpha v\beta 3$ deserves special attention among the other particular mediators under investigation for antiangiogenic therapy. In animal models, it has been demonstrated that inhibiting αvβ3 integrin reduces synovial angiogenesis have shown promise in the treatment of inflammatory arthritis. These systems deserve further study to fully assess their efficacy and toxicities *in vivo*. Additionally, brand new antiangiogenic targets as HIF-α are still being discovered and should be taken into account. It needs to be seen if antiangiogenic therapy focused on a single factor or pathway will have a long-lasting effect or whether it will need to be coupled with other medications for maintaining efficacy [23].

5.3 Solid Lipid Nanoparticles for RA Treatment

Solid lipid nanoparticles (SLNs), which integrate the uses of polymeric nanoparticles and o/w emulsions, are colloidal carriers that have particle sizes between 120 and 200 nm, which can be often used for controlled drug transport [24, 25]. The outstanding properties of SLNs consist of their excessive drug loading capacity, proper tolerability, safety of integrated energetic compounds from chemical degradation, better bioavailability by the incorporation of both lipophilic and hydrophilic drugs and relative protection for organic applications [26]. Due to their distinct size range, SLNs are hardly ever cleared from the stream through the reticuloendothelial device. SLNs generally comprise physiological lipids along with phospholipids, fatty acids, mono, di and triglycerides. SLNs may be made with the use of numerous processes, which include excessive shear homogenization, excessive pressure homogenization, bloodless homogenization, ultrasound, warm homogenization and evaporation methods. Greater attention has been positioned on lipid-based formulations in latest years so as to increase the oral bioavailability of drug treatments which might be poorly water-soluble using SLNs [27]. Because of its superior physical stability, ease of scale-up, reasonably priced and production, the drug service combines the benefits of polymeric nanoparticles, fats emulsions and liposomes [28]. Arora et al. created curcumin-loaded stable lipid nanoparticles (C-SLNs) to deal with irritation through overcoming curcumin's low bioavailability problems [29]. They confirmed that SLNs have been the premiere drug transport device for drug encapsulation and controlled release. By decreasing the discharge of inflammatory cytokines, Piroxicam-SLNs confirmed the anti-inflammatory outcomes in edematous sites.

For the remedy of RA, the significance of stable lipid nanoparticle-based formulations can also additionally provide a controlled and sustained release sample with reducing dose frequencies. These stable lipid-based nanoparticles will also be capable of increasing the bioavailability of the drugs contained inside them when used to treat RA.

5.4 Recent Advancements for RA Therapy

The effective treatment of RA has recently been attempted using siRNA, peptides and targeted nanoformulation methods.

(a) siRNA-based nanoparticulate system: RNA interference (RNAi) is defined as a cellular process that silences messenger RNA(mRNA)-based genes post transcriptionally. Small interference RNA (siRNA)-based silencing is only temporary, hence new methods have been devised and described to produce silencing that is more long-lasting. Short hairpin RNA (shRNA), is a vector-encoded technique that can be employed for long-lasting, reliable cell silencing. RNAi has a great potential for gene silencing and has gained popularity because of its high specificity, considerable impact, few side effects and ease of production. A particular gene of interest can be silenced with siRNA. When naked siRNA was administered systemically, the difficulty was that it was degraded by nucleases, which shortened the time that siRNA spent circulating in the blood. Additionally, siRNA is taken up by receptor-mediated endocytosis and escaping from the endosomal compartment, which reduces the healing efficacy of the naked siRNA. The development of products based on nanotechnology, however, has lately overcome these problems. The siRNA had been enclosed in positively charged particles in order to provide better protection. This successfully shields the siRNA from degradation of serum and off-target immunological effects. In latest years, the delivery systems based on siRNA were used to deal with RA, mainly due to the fact they will successfully reach peripherally inflamed tissues. Small interference RNA (siRNA), which has a high degree of specificity and the ability to silence genes, is a key player in the important phenomenon known as RNA interference. Komano et al. conducted a study in which they came to the conclusion that TNF-α siRNA/WS therapy lowers TNF-αmRNA levels in the joints when compared to the controlled group. The effective transport of siRNA to arthritic joints was highlighted lastly [30].

RGD functionalized siRNA-loaded poly (lactide-co-glycolide) (PLGA) nanoparticles (NPs) have been created by Scheinman et al. as a nanosystem for STAT1 siRNA transport to joint tissues of CIA mice model. After siRNA encapsulation, they found the stability and the nanoparticle properties. For the remedy of arthritis, RGD functionalized PLGA nanoparticles encapsulating STAT1-focused siRNAs can be extra efficient, probably through selectively inhibiting macrophages and dendritic cell activation [31].

Park et al. created PLGA nanoparticles that were loaded with siRNA and dexamethasone in RA therapy. Here, PLGA nanoparticles were first loaded with dexamethasone before being combined with poly(-ethyleneimine) (PEI)/siRNA. They concluded that COX-2 siRNA – complexed PLGA nanoparticles loaded with dexamethasone effectively reduced the expression of genes and protein linked to arthritic diseases [32].

For the successful remedy of arthritis, Duan et al. created core-shell NPs that had been loaded with siRNA. For delivering siRNA, they created the nanocarrier using (polyethyleneimine [PEI] superparamagnetic iron oxide nanoparticle [SPIO]), which combines an iron oxide core with a PEI shell. According to *in vitro* investigations, siRNA-loaded PEI-SPIOs confirmed no cytotoxicity, better siRNA stability, and brought about focused gene silencing. When an outside magnetic field is applied, PEI-functionalized SPIOs utilized for systemic siRNA administration in RA provide an extra healing benefit [33].

(b) Targeted nanoparticulate system: Active targeting ligands including antibodies, peptides and polysaccharides can be used to further increase drug delivery systems' therapeutic efficacy and specificity for treating a variety of illnesses. Both active and passive targeting were used. The nanoparticulate formulation has been specifically designed to target the preferentially expressed CD44 surface receptors for the treatment of RA. Growth factors, chemokines, pro-inflammatory cytokines, cell adhesion molecules and proteases are mediating factors that are crucial to the development of RA. Angiogenesis and inflammation were the factors in this plan that contributed to the development of RA. A nanoparticle made of alginate and encapsulated with plasmid DNA that codes for the anti-inflammatory cytokine IL-10 was created by Jain et al. Therefore, they found that these IL-10 plasmid DNA-loaded targeted alginate nanoparticles may effectively repolarize macrophages from M1 to M2 state, providing a novel cure for chronic inflammatory disorders [34].

Synovial joints have been described by Yang et al. It is specifically attacked in autoimmune arthritis of the articular vasculature. They used a human RA model of adjuvant-induced arthritis to profile the synovial vasculature (both ex vivo and *in vivo*) of specific phage peptide display libraries. They discovered that synthesized peptides have specificity in preventing the binding of each phage to the synovial vasculature as well as binding to the endothelial cells originating from joints. It's interesting to note that using one of these peptides to treat arthritis-prone animals effectively stopped the disease's progression. However, peptide-induced reduction of T-cell trafficking into the joints and preventing angiogenesis were used to reduce arthritis. Additionally, the peptide was different from a previously studied peptide which contained arginine-glycine-aspartic acid in terms of sequence, receptor binding selectivity and inflammation-related cell signaling. They demonstrated how peptides could be further used to distribute anti-arthritic medications only to the affected joints, increasing their effectiveness and lowering systemic toxicity [35].

(c) Peptide-based nanoparticulate system: Recently, peptides have attracted significant for use in medication delivery for a variety of treatment modalities. After being subjected to enzymatic proteolysis, bioactive peptides generated from naturally occurring sources of protein have biological effects for a variety of diseases. The majority of peptides have antibacterial, anti-inflammatory, antioxidant, anti-cancer, antidiabetic and antihypertensive effects. Peptides had limited bioavailability, metabolic liability, gastrointestinal tract breakdown, minimal absorption, and an inability of crossing the epithelial barriers. Protein engineering, solid-phase peptide synthesis, and ring-opening polymerization were used to insert the peptides into the nanostructures. Dipeptides, amphiphilic peptides, α-helical peptides, cyclic peptides, and β-sheet peptides have all been employed as nanoparticulate self-assemblies. Peptide-based delivery systems, including those derived from synthetic and natural peptides, have recently been employed to treat RA.

According to Zhou et al., a cationic amphipathic peptide generated from Mellitin combined with siRNA works as an efficient targeting agent for the NF-KB p65 subunit (p5RHH-p65). According to their findings, self-constructed p5RHH-p65 siRNA nanocomplexes serve as a safe delivery vehicle for siRNA that is meant to target and modulate inflammatory processes in the treatment of a variety of illnesses [36].

Shen et al. created an immunomodulatory peptide which targeted the T-cell receptor (TCR), which is crucial in immunological disorders like autoimmune arthritis. They employed the SCHOOL (signaling chain honi oligomerization) strategy and the SARS-CoV fusion peptide sequence to target TCR. They discovered that peptide prevents bone and cartilage degradation and alleviates collagen-induced arthritis in DBA/1J mice [37].

Rush et al. created cell-penetrating anti-inflammatory peptide (KAFAK)-encapsulated degradable and non-degradable poly (NIPAm-AMPS) nanoparticles loaded with KAFAK that might become useful in the treatment of osteoarthritis [38]. The triad associating various advancements for RA therapy is depicted in Fig. 5.2.

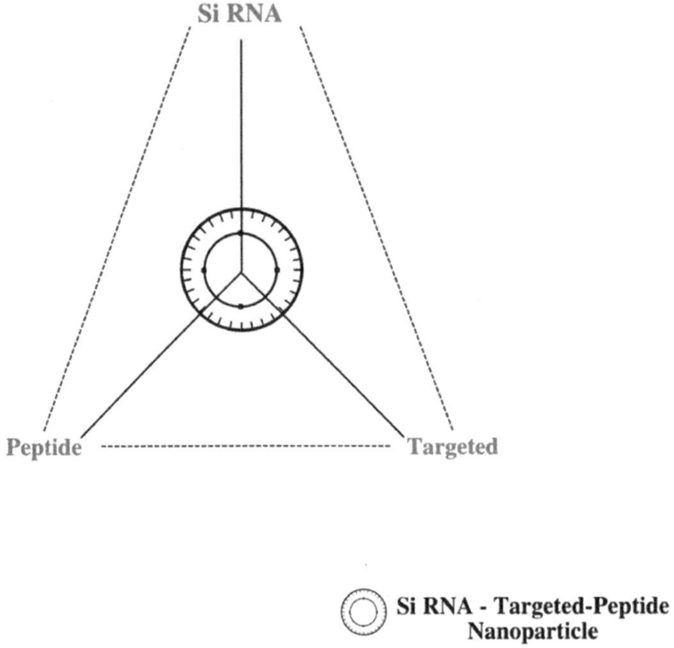

Figure 5.2 The triad associating various advancements for RA therapy.

5.5 Nanotechnology for OA Therapy

Sunscreens, cosmetics, textiles and sports equipment are a few examples of many areas of our daily lives where nanotechnology has proven to be extremely useful. Nanotechnology is also applied in biomedicine, and some of these applications have reached the clinical stage. Drug delivery of therapeutics for OA is more advantageous by nanotechnology in four specific ways:

1. Enhancing drug solubility and stability
2. Improving the targeting and effective delivery of drug
3. Increasing efficacy of drug and minimizing its adverse reactions
4. Reducing medication dispersion and degradation in bodily fluids and increasing drug circulation and retention duration [39–41]

New concepts and techniques for treating OA have emerged as a result of the rapid development of nanotechnology in medication delivery systems in recent years.

(a) Liposomes

A phospholipid bilayer surrounds an aqueous core spherical vesicle called a liposome. The FDA's first licensed nano drug carrier, liposomes are regarded as the most optimal drug delivery mechanism [42]. Liposomal compositions have been used in clinical practice in a variety of ways. Similarly, in Germany, Lipotalon (dexamethasone palmitate) is used therapeutically for treating OA via intra-articular (IA) administration [43].

For the preservation of cartilage homeostasis, adenosine plays a crucial autocrine role. Adenosine has multiple receptor subtypes, including the A2A receptor [44]. Adenosine and an A2A receptor agonist were originally combined into liposomes by Corciulo et al., who subsequently used interperitoneal injections of these liposomes to stop the progression of OA in both obesity-induced OA in mice and post-traumatic OA in rats [45]. The findings imply that the A2A receptor is a useful target for the therapy of osteoarthritis.

Rapamycin is a particular inhibitor of the rapamycin's mammalian target (mTOR). A potential therapeutic target for OA is mTOR. The PI3/Akt/ mTOR signaling cascade is how rapamycin potentially accomplishes its therapeutic benefits [46]. According to a recent study by Chen et al., IA administration of liposome-encapsulated rapamycin significantly reduces inflammation in guinea pigs with spontaneous OA [47].

(b) Micelles

Micelles are amphiphilic nanoscale structures with a hydrophobic core and a hydrophilic exterior [48]. Polymeric micelles are the most popular type of micelles employed in drug delivery systems [49]. Block-copolymers with both hydrophilic and hydrophobic chains make up their structure. Polymeric micelles are more stable and have longer circulation duration than other micelles because of their low critical micelle concentration (CMC) [50]. The minimal amphiphilic concentration required for micelle production is known as the CMC. Poly (β-amine ester) (PAE) is a cationic polymer with minimal cytotoxicity. By changing the ionization and deionization transition of the tertiary amine, pH can modify the hydrophobic/hydrophilic block transition of PAE [51]. By electrostatically interacting with cartilage GAGs, the positive charges of PAE are advantageous in drug delivery with a particular target [52]. Kang et al. designed an acid-activatable curcumin polymer (ACP), by using two characteristics of PAE which was covalently integrated with curcumin. In animal models of monoiodoacetic acid (MIA)-induced OA, the therapeutic benefits of ACP micelles were examined. The outcomes demonstrated that ACP micelles dramatically reduced TNF-α and IL-1β expression, protecting the articular cartilage against OA [53]. Micelles have various advantageous features including improved solubility of highly lipophilic medicines, allowing controlled drug release and tunable chemical and physical properties. However, they have several drawbacks such as non-encapsulating hydrophilic drugs, toxicity issues and dependence on CMC which need to be overcome by modifying the micelles.

(c) PNPs

PNPs comprise biocompatible and biodegradable synthetic polymers as well as natural polymers such as alginate, albumin, chitosan, and others [54]. PNPs can assume two different structural forms: nanospheres and nanocapsules. While nanocapsules are nanostructures with a reservoir core and a polymeric membrane enclosing the medicine, nanospheres are constructed of a polymer matrix over which the drug is equally distributed [55]. PNPs are frequently employed in the field of nanomedicine because they can be made comparatively easily as compared to other NPs. PNPs often serve the following purposes for nano drug delivery:

(1) prolonging drug half-life
(2) regulating drug release

Important biological polymers called polyurethanes have urethane linkages in their main chains. These were initially utilized commercially for biomedical reasons in 1960 [56]. Fan et al. first synthesized amphiphilic polyurethane NPs with a pendant amino group, then formed a covalent bond between the polyurethane's amine group and Khan's carboxyl group to form the polyurethane-KGN conjugate. According to the treatment outcomes in osteoarthritic rat models, intra-articular injection of polyurethane-KGN NPs might preserve more cartilage matrix and prevent the onset of osteoarthritis [57]. Nanocrystal technology, such as KGN, has the ability to deliver poorly soluble medicines with sizes between 100 to 1000 nm [58]. PNPs have a number of benefits, including better stability, the integration of hydrophilic and hydrophobic pharmaceuticals and regulated drug release. However, they also have some disadvantages, such as inadequate drug loading and toxicity issues which are yet to be overcome.

(d) Inorganic NPs

The human body contains three major antioxidant enzymes: peroxidase, catalase, and superoxide dismutase (SOD) [59]. By scavenging reactive oxygen species (ROS), they mitigate the harm brought on by oxidative stress. However, the activity of these endogenous enzymes gets lost easily due to the impact of the surrounding microenvironment, which includes proteases, pH, temperature, and other factors. As a result, several studies are being conducted on the production of nanozymes. A nanozyme is an example of an NP having activity like that of natural enzymes [60]. Because of their multi-enzymatic activity, inorganic NPs like as cerium oxide (CeO_2), manganese dioxide (MnO_2), platinum (Pt), and others have piqued the interest of researchers in the field of biomedicine. SOD, catalase, and peroxidase-like activities, for example, are mimicked by CeO_2, Pt, and MnO_2 nanoparticles, whereas SOD and catalase-like activities are mimicked by SOD and MnO_2 nanoparticles.

Chloroplatinic acid and chondroitin sulfate were employed by Yin et al. to biosynthesize PtNPs that ranged in size from 3 to 5 nm. PtNPs are biocompatible with human OA chondrocytes up to an *in vitro* bioactivity investigation. The findings imply that PtNPs may be used for treating OA [61]. Inorganic NPs' main problem is their toxicity, which is a result of inadequate toxicological evaluation in the literature. Therefore, it has become necessary to strengthen toxicology research in order to provide trustworthy experimental data for treating OA.

(e) Dendrimers

Dendrimers are macromolecules that are repeatedly branched and have topological nanostructures and they resemble trees. Dendrimers are made up of three parts: core, branches, and shell. The shell provides the dendrimer's outer surface, which can be used for conjugation with cargo or specific ligands. The cargo can be carried by the hydrophobic core. The number of generations contained in the structure of a dendrimer influences its size [62]. Dendrimers' cargo payload efficiency, monodispersity, and well-defined number of surface functional groups are all advantages as a drug delivery mechanism [63, 64]. The use of dendrimers has been studied extensively in pre-clinical literature. Dendrimers can be administered by intravenous, cutaneous, oral and other routes [65] as drug carriers. However, dendrimers are no longer researched as an OA treatment. Catabolism exceeding anabolism in chondrocytes is the cause of the deterioration of OA cartilage. The anabolic growth factor insulin-like growth factor 1 (IGF-1) has anti-inflammatory properties and encourages the manufacture of cartilage matrix [66]. Geiger et al. [67] created cationic PEGylated PAMAM combined with IGF-1 for targeting OA anionic cartilage tissue. According to the *in vivo* investigation, through electrostatic interactions, PEGylated Dendrimer-IGF-1 successfully infiltrated the entire thickness of rat articular cartilage and prevented cartilage degeneration in rat models of medically induced osteoarthritis. For the development of novel drugs for OA therapy, the results of these studies were helpful. Dendrimers have a number of benefits, including the ability to increase the solubility of hydrophobic drugs, and have tunable physicochemical properties. However, they also have some drawbacks, including the inability to entrap hydrophilic drugs and cellular toxicity comparable to that of micelles. Multiple functional groups in the structure of dendrimers are one of its distinctive characteristics. Dendrimers are therefore thought of as potential drug delivery vehicles for specific drug delivery.

(f) Exosomes

Exosomes are defined as membrane-bound phospholipid bilayer vesicles which have diameters between 50 to 150 nm that develop from endosomes. Exosomes carry proteins that can move between cells, bioactive lipids and nucleic acids (mRNAs, DNAs and micro RNAs, and Inc RNA) [68]. Almost all cell types, both diseased and normal cells, have the ability to produce exosomes. They are found in body fluids such as urine, saliva, blood, breast milk, and synovial fluids *in vivo*. *In vitro*, they are found in the conditional medium of all different kinds of cells [69, 70]. MSCs may be effective as a treatment for OA, according to numerous studies. MSC-secreted secret one and exosomes are mostly blamed for the consequences. Growth factors, hormones, cytokines and other proteins are all part of the MSC secretome [71]. Exosomal miRNAs and IncRNAs have recently been revealed to be essential for anti-OA efficacy.

5.6 Functional Nanotherapeutic Strategies for OA

Even though several nanomaterial-based medicines and nanotherapeutic techniques have been researched for the treatment of OA, and multiple clinical trials on nanotherapeutic approaches are now underway. The bulk of nanomedicines in clinical trials at present are non-functional nanoscale/microscale materials loaded with out-of-date pharmaceuticals for the treatment of OA that are already commercially accessible [72–74]. Wang et al. [75] claim that they predominantly increase medication retention time while decreasing systemic diffusion.

(a) Therapeutic strategies based on stimuli-responsive NPs

The agents of stimuli-responsive NPs are only released in response to a sufficient trigger or a set of predetermined circumstances. These types of nanocarriers with specific activities can be designed with help from disease-related local microenvironments like pH, temperature and oxidative stress or external stimuli like NIR light [76]. Zhao et al. reported the light-responsive dual functional biodegradable mesoporous silica NPs to treat OA. These particles were made by supramolecular interactions b/w cyclodextrin-modified poly(2-methacryloyloxyethyl phosphorylcholine) (CD-PMPC) and nonporous silica nanoparticles that had been modified with azobenzene [77]. For the treatment of OA to have a synergistic impact, the technique combining light-responsive local medication release with lubrication augmentation is necessary [78]. The isomerization of azobenzene, which can be activated by visible light, can be used to promote drug release after the nanoparticles have transversed the dermal tissue. Additionally, ND-Hb@siRNA@PLGA-PEG (NHsPP), a photothermal-induced nitric nanogenerator in combination with siRNA, can inhibit macrophage inflammation by effective conversion of absorbed NIR light energy to enough heat for activating the production of NO [79].

(b) Therapeutic strategies based on multifunctional NPs

An innovative method for increasing the effectiveness of therapy is the multifunctionalization of nanocarriers, which involves combining various functions into a single nanovehicle. This approach can enhance biological activity, targeted efficacy, for instance. Numerous different functional combinations, including targeted and stimuli-responsive nanotherapies, have also been researched for the treatment of OA [75]. OA therapy requires the targeted reduction of activated macrophage growth and the removal of high concentrations of ROS generated with the help of macrophages [80, 81].

According to studies, ROS and reactive nitrogen species (RNS) both have a substantial role in the onset and progression of OA. Antioxidants may therefore be useful in the treatment of OA [82]. Research on several antioxidants revealed that they are only temporarily kept in the joint, like melatonin and N-acetylcystein (NAC) [83, 84] The surface quinone residues of natural melanin shield the skin from ultraviolet (UV) light. Research into the antioxidant process of synthetic melanin nanoparticles revealed that these substances may scavenge a wide range of radicals [85, 86]. Dopamine melanin (DM) nanoparticles were studied by Zhong et al. to scavenge ROS and RNS for osteoarthritic treatment [87]. Following intra-articular injection, these Dopamine melanin nanoparticles remained at the injection site and showed a potent ability to scavenge ROS and RNS with a minimal deleterious effect. On IL-1-induced chondrocytes, the DM nanoparticles had anti-inflammatory and chondroprotective properties. These nanoparticles mitigated the loss of proteoglycans and reduced the production of inflammatory cytokines when tested *in vivo* in an osteoarthritic model, which decreased cartilage deterioration. Additional mechanistic studies demonstrated that Dopamine melanin nanoparticles dramatically raised autophagy marker expression levels in IL-1-stimulated chondrocytes and promoted autophagy for chondrocyte protection, which aided in the management of OA [88].

5.7 Future Perspectives and Conclusion

Physical therapy and psychological therapy are examples of natural therapies that are now helpful in treating autoimmune inflammatory disorders like RA. Even though combinatorial medications have a higher response rate, selectivity and toxicity to healthy cells are significant issues. In addition to nanoparticulate formulations, the discovery of targeted inhibitors of pro-inflammatory cytokines using monoclonal antibodies, bioactive peptides, and the delivery techniques based on siRNA may be the focus of future RA therapeutic alternatives. A more effective approach for creating formulations that particularly target pro-inflammatory cytokines may be to focus on molecular biology and computational chemistry.

As a result of continued nanotechnological advancements and a growing understanding of the pathogenic mode of actions underlying OA, several nanoparticles have been widely researched in the treatment of OA and other disorders. The capacity of these drug delivery systems based on various nanoparticles to release drugs over an extended length of time, enhanced drug retention in joints, and higher therapeutic efficacy as a result of functional regulatory techniques are the primary advantages. These strategies can be used to reduce the therapeutic dose, as well as the administration frequency, pharmacological efficacy, and off-target toxicity. Furthermore, as a result of the fast development and ongoing nanomaterials' optimization, synthetic techniques, and relative ligands, much more widespread problems such as stability of nanocarriers, satisfactory retention time, minor side effects in tissues other than the target, and systemic biosafety may be addressed. Future nanotherapeutic treatments for OA will be more effective.

References

1. Senthelal S, Li J, Ardeshirzadeh S, et al. Arthritis. [Updated 2022 Jun 19]. In: StatPearls [Internet]. Treasure Island (FL): StatPearls Publishing. 2022 Jan.
2. Ma L, Cranney A, Holroyd-Leduc JM. Acute monoarthritis: what is the cause of my patient's painful swollen joint? *CMAJ*. 2009 Jan 06; 180(1): 59–65.
3. Reginato AM, Olsen BR. The role of structural genes in the pathogenesis of osteoarthritic disorders. *Arthritis Res*. 2002; 4(6): 337–45.
4. Siva C, Velazquez C, Mody A, Brasington R. Diagnosing acute monoarthritis in adults: a practical approach for the family physician. *Am Fam Physician*. 2003 Jul 01; 68(1): 83–90.
5. Hazes JM, Luime JJ. The epidemiology of early inflammatory arthritis. *Nat Rev Rheumatol*. 2011 Jun 14; 7(7): 381–90.
6. Hart DJ, Spector TD. The relationship of obesity, fat distribution and osteoarthritis in women in the general population: the Chingford Study. *J Rheumatol*. 1993 Feb; 20(2): 331–5.
7. Heliövaara M, Mäkelä M, Impivaara O, Knekt P, Aromaa A, Sievers K. Association of overweight, trauma and workload with coxarthrosis. A health survey of 7,217 persons. *Acta Orthop Scand*. 1993 Oct; 64(5): 513–8.
8. Crowson CS, Matteson EL, Myasoedova E, Michet CJ, Ernste FC, Warrington KJ, Davis JM, Hunder GG, Therneau TM, Gabriel SE. The lifetime risk of adult-onset rheumatoid arthritis and other inflammatory autoimmune rheumatic diseases. *Arthritis Rheum*. 2011 Mar; 63(3): 633–9.
9. Struglics A, Larsson S, Kumahashi N, Frobell R, Lohmander LS. Changes in Cytokines and Aggrecan ARGS Neoepitope in Synovial Fluid and Serum and in C-Terminal Crosslinking Telopeptide of Type II Collagen and N-Terminal Crosslinking Telopeptide of Type I Collagen in Urine Over Five Years After Anterior Cruciate Ligament Rupture: An Exploratory Analysis in the Knee Anterior Cruciate Ligament, Nonsurgical Versus Surgical Treatment Trial. *Arthritis Rheumatol*. 2015 Jul; 67(7): 1816–25.

10. De Hair MJ, van de Sande MG, Ramwadhdoebe TH, Hansson M, Landewé R, van der Leij C, Maas M, Serre G, van Schaardenburg D, Klareskog L, Gerlag DM, van Baarsen LG, Tak PP. Features of the synovium of individuals at risk of developing rheumatoid arthritis: implications for understanding preclinical rheumatoid arthritis. *Arthritis Rheumatol.* 2014 Mar; 66(3): 513–22.

11. Ahuja NK, Rajawat JS, Novel nano therapeutic materials for the effective treatment of rheumatoid arthritis-recent insights. *Int J Appl Pharm.* 2021; 13(6): 31–40.

12. Bahadar H, Maqbool F, Niaz K, Abdollahi M. Toxicity of nanoparticles and an overview of current experimental models. *Iran Biomed J.* 2016; 20(1):1–11. Doi: 10.7508/ibj.2016.01.001, PMID 26286636.

13. Panahi Y, Farshbaf M, Mohammadhosseini M, Mirahadi M, Khalilov R, Saghfi S, Akbarzadeh A. Recent advances on liposomal nanoparticles: synthesis, characterization and biomedical applications. *Artif Cells Nanomed Biotechnol.* 2017; 45(4): 788–99. doi: 10.1080/21691401.2017.1282496, PMID 28278586.

14. Pham CTN. Nanotherapeutic approaches for the treatment of rheumatoid arthritis. *Wiley Interdiscip Rev Nanomed Nanobiotechnol.* 2011; 3(6): 607–619. doi:10.1002/wnan.157.

15. Bongartz T, Sutton AJ, Sweeting MJ, Buchan I, Matteson EL, Montori V. Anti-TNF antibody therapy in rheumatoid arthritis and the risk of serious infections and malignancies: systematic review and meta-analysis of rare harmful effects in randomized controlled trials. *JAMA.* 2006; 295: 2275–2285.

16. Putnam D. Polymers for gene delivery across length scales. *Nat Mater.* 2006; 5: 439–451.

17. Lundin KE, Simonson OE, Moreno PM, Zaghloul EM, Oprea II, et al. Nanotechnology approaches for gene transfer. *Genetica.* 2009; 137: 47–56.

18. Pathak A, Patnaik S, Gupta KC. Recent trends in non-viral vector-mediated gene delivery. *Biotechnol J.* 2009; 4: 1559–1572.

19. Parveen S, Misra R, Sahoo SK. Nanoparticles: a boon to drug delivery, therapeutics, diagnostics and imaging. Nanomedicine. 2011.

20. Costa C, Incio J, Soares R. Angiogenesis and chronic inflammation: cause or consequence? *Angiogenesis.* 2007; 10: 149–166.

21. Szekanecz Z, Besenyei T, Szentpetery A, Koch AE. Angiogenesis and vasculogenesis in rheumatoid arthritis. *Curr Opin Rheumatol.* 2010; 22: 299–306.

22. Nagashima M, Wauke K, Hirano D, Ishigami S, Aono H, et al. Effects of combinations of anti-rheumatic drugs on the production of vascular endothelial growth factor and basic fibroblast growth factor in cultured synoviocytes and patients with rheumatoid arthritis. *Rheumatology (Oxford)*. 2000; 39: 1255–1262.

23. Mukherjee P, Bhattacharya R, Wang P, Wang L, Basu S, et al. Antiangiogenic properties of gold nanoparticles. *Clin Cancer Res.* 2005; 11: 3530–3534.

24. Janakiraman K, Krishnaswami V, Rajendran V, Natesan S, Kandasamy R, Novel nano therapeutic materials for the effective treatment of rheumatoid arthritis-recent insights. *Mater Today Commun.* 2018; 17: 200–213.

25. Kumar R, Singh A, Garg N, Siril PF. Solid lipid nanoparticles for the controlled delivery of poorly water soluble non-steroidal anti-inflammatory drugs. *Ultrason Sonochem.* 2018; 40(Pt A): 686–696.

26. Moritz MG, Moritz M. Solid lipid nanoparticles as attractive drug vehicles composition, properties and therapeutic strategies. *Mater Sci Eng C.* 2016; 68: 982–994.

27. Garg NK, Singh B, Tyagi RK, Sharma G, Katare OP, Effective transdermal delivery of methotrexate through nanostructured lipid carriers in an experiment tally induced arthritis model. *Colloids Surf B Biointerfaces.* 2016; 147: 17–24.

28. Chavan D, Gangode B, Jadhav A, Patil M, Kshirsagar S, Solid lipid nanoparticles: a modern formulation approach in drug delivery system. *IJOD.* 2017; 5(2): 56–70.

29. Arora R, Kuhad A, Kaur IP, Chopra K. Curcumin loaded solid lipid nanoparticles ameliorate adjuvant-induced arthritis in rats. *Eur J Pain.* 2014; 19(7): 940–952.

30. Komano Y, Yagi N, Onoue I, Kaneko K, Miyasaka N, Nanki T, Arthritic joint-targeting small interfering rna-encapsulated liposome: implication for treatment strategy for rheumatoid arthritis. *J Pharmacol Exp Ther.* 2012; 340(1): 109–113.

31. Scheinman RI, Trivedi R, Vermillion S, Kompella UB. Functionalized STAT1 siRNA nanoparticles regress rheumatoid arthritis in a mouse model. *Nanomedicine.* 2011; 6(10): 1669–1682.

32. Park JS, Yang HN, Jeon SY, Woo DG, Kim MS, Park KH. The use of anti-COX_2 siRNA coated onto PLGA nanoparticles loading dexamethasone in the treatment of rheumatoid arthritis. *Biomaterials.* 2012; 33: 8600–8612.

33. Duan J, Dong J, Zhang T, Su Z, Ding J, Zhang Y, Mao X. Polyethyleneimine-functionalized iron oxide nanoparticles for systemic siRNA delivery in experimental arthritis. *Nanomedicine.* 2014; 9(6): 789–801.

34. Jain S, Tran TH, Amiji M. Macrophage repolarization with targeted alginate Nanoparticles containing IL-10 plasmid DNA for the treatment of experimental arthritis. *Biomaterials.* 2015; 61: 162–177.

35. Yanga YH, Rajaiaha R, Ruoslahtib E, Moudgil KD, Peptides targeting inflamed synovial vasculature attenuate autoimmune arthritis. *PNAS.* 2011; 108(31): 12857–12862.

36. Zhou HF, Yan H, Pan H, Hou KK, Akk A, Springer LE, Hu Y, Allen JS, Wickline SA, Pham CTN. Peptide-siRNA nanocomplexes targeting NF-κB subunit p65 suppress nascent experimental arthritis. *J Clin Invest.* 2014; 124(10): 4363–4374.

37. Shen ZT, Sigalov AB, SARS coronavirus fusion peptide-derived sequence suppresses collagen-induced arthritis in DBA/1J Mice. *Sci. Rep.* 2016; 28(6): 28672.

38. Bartlett II RL, Sharma S, Panitch A. Cell-penetrating peptides released from thermo sensitive nanoparticles suppress pro-inflammatory cytokine response by specifically targeting inflamed cartilage explants. *Nanomed.: Nanotechnol. Biol Med.* 2013; 9: 419–427.

39. Jin G-Z, Current nanoparticle-based technologies for osteoarthritis therapy. *Nanomaterials.* 2020; 10: 2368; doi:10.3390/nano-10122368.

40. Lawson TB, Mäkelä JTA, Klein T, Snyder BD, Grinstaff MW. Nanotechnology and osteoarthritis; part 1: Clinical landscape and opportunities for advanced diagnostics. *J Orthop Res.* 2020.

41. Gu W, Wu C, Chen J, Xiao Y. Nanotechnology in the targeted drug delivery for body diseases and bone regeneration. *Int J Nanomed.* 2013; 8: 2305–2317.

42. Adler-Moore J, Proffitt RT. AmBisome: Liposomal formulation, structure, mechanism of action and pre-clinical experience. *J Antimicrob Chemother.* 2002; 49: 21–30.

43. Evans CH, Kraus VB, Setton LA. Progress in intra-articular therapy. *Nat Rev Rheumatol.* 2014; 10: 11–22.

44. Corciulo C, Lendhey M, Wilder T, Schoen H, Cornelissen AS, Chang G, Kennedy OD. Cronstein, BN. Endogenous adenosine maintains cartilage homeostasis and exogenous adenosine inhibits osteoarthritis progression. *Nat. Commun.* 2017; 8: 15019.

45. Corciulo C, Castro CM, Coughlin T, Jacob S, Li Z, Fenyö D, Rifkin DB, Kennedy OD, Cronstein, BN. Intraarticular injection of liposomal adenosine reduces cartilage damage in established murine and rat models of osteoarthritis. *Sci Rep.* 2020; 10: 13477.

46. Pal B, Endisha H, Zhang Y, Kapoor M. mTOR: a potential therapeutic target in osteoarthritis? *Drugs R D.* 2015; 15: 27–36.

47. Chen CH, Kuo SM, Tien YC, Shen PC, Kuo YW, Huang HH. Steady augmentation of anti-osteoarthritic actions of rapamycin by liposome-encapsulation in collaboration with low-intensity pulsed ultrasound. *Int J Nanomed.* 2020; 15: 3771–3790.

48. Oerlemans C, Bult W, Bos M, Storm G, Nijsen JF, Hennink WE. Polymeric micelles in anticancer therapy: Targeting, imaging and triggered release. *Pharm. Res.* 2010; 27: 2569–2589.

49. Movassaghian S, Merkel OM, Torchilin VP. Applications of polymer micelles for imaging and drug delivery. *Wiley Interdiscip Rev Nanomed Nanobiotechnol.* 2015; 7: 691–707.

50. Adams ML, Lavasanifar A, Kwon GS. Amphiphilic block copolymers for drug delivery. *J Pharm Sci.* 2003; 92: 1343–1355.

51. Koo H, Lee H, Lee S, Min KH, Kim MS, Lee DS, Choi Y, Kwon IC, Kim K, Jeong SY. *In vivo* tumor diagnosis and photodynamic therapy via tumoral pH-responsive polymeric micelles. *Chem. Commun.* 2010; 46: 5668–5670.

52. Perni S, Prokopovich P. Poly-beta-amino-esters nano-vehicles based drug delivery system for cartilage. *Nanomedicine.* 2017; 13: 539–548.

53. Kang C, Jung E, Hyeon H, Seon S, Lee D. Acid-activatable polymeric curcumin nanoparticles as therapeutic agents for osteoarthritis. *Nanomedicine.* 2020; 23: 102104.

54. Zazo H, Colino CI, Lanao JM. Current applications of nanoparticles in infectious diseases. *J Control Release.* 2016; 224: 86–102.

55. Steichen SD, Caldorera-Moore M, Peppas NA. A review of current nanoparticle and targeting moieties for the delivery of cancer therapeutics. *Eur J Pharm Sci.* 2013; 48: 416–427.

56. Guelcher SA. Biodegradable polyurethanes: Synthesis and applications in regenerative medicine. *Tissue Eng. Part B Rev.* 2008; 14: 3–17.

57. Fan W, Li J, Yuan L, Chen J, Wang Z, Wang Y, Guo C, Mo X, Yan Z. Intra-articular injection of kartogenin-conjugated polyurethane

nanoparticles attenuates the progression of osteoarthritis. *Drug Deliv.* 2018; 25: 1004–1012.

58. Mohammad IS, Hu H, Yin L, He W. Drug nanocrystals: Fabrication methods and promising therapeutic applications. *Int J Pharm.* 2019; 562: 187–202.

59. Sindhu RK, Najda A, Kaur P, Shah M, Singh H, Kaur P, Cavalu S, Jaroszuk-Sierocińska M, Rahman MH. Potentiality of nanoenzymes for cancer treatment and other diseases: current status and future challenges. *Materials.* 2021; 14: 5965. https://doi.org/10.3390/ma14205965.

60. Wu J, Wang X, Wang Q, Lou Z, Li S, Zhu Y, Qin L, Wei H. Nanomaterials with enzyme-like characteristics (nanozymes): Next-generation artificial enzymes (II). *Chem Soc Rev.* 2019; 48: 1004–1076.

61. Yin XF, Wang LL, Chu XC. A novel chondroitin sulfate decorated nano platinum for the treatment of osteoarthritis. *Mater Sci Eng C Mater Biol Appl.* 2017; 78: 452–456.

62. Abbasi E, Aval SF, Akbarzadeh A, Milani M, Nasrabadi HT, Joo SW, Hanifehpour Y, Nejati-Koshki K, Pashaei-Asl R. Dendrimers: synthesis, applications, and properties. *Nanoscale Res Lett.* 2014; 9: 247.

63. Li J, Liang H, Liu J, Wang Z. Poly (amidoamine) (PAMAM) dendrimer mediated delivery of drug and pDNA/siRNA for cancer therapy. *Int J Pharm.* 2018; 546: 215–225.

64. Abedi-Gaballu F, Dehghan G, Ghaffari M, Yekta R, Abbaspour-Ravasjani S, Baradaran B, Dolatabadi JEN, Hamblin MR. PAMAM dendrimers as efficient drug and gene delivery nanosystems for cancer therapy. *Appl Mater Today.* 2018; 12: 177–190.

65. Dave K, Krishna Venuganti VV. Dendritic polymers for dermal drug delivery. *Ther Deliv.* 2017; 8: 1077–1096.

66. Li Y, Wang Y, Chubinskaya S, Schoeberl B, Florine E, Kopesky P, Grodzinsky AJ. Effects of insulin-like growth factor-1 and dexamethasone on cytokine-challenged cartilage: Relevance to post-traumatic osteoarthritis. *Osteoarthr Cartil.* 2015; 23: 266–274.

67. Geiger BC, Wang S, Padera RF Jr, Grodzinsky AJ, Hammond PT. Cartilage-penetrating nanocarriers improve delivery and efficacy of growth factor treatment of osteoarthritis. *Sci Transl Med.* 2018; 10: eaat8800.

68. Mathieu M, Martin-Jaular L, Lavieu G, Théry C. Specificities of secretion and uptake of exosomes and other extracellular vesicles for cell-to-cell communication. *Nat Cell Biol.* 2019; 21: 9–17.

69. Théry C, Zitvogel L, Amigorena S. Exosomes: Composition, biogenesis and function. *Nat Rev Immunol.* 2002; 2: 569–579.

70. Tkach M, Théry C. Communication by extracellular vesicles: where we are and where we need to go. *Cell.* 2016; 164: 1226–1232.

71. Bousnaki M, Bakopoulou A, Kritis A, Koidis P. The efficacy of stem cells secretome application in osteoarthritis: a systematic review of *in vivo* studies. *Stem Cell Rev Rep.* 2020; 16: 1222–1241.

72. Guo X, Lou J, Wang F, Fan D, Qin Z. Recent advances in nanotherapeutic strategies for osteoarthritis. *Front Pharmacol.* 2022; 13: 924387. doi: 10.3389/fphar.2022.924387.

73. Dejulius CR, Gulati S, Hasty KA, Crofford LJ, and Duvall CL. Recent advances in clinical translation of intra-articular osteoarthritis drug delivery systems. *Adv Ther (Weinh).* 2021; 4(1): 2000088. doi:10.1002/adtp.202000088.

74. Hunter DJ, Chang CC, Wei JC, Lin HY, Brown C, Tai TT, et al. TLC599 in patients with osteoarthritis of the knee: a phase IIa, randomized, placebo-controlled, dose-finding study. *Arthritis Res Ther.* 2022; 24(1): 52. doi:10.1186/s13075-022-02739-4.

75. Wang Z, Wang S, Wang K, Wu X, Tu C, and Gao C. Stimuli-sensitive nanotherapies for the treatment of osteoarthritis. *Macromol Biosci.* 2021; 21(11): e2100280. doi:10.1002/mabi.202100280.

76. Lawson TB, Mäkelä JTA, Klein T, Snyder BD, and Grinstaff MW. Nanotechnology and osteoarthritis. Part 2: opportunities for advanced devices and therapeutics. *J Orthop Res.* 2021; 39(3): 473–484. Doi:10.1002/jor. 24842.

77. Zhao W, Wang H, Wang H, Han Y, Zheng Z, Liu X, et al. Light responsive dual-functional biodegradable mesoporous silica nanoparticles with drug delivery and lubrication enhancement for the treatment of osteoarthritis. *Nanoscale.* 2021; 13(13): 6394–6399. doi:10.1039/ d0nr08887k.

78. Moro T, Takatori Y, Ishihara K, Konno T, Takigawa Y, Matsushita T, et al. Surface grafting of artificial joints with a biocompatible polymer for preventing periprosthetic osteolysis. *Nat Mat.* 2004; 3(11): 829–836. doi:10.1038/ nmat1233.

79. Chen X, Liu Y, Wen Y, Yu Q, Liu J, Zhao Y, et al. A photothermal triggered nitric oxide nanogenerator combined with siRNA for precise therapy of osteoarthritis by suppressing macrophage inflammation. *Nanoscale.* 2019; 11(14): 6693–6709. doi:10.1039/c8nr10013f.

80. Pu HL, Chiang WL, Maiti B, Liao ZX, Ho YC, Shim MS, et al. Nanoparticles with dual responses to oxidative stress and reduced Ph for drug

release and anti-inflammatory applications. *ACS Nano*. 2014; 8(2): 1213–1221. doi:10.1021/nn4058787.

81. Yang W, Tao Y, Wu Y, Zhao X, Ye W, Zhao D, et al. Neutrophils promote the development of reparative macrophages mediated by ROS to orchestrate liver repair. *Nat Commun*. 2019; 10(1): 1076. doi:10.1038/s41467-019-09046-8.

82. Mazzetti I, Grigolo B, Pulsatelli L, Dolzani P, Silvestri T, Roseti L, et al. Differential roles of nitric oxide and oxygen radicals in chondrocytes affected by osteoarthritis and rheumatoid arthritis. *Clin Sci (Lond)*. 2001; 101(6): 593–599. doi:10.1042/cs20010030.

83. Schreck R, Rieber P, and Baeuerle PA. Reactive oxygen intermediates as apparently widely used messengers in the activation of the NF-kappa B transcription factor and HIV-1. *EMBO J*. 1991; 10(8): 2247–2258. doi:10.1002/j. 1460-2075.1991.tb07761.x.

84. Lim HD, Kim YS, Ko SH, Yoon IJ, Cho SG, Chun YH, et al. Cytoprotective and anti-inflammatory effects of melatonin in hydrogen peroxide-stimulated CHON-001 human chondrocyte cell line and rabbit model of osteoarthritis via the SIRT1 pathway. *J Pineal Res*. 2012; 53(3): 225–237. doi:10.1111/j.1600-079X.2012.00991.x.

85. Liu Y, Ai K, Liu J, Deng M, He Y, and Lu L. Dopamine-melanin colloidal nanospheres: an efficient near-infrared photothermal therapeutic agent for *in vivo* cancer therapy. *Adv Mat*. 2013; 25(9): 1353–1359. doi:10.1002/ adma.201204683.

86. Liu Y, Ai K, Ji X, Askhatova D, Du R, Lu L, et al. Comprehensive insights into the multi-antioxidative mechanisms of melanin nanoparticles and their application to protect brain from injury in ischemic stroke. *J Am Chem Soc*. 2017; 139(2): 856–862. doi:10.1021/jacs.6b11013.

87. Zhong G, Yang X, Jiang X, Kumar A, Long H, Xie J, et al. Dopamine melanin nanoparticles scavenge reactive oxygen and nitrogen species and activate autophagy for osteoarthritis therapy. *Nanoscale*. 2019; 11(24): 11605–11616. doi:10.1039/c9nr03060c.

88. Mi B, Wang J, Liu Y, Liu J, Hu L, Panayi AC, et al. Icariin activates autophagy via down-regulation of the NF-κB signaling-mediated apoptosis in chondrocytes. *Front Pharmacol*. 2018; 9: 605. doi:10.3389/fphar. 2018.00605.

Chapter 6

Novel Drug Delivery System for Ocular Target

Astha Mishra,[a] Shaima K. A.,[b] and Rakesh K. Sindhu[c]

[a]*Optometry department, Chitkara School of Health Sciences, Chitkara University, Punjab, India*
[b]*Shambhunath Institute of Pharmacy, Jhalwa, Paryagraj, Uttar Pradesh, India*
[c]*School of Pharmacy, Sharda University, Greater Noida, Uttar Pradesh, India*

rakeshsindhu16@gmail.com

Because of numerous barriers like anatomical and physiological, ocular pharmacokinetics and pharmacodynamics have been always associated with drawbacks. For example, apart from the cartilage, the cornea and crystalline lens are the only tissues in the body that do not have blood supply. This has caused ophthalmologists to experience a bottleneck. When a mild ocular disease remains untreated or becomes severe, it has the potential to impair vision to the point of blindness in various ocular diseases like – corneal ulcer, dry eyes and posterior segment diseases, etc., whereas the traditional therapies are yet to deliver absolute therapy because of a number of constraints like poor bioavailability and because of blood-retinal barrier. Nowadays modern lifestyle has increased the prevalence of some ocular diseases. That is why a major focus of pharmaceutical scientists

Nanotechnology and Drug Delivery: Principles and Applications
Edited by Rakesh K. Sindhu

ISBN 978-981-4968-83-6 (Hardcover), 978-1-003-43040-7 (eBook)
www.jennystanford.com

is on developing appropriate medication delivery methods for ocular disorders. Thanks to nanoparticles like niosomes, liposomes, micelles, dendrimers, and other polymeric vesicles, nanotechnology plays a significant role in ophthalmology and the ocular medicine delivery system. Niosomes, which are nanovesicles made of nonionic surfactants, are becoming nanocarriers in drug delivery applications due to their solution/strong stability and cost-effectiveness. So specifically, this review focuses on the importance of designing novel delivery systems like nanomedicine applications, it offers various important benefits such as prolonged medication release and targeted tissue targeting. In this book, we discussed the development of various inorganic and organic nanoparticles for ocular applications, as well as unique approaches in the new ocular drug delivery system.

6.1 Introduction

The human eye is a very complicated organ. It consists of two chambers—the anterior chamber and the posterior chamber—and two segments—the anterior segment and the posterior segment, which are highly prone to disease. If we talk about the most common anterior chamber disorders, those are dry eye, glaucoma, allergic conjunctivitis, uveitis, cataract and infections and if we talk about the most common and frequent posterior segment disorders, those are diabetic retinopathy (DR), age-related macular degeneration (ARMD), etc. Earlier the topical instillation of medications was the recommended technique of therapy for the treatment of numerous ocular illnesses, since it is straightforward, convenient and noninvasive. Because of their ease of use, traditional eye drops are the most often used topical ophthalmic dose type [1, 2]. However, because of low bioavailability and medication absorption into the ocular tissues as a consequence of turnover of tear, nasolacrimal drainage and blinking process, it is less effective in specific scenarios or treatments [3]. For example, infections affecting the posterior portion of the eye are substantially more difficult to treat. Eye membranes hinder drug entry to the posterior portion, such as the cornea, conjunctiva and sclera; because of this, limited penetration further restricts the utility of the topical administration as a method for treating disorders affecting the retina, choroid or vitreous humor. These obstacles were taken into account when improving the topical ophthalmic dosage form's efficacy [4–6]. Previous literature has concluded that therapeutic substances are difficult to distribute due to the structure of the eye. Because of the barriers like blood-retinal barriers (BRB), the eye is resistant to foreign material exposure, and pharmaceutical agents trying to reach the intended ocular tissues [7, 8]. A barrier like BRB is made up of an inner and outer barrier. Because of the tight connections, the retinal vascular endothelium, the iris vascular epithelium and the nonpigmented ciliary epithelium keep the blood-retinal barrier in place, which is very necessary for sustaining the homoeostasis of the retina [9]. However, the outer part of BRB consists of functional complexes of retinal pigment epithelium (RPE) and pigment epithelial cells of the pars plana. Whereas the inner segment is made up of the tight connections between the endothelial cells of the retinal capillaries.

There is very less molecular convection as the blood-retinal barrier lacks cellular components and it is preferentially permeable to more lipophilic molecules [10]. As a result, systemic drug administration is very critical for treating posterior segment diseases, only 1% to 2% of injected drug reaches the vitreous cavity; that is why massive doses of the medicine must be administered, resulting in a slew of systemic adverse effects [11–14]. So intravitreous injections are a good way to boost medication bioavailability in this eye segment [15–18]. However, problems linked with this method of administration include retinal detachment. Endophthalmitis and intravitreous hemorrhages [19]. For overcoming these difficulties, we can use topical medicine distribution if the therapeutic window could be achieved and also maintained for an extended period of time. However, developing an effective topical dosage from that can deliver the medicine at the precise amount without requiring frequent instillation is a huge issue for pharmaceutical science and technology. The development of medication delivery methods that do not require large dosage or repeated administrations is an essential technique for treating illness affecting the front part of the eye, Although several recent studies have emphasized different delivery methods, particularly these evaluations do not focus on the both eye segments, nanoparticle systems, which aims to boost the drugs delivery to both segments of the eye [4, 20–26]. Whereas traditional topical ocular therapies have substantial drawbacks, currently one approach is to use nanotechnology in the production process. Nanomicelles are nanoparticle-based ocular medication delivery systems. nanoparticles such as niosomes, liposomes, micelles, dendrimers, and other polymeric vesicles. Because of their solution/strong stability and cost-effectiveness, niosomes, which are nanovesicles consisting of nonionic surfactants, are becoming nanocarriers in drug delivery applications [2].

6.2 Revolution from Traditional to Nanodrug Delivery System in Delivery of Drugs to the Eye

6.2.1 Traditional System of Delivery of Drug and Drawbacks to the "Anterior Segment of the Eye"

6.2.1.1 Topical eye drop solutions

Traditional eye drops solutions are patient-friendly, instant-acting and also a noninvasive pharmaceutical formulation. The traditional method of delivering eye drop solutions to the cornea and conjunctiva involves delivering them via a cul-de-sac, followed by rapid first-order absorption. Modifying the drug characteristics or the qualities of the drug delivery device can boost drug penetration and bioavailability [25]. Because to reflux blinking or nasolacrimal drainage, the majority of the topically applied dosage, regardless of the amount injected, is quickly lost during the first 6 min after delivery. Just 20% (roughly 7 L) of the fluid is maintained in the conjunctival pocket, with only 1 to 3% reaching the intraocular tissue [1, 27–30]. Traditionally eye drops in the form of solutions, suspensions and emulsions have been utilized for treating diseases those are related to anterior segments. The prodrug technique little bit alters the drug's physiochemical characteristics to improve absorption via passive or active diffusion [31].

6.2.1.2 Suspensions

Routine ocular suspensions are usually insoluble drug dispersion in an aqueous medium that contains dispersing and solubilizing agents. The precorneal cavity keeps drug particles suspended, extending the medication's contact duration. The time it takes for drug molecules to diffuse into corneal tissue is regulated by drug particle size, which influences drug bioavailability. Alcon, Inc's Tobra-Dex ST is a suspension containing (0.3%) tobramycin and (0.05%) dexamethasone for ocular infections caused by bacteria [20]. They transport the medicines as a dispersion in an aqueous solvent. In suspensions, particles are maintained within the conjunctival pocket, and their size determines the effect's duration [28, 32–34]. The active pharmaceutical ingredients were shown to be more concentrated in tissues and more effective against *Staphylococcus aureus* and *pseudomonas aeruginosa* [35–37].

6.2.1.3 Emulsions

Routine ophthalmic emulsions can increase the bioavailability and solubility of water-insoluble medicines. The two most prevalent varieties of pharmaceutical emulsions are "water in oil" (w/o) and "oil in water" (o/w) [20]. When applied to the vitreous, retina, and choroid of rabbit eyes following not only one but multiple topical drop instillations, [3H]-difluprednate, a prednisolone derivate, can treat anterior ocular inflammation [1, 38, 39].

6.2.1.4 Ointments

Ophthalmic ointments are a topical carrier system with improved bioavailability and long-term drug release. In this case, they are composed of hydrocarbon molecules (paraffins) that are solid and semisolid with a melting point of 340°C (the physiological ocular temperature) [1]. Ointments are widely tolerated, relatively safe and a great way to extend ocular contact duration. Improved contact time increases ocular medication levels in the case of some antibiotics. Ophthalmic ointments should not be used on open sores in the eyes. Ointment instillation into postoperative eyes with a tight wound closure appears to be safe and beneficial [40].

6.2.2 Traditional Drug Delivery System and Drawbacks to the "Posterior Segment of the Eye":

6.2.2.1 Intravitreal injections of anti-VEGF agents

Anti-VEGF (vascular endothelial growth factor) treatments are administered intravitreally to treat a number of retinal illnesses, such as diabetic retinopathy, age-related macular degeneration, retinal vascular occlusions, and retinopathy of prematurity [41, 42]. Apart from regulating angiogenesis, VEGF (vascular endothelial growth factor) is a survival factor for endothelial cells, causing abnormal blood vessel phenotypes in wet age-related macular degeneration (AMD), diabetic macular edema (DME), and retinal vein occlusion (RVO). Angiogenesis and neovascularization cause slow and persistent central vision distortion and blurring, affecting the quality of life significantly. Many individuals with this illness have improved their quality of life—a result of anti-VEGF therapy and knowledge of VEGF's important role in angiogenesis [43, 44]. Aflibercept and ranibizumab are two kinds of VEGF inhibitors that have been authorized, and the number of IVIs done each year has grown dramatically. Endophthalmitis is the most significant consequence following IVI. It is uncommon, with a rate ranging from 0.01 to 0.26% [45, 46]. Several investigations in recent years have found negative effects ranging from increased intraocular pressure to visually unpleasant silicone oil vesicles in the vitreous cavity, because of very long-term use of anti-VEGF drugs, and a greater number of injections worldwide several investigations have discovered that the medication, as well as its manufacture, storage, environmental factors, and syringe material and design, all have a major impact on these side effects [47–50].

6.2.3 Other Ocular Drug Delivery Technologies

For overcoming the limitations associated with conventional formulations, novel techniques for ocular medication administration are now being explored and developed (such as other systemic complications because of increased systemic API availability following chronic administration and adverse reactions induced by preservatives) [1, 51].

6.2.3.1 Contact lens

Multiple studies have found that immersing soft contact lenses in a pharmaceutical solution increases the length of drug interaction with ocular tissues all the way across the cornea. It also increases the drug's absorption while decreasing its loss through lacrimal drainage [52–55]. The lenses were immersed in a 1% homatroine aqueous solution, causing patient's pupils to dilate completely for a longer period than eye drop alone. Vistakon pharmaceuticals conducted a study to explore if a pre-soaked contact lens that produced ketotifen, an antihistamine, could be effective medication, after application may prevent allergic conjunctivitis in contact lens wearers [56, 57]. When dexamethasone was released through contact lenses, it had a greater bioavailability than when it was released from eye drops. According to Kim et al., contact lenses that include liposomes or disperse pharmaceuticals into micelles have been created to selectively release medications into the eye based on specified variables such as pH or temperature. This method efficiently eliminates medication loss during storage while also ensuring focused drug administration to the eye [58–61].

In the case of timolol, molecularly imprinted contact lenses demonstrated increased drug-loading capacity and also extended drug administration [62]. Piggyback contact lenses with ion ligand-containing polymeric hydrogels and drug plate or drug solution combinations are also being investigated [63, 64]. Hence the new technology can deliver hours to days of medication release. Drug-eluting contact lenses have been proved to be safe and efficacious *in vivo* and clinical studies, with significant advantages over eye drops. Although the future seems bright, some obstacles remain, including processing and storage concerns, regulatory impediments, costly clinical study costs, probable lack of acceptability by the elderly, and so on [52, 62–67].

6.2.3.2 Ocular inserts

Ophthalmic inserts are specific sizes and forms of sterile preparations having a solid or semisolid consistency for use in the eyes. The drugs contained in the polymeric support of ocuserts can be used topically or systemically to treat the eyes. The primary goal of using ophthalmic inserts is to increase the active form of a drug's retention duration in the eye, resulting in a more consistent release [68–71]. Ocular inserts were created to satisfy the growing number of patients who require therapy with the fewest possible adverse effects. Ocuserts decreased the number of doses administered, resulting in improved patient compliance. It increases bioavailability by extending contact time. Systemic side effects can be decreased, which reduces undesirable consequences. Preservatives are not allowed, lowering the likelihood of allergic responses. Ocular implants are made in a variety of ways and may be assessed using a variety of metrics. Ocuserts are emerging ways in the era of ocular medication delivery [71]. Patient noncompliance with these inserts is widespread, resulting in symptoms such as foreign body sensations in the eye, difficulties with self-insertions, and the impression that the insert has been lost from the eye. To make ocular inserts soluble, erodible and hydrogel-like, many methods are applied [72].

6.2.3.3 Punctal plugs

Punctal plugs have been used to enhance retention duration and hence the absorption of eye drops by blocking the nasolacrimal drainage system. A decrease in the intraocular pressure of around 2 mmHg was found in the plugged eye when compared with unplugged eye following routine topical instillation of ocular hypotensive eye drops [73]. Punctal plugs are useful not only for treating aqueous-deficient dry eye but also for treating a range of other ocular surface disorders, where they act as therapeutic adjuvants. They may now be utilized in most cases thanks to new versions that have been created to increase tolerance and efficacy. Each model has its own safety profile, which the prescriber must be aware of. Because late issues are conceivable, long-term monitoring is required. Hence, punctal plugs obliterate the lacrimal punctum completely. At the slit light, they are visible and easily separable. They have a low probability of migrating into the lacrimal channels but a high probability of extrusion loss. Punctal plugs have been designed in a variety of ways to improve their efficacy and reduce problems [74–77]. Canalicular plugs have the following major disadvantages: (i) difficulty in seeing them and determining their placement. (ii) difficulty in removing them, and (iii) greater risk of canaliculitis [77]. Patients who are allergic to plug material or who have blockage of the lacrimal canals, ectropion, or an active ocular infection should not use punctal or canalicular plugs (conjunctivitis and keratitis). Very severe ocular surface conditions and lid irritation such as blepharitis must be treated before putting punctal plugs [78].

6.2.3.4 Episcleral implants

Transscleral administration has been found to be an effective approach to attaining therapeutic medication concentrations in the posterior region of the eye [79, 80]. For example, LX201 is an episcleral implant consisting of a silicone matrix that provides possibly therapeutic cyclosporine dosage to the lacrimal gland on a continuous basis in preclinical studies with rabbits and dogs [81, 82]. A subconjunctival insert was developed by Pfizer, Inc. of a poly tube with a latanoprost core. The active pharmaceutical component is released through the permeable end of the tube after 3 to 6 months. The release rate is controlled by the PGLA tube's internal diameter [27, 83]. MEMS (Microelectromechanical Systems) are devices for drug delivery made of parylene ("biocompatible and flexible") that are implanted in the subconjunctival area and connected to a cannula via an incision in the anterior or posterior segments of the eye. Electrolysis (powered by a battery and wireless inductive power transmission) creates pressure inside the reservoir, forcing the medication through the cannula as water is electrochemically converted into hydrogen and oxygen gas. This enables the exact administration of the required dose volume, addressing the limitations of the previous generation of manually controlled MEMS, which includes fluctuations in drug release time and depressing force. The MEMS device enables medication solution replenishment, allowing for long-term drug therapy and avoiding several operations. After three months, no problems were identified in a trial employing subconjunctival device implantation, highlighting the safety of this method. Furthermore, utilising travoprost-loaded MEMS devices, a constant drop in intraocular pressure (IOP) was obtained in dogs for up to

8 hours. MEMS medicine delivery devices are investigated for the treatment of chronic and resistant eye diseases such as glaucoma and age-related macular degeneration [27]. To address these problems, several tactics can be applied, such as tailoring a basic material's properties using molecules. The creation of unique forms that depart from conventional geometry and permit the use of bigger surface areas on devices, the application of novel technologies to fit new designs, and the use of previously undiscovered materials with the potential to create ocular implants [84].

6.2.4 Nanotechnology: Recent Approach for Ocular Drug Delivery Systems

"Combining science and technology, nanotechnology allows for the modification of properties and structures at the nanoscale (1 to 100 nm)". There are many applications of nanotechnology like science as well as clinical medicine, diagnostics and disease management those have an ability to control molecules at such a microscopic level [85]. Nanotechnology has been employed in medicine delivery systems to treat ocular disorders since the 1980s. For increasing the retention period, better interaction with ocular mucosa of the associated drug and as well as for increasing its permeability across the epithelium of conjunctiva and cornea the nanocarriers have been discovered recently. Nanodrug delivery and nanotherapies are introduced to treat some of the most common ocular conditions like infections, inflammation, glaucoma, dry eyes and retinopathies [86]. Nanoparticles, both organic and inorganic, are a fresh approach to meeting unmet therapeutic needs, notably in the ocular sector, by altering and boosting medicine delivery [85]. As a result of that till now several nanoparticles have been discovered and developed, like "lipid-based nanoparticles, nanosuspensions, nanoemulsion and metal-based nanoparticles". In this review, we will focus on the advances in nanocarrier-based drug delivery systems. We will also cover new issues and an overview of future trends of nano-based ocular drug delivery systems and strategies in ophthalmology, with the goal of eventually providing practical applications for treating ocular illness [87].

6.2.5 Ocular Medication Delivery System Based on Nanotechnology:

6.2.5.1 Organic nanoparticles

Examples of nanocarriers include liposomes, niosome, dendrimers, solid lipid nanoparticles, polymers, and protein/peptide-based nanoparticles. Made of proteins, lipids, carbohydrates, or other organic materials, organic nanoparticles seem to have a number of medical advantages [88]. The potential organic and inorganic nanoparticles for ophthalmic drug delivery are depicted in Fig. 6.1.

6.2.5.2 'Liposomes'

Liposomes are a new approach in new drug delivery systems that are nonirritating to the eye and also have a long retention time on the ocular surface, providing greater efficacy and bioavailability. Liposome-based methods for ocular medication administration are advantageous because they can entrap both hydrophobic and hydrophilic medications and deliver them to both the anterior and posterior portions of the eye [89]. Liposomes are lipid vesicles composed of one or more phospholipid bilayers encircling an aqueous core and having sizes from 0.08 to 10.00 m. Liposomes are divided into tiny unilamellar vesicles with diameters of 100 to 300 nm, and multilamellar vesicles with more than a single phospholipid bilayer [1, 90]. The positive charge of liposomes can increase corneal drug permeability, existing drug release. Li et al. created formulations like diclofenac sodium-loaded with low-molecular-weight chitosan (LCH) coating. The findings revealed a little increase in particle size with prolonged drug release, the stability test findings were satisfactory, and the preservation and penetration of LCH-coated liposomes across the cornea were improved [90, 91]. Other studies also found there was no eye irritation or toxicity and investigated the therapeutic impact of liposome formulation for delivering latanoprost by subconjunctival injection to treat glaucoma. In the subconjunctival area, the liposomal formulation improved medication targeting and sustainability. Furthermore, compared to traditional topical

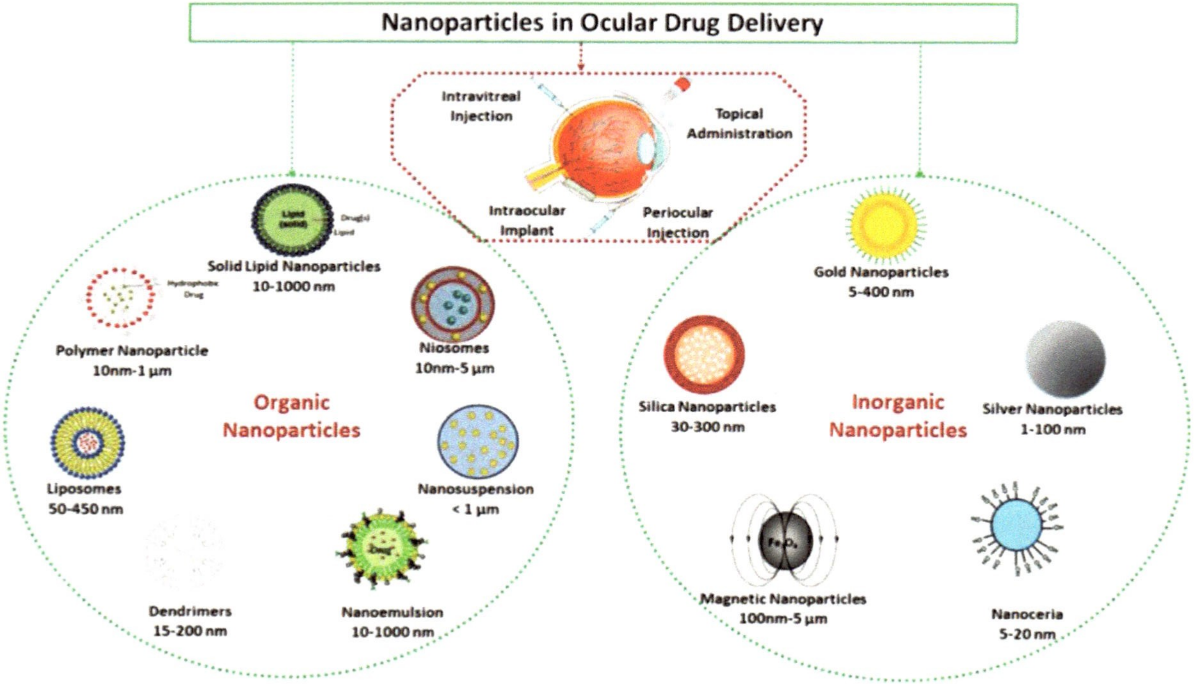

Figure 6.1 The potential organic and inorganic nanoparticles for ophthalmic drug delivery [88].

eyedrops, latanoprost-encapsulated liposomes showed a 50-day decrease in the IOP in the rabbit eye [92, 93]. Tears again® is a spray that treats dry eye disease with phospholipid liposomes [94, 95]. Endophthalmitis, vitreous hemorrhage, and retinal detachment are among the side effects associated with intravitreal instillation, since liposomes offer targeted medication administration at the site of action and overcome the limitation in terms of bioavailability [96]. In another research, Vallejo et al. utilized triamcinolone acetonide-loaded liposomes for vitreous cavity and retina injection in the rabbit eye, there was no increase in intraocular pressure [97].

6.2.5.3 Niosomes

Many studies and pharmaceutical companies are looking into niosomes as bi/multi-layer nanoparticles for a number of applications. Some important studies look for the best ways of drug encapsulation as well as drug/protein loading and release kinetics. Because they can increase bioavailability and effectiveness and treat serious illnesses like cancer, researchers are interested in using niosomal drug delivery systems to treat severe inflammations [98, 99]. Niosomes, which are nanovesicles made of nonionic surfactants, are becoming nanocarriers for drug administration due to their cost-effectiveness and solution/storage stability. They are also biocompatible, biodegradable, have a flexible shape, and can hold both hydrophobic and hydrophilic medicines. Niosomes are attractive nanocarriers in the treatment of eye disorders because of their features [100]. Currently, niosomes are being studied for glaucoma therapy as a drug delivery vehicle, because of several benefits like no need for frequent administration, longer intraocular-pressure-lowering efficacy, very high corneal permeability and very few ocular toxicities currently niosomal drug delivery becoming popular. "Aggarwal and Kaur synthesized timolol maleate using reverse phase evaporation (REV), ether injection, and film hydration techniques" (a water-soluble medication used to treat open-angle glaucoma) encapsulated chitosan or carbopol-coated niosome formulations [101]. Due to the production of large unilamellar vesicles (LUVs) that could effectively encapsulate a water-soluble medication in large numbers, niosomes made using the REV technique showed the highest ratio of entrapment efficacy when compared to others. Compared to carbopol-coated niosomal formulations, chitosan-coated formulations showed superior control over IOP [102]. Recently Hashim et al. demonstrated the potential of niosomal in situ gel as an ocular delivery vehicle for atenolol, a 1 adrenoceptor blocker, for treating glaucoma. To produce niosomes with different Span 60 and cholesterol molar ratios, the thin film-hydration (TFH) methodology was employed. The produced niosomes' highest entrapment efficiency (EE percent) was 80.7%. When niosomes were introduced into the in situ gel, they enhanced drug release and IOP-lowering activity by more than 8 h, suggesting that niosomal in situ gel had the longest drug release and IOP-lowering activity [103]. Abdelkader and coworkers set out to create and test niosomes based on Span 60 for naltrexone topical application (NTX). Dicetyl phosphate (DCP) and stearyl amine (STA) were investigated as bilayer membrane additives in four different ways. They placed niosomal formulations on the surface of 10-day-old chicken's chorioallantoic membrane they found no irritation. NTX's ocular permeability was enhanced by modulating its release from a niosomal formulation [104]. When in another study they used solvent injection to make chitosan-coated Span 60 niosomes containing gatifloxacin, an ocular drug for treating bacterial eye infections. No toxicity was deducted and the drug transition through the cornea was greatly improved when chitosan-coated niosomes were compared to untreated niosomes [105]. Utilizing tween 80 as a surfactant, cationic lipid 2,3-di(tetradecycloxy)propan-1-amine as an additive, and cationic lipid 2,3-di(tetradecycloxy) propan-1-amine as an additive, a formulation was created using the pCMS-EGFP plasmid. An original cationic niosome was created by Puras and colleagues for the delivery of retinal genes. The pCMS-EGFP plasmid was used for formulation through O/W (oil in water) emulsification. Tween 80 was employed as a surfactant, 2,3-di(tetradecycloxy)propan-1-amine and squalene were used as cationic lipids, and other ingredients included cationic lipids. To assess the efficacy and internalization process of transfections in HEK-293 and ARPE-19 cells, as well as in rats following injection into the retina, researchers have carried out *in vitro* and *in vivo* studies. Nioplexes showed better cell survival than Lipofectamine 2000; however, they performed less effectively during transfection. Depending on the delivery method, subretinal injections have been shown to successfully transfect RPE *in vivo* [106]. Rat retinas have been used to examine the impact of a nonionic surfactant on the efficiency of niosome transfection. Three niosome formulations were made, each of which differed only in terms of nonionic tensioactives. Niosomes contained beneficial lipids including squalene and polysorbate 20 or 85 in addition to 1,2-di-octadecenyl-3-trimethyl-ammonium propane (DOTMA). Consequently, polysorbate 20 niosome-based nioplexes were more effective *in vitro* at transfecting ARPE-19 retinal cells. Further, because the transgenes were administered intravitreal and subretinal, substantial levels of transgene expression were seen in the retinas of rats. Consequently, this formulation stands out as a potential nonviral candidate for efficiently transferring particular therapeutic genes [107]. In 2017, Paradkar et al. created and tested a natamycin-loaded niosomal in situ gel for ocular medication delivery in the treatment of fungal keratitis. Niosome formulations had a high EE (>65 and gel niosome formulations extended drug release to 24 h with greater corneal penetration [108].

For the treatment of keratitis, niosomes containing voriconazole were mixed into gelling ocular implants. Surfactants were used to make the niosomes such as Span 60 and Span 40 using pluronic L64 and F127. EE was found to be greater than 49% in the formulations produced. The drug release of niosomes and niosomal gel formulations was further extended by up to 8 h using niosomes [109]. As nanocarriers, niosomes are available in a variety of sizes, ranging from micrometers to nanometers. By enhancing corneal permeability, increasing ocular bio-availability, and ensuring longer drug release, niosomes deliver medications and genes to the front and back of the eye.

Furthermore, niosomes can be embedded in gels or covered with mucoadhesive polymers such as carbopol, chitosan to enhance their benefits [102, 110–112]. Niosomes have greater chemical stability and are more widely distributed on the eye's surface, thus offering excellent bioavailability compared to other nanostructures used in ocular drug delivery formulations [23].

Niosomes have a higher penetration rate than the others. Niosomes and liposomes have comparable structural properties; however, niosomes are formed of more stable materials [113].

6.2.5.4 Solid lipid nanoparticles

To increase medication absorption, solid lipid nanoparticles (SLNs) are commonly used as topical carriers. SLNs were created using high-speed stirring and the ultrasonication process. As a result of solubility experiments, stearic acid was selected as the lipid former, Tween 80 as the surfactant, and Transcutol P as the cosurfactant. Clarithromycin-loaded SLN was optimized using fractional factorial screening and 32 complete factorial designs.

The morphology, penetration, irritation, and ocular pharmacokinetics of stable SLNs (CL10) were studied in rabbits [114]. Because they have the capacity to improve ocular absorption and hence improve bioavailability along with prolonged and regulate drug release characteristics for lipophilic and hydrophilic drugs, SLNs have recently gained a lot of interest as possible candidates for drug delivery to ocular surfaces [115, 116]. Solid lipid nanoparticles for the application of tobramycin were researched by Cavalli et al., topically applied to New Zealand albino rabbits, the formulation demonstrated improved ocular bioavailability and extended preocular drug retention [117]. Using synthesized SNL coupled with a phospholipid and a homolipid produced from goat fat, Attama et al. studied the ocular penetration and sustained release impact of diclofenac sodium. Diclofenac penetration tests in cell culture through a human cornea construct demonstrated an increase in cornea permeability capabilities when drugs were loaded with SNL [118].

6.3 Polymeric Nanoparticles

These monomers can take any shape as long as they share two reactive functional groups with another monomer. By selecting the suitable monomer/s, a polymer with certain properties might be formed. Polymers are not only a one-of-a-kind material that can have all of the aforementioned characteristics, but their great synthetic flexibility also allows researchers to modify them to their specific demands or aims. To obtain specific properties, polymeric tailoring might be performed directly on biopolymers by chemical derivatization [119, 120]. Another option is to synthesize polymers from monomers, which can result in a broad range of structures and uses [121–124]. Polymeric materials are becoming increasingly relevant in nanotechnology. Surfactants may be necessary for the preparation of polymeric NPs. The combination of hydrophobic and hydrophilic molecules produces nonionic surfactants with amphiphilic characteristics [125]. Because they have the capability to entrap hydrophilic/hydrophobic drug molecules with delayed drug release, poly(lactic-co-glycolic acid) (PLGA) nanoparticles, a biodegradable copolymer, have been employed in ocular drug delivery [126]. Cerium oxide nanoparticles encapsulated in glycol chitosan were used to study dry eye conditions. According to a study, the drug can infiltrate corneal and conjunctival cells and increase SOD2 expression [127]. During *in vivo* investigations, Sharma et al. observed that chloro trimethyl-ammonium methyl methacrylate (Eudragit RS 100/RL 100) polymeric nanoparticles with amikacin sulfate formulation caused strong corneal adhesion, leading in higher drug retention and drug controlled release efficiency [128]. Li et al. conducted another significant contribution to the field on the effectiveness of combining hydroxypropyl-beta-cyclodextrin (HP–CD) and PLGA (PLGA) nanoparticles for triamcinolone acetonide encapsulation in ocular application. Drug-loaded PLGA with hydroxypropyl-beta-cyclodextrin (HP–CD) nanoparticles released medications faster than drug-loaded PLGA without-CD solution, according to *in vitro* drug release experiments. Furthermore, increasing drug concentration in the aqueous humor was correlated with enhanced drug penetration of HP–CD/PLGA in the trans corneal location, indicating that an HP–CD/PLGA nanoparticle-loaded triamcinolone acetonide eye drop formulation might be a feasible choice [129].

6.4 Dendrimers

Dendrimers are monodisperse macromolecules with logically defined sizes and a molecular structure made of three primary components: (i) an inner core within the dendrimer's central molecule, (ii) a highly branching unit termed generation that links to the core, and (iii) an exterior surface with many valent functional groups [130]. The pharmaceutical industry is interested in dendrimers because of their tree-like branching structure with many covalent connections, which allows them to attach several functional groups, including medications, within dendrimers and conjugate them to the surface via covalent bonds. Their advantages include hydrophilic or lipophilic qualities that provide control insolubility, and dendrimers, which can entrap tiny drug molecules inside their branches due to their global shape [131, 132].

Polycationic polyamidoamine (PAMAM) dendrimers have been proven to be cytotoxic, with toxicity rising with generation; however, hydroxy-terminated G4 PAMAM dendrimers are expected to be harmless due to their near-neutral surface charge, which lowers nonspecific retention and interactions in tissues [133]. PAMAM dendrimers with a primary amine and carboxylate surface groups were employed in another investigation to boost drug corneal penetration and characteristics during *in vitro* release. Puerarin medication administration was effectively evaluated on the albino rabbit model for ocular hypertension and cataracts glaucoma treatment using a dendrimer-based formulation [134]. Dendrimer conjugated ODN-1 was found to considerably slow the growth of choroidal neovascularization (CNV), with no negative side effects detected during the trial [135]. Because of their numerous benefits, dendrimer compositions have the potential to increase the efficacy of ophthalmic medications.

6.5 Nanosuspensions

Nanosuspensions are part of nanotechnology. Many of the drug possibilities have low water solubility. The use of medicine nanosuspension is a universal formulation strategy for increasing the therapeutic efficacy of these medications in any route of administration. A pharmaceutical nanosuspension is defined as very finely colloid, biphasic, dispersed, solid drug particles in an aqueous vehicle, size less than 1 m, without any matrix material, stabilized by surfactants and polymers, prepared by suitable methods for Drug Delivery applications, and administered via various routes such as oral, topical, parenteral, ocular, and pulmonary [136]. Nanosuspensions might be useful for drugs that are poorly soluble in lachrymal fluids. Nanosuspensions are an ideal alternative for the ocular distribution of hydrophobic medications due to their inherent ability to enhance pharmaceutical saturation solubility. The medication's nanoparticulate shape permits it to remain in the cul-de-sac for a longer length of time, allowing for continuous drug release [137]. Pignatello et al. created eudragit delay cloricromene nanosuspensions for intraocular injection [138]. A previous research has found that the topical administration of an ibuprofen sodium salt (IBU) sodium salt-coated chloro trimethyl-ammonium methyl methacrylate nanosuspension (Eudragit RS 100) polymer improved penetration to the anterior segment of the eye, extended drug release, and increased drug level in the aqueous humor [139]. Some glucocorticoids, such as dexamethasone, hydrocortisone, and prednisolone, used topically to treat eye irritation, have been nanoformulated, resulting in longer drug absorption and enhanced drug bioavailability in ocular drug delivery, minimizing the need for frequent drug administration [140, 141].

6.6 Nanoemulsion

Cationic nanoemulsions can be utilized topically to deliver active compounds to the eye. Over the previous decade, Novagali Pharma has successfully developed and released Novasorb, a complex pharmaceutical technology for the treatment of eye disorders [142]. Because of their multiple benefits, including prolonged activity and efficient drug penetration into the deeper layers of the ocular structure and the aqueous humor, dilutable nanoemulsions are useful drug delivery vehicles for ophthalmic application [143]. Droplets' tiny size provides a wide surface area, which has the potential to increase ophthalmic medicine delivery effectiveness by enhancing ocular permeability and bioavailability [144]. The low surface tension of nanoemulsions is hypothesized to allow for improved medicine distribution on the cornea and mixing with the precorneal contents. This increases the amount of time the medicine is in contact with the corneal epithelium [145]. Ismail et al. discovered that the antiglaucoma medicine dorzolamide hydrochloride nanoemulsion showed excellent results in ocular treatment. The pharmacological formulation produced a long-lasting impact with an early beginning of action, eliminating the requirement for recurrent administration of eye drops [146]. Mahboobian et al. assessed the absorption of acyclovir nanoemulsion in the bovine cornea after trans corneal permeation in a clinical study. The results demonstrated better acyclovir permeability across the corneal membrane cells and no irritation in the rabbit eye, indicating that the formulation is safe for treating ocular infection [147].

Table 6.1 Organic nanoparticles applications for ophthalmic drug delivery

Nanomaterials	Drug	Application	Animal model	Function	Ref.
Liposomes	Acyclovir	Topical	Rabbit	Prolong drug penetration	[148]
Niosomes	Tacrolimus	Topical	Rabbit	Increased precorneal drug retention	[149]
Solid lipid nanoparticle	Tobramycin	Topical	Rabbit	Increased drug retention	[150]
Polymeric NPs	Amikacin	Topical	Rabbit	Improved ocular penetration Controlled release	[151]
Dendrimers	Acetazolamide	Topical	Rabbit	Enhanced drug residence time	[152]
Nanosuspension	IBU sodium salt	Topical	Rabbit	Increased penetration Prolonged drug release	[139]
Nanoemulsion	Acyclovir	Topical	Rabbit	Increased corneal permeation	[147]

6.7 Inorganic Nanoparticles

The most prevalent inorganic nanoparticles are metallic nanoparticles and quantum dots. Metallic nanoparticles have sparked a lot of attention since Faraday revealed that they can survive in solution over a decade ago [35]. Metal nanoparticles, metal oxide nanoparticles, doped metal–metal/oxide–metal nanoparticles, metal sulfide, and metal–organic frameworks are the four families. Metal nanoparticles (MNPs) such as silver (Ag), gold (Au), copper (Cu), magnesium (Mg), titanium (Ti), platinum (Pt), zinc (Zn), and iron (Fe) have been studied in numerous fields and have proven to be effective, stable drug delivery platforms with fewer side effects, as well as potent imaging probes. Single metals with better characteristics were discovered to be less hazardous than doped metallic nanoparticles, such as ZnO doped with Co.60.61. Metals like cerium oxide (CeO_2) nanoparticles and gold nanoparticles have shown potential antioxidant properties in the ocular medicine and gene delivery sectors, with a high safety profile following eye administration and significant antioxidant activity.

6.8 Gold NPs (AuNPs)

Several studies are being undertaken to enhance ophthalmology diagnosis and therapy. Indeed, 285 million individuals worldwide suffer from visual acuity issues, and several ways to improve patient treatment are being researched. One of these alternatives is to employ gold nanoparticles (GNP), which have a wide range of properties and may be used for both diagnostic and therapeutic purposes [153].

In previous studies rod-shaped particles were found to be less biocompatible than 50 and 100 nm spheres and cubes, which showed minimal cytotoxicity and excellent internalization [154]. Dong et al. demonstrated that giving streptozotocin-induced diabetic rats resveratrol-coated AuNPs with a median size of 20 nm and dosages of 200–300 mg/kg for 3 months may protect against diabetic retinopathy. The inhibitory effects of the ERK1/2 pathway and nuclear factor kappa B (NF-kb) expression in diabetic rats, which may reduce inflammation and permeability of the blood-retinal barrier, may aid in restoring the balance of angiogenesis stimulators and inhibitors.

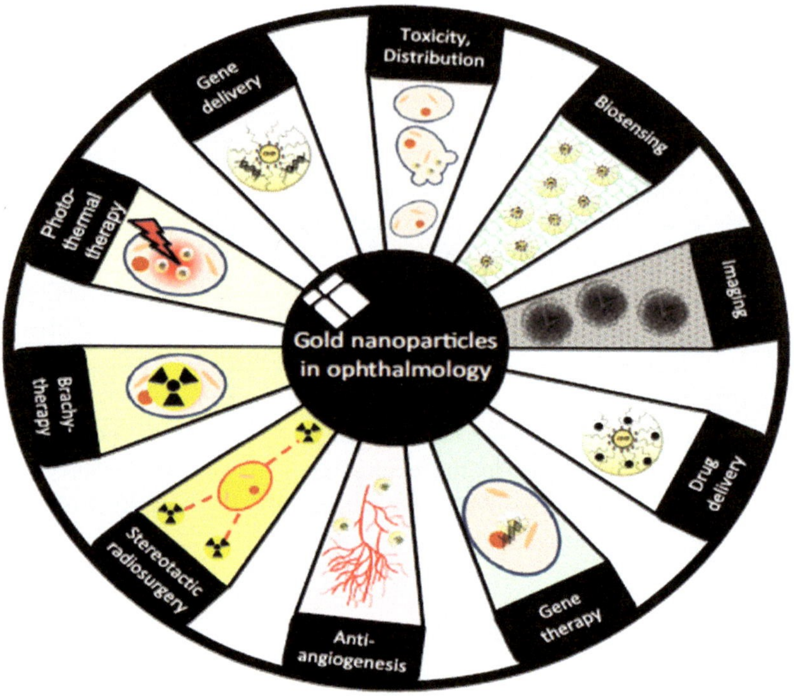

Figure 6.2 Illustration of the uses of the GNP in ophthalmology [153].

Furthermore, VEGF-1, TNF, and IL-6 mRNA expression in the retina was significantly decreased [155]. VEGF-induced RF/6A cell migration in choroid-retina endothelial (RF/6A) cells was substantially suppressed by AuNPs of 3–5 nm via the Akt/eNOS pathways. They found no cytotoxic effects on AuNPS on RF/6A or negative effects on normal physiological cell attachment to fibronectin in their cell viability and cell adhesion assays [156]. According to Kim et al., the passage of AuNPs of 20 nm increased cell mortality compared to cells lacking NPs enhances the possibility of future therapeutic studies [157].

6.9 Silver Nanoparticles (AgNPs)

Silver nanoparticles (AgNPs), a well-known nanotechnology product, have generated attention as a nanomedicine in recent years due to their unique properties and numerous therapeutic uses [158]. Hippocrates, the father of modern medicine, believed silver powder had medicinal powers and recommended it as an ulcer treatment. Prior to the discovery of sulfadiazine cream in the nineteenth century, weak solutions of silver nitrate were used to treat infections. Before the discovery of sulfadiazine cream, weak silver nitrate solutions were used to treat infections in the nineteenth century [159]. Silver nanoparticles (AgNPs) have been widely used in nanomedicine because to their unique chemical and physical characteristics, huge surface area to volume ratio, low manufacturing cost, and biocompatibility [160]. Because of their unique chemical and physical features, large surface area to volume ratio, cheap manufacturing cost, and biocompatibility, silver nanoparticles (AgNPs) have been widely employed as drug delivery vehicles in nanomedicine [161]. Because of their strong tumor-killing and antibacterial properties, AgNPs have been described as useful nanoparticles in the treatment of cancer and infections. AgNPs have been utilized to carry medications to the eyes and as an ocular contact lens coating agent. Furthermore, in a number of cell culture systems and animal models for ocular disorders, AgNPs, alone or in combination with natural plant extracts, demonstrated substantial anti-angiogenic, antioxidant, anti-glycation end products, and anti-cataractogenic activities [162]. Anbukkarasi et al. assessed the antioxidant and anti-cataractogenic effects of AgNPs varying in diameter from 15 to 50 nm generated from an ethanolic extract of T. divaricate leaves, which is known to exhibit antioxidant and anti-cataractogenic pharmacological action. The researchers created an *in vitro* selenite-induced cataractogenic model to investigate the effect of AgNPs on dense opacification of Wistar rat lenses. The findings showed that the AgNPs created worked as a powerful antioxidant by scavenging the free radicals DPPH and H_2O_2, which are the primary culprits of cataract development [163]. Despite the fact that AgNPs have antifungal, antioxidant, anti-angiogenic, and anti-inflammatory properties, their poor success in the field of ocular drug delivery can be attributed to their toxicity in multiple investigations. The release of silver ions from the nanoparticle surface induces irritation in various ocular regions, which is the most commonly reported toxicity. Jun et al. studied the toxicity of silver nanoparticles at 0.4 mg/L and observed that cell death or a blockade of nuclear DNA or RNA export induced downregulation of numerous lens crystalline genes [164]. AgNPs with diameters of 22.4 and 42.5 nm produced cytotoxicity in bovine retinal endothelial cells (BRECs) and activated the reactive oxygen species (ROS) system in one investigation [165].

6.10 Cerium Oxide Nanoparticles (Nanoceria-CeO_2-NPs)

Cerium is a rare earth element in the periodic table's lanthanide series that is considered a potent antioxidant. CeO_2-NPs with 3–5 nm diameters catalyze antioxidant reactions via two oxidation states: The reduction of Ce^{4+} to Ce^{3+} and the loss of an oxygen atom [166]. This process fills cell gaps with reactive oxygen species (ROS), mimicking the antioxidant enzymatic functions of superoxide dismutase (SOD) and catalase [167]. In the realm of ophthalmology, CeO_2-NPs have been studied in many animal models of AMD and have shown potential antioxidant, anti-inflammatory, and anti-angiogenic properties. They were also demonstrated to provide long-term neuroprotection for photoreceptors in RP mice with minimal side effects. They were also discovered to be safe for lens cells and employed as an efficient anti-cataractogenicagent [168]. In rat retinal primary cell cultures, Chen et al. reported that 20 nm CeO_2-NPs could prevent an increase in free radical concentrations. They decided to test the NPs *in vivo* by exposing albino rats to 2700 lux of light for 6 h. Light exposure generally kills 50–60% of photoreceptors; however, electroretinogram (ERG) data showed that a large percentage of photoreceptor cells were preserved following posttreatment with CeO_2-NPs [169]. Pretreatment of albino Sprague–Dawley rats with intravenous and intravitreal injections of CeO_2-NPs for 3 weeks decreased neuronal mortality induced by 1000 lux light for 24 h and helped maintain the integrity of the outer nuclear layer, according to Fiorani et al. The study also found that nanoceria can prevent microglial activation and migration to the outer nuclear layer for a prolonged length of time. Nanoceria of 5–10 nm, according to Bhargava et al., might increase the lifetime of rod and cone photoreceptors in culture by aiding with cell line maintenance, allowing for enhanced drug screening trials on these cell lines [170].

6.11 Magnetic Nanoparticles (MNPs)

Magnetic nanoparticles (MNPs) are nanotechnology-based materials that contain magnetic elements such as iron, cobalt, chromium, and manganese. Its biological uses include medication delivery, magnetic resonance imaging, tissue healing, transfection, and tissue targeting [171]. Because its reactive surface may be functionalized with biocompatible coatings or bioactive chemicals, it yields a powerful drug delivery system with increased selectivity for biological targets while avoiding interactions with healthy cells [172]. Iron oxide magnetic particles are the most often used MNPs. Coating iron oxide magnetic particles with biocompatible material inhibits particle aggregation, biodegradation, and change from their original condition, allowing the bioactive component to be entrapped on the particle via covalent attachment or adsorption [173]. Therapeutic chemicals are bound to the magnetic nanoparticle shell. The fundamental advantage of employing magnetic iron oxide nanoparticles is that they can be viewed via magnetic resonance imaging, and drug-loaded nanoparticles may be kept in place with the help of a magnetic field. Fluid MAG-D labeled mesenchymal stem cells (MSCs) were implanted intravitreally into a retinal degenerative transgenic rat. This approach may give the most help in outer retinal illnesses such as AMD where controlled distribution to target cells is necessary since it can deliver a greater drug load to the region of interest and has resulted in therapeutically beneficial biochemical alterations in the dystrophic retina [174]. After injecting magnetic nano- and microparticles, measurements of IOP, ERG, and histology revealed no damage. Microparticles were relatively safe in terms of ocular endothelial cell numbers and iron accumulation in tissues. Another study found polymer-coated MNPs to be histologically and electro-physiologically safe for photoreceptors. IOP, ERG, and histopathology measurements following magnetic nano- and microparticle injection revealed no harm. Microparticles were relatively safe in terms of ocular endothelial cell numbers and iron accumulation in tissues. Another study found that polymer-coated MNPs are both histologically and electro-physiologically safe for photoreceptors [175].

Table 6.2 Applications of inorganic nanoparticles for drug delivery to ocular surfaces

Nanomaterials	Drug	Application	Animal model	Function	Ref.
AuNPs	Resveratrol	Injection	Rabbit	Reduced retinal inflammation	[65]
AgNPs			Rat	Produced antioxidants that exhibit anticataractogenic properties, indicating their potential in preventing cataract formation.	[75]
Cerium oxide NPs		Intravenous injection	Rat	Decrease neurodegenerative	[89]
MNPs	Mesenchymal stem cells (MSCs)	Intravitreal injection	Rat	Increase tenfold in delivery of drug load to the site of interest	[98]

6.12 Implant Devices

Drugs can be administered by implant devices made of polymeric materials. Ozurdex (dexamethasone biodegradable implant; Allergan, Inc., Irvine, CA, USA), Trivaris (triamcinolone acetonide suspension; Allergan, Inc.), Kenalog (triamcinolone acetonide suspension; Bristol-Myers Squibb, Princeton, NJ, USA), and Triesence (triamcinolone acetonide suspension; Bristol-Myers Squibb, Princeton, NJ (triamcinolone acetonide suspension; Alcon, Fort Worth, TX, USA). Nonbiodegradable implants provided more precise medication release control and longer release periods as compared to biodegradable implants. Nonbiodegradable implant removal, on the other hand, may cause issues for the patient. Medication release in the retina might take anywhere from five weeks to six months, depending on where it is put [176].

6.13 Clinical Trials and Commercialization of Ocular Nanomedicine

The first nanomedicine product entered the market over two decades ago. In 2012, there were 33 nanotherapies on the market, with over 100 treatments in development, and the United States was home to more than half of the nanomedicine businesses [177, 178]. The fast progress of nanotechnology in the drug delivery sector has resulted in the advancement of formulations for ocular medicine administration, many of which are now in clinical trials or on the market. Despite the approval of a drug-free nanoemulsion to treat dry eye, other formulations, such as drug-loading emulsions, are still behind in terms of therapeutic progress. Restasis®, a nanoemulsion containing cyclosporin A, was the first drug to be licenced for the treatment of chronic dry eye condition, and Durezol®, a nanoemulsion containing the chemical difluprednate, is approved to treat eye inflammation [179]. According to Grumezescu, many ophthalmic nanoformulations are in clinical trials, including TLC399 (ProDex), which contains dexamethasone sodium phosphate and is now in phase II for the treatment of macular edema induced by retinal vein occlusion. A phase II clinical trial with latanoprost coated liposomes (POLAT-001) for the treatment of ocular hypertension and primary open-angle glaucoma has also been completed [180]. "According to clinicaltrials.gov, a website developed by the United States National Institutes of Health, Department of Health and Human Services, SYSTANE®, a propylene glycol-based eye drops nanoemulsion that has completed phase IV for dry eye disease treatment, is one current ocular nanomedicine under clinical trial in 2020". Despite the need for more research and studies on nanostructure dispersion to the eye, the progress of nanotechnology in ocular therapeutics appears to be a viable method, with a rising number of nano-based formulations in clinical trials and on the market [181].

Table 6.3 Nanomedicine for ocular diseases under clinical trial and approved by the Food and Drug Administration (FDA)

Product	Nanoformulation	Indication	FDA approval status	Ref.
Restasis®	Nanoemulsion	Dry eye	Approved	[7]
Ozurdex	Dexamethasone biodegradable implant	Macular edema Noninfectious uveitis	Approved	[69]
Triesence	Triamcinolone acetonide suspension	Macular edema	Approved	[69]
Visudyne®	Liposome	AMD	Approved	[106]
TLC399 (ProDex)	Lipid-based nanoparticle	Madular edema	Phase II	[107]

6.14 Conclusion

Nanoparticles have attracted great attention in drug distribution pathway research over the last few decades, with scientists attempting to create drug-filled nanoparticles for transmission to the anterior and posterior portions of the eye. Traditional drug delivery formulations have shown success in the treatment of anterior eye part problems, but are less effective in the treatment of posterior eye part illnesses, even with frequent dosage. Although eye drops, suspensions, and ointments are convenient, instantly active, and safe ways of ocular medication delivery, the truth is that topically applied doses are rapidly lost after 5 to 6 min of administration owing to reflex blinking and nasolacrimal drainage. Because of their small size, nanoparticles are good candidates for ocular application. To address the issues associated with traditional medicine delivery in ocular formulations, several organic and inorganic nanoparticles have been produced. The nanomedicine market is still in its early stages, with numerous drug delivery technologies in clinical studies. Several intravitreal polymeric medicine delivery implants for eye problems have been authorized by the Food and Drug Administration (FDA). The use of nanotechnology in ocular nanomedicine research has shown tremendous promise. Nanomaterials have the potential to improve the bioavailability of a wide range of pharmaceuticals. Liposomes, dendrimers, niosomes, and metal nanoparticles are some examples of nanomaterials. Several studies are focusing on the combination of hybrid systems with hydrogels using micelles, dendrimers, and cyclo-dextrins [109]. AR 13,503 is now undergoing clinical studies and is likely to be utilized to treat DME and wet AMD. Another advanced nanofabrication technology is the hydrogel template approach, which may be utilized to create huge quantities of homogeneous nanoparticles and microparticles [111].

References

1. Patel, A., Cholkar, K., Agrahari, V., and Mitra, A. K. (2013). Ocular drug delivery systems: an overview. *World Journal of Pharmacology*, 2(2), 47.
2. Mehrandish, S., and Mirzaeei, S. (2021). A review on ocular novel drug delivery systems of antifungal drugs: functional evaluation and comparison of conventional and novel dosage forms. *Advanced Pharmaceutical Bulletin*, 11(1), 28.
3. Souza, J. G., Dias, K., Pereira, T. A., Bernardi, D. S., and Lopez, R. F. (2014). Topical delivery of ocular therapeutics: carrier systems and physical methods. *Journal of Pharmacy and Pharmacology*, 66(4), 507–530.
4. Gaudana, R., Jwala, J., Boddu, S. H., and Mitra, A. K. (2009). Recent perspectives in ocular drug delivery. *Pharmaceutical Research*, 26(5), 1197–1216.
5. Le Bourlais, C., Acar, L., Zia, H., Sado, P. A., Needham, T., and Leverge, R. (1998). Ophthalmic drug delivery systems—recent advances. *Progress in Retinal and Eye Research*, 17(1), 33–58.
6. Kang-Mieler, J. J., Rudeen, K. M., Liu, W., and Mieler, W. F. (2020). Advances in ocular drug delivery systems. *Eye*, 34(8), 1371–1379.
7. Cunha-Vaz, J., Bernardes, R., and Lobo, C. (2011). Blood-retinal barrier. *European Journal of Ophthalmology*, 21(6 suppl), 3–9.
8. Campbell, M., and Humphries, P. (2013). The blood-retina barrier. In *Biology and Regulation of Blood-Tissue Barriers*, Springer, New York, NY, pp. 70–84.
9. Janoria, K. G., Gunda, S., Boddu, S. H., and Mitra, A. K. (2007). Novel approaches to retinal drug delivery. *Expert Opinion on Drug Delivery*, 4(4), 371–388.

10. Yasukawa, T., Ogura, Y., Tabata, Y., Kimura, H., Wiedemann, P., and Honda, Y. (2004). Drug delivery systems for vitreoretinal diseases. *Progress in Retinal and Eye Research*, 23(3), 253–281.
11. Himawan, E., Ekström, P., Buzgo, M., Gaillard, P., Stefánsson, E., Marigo, V., ... and Paquet-Durand, F. (2019). Drug delivery to retinal photoreceptors. *Drug Discovery Today*, 24(8), 1637–1643.
12. Nagai, N., Saijo, S., Song, Y., Kaji, H., and Abe, T. (2019). A drug refillable device for transscleral sustained drug delivery to the retina. *European Journal of Pharmaceutics and Biopharmaceutics*, 136, 184–191.
13. Patel, J. K., Sutariya, V., Kanwar, J. R., and Pathak, Y. V., eds. (2018). *Drug Delivery for the Retina and Posterior Segment Disease*. Springer.
14. Kim, H. M., and Woo, S. J. (2021). Ocular drug delivery to the retina: current innovations and future perspectives. *Pharmaceutics*, 13(1), 108.
15. Yadav, D., Varma, L. T., and Yadav, K. (2018). Drug delivery to posterior segment of the eye: conventional delivery strategies, their barriers, and restrictions. In *Drug Delivery for the Retina and Posterior Segment Disease*, Springer, Cham, pp. 51–67.
16. Varela-Fernández, R., Díaz-Tomé, V., Luaces-Rodríguez, A., Conde-Penedo, A., García-Otero, X., Luzardo-Álvarez, A., ... and Otero-Espinar, F. J. (2020). Drug delivery to the posterior segment of the eye: biopharmaceutic and pharmacokinetic considerations. *Pharmaceutics*, 12(3), 269.
17. Navarro-Partida, J., Castro-Castaneda, C. R., Cruz-Pavlovich, S., Francisco, J., Aceves-Franco, L. A., Guy, T. O., and Santos, A. (2021). Lipid-based nanocarriers as topical drug delivery systems for intraocular diseases. *Pharmaceutics*, 13(5), 678.
18. Cabrera, F. J., Wang, D. C., Reddy, K., Acharya, G., and Shin, C. S. (2019). Challenges and opportunities for drug delivery to the posterior of the eye. *Drug Discovery Today*, 24(8), 1679–1684.
19. Maroñas, O., García-Quintanilla, L., Luaces-Rodríguez, A., Fernández-Ferreiro, A., Latorre-Pellicer, A., Abraldes, M. J., ... and Carracedo, A. (2020). Anti-VEGF treatment and response in age-related macular degeneration: disease's susceptibility, pharmacogenetics and pharmacokinetics. *Current Medicinal Chemistry*, 27(4), 549–569.
20. Gote, V., Sikder, S., Sicotte, J., and Pal, D. (2019). Ocular drug delivery: present innovations and future challenges. *Journal of Pharmacology and Experimental Therapeutics*, 370(3), 602–624.

21. de Vries, J. W., Schnichels, S., Hurst, J., Strudel, L., Gruszka, A., Kwak, M., ... and Herrmann, A. (2018). DNA nanoparticles for ophthalmic drug delivery. *Biomaterials*, 157, 98–106.

22. Maccarone, R., Tisi, A., Passacantando, M., and Ciancaglini, M. (2020). Ophthalmic applications of cerium oxide nanoparticles. *Journal of Ocular Pharmacology and Therapeutics*, 36(6), 376–383.

23. Omerović, N., and Vranić, E. (2020). Application of nanoparticles in ocular drug delivery systems. *Health and Technology*, 10(1), 61–78.

24. Chen, F., Si, P., de la Zerda, A., Jokerst, J. V., and Myung, D. (2021). Gold nanoparticles to enhance ophthalmic imaging. *Biomaterials Science*, 9(2), 367–390.

25. Huang, H., Yang, X., Li, H., Lu, H., Oswald, J., Liu, Y., ... and Song, X. (2020). iRGD decorated liposomes: a novel actively penetrating topical ocular drug delivery strategy. *Nano Research*, 13(11), 3105–3109.

26. Gote, V., Sikder, S., Sicotte, J., and Pal, D. (2019). Ocular drug delivery: present innovations and future challenges. *Journal of Pharmacology and Experimental Therapeutics*, 370(3), 602–624.

27. Kuno, N., and Fujii, S. (2011). Recent advances in ocular drug delivery systems. *Polymers*, 3(1), 193–221.

28. Agrahari, V., Mandal, A., Agrahari, V., Trinh, H. M., Joseph, M., Ray, A., ... and Mitra, A. K. (2016). A comprehensive insight on ocular pharmacokinetics. *Drug Delivery and Translational Research*, 6(6), 735–754.

29. Durairaj, C. (2016). Ocular pharmacokinetics. In *Pharmacologic Therapy of Ocular Disease*, Springer, Cham, pp. 31–55.

30. Schoenwald, R. D. (1990). Ocular drug delivery. *Clinical Pharmacokinetics*, 18(4), 255–269.

31. Mandal, A., Patel, M., Sheng, Y., and K Mitra, A. (2016). Design of lipophilic prodrugs to improve drug delivery and efficacy. *Current Drug Targets*, 17(15), 1773–1798.

32. Yasueda, S. I., Inada, K., Matsuhisa, K., Terayama, H., and Ohtori, A. (2004). Evaluation of ophthalmic suspensions using surface tension. *European Journal of Pharmaceutics and Biopharmaceutics*, 57(2), 377–382.

33. Bachu, R. D., Chowdhury, P., Al-Saedi, Z. H., Karla, P. K., and Boddu, S. H. (2018). Ocular drug delivery barriers—role of nanocarriers in the treatment of anterior segment ocular diseases. *Pharmaceutics*, 10(1), 28.

34. Kheirkhah, A., Dohlman, T. H., Amparo, F., Arnoldner, M. A., Jamali, A., Hamrah, P., and Dana, R. (2015). Effects of corneal nerve density on the response to treatment in dry eye disease. *Ophthalmology*, 122(4), 662–668.

35. Farkouh, A., Frigo, P., and Czejka, M. (2016). Systemic side effects of eye drops: a pharmacokinetic perspective. *Clinical Ophthalmology (Auckland, NZ)*, 10, 2433.

36. Andrew, R., Luecke, G., Dozier, S., and Diven, D. G. (2012). A pilot study to investigate the efficacy of Tobramycin–Dexamethasone ointment in promoting wound healing. *Dermatology and Therapy*, 2(1), 1–6.

37. Cagini, C., Mariniello, M., Messina, M., Muzi, A., Balducci, C., Moretti, A., ... and Mencacci, A. (2020). The role of ozonized oil and a combination of tobramycin/dexamethasone eye drops in the treatment of viral conjunctivitis: a randomized clinical trial. *International Ophthalmology*, 40(12), 3209–3215.

38. Souto, E. B., Dias-Ferreira, J., López-Machado, A., Ettcheto, M., Cano, A., CaminsEspuny, A., ... and Sánchez-López, E. (2019). Advanced formulation approaches for ocular drug delivery: state-of-the-art and recent patents. *Pharmaceutics*, 11(9), 460.

39. Kesavan, K., Kant, S., Singh, P. N., and Pandit, J. K. (2011). Effect of hydroxypropyl-β-cyclodextrin on the ocular bioavailability of dexamethasone from a pH-induced mucoadhesive hydrogel. *Current Eye Research*, 36(10), 918–929.

40. Robin, J. S., and Ellis, P. P. (1978). Ophthalmic ointments. *Survey of Ophthalmology*, 22(5), 335–340.

41. Falavarjani, K. G., and Nguyen, Q. D. (2013). Adverse events and complications associated with intravitreal injection of anti-VEGF agents: a review of literature. *Eye*, 27(7), 787–794.

42. Sachdeva, M. M., Moshiri, A., Leder, H. A., and Scott, A. W. (2016). Endophthalmitis following intravitreal injection of anti-VEGF agents: long-term outcomes and the identification of unusual micro-organisms. *Journal of Ophthalmic Inflammation and Infection*, 6(1), 1–7.

43. Semeraro, F., Morescalchi, F., Duse, S., Gambicorti, E., Cancarini, A., and Costagliola, C. (2015). Pharmacokinetic and pharmacodynamic properties of anti-VEGF drugs after intravitreal injection. *Current Drug Metabolism*, 16(7), 572–584.

44. Good, T. J., Kimura, A. E., Mandava, N., and Kahook, M. Y. (2011). Sustained elevation of intraocular pressure after intravitreal injections of anti-VEGF agents. *British Journal of Ophthalmology*, 95(8), 1111–1114.

45. Morioka, M., Takamura, Y., Nagai, K., Yoshida, S., Mori, J., Takeuchi, M., ... and Inatani, M. (2020). Incidence of endophthalmitis after intravitreal injection of an anti-VEGF agent with or without topical antibiotics. *Scientific Reports*, 10(1), 1–6.

46. Menchini, F., Toneatto, G., Miele, A., Donati, S., Lanzetta, P., and Virgili, G. (2018). Antibiotic prophylaxis for preventing endophthalmitis after intravitreal injection: a systematic review. *Eye*, 32(9), 1423–1431.

47. Schargus, M., and Frings, A. (2020). Issues with intravitreal administration of anti-VEGF drugs. *Clinical Ophthalmology (Auckland, NZ)*, 14, 897.

48. Berg, K., Hadzalic, E., Gjertsen, I., Forsaa, V., Berger, L. H., Kinge, B., ... and Bragadóttir, R. (2016). Ranibizumab or bevacizumab for neovascular age-related macular degeneration according to the lucentis compared to avastin study treat-and-extend protocol: two-year results. *Ophthalmology*, 123(1), 51–59.

49. Sun, J. K., Glassman, A. R., Beaulieu, W. T., Stockdale, C. R., Bressler, N. M., Flaxel, C., ... and Diabetic Retinopathy Clinical Research Network. (2019). Rationale and application of the protocol S anti–vascular endothelial growth factor algorithm for proliferative diabetic retinopathy. *Ophthalmology*, 126(1), 87–95.

50. Kiddee, W., and Montriwet, M. (2015). Intraocular pressure changes in non-glaucomatous patients receiving intravitreal anti-vascular endothelial growth factor agents. *PLOS One*, 10(9), e0137833.

51. Macovei, L., Gheorghe, A., Schmitzer, S., Burcea, M., and Morosanu, M. (2021). Ocular drug delivery systems: a review. *Farmacia*, 69(6), 1018–1031.

52. Bengani, L. C., Hsu, K. H., Gause, S., and Chauhan, A. (2013). Contact lenses as a platform for ocular drug delivery. *Expert Opinion on Drug Delivery*, 10(11), 1483–1496.

53. Guzman-Aranguez, A., Colligris, B., and Pintor, J. (2013). Contact lenses: promising devices for ocular drug delivery. *Journal of Ocular Pharmacology and Therapeutics*, 29(2), 189–199.

54. Maulvi, F. A., Soni, T. G., and Shah, D. O. (2016). A review on therapeutic contact lenses for ocular drug delivery. *Drug Delivery*, 23(8), 3017–3026.

55. Xu, J., Xue, Y., Hu, G., Lin, T., Gou, J., Yin, T., ... and Tang, X. (2018). A comprehensive review on contact lens for ophthalmic drug delivery. *Journal of Controlled Release*, 281, 97–118.

56. CinicalTrials.gov. Evaluation of efficacy and safety of an anti-allergy drug with a contact lens in allergic conjunctivitis. http://clinicaltrials.gov/ct2/show/NCT00432757?term=vistakon+AND+contact+lens&rank=6.

57. ClinicalTrials.gov. Evaluation of efficacy and safety of an anti-allergy drug with a contact lens in the treatment of allergic conjunctivitis. http://clinicaltrials.gov/ct2/show/NCT00445874?term=vistakon+AND+contact+lens&rank=7.

58. Kim, J., and Chauhan, A. (2008). Dexamethasone transport and ocular delivery from poly (hydroxyethyl methacrylate) gels. *International Journal of Pharmaceutics*, 353(1–2), 205–222.

59. Sato, T., Uchida, R., Tanigawa, H., Uno, K., and Murakami, A. (2005). Application of polymer gels containing side-chain phosphate groups to drug-delivery contact lenses. *Journal of Applied Polymer Science*, 98(2), 731–735.

60. Danion, A., Brochu, H., Martin, Y., and Vermette, P. (2007). Fabrication and characterization of contact lenses bearing surface-immobilized layers of intact liposomes. *Journal of Biomedical Materials Research Part A*, 82(1), 41–51.

61. Danion, A., Brochu, H., Martin, Y., and Vermette, P. (2007). Fabrication and characterization of contact lenses bearing surface-immobilized layers of intact liposomes. *Journal of Biomedical Materials Research Part A*, 82(1), 41–51.

62. Hiratani, H., Fujiwara, A., Tamiya, Y., Mizutani, Y., and Alvarez-Lorenzo, C. (2005). Ocular release of timolol from molecularly imprinted soft contact lenses. *Biomaterials*, 26(11), 1293–1298.

63. Sano, K., Tokoro, T., and Imai, Y. (1996). A new drug delivery system utilizing piggyback contact lenses. *Acta Ophthalmologica Scandinavica*, 74(3), 243–248.

64. Uchida, R., Sato, T., Tanigawa, H., and Uno, K. (2003). Azulene incorporation and release by hydrogel containing methacrylamide-propyltrimenthylammonium chloride, and its application to soft contact lens. *Journal of Controlled Release*, 92(3), 259–264.

65. Xinming, L., Yingde, C., Lloyd, A. W., Mikhalovsky, S. V., Sandeman, S. R., Howel, C. A., and Liewen, L. (2008). Polymeric hydrogels for novel contact lens-based ophthalmic drug delivery systems: a review. *Contact Lens and Anterior Eye*, 31(2), 57–64.

66. Alvarez-Lorenzo, C., Yañez, F., and Concheiro, A. (2010). Ocular drug delivery from molecularly-imprinted contact lenses. *Journal of Drug Delivery Science and Technology*, 20(4), 237–248.

67. Choi, S. W., and Kim, J. (2018). Therapeutic contact lenses with polymeric vehicles for ocular drug delivery: a review. *Materials*, 11(7), 1125.

68. Devhadrao, N. V., and Siddhaia, M. (2018). Review on ocular insert drug delivery system. *Journal of Drug Delivery and Therapeutics*, 8(5-s), 115–121.

69. Khan, A., Raza, S. N., Itoo, A., Bashir, S., Wani, T. U., and Khan, N. A. (2019). Ocular inserts-a novel approach in ocular drug delivery. *Journal of Drug Delivery and Therapeutics*, 9(4), 693–703.

70. Kriti, D., and Yashika, U. (2019). Ocular inserts: novel approach for drug delivery into eyes. *GSC Biological and Pharmaceutical Sciences*, 7(3), 01–07.

71. Pawar P, Kashyap H, Malhotra S, Sindhu R (2013). Hp-β-CD-voriconazole in situ gelling system for ocular drug delivery: *in vitro*, stability, and antifungal activities assessment. *Biomed Res Int.*, 2013, 341218.

72. Snehaprabha, Bajaj A. (2016). Design of ocular controlled release ocuserts of brinzolamide. *International Journal of Pharmacy*, 6, 191–202.

73. Comez, A. T., Karakilic, A. V., and Yildiz, A. (2019). Silicone perforated punctal plugs for the treatment of punctal stenosis. *Arquivos Brasileiros de Oftalmologia*, 82, 394–399.

74. Ervin, A. M., Law, A., and Pucker, A. D. (2019). Punctal occlusion for dry eye syndrome: summary of a Cochrane systematic review. *British Journal of Ophthalmology*, 103(3), 301–306.

75. Sherwin, J. C., Ratnarajan, G., Elahi, B., Bilkiewicz-Pawelec, A., and Salmon, J. F. (2018). Effect of a punctal plug on ocular surface disease in patients using topical prostaglandin analogues: a randomized controlled trial. *Clinical & Experimental Ophthalmology*, 46(8), 888–894.

76. Song, J. S., Woo, I. H., Eom, Y., and Kim, H. M. (2018). Five misconceptions related to punctal plugs in dry eye management. *Cornea*, 37, S58–S61.

77. Best, A. L., Labetoulle, M., Legrand, M., M'garrech, M., Barreau, E., and Rousseau, A. (2019). Punctal and canalicular plugs: indications, efficacy and safety. *Journal Françaisd'Ophtalmologie*, 42(3), e95–e104.

78. Craig, J. P., Nichols, K. K., Akpek, E. K., Caffery, B., Dua, H. S., Joo, C. K., ... and Stapleton, F. (2017). TFOS DEWS II definition and classification report. *The Ocular Surface*, 15(3), 276–283.

79. Ambati, J., Canakis, C. S., Miller, J. W., Gragoudas, E. S., Edwards, A., Weissgold, D. J., ... and Adamis, A. P. (2000). Diffusion of high molecular weight compounds through sclera. *Investigative Ophthalmology & Visual Science*, 41(5), 1181–1185.

80. Geroski, D. H., and Edelhauser, H. F. (2001). Transscleral drug delivery for posterior segment disease. *Advanced Drug Delivery Reviews*, 52(1), 37–48.

81. Kim, H., Csaky, K. G., Gilger, B. C., Dunn, J. P., Lee, S. S., Tremblay, M., ... and Robinson, M. R. (2005). Preclinical evaluation of a novel episcleral cyclosporine implant for ocular graft-versus-host disease. *Investigative Ophthalmology & Visual Science*, 46(2), 655–662.

82. Gilger, B. C., Moore, C. P., Narfstrom, K., Liu, J., Lawson, C., Cacek, T., ... and Velagaleti, P. (2008). Preclinical acute toxicity and pharmacokinetics of episcleral LX201 implants in rabbits. *Investigative Ophthalmology & Visual Science*, 49(13), 1964–1964.

83. Kuno, N., and Fujii, S. (2011). Recent advances in ocular drug delivery systems. *Polymers*, 3(1), 193–221.

84. García-Estrada, P., García-Bon, M. A., López-Naranjo, E. J., Basaldúa-Pérez, D. N., Santos, A., and Navarro-Partida, J. (2021). Polymeric implants for the treatment of intraocular eye diseases: trends in biodegradable and non-biodegradable materials. *Pharmaceutics*, 13(5), 701.

85. Sim, S., and Wong, N. K. (2021). Nanotechnology and its use in imaging and drug delivery. *Biomedical Reports*, 14(5), 1–9.

86. Reimondez-Troitiño, S., Csaba, N., Alonso, M. J., and De La Fuente, M. (2015). Nanotherapies for the treatment of ocular diseases. *European Journal of Pharmaceutics and Biopharmaceutics*, 95, 279–293.

87. Zhang, J., Jiao, J., Niu, M., Gao, X., Zhang, G., Yu, H., ... and Liu, L. (2021). Ten years of knowledge of nano-carrier based drug delivery systems in ophthalmology: current evidence, challenges, and future prospective. *International Journal of Nanomedicine*, 16, 6497.

88. Khiev, D., Mohamed, Z. A., Vichare, R., Paulson, R., Bhatia, S., Mohapatra, S., ... and Biswal, M. R. (2021). Emerging nano-formulations and nanomedicines applications for ocular drug delivery. *Nanomaterials*, 11(1), 173.

89. Sahoo, S. K., Dilnawaz, F., and Krishnakumar, S. (2008). Nano-technology in ocular drug delivery. *Drug Discovery Today*, 13(3–4), 144–151.

90. Kaur, I. P., Garg, A., Singla, A. K., and Aggarwal, D. (2004). Vesicular systems in ocular drug delivery: an overview. *International Journal of Pharmaceutics*, 269(1), 1–14.

91. Asasutjarit, R., Managit, C., Phanaksri, T., Treesuppharat, W., and Fuongfuchat, A. (2020). Formulation development and *in vitro* evaluation of transferrin-conjugated liposomes as a carrier of ganciclovir targeting the retina. *International Journal of Pharmaceutics*, 577, 119084.

92. Li, N., Zhuang, C., Wang, M., Sun, X., Nie, S., and Pan, W. (2009). Liposome coated with low molecular weight chitosan and its potential use in ocular drug delivery. *International Journal of Pharmaceutics*, 379(1), 131–138.

93. Natarajan, J. V., Chattopadhyay, S., Ang, M., Darwitan, A., Foo, S., Zhen, M., ... and Venkatraman, S. S. (2011). Sustained release of an anti-glaucoma drug: demonstration of efficacy of a liposomal formulation in the rabbit eye. *PLOS ONE*, 6(9), e24513.

94. Dieter, D., Suwan, L., Sabine, D., Chan, K. J., Gregor, S., and Wanda, M. (2006). Comparative study of treatment of the dry eye syndrome due to disturbances of the tear film lipid layer with lipid-containing tear substitutes Efficacy of lipid-containing tear substitutes. *Klin Monatsbl Augenheilkd*, 223, 974–983.

95. Lee, S., Dausch, S., Maierhofer, G., and Dausch, D. (2004). A new therapy concept for the treatment of dry eye--the usefulness of phospholipid liposomes. *Klinische Monatsblatter fur Augenheilkunde*, 221(10), 825–836.

96. Geroski, D. H., and Edelhauser, H. F. (2000). Drug delivery for posterior segment eye disease. *Investigative Ophthalmology & Visual Science*, 41(5), 961–964.

97. Altamirano-Vallejo, J. C., Navarro-Partida, J., Gonzalez-De la Rosa, A., Hsiao, J. H., Olguín-Gutierrez, J. S., Gonzalez-Villegas, A. C., ... and Santos, A. (2018). Characterization and pharmacokinetics of triamcinolone acetonide-loaded liposomes topical formulations

for vitreoretinal drug delivery. *Journal of Ocular Pharmacology and Therapeutics*, 34(5), 416–425.

98. Bidram, E., Esmaeili, Y., Ranji-Burachaloo, H., Al-Zaubai, N., Zarrabi, A., Stewart, A., and Dunstan, D. E. (2019). A concise review on cancer treatment methods and delivery systems. *Journal of Drug Delivery Science and Technology*, 54, 101350.

99. Ge, X., Wei, M., He, S., and Yuan, W. E. (2019). Advances of non-ionic surfactant vesicles (niosomes) and their application in drug delivery. *Pharmaceutics*, 11(2), 55.

100. Durak, S., Esmaeili Rad, M., Alp Yetisgin, A., Eda Sutova, H., Kutlu, O., Cetinel, S., and Zarrabi, A. (2020). Niosomal drug delivery systems for ocular disease—recent advances and future prospects. *Nanomaterials*, 10(6), 1191.

101. Sahoo, R. K., Biswas, N., Guha, A., Sahoo, N., and Kuotsu, K. (2014). Nonionic surfactant vesicles in ocular delivery: innovative approaches and perspectives. *BioMed research international*, 2014, 263604.

102. Aggarwal, D., and Kaur, I. P. (2005). Improved pharmacodynamics of timolol maleate from a mucoadhesive niosomal ophthalmic drug delivery system. *International Journal of Pharmaceutics*, 290(1–2), 155–159.

103. Hashim, I. I. A., El-Dahan, M. S., Yusif, R. M., Abd-ElGawad, A. E. H., and Arima, H. (2014). Potential use of niosomal hydrogel as an ocular delivery system for atenolol. *Biological and Pharmaceutical Bulletin*, 37(4), 541–551.

104. Abdelkader, H., Ismail, S., Kamal, A., and Alany, R. G. (2011). Design and evaluation of controlled-release niosomes and discomes for naltrexone hydrochloride ocular delivery. *Journal of Pharmaceutical Sciences*, 100(5), 1833–1846.

105. Zubairu, Y., Negi, L. M., Iqbal, Z., and Talegaonkar, S. (2015). Design and development of novel bioadhesiveniosomal formulation for the transcorneal delivery of anti-infective agent: *in vitro* and ex vivo investigations. *Asian Journal of Pharmaceutical Sciences*, 10(4), 322–330.

106. Puras, G., Mashal, M., Zárate, J., Agirre, M., Ojeda, E., Grijalvo, S., ... and Pedraz, J. L. (2014). A novel cationic niosome formulation for gene delivery to the retina. *Journal of Controlled Release*, 174, 27–36.

107. Villate-Beitia, I., Gallego, I., Martínez-Navarrete, G., Zárate, J., López-Méndez, T., Soto-Sánchez, C., ... and Pedraz, J. L. (2018). Polysorbate 20 non-ionic surfactant enhances retinal gene delivery efficiency of

cationic niosomes after intravitreal and subretinal administration. *International Journal of Pharmaceutics*, 550(1–2), 388–397.

108. Paradkar, M. U., and Parmar, M. (2017). Formulation development and evaluation of Natamycin niosomal in situ gel for ophthalmic drug delivery. *Journal of Drug Delivery Science and Technology*, 39, 113–122.

109. Shukr, M. H. (2016). Novel in situ gelling ocular inserts for voriconazole-loaded niosomes: design, *in vitro* characterisation and *in vivo* evaluation of the ocular irritation and drug pharmacokinetics. *Journal of Microencapsulation*, 33(1), 71–79.

110. Zeng, W., Li, Q., Wan, T., Liu, C., Pan, W., Wu, Z., ... and Xu, Y. (2016). Hyaluronic acid-coated niosomes facilitate tacrolimus ocular delivery: mucoadhesion, precorneal retention, aqueous humor pharmacokinetics, and transcorneal permeability. *Colloids and Surfaces B: Biointerfaces*, 141, 28–35.

111. Kaur, I. P., Aggarwal, D., Singh, H., and Kakkar, S. (2010). Improved ocular absorption kinetics of timolol maleate loaded into a bioadhesiveniosomal delivery system. *Graefe's Archive for Clinical and Experimental Ophthalmology*, 248(10), 1467–1472.

112. Verma, A., Sharma, G., Jain, A., Tiwari, A., Saraf, S., Panda, P. K., ... and Jain, S. K. (2019). Systematic optimization of cationic surface engineered mucoadhesive vesicles employing Design of Experiment (DoE): a preclinical investigation. *International Journal of Biological Macromolecules*, 133, 1142–1155.

113. More, V. V. (2018). Niosomal drug delivery-a comprehensive review. *Asian Journal of Pharmaceutics (AJP) Free Full Text Articles from Asian J Pharm*, 12(04), S1159–S1164.

114. Nair, A. B., Shah, J., Al-Dhubiab, B. E., Jacob, S., Patel, S. S., Venugopala, K. N., ... and Shinu, P. (2021). Clarithromycin solid lipid nanoparticles for topical ocular therapy: optimization, evaluation and *in vivo* studies. *Pharmaceutics*, 13(4), 523.

115. Seyfoddin, A., Shaw, J., and Al-Kassas, R. (2010). Solid lipid nanoparticles for ocular drug delivery. *Drug Delivery*, 17(7), 467–489.

116. Kumar, N., and Goindi, S. (2021). Development and optimization of itraconazole-loaded solid lipid nanoparticles for topical administration using high shear homogenization process by design of experiments: *in vitro*, ex vivo and *in vivo* evaluation. *AAPS PharmSciTech*, 22(7), 1–21.

117. Cavalli, R., Gasco, M. R., Chetoni, P., Burgalassi, S., and Saettone, M. F. (2002). Solid lipid nanoparticles (SLN) as ocular delivery system

for tobramycin. *International Journal of Pharmaceutics*, 238(1–2), 241–245.

118. Attama, A. A., Reichl, S., and Müller-Goymann, C. C. (2008). Diclofenac sodium delivery to the eye: *in vitro* evaluation of novel solid lipid nanoparticle formulation using human cornea construct. *International Journal of Pharmaceutics*, 355(1–2), 307–313.

119. Liu, R., Zhao, J., Han, Q., Hu, X., Wang, D., Zhang, X., and Yang, P. (2018). One-step assembly of a biomimetic biopolymer coating for particle surface engineering. *Advanced Materials*, 30(38), 1802851.

120. Pla, D., and Gomez, M. (2016). Metal and metal oxide nanoparticles: a lever for C–H functionalization. *ACS Catalysis*, 6(6), 3537–3552.

121. Begines, B., de-Paz, M. V., Alcudia, A., and Galbis, J. A. (2016). Synthesis of reduction sensitive comb-like polyurethanes using click chemistry. *Journal of Polymer Science Part A: Polymer Chemistry*, 54(24), 3888–3900.

122. He, Y., Zhang, F., Saleh, E., Vaithilingam, J., Aboulkhair, N., Begines, B., ... and Wildman, R. D. (2017). A tripropylene glycol diacrylate-based polymeric support ink for material jetting. *Additive Manufacturing*, 16, 153–161.

123. Begines, B., Zamora, F., de Paz, M. V., Roffé, I., Mancera, M., and Galbis, J. A. (2013). Synthesis and characterization of new carbohydrate-based polyureas. *Journal of Renewable Materials*, 1(3), 212–221.

124. Begines, B., Alcudia, A., Aguilera-Velazquez, R., Martinez, G., He, Y., Trindade, G. F., ... and Prado-Gotor, R. (2019). Design of highly stabilized nanocomposite inks based on biodegradable polymer-matrix and gold nanoparticles for Inkjet Printing. *Scientific Reports*, 9(1), 1–12.

125. Sakamoto, K., Lochhead, H., Maibach, H., and Yamashita, Y., eds. (2017). *Cosmetic Science and Technology: Theoretical Principles and Applications*. Elsevier.

126. Rupenthal, I. D. Nanotechnology for ocular drug delivery. In *Design of Nanostructures for Versatile Therapeutic Applications*, Elsevier.

127. Yu, F., Zheng, M., Zhang, A. Y., and Han, Z. (2019). A cerium oxide loaded glycol chitosan nano-system for the treatment of dry eye disease. *Journal of Controlled Release*, 315, 40–54.

128. Sharma, U. K., Verma, A., Prajapati, S. K., Pandey, H., and Pandey, A. C. (2015). *In vitro, in vivo* and pharmacokinetic assessment of amikacin sulphate laden polymeric nanoparticles meant for controlled ocular drug delivery. *Applied Nanoscience*, 5(2), 143–155.

129. Li, F., Wen, Y., Zhang, Y., Zheng, K., Ban, J., Xie, Q., ... and Lu, Z. (2019). Characterisation of 2-HP-β-cyclodextrin-PLGA nanoparticle complexes for potential use as ocular drug delivery vehicles. *Artificial Cells, Nanomedicine, and Biotechnology*, 47(1), 4097–4108.

130. Kalomiraki, M., Thermos, K., and Chaniotakis, N. A. (2016). Dendrimers as tunable vectors of drug delivery systems and biomedical and ocular applications. *International Journal of Nanomedicine*, 11, 1.

131. Chaplot, S. P., and Rupenthal, I. D. (2014). Dendrimers for gene delivery—a potential approach for ocular therapy? *Journal of Pharmacy and Pharmacology*, 66(4), 542–556.

132. Villanueva, J. R., Navarro, M. G., and Villanueva, L. R. (2016). Dendrimers as a promising tool in ocular therapeutics: latest advances and perspectives. *International Journal of Pharmaceutics*, 511(1), 359–366.

133. Nance, E., Zhang, F., Mishra, M. K., Zhang, Z., Kambhampati, S. P., Kannan, R. M., and Kannan, S. (2016). Nanoscale effects in dendrimer-mediated targeting of neuroinflammation. *Biomaterials*, 101, 96–107.

134. Yao, W. J., Sun, K. X., Liu, Y., Liang, N., Mu, H. J., Yao, C., ... and Wang, A. P. (2010). Effect of poly (amidoamine) dendrimers on corneal penetration of puerarin. *Biological and Pharmaceutical Bulletin*, 33(8), 1371–1377.

135. Marano, R. J., Toth, I., Wimmer, N., Brankov, M., and Rakoczy, P. E. (2005). Dendrimer delivery of an anti-VEGF oligonucleotide into the eye: a long-term study into inhibition of laser-induced CNV, distribution, uptake and toxicity. *Gene Therapy*, 12(21), 1544–1550.

136. Krishna, K. B., and Prabhakar, C. (2011). A review on nanosuspensions in drug delivery. *International Journal of Pharma and Bio Sciences*, 2(1), 549–58.

137. Chen, Y., Liu, J., Yang, X., Zhao, X., and Xu, H. (2005). Oleanolic acid nanosuspensions: preparation, in-vitro characterization and enhanced hepatoprotective effect. *Journal of Pharmacy and Pharmacology*, 57(2), 259–264.

138. Schöler, N., Krause, K., Kayser, O., Müller, R. H., Borner, K., Hahn, H., and Liesenfeld, O. (2001). Atovaquone nanosuspensions show excellent therapeutic effect in a new murine model of reactivated toxoplasmosis. *Antimicrobial Agents and Chemotherapy*, 45(6), 1771–1779.

139. Pignatello, R., Bucolo, C., Ferrara, P., Maltese, A., Puleo, A., and Puglisi, G. (2002). Eudragit RS100® nanosuspensions for the

ophthalmic controlled delivery of ibuprofen. *European Journal of Pharmaceutical Sciences*, 16(1–2), 53–61.

140. Kassem, M. A., Rahman, A. A., Ghorab, M. M., Ahmed, M. B., and Khalil, R. M. (2007). Nanosuspension as an ophthalmic delivery system for certain glucocorticoid drugs. *International Journal of Pharmaceutics*, 340(1–2), 126–133.

141. Kamaleddin, M. A. (2017). Nano-ophthalmology: applications and considerations. *Nanomedicine: Nanotechnology, Biology and Medicine*, 13(4), 1459–1472.

142. Lallemand, F., Daull, P., Benita, S., Buggage, R., and Garrigue, J. S. (2012). Successfully improving ocular drug delivery using the cationic nanoemulsion, novasorb. *Journal of Drug Delivery*, 2012, 604204.

143. Ammar, H. O., Salama, H. A., Ghorab, M., and Mahmoud, A. A. (2009). Nanoemulsion as a potential ophthalmic delivery system for dorzolamide hydrochloride. *AAPS PharmSciTech*, 10(3), 808–819.

144. Ismail, A., Nasr, M., and Sammour, O. (2020). Nanoemulsion as a feasible and biocompatible carrier for ocular delivery of travoprost: improved pharmacokinetic/pharmacodynamic properties. *International Journal of Pharmaceutics*, 583, 119402.

145. Morsi, N., Ibrahim, M., Refai, H., and El Sorogy, H. (2017). Nanoemulsion-based electrolyte triggered in situ gel for ocular delivery of acetazolamide. *European Journal of Pharmaceutical Sciences*, 104, 302–314.

146. Pahuja, P., Kashyap, H., and Pawar P. (2014). Design and evaluation of HP-β-CD based voriconazole formulations for ocular drug delivery. *Curr Drug Deliv.*, 11(2), 223–32.

147. Mahboobian, M. M., Mohammadi, M., and Mansouri, Z. (2020). Development of thermosensitive in situ gel nanoemulsions for ocular delivery of acyclovir. *Journal of Drug Delivery Science and Technology*, 55, 101400.

148. Law, S. L., Huang, K. J., and Chiang, C. H. (2000). Acyclovir-containing liposomes for potential ocular delivery: corneal penetration and absorption. *Journal of Controlled Release*, 63(1–2), 135–140.

149. Zeng, W., Li, Q., Wan, T., Liu, C., Pan, W., Wu, Z., ... and Xu, Y. (2016). Hyaluronic acid-coated niosomes facilitate tacrolimus ocular delivery: mucoadhesion, precorneal retention, aqueous humor pharmacokinetics, and transcorneal permeability. *Colloids and Surfaces B: Biointerfaces*, 141, 28–35.

150. Cavalli, R., Gasco, M. R., Chetoni, P., Burgalassi, S., and Saettone, M. F. (2002). Solid lipid nanoparticles (SLN) as ocular delivery system for tobramycin. *International Journal of Pharmaceutics*, 238(1–2), 241–245.

151. Sharma, U. K., Verma, A., Prajapati, S. K., Pandey, H., and Pandey, A. C. (2015). *In vitro, in vivo* and pharmacokinetic assessment of amikacin sulphate laden polymeric nanoparticles meant for controlled ocular drug delivery. *Applied Nanoscience*, 5(2), 143–155.

152. Mishra, V., and Jain, N. K. (2014). Acetazolamide encapsulated dendritic nano-architectures for effective glaucoma management in rabbits. *International Journal of Pharmaceutics*, 461(1–2), 380–390.

153. Masse, F., Ouellette, M., Lamoureux, G., and Boisselier, E. (2019). Gold nanoparticles in ophthalmology. *Medicinal Research Reviews*, 39(1), 302–327.

154. Karakoçak, B. B., Raliya, R., Davis, J. T., Chavalmane, S., Wang, W. N., Ravi, N., and Biswas, P. (2016). Biocompatibility of gold nanoparticles in retinal pigment epithelial cell line. *Toxicology in vitro*, 37, 61–69.

155. Dong, Y., Wan, G., Yan, P., Qian, C., Li, F., and Peng, G. (2019). Fabrication of resveratrol coated gold nanoparticles and investigation of their effect on diabetic retinopathy in streptozotocin induced diabetic rats. *Journal of Photochemistry and Photobiology B: Biology*, 195, 51–57.

156. Boken, J., Khurana, P., Thatai, S., Kumar, D., and Prasad, S. (2017). Plasmonic nanoparticles and their analytical applications: a review. *Applied Spectroscopy Reviews*, 52(9), 774–820.

157. Kim, J. H., Kim, J. H., Kim, K. W., Kim, M. H., and Yu, Y. S. (2009). Intravenously administered gold nanoparticles pass through the blood–retinal barrier depending on the particle size, and induce no retinal toxicity. *Nanotechnology*, 20(50), 505101.

158. Bhattacharya, R., and Mukherjee, P. (2008). Biological properties of "naked" metal nanoparticles. *Advanced Drug Delivery Reviews*, 60(11), 1289–1306.

159. Ewald, A., Glückermann, S. K., Thull, R., and Gbureck, U. (2006). Antimicrobial titanium/silver PVD coatings on titanium. *Biomedical Engineering Online*, 5(1), 1–10.

160. Mathew, T. V., and Kuriakose, S. (2013). Photochemical and antimicrobial properties of silver nanoparticle-encapsulated

chitosan functionalized with photoactive groups. *Materials Science and Engineering C*, 33(7), 4409–4415.

161. Iravani, S., Korbekandi, H., Mirmohammadi, S. V., and Zolfaghari, B. (2014). Synthesis of silver nanoparticles: chemical, physical and biological methods. *Research in Pharmaceutical Sciences*, 9(6), 385.
162. Ge, L., Li, Q., Wang, M., Ouyang, J., Li, X., and Xing, M. M. (2014). Nanosilver particles in medical applications: synthesis, performance, and toxicity. *International Journal of Nanomedicine*, 9, 2399.
163. Anbukkarasi, M., Thomas, P. A., Sheu, J. R., and Geraldine, P. (2017). *In vitro* antioxidant and anticataractogenic potential of silver nanoparticles biosynthesized using an ethanolic extract of Tabernaemontanadivaricata leaves. *Biomedicine & Pharmacotherapy*, 91, 467–475.
164. Zhang, Y., Wang, Z., Zhao, G., and Liu, J. X. (2018). Silver nanoparticles affect lens rather than retina development in zebrafish embryos. *Ecotoxicology and Environmental Safety*, 163, 279–288.
165. Maneewattanapinyo, P., Banlunara, W., Thammacharoen, C., Ekgasit, S., and Kaewamatawong, T. (2011). An evaluation of acute toxicity of colloidal silver nanoparticles. *Journal of Veterinary Medical Science*, 73(11), 1417–1423.
166. Patil, S., Seal, S., Guo, Y., Schulte, A., and Norwood, J. (2006). Role of trivalent La and Nd dopants in lattice distortion and oxygen vacancy generation in cerium oxide nanoparticles. *Applied Physics Letters*, 88(24), 243110.
167. Korsvik, C., Patil, S., Seal, S., and Self, W. T. (2007). Superoxide dismutase mimetic properties exhibited by vacancy engineered ceria nanoparticles. *Chemical Communications*, (10), 1056–1058.
168. Maccarone, R., Tisi, A., Passacantando, M., and Ciancaglini, M. (2020). Ophthalmic applications of cerium oxide nanoparticles. *Journal of Ocular Pharmacology and Therapeutics*, 36(6), 376–383.
169. Chen, J., Patil, S., Seal, S., and McGinnis, J. F. (2006). Rare earth nanoparticles prevent retinal degeneration induced by intracellular peroxides. *Nature Nanotechnology*, 1(2), 142–150.
170. Bhargava, N., Shanmugaiah, V., Saxena, M., Sharma, M., Sethy, N. K., Singh, S. K., ... and Das, M. (2016). Nanocerium oxide increases the survival of adult rod and cone photoreceptor in culture by abrogating hydrogen peroxide-induced oxidative stress. *Biointerphases*, 11(3), 031016.

171. Gupta, A. K., Naregalkar, R. R., Vaidya, V. D., and Gupta, M. (2007). Recent advances on surface engineering of magnetic iron oxide nanoparticles and their biomedical applications. *Nanomedicine (Lond)*, 2(1), 23–39.

172. Giannaccini, M., Giannini, M., Calatayud, M. P., Goya, G. F., Cuschieri, A., Dente, L., and Raffa, V. (2014). Magnetic nanoparticles as intraocular drug delivery system to target retinal pigmented epithelium (RPE). *International Journal of Molecular Sciences*, 15(1), 1590–1605.

173. Bruschi, M. L., and de Toledo, L. D. A. S. (2019). Pharmaceutical applications of iron-oxide magnetic nanoparticles. *Magnetochemistry*, 5(3), 50.

174. Yanai, A., Häfeli, U. O., Metcalfe, A. L., Soema, P., Addo, L., Gregory-Evans, C. Y., ... and Gregory-Evans, K. (2012). Focused magnetic stem cell targeting to the retina using superparamagnetic iron oxide nanoparticles. *Cell Transplantation*, 21(6), 1137–1148.

175. Häfeli, U. O., Riffle, J. S., Harris-Shekhawat, L., Carmichael-Baranauskas, A., Mark, F., Dailey, J. P., and Bardenstein, D. (2009). Cell uptake and *in vitro* toxicity of magnetic nanoparticles suitable for drug delivery. *Molecular Pharmaceutics*, 6(5), 1417–1428.

176. Shen, H. H., Chan, E. C., Lee, J. H., Bee, Y. S., Lin, T. W., Dusting, G. J., and Liu, G. S. (2015). Nanocarriers for treatment of ocular neovascularization in the back of the eye: new vehicles for ophthalmic drug delivery. *Nanomedicine*, 10(13), 2093–2107.

177. Weissig, V., Pettinger, T. K., and Murdock, N. (2014). Nanopharmaceuticals (part 1): products on the market. *International Journal of Nanomedicine*, 9, 4357.

178. Wagner, V., Dullaart, A., Bock, A. K., and Zweck, A. (2006). The emerging nanomedicine landscape. *Nature Biotechnology*, 24(10), 1211–1217.

179. Reimondez-Troitiño, S., Csaba, N., Alonso, M. J., and De La Fuente, M. (2015). Nanotherapies for the treatment of ocular diseases. *European Journal of Pharmaceutics and Biopharmaceutics*, 95, 279–293.

180. Grumezescu, A. M., ed. (2018). *Design of Nanostructures for Versatile Therapeutic Applications*. William Andrew.

181. Medicine USNLo. Study of Efficacy and Tolerability of SYSTANE Complete in Patients with Dry Eye Disease. Available online: https://clinicaltrials.gov/ct2/show/NCT03492541?term=nano&cond=ocular&cntry=US&draw=2&rank=1 (accessed on 27 June 2020).

Chapter 7

Nanotechnology-Based Drug Delivery Systems for the Treatment of Pulmonary Diseases

Shristhi Rawat, Arya Rai, Simrandeep Kaur, Ayushi Goyal, and Inderbir Singh

Chitkara College of Pharmacy, Chitkara University, Punjab, India

inderbir.singh@chitkara.edu.in

Pulmonary delivery is the most promising route for drug delivery as the lungs are capable of absorbing drugs for both local depositions as well as for systemic delivery. Pulmonary disorders are the leading cause of mortality worldwide, major chronic disorders include asthma, chronic obstructive pulmonary disease (COPD), tuberculosis, lung cancer, and cystic fibrosis. Pulmonary barriers (behavioral, mechanical, chemical, and immunological), as well as the diverse mechanisms of particle deposition within the lungs, are the crucial parameters for achieving the therapeutic efficacy of the drug. To conquer all such barriers various nanosystems (liposomes, microparticles, solid lipid nanoparticles, polymeric nanoparticles, carbon nanotubes, and dendrimers) are developed. Some of the patents associated with targeted pulmonary drug delivery are explained in detail in the given chapter.

Nanotechnology and Drug Delivery: Principles and Applications
Edited by Rakesh K. Sindhu

ISBN 978-981-4968-83-6 (Hardcover), 978-1-003-43040-7 (eBook)
www.jennystanford.com

7.1 Introduction

Pharmaceutical researchers and developers have faced challenges with pulmonary drug delivery. The intricate defense system of the human respiratory system frequently prevents drugs from entering circulation and providing the body with a therapeutic dosage. Even if medicine can successfully travel via the nasal passages, it can be challenging to cross the lungs, the circulation, and the intricate web of blood arteries and capillaries. The bloodstream, on the other hand, frequently provides a faster and more direct path to the bloodstream and can get over the defenses [1].

Pulmonary disease conditions such as asthma, cystic fibrosis, pulmonary hypertension, a chronic obstructive pulmonary disorder, and lung tumor have become one of the leading reasons for death. Researchers have made several attempts to create a reliable drug delivery device. Nasal drops and other traditional methods have been replaced by cutting-edge formulation methods including liposomes, nanoparticles, dendrimers, and carbon nanotubes as well as devices like nebulizers and metered drug inhalers. These innovative methods offer a new method for delivering drugs to the lungs' target sites. Such innovative drug delivery methods have the potential to offer prolonged drug release, target delivery, quick onset, and enhanced bioavailability [2].

7.2 Respiratory Tract: Anatomy

The respiratory system encompasses disparate elements: the respiratory tract, the chest wall, central nervous system, and pulmonary circulation [3]. The respiratory tract is fractionated into four pivotal distinct segments: the alveoli, the respiratory bronchioles, the conducting airways, the respiratory bronchioles, and the nasal oropharynx [4]. Naso-oropharynx region embodies the nose, mouth (oral/buccal cavity), pharynx, and larynx (all comprise upper airways). This upper airway region heats, humidifies, warms and filter/purify the inhaled air ante it reaches to alveoli [5]. The lower airways comprehend trachea (conducting airways), bronchi, and bronchioles (secondary, tertiary terminal bronchioles) alveoli. The lower airway region equips mucous protection and immunological characteristics to the lungs [6]. Gas commutation takes place at the alveoli level, thereupon alveoli supply oxygen to the body organs as obligatory for regular day-to-day activities [4] (Fig. 7.1). The total surface area of human lungs is approx. 130–180 m^2. Nearby billions of alveoli are immersed amid the capillaries to establish an air-blood interface. Alveoli's surface is the major primary area for O_2 and CO_2 gas diffusion and exchange. In the alveolar region, gases and blood are in close contact with each other across a large surface area [7, 8]. The right lung is demarcated into lower, middle, and upper lobes, which are additionally sub-partitioned into divergent fragments, whereas the left lung embodies upper and lower lobes [4]. Lungs perform a key role in breathing, transporting oxygen to body tissues (this phenomenon is christened as inspiration/inhalation), and displacing carbon dioxide out of the body tissues (labeled as expiration/exhalation). The respiratory system conducts/transports oxygen from the outside environment to the mitochondria in the cells across the entire body and thereby a major route for the entrance of toxic and foreign substances from outside air into the human body [9, 10]. The entire respiratory tract is divided with a thin layer (having a thickness of about 0.1–0.2 μm) capillary network of the alveolar vascular epithelium [5]. There are four pivotal histological layers within the respiratory system: The respiratory mucosa consists of the epithelium and lamina propriety (supporting layer), cartilage or muscular layer, submucosa, and adventitia. The larger segment of the respiratory tract, extending from the nasal cavity to the bronchi, is covered with pseudostratified columnar ciliated epithelium. The bronchioles are covered by cuboidal epithelium to simple columnar cells. The alveoli, which are responsible for gaseous exchange, are lined with squamous epithelium. The major part of the respiratory tract is webbed with ciliated pseudostratified columnar epithelium except for the larynx and pharynx segments. The function of ciliated pseudostratified columnar epithelium is to protect against foreign particles and pathogens, furthermore curtails/lessens the infections and tissue injury via utilization of mucociliary elevator [11].

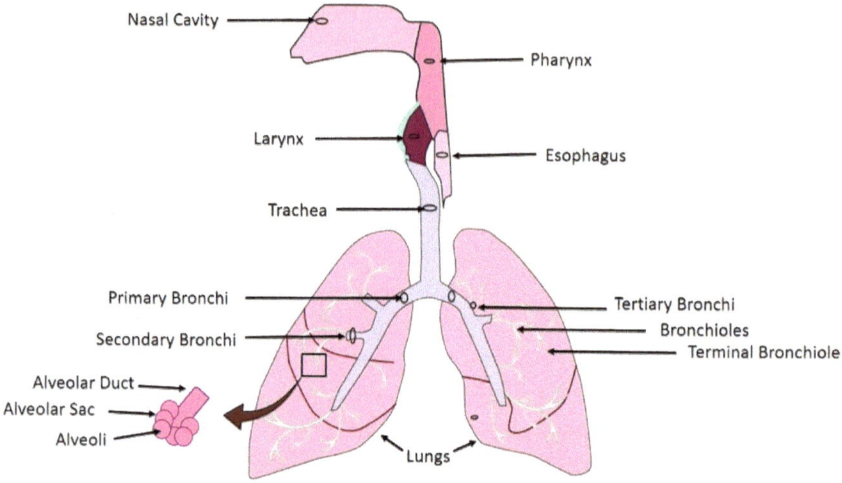

Figure 7.1 Organ and structure of respiratory system.

7.3 Primary Pulmonary Disorders Targeted by Potential Drug Delivery Systems

Among all the diseases occurring worldwide, pulmonary diseases are the third most common cause of mortality. They range from bronchiolitis, cough, common cold, and irregular breathing to more life-threatening diseases such as asthma, cystic fibrosis, pulmonary hypertension, chronic obstructive pulmonary disease, and lung cancer. A decisive method is pulmonary drug delivery, which is appropriate for local and systemic effects. Factors that construct the pulmonary system as a standard delivery target comprise thin alveolar absorptive membranes, high solute exchange capacity, vast epithelial surface area, and high vascularization [12]. The pulmonary route is an appropriate system for the delivery of drugs that have poor oral absorption and are broken down by stomach acid and first-pass metabolism in the liver [13]. Evidence supports the application of a targeted drug delivery system in the cure of pulmonary-related diseases. They cover lung cancer, cystic fibrosis, asthma, and pneumonia [14].

Firstly, cystic fibrosis is an autosomal recessive genetic disorder in which there is enormous production of mucous that causes respiratory infections, respiratory breakdown, and pulmonary blockage [15]. The exchange of gases in the lungs is affected in the case of pneumonia which is a lung parenchymal infection. It is initiated by toxic chemicals or other catastrophic foreign particulates or protozoal, bacteria, fungal and viral infection. Fatigue, shortness of breath, chest pain, confusion, and fever are the prevailing indications of this disease. To cure pneumonia, various classes of drugs are used, including cough suppressants, antibiotics, and antifungals.

Bronchial asthma is considered a type of COPD, distinguished by airflow hindrance because of numerous stimuli comprising environmental allergy, psychological components, and infection. Drugs that are used commonly for the treatment include immunomodulators, mast cell stabilizers, bronchodilators, corticosteroids, and leukotriene modifiers [12].

Further, lung cancer is a notably persistent malignant tumor occurring globally with a high fatality rate [12]. Unbalanced diet, susceptibility, occupational exposure, tobacco, and air pollution are some of the common causes of lung cancer [16]. Tuberculosis is a major health concern around the globe. Pulmonary tuberculosis arises due to lungs infection where a massive amount of infectious bacilli are present in the alveoli. Pulmonary tuberculosis can be cured by effective therapies like directly observed therapy (DOTs) and multi-drug therapy is currently used therapy for the treatment of pulmonary tuberculosis [19]. Toxicity, side effects, and adverse reactions are various drawbacks of various drug combinations. However, targeted carrier systems provide less toxicity and fewer adverse drug reactions, and more therapeutic efficacy [17].

Chronic obstructive pulmonary disorder modulates a chronic lung disorder majorly chronic obstructive bronchitis and emphysema. It is identified by respiratory muscle dysfunction, hyperinflammation, airflow limitation, and bronchial inflammation [19]. Various components that initiate the pathogenesis of COPD include genetic predisposition environmental exposure, and cigarette smoking. For the treatment of COPD corticosteroids, anticholinergics, beta-agonists, and long-acting bronchodilators are targeted [18].

7.4 Mechanism of Novel Drug Carrier Administered by Naso-Pulmonary Route

Nanoparticulate systems such as microparticles, solid lipid nanoparticles (SLNs), liposomes, nanosuspensions, Dendrimers, polymeric nanosystems, and inorganic nanoparticles are extensively employed for pulmonary drug delivery to treat local respiratory infections and diseases(such as bronchitis, COPD, asthma, lung cancer). Nanocarriers encapsulate drugs such as toxic anticancer agents (doxorubicin utilized to treat lung cancer) and lessen systemic toxicity. These nanoparticulate systems are having the size dimensions of nano or microns (1–5 μm) and have the capability to penetrate profoundly into the lungs thus efficiently and effectively providing target site-specific drug distribution. These nanosystems are inhaled into the respiratory route with disparate devices such as aerosols, nebulizers, metered-dose inhalers (MDI), and pressurized metered-dose inhalers (pMDI). Nanopariculates after inhalation (by using different inhalation devices) contact with the mucosal membrane, this association between inhaled nano particulates and the mucosal layer causes the dissolution of the nanosystem. Particles having smaller diameters exhibit better interaction with mucosal membrane and displayed a high dissolution rate and ultimately leading to drug release at a specific site, dwindling systemic adverse effects, and ameliorating the bioavailability of active drug molecules. Nanocarriers are readily uptaken by tumor cells within the lungs by endocytosis, contributing towards the enhancement of antitumor efficacy of active therapeutic agents [19, 20].

Pulmonary drug deposition is a complicated process that is influenced by particle size, velocity, respiratory tract location, and lung capacity. Due to impaction, large particles (>10 μm) get deposited in the oropharynx and larynx. Usually, very tiny particles (less than 0.5 μm) are generally not deposited and are expelled upon exhalation [21].

Impaction

The bronchial region experiences the most impaction deposition and is a widely observed phenomenon with bigger particles. The particles deposit by their aerodynamic diameter and inertia. Due to impaction at the airway surface and inertia, particle movement occurs with the airflow. The bronchial area experiences increased particle deposition due to impactions.

Sedimentation

It is a process of particles settling in the bronchi, bronchioles as well as in alveoli based on the rate of sedimentation depending on the particles' diameter and settling rate. The size of hygroscopic particles may enhance as they migrate through the moist airway sedimentation-related deposits.

Interception

Due to the physical size and shape of the particles, contact between the airway surface and the particles may result in an interception. Fibrous particles typically involve interception in the respiratory airways because of their length.

Diffusion

Due to Brownian motion, diffusion is the process of moving particles from a location of higher concentration to a region of lower concentration. The diffusion deposition phenomenon occurs from the nasopharynx also in the smaller airways of the pulmonary region, where airflow is less [22].

Absorption

The drug particle absorption is regulated by epithelial cells that cover the lungs. The thickness of epithelial cells in the trachea is about 50–70 μm and approximately 0.2 μm in the alveoli region of the lungs. These are regions that are important and targeted for the absorption of the drug in the lungs [23].

7.5 Pulmonary Barrier

Given the most recent developments in the post-genomic age, physiology, associated areas of molecular biology, morphology, a deeper knowledge of the molecular and biochemical makeup of the lung tissue is crucial. Following such advancements would primarily aid in understanding issues related to the molecular basis of illnesses and obstacles to therapeutic delivery [24]. Due to several sorts of obstacles, including behavioral, chemical, mechanical, and immunological barriers, drug administration via the pulmonary route is highly difficult. Drug distribution to the lungs was a difficult problem up until the second half of the 20th century because the pulmonary defense mechanisms were not well understood back then [25]. However, by properly resolving these issues, pharmaceutical scientists can design efficient medication delivery methods for targeting the lungs (Fig. 7.2).

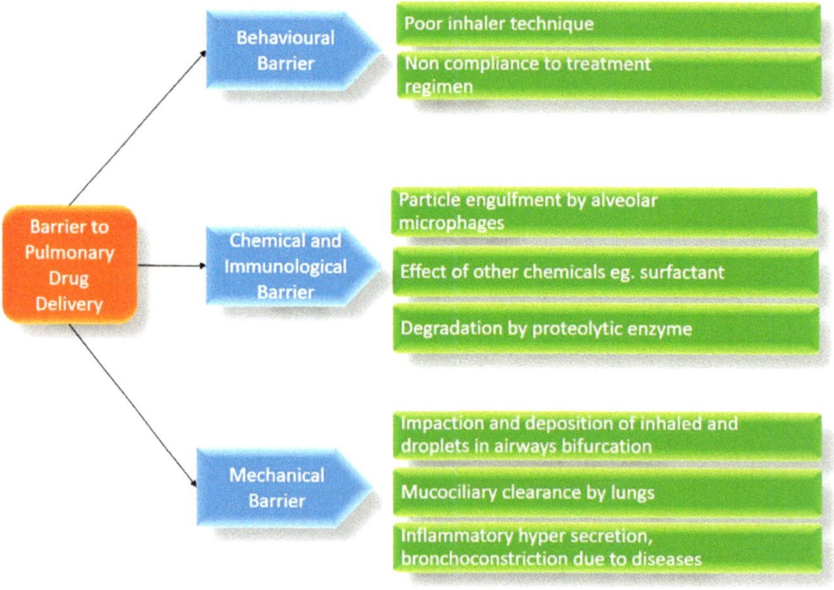

Figure 7.2 Different types of barriers for pulmonary target drug delivery.

Mechanical barrier: the bronchial tree, a sophisticated network of airway tissues, makes up the lungs. There are various airway bifurcations that a particle proceeds from the alveolar area to the epithelial target sites may deposit in. Because of disease-related inflammation, bronchoconstriction, or mucous hyper secretion, the pulmonary region's mechanical barrier becomes more prominent. By clearing the accumulated particles from the airways, lung mucociliary clearance also provides important mechanical barrier properties [25].

Chemical and immunological: chemical and immunological obstacles in the administration of pulmonary drugs include alveolar macrophage, surfactants, and proteolytic enzymes. The hydrolysis of protein and peptides in the lungs is carried out by proteolytic enzymes such as endopeptidase and cathepsin H [26]. Phosphocytic cells called alveolar macrophages absorb toxic particles and eliminate them from the lungs. Surfactants facilitate the elimination of inhaled particles by macrophages by preventing them from adhering to the epithelial membrane of the lungs [27].

Behavioral barrier: patient characteristics such as non-adherence to the therapeutic regimen, which might be intentional or unintentional, can have a substantial impact on the therapy's outcome. Furthermore, cultural variables may contribute to patients' non-compliance. Suboptimal and unpredictable medication deposition in the lungs could result from poor inhaler technique and handling errors [28].

7.6 Strategies for Pulmonary Target Drug Delivery

Inhalation drug delivery has the potential to improve the efficacy and safety of inhaled therapies for respiratory disorders. The principal advantages of inhaled administration are rapid drug absorption and elimination from the blood, which is less likely to be affected by gastrointestinal side effects than oral administration. Inhaled dosage forms are also convenient, portable, and can be used anywhere, making them an attractive alternative to oral administration for some indications. However, inhaled dosage forms are limited to use only in the lung, which is not always an adequate site for *in vivo* drug delivery [29].

Approaches

Drug delivery at the pulmonary region is acquired by different types of approaches. The aim is to convey the drug at the target region to attain maximum bioavailability of it. The required bioavailability is achieved by increasing the drug retention time at the target site. The major factor that determines the type drug release system is the type of polymer used.

1. Immediate drug release system.
2. Controlled drug release systems – such as liposomes, nanoparticles, microparticles and micelles.
3. Sustained drug release system – such as microspheres.

The control and sustained drug release system comes with several advantages such as increased duration of action, reduced dosing frequency, aided patient compliance, economical and increased bioavailability. The selection of carrier polymer plays an important role and is made according to the disease. Formulations, method of preparation, and delivery device are considered according to the disease state and target site [30].

Naso-Pulmonary Route for Drug Delivery is the ideal non-invasive route for a local and systemic therapeutic action of drug molecules, this route displays a wide surface area for drug absorption, eventually leads to augmented bioavailability, efficacy, and accelerated therapeutic efficacy, dwindles the amount of dose administered, lessened undesirable systemic adverse effects. The pulmonary route exhibits high vascularization, a non-invasive pathway, and bypasses the first-pass metabolism [31]. Pulmonary Route is appropriate pathway for targeting alveolar macrophages, maintaining sustained and controlled drug release, and abating drug toxicity [32].

7.6.1 Liposomes

Liposomes are small, spherical-shaped vesicles having single or multiple concentric lipoidal bilayers (of natural non-toxic phospholipids and cholesterol, non-polar and lipophilic drugs are entrapped in lipoidal bilayer) that surround an aqueous compartment (Polar/Hydrophilic drugs are loaded in the aqueous core) (Fig. 7.3). Prevalent methods of liposome preparations are the **mechanical dispersion method** (sonication, membrane extrusion, lipid film hydration, micro emulsification methods), **solvent dispersion method** (Ether injection, reverse phase evaporation, ethanol injection, method), **and detergent removal method**.

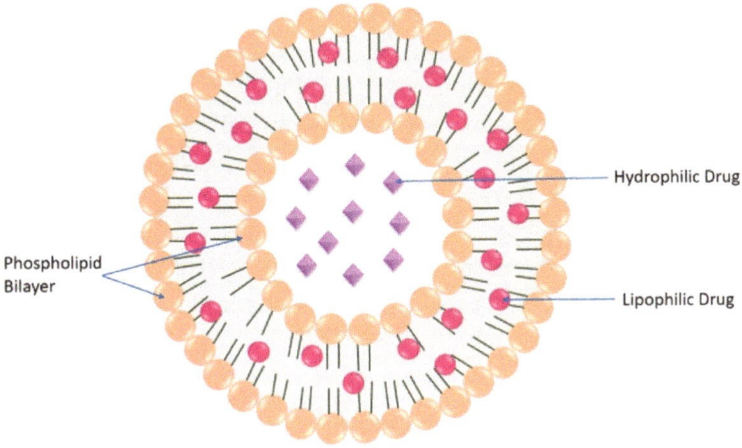

Figure 7.3 Structure of liposome.

Liposomes are extensively used as a drug delivery system owing to their similarity with cell membranes as well as their capability to load both hydrophobic and hydrophilic drug molecules, in the treatment of disparate diseases such as diverse types of cancer (Lung cancer, Breast cancer, Prostate cancer cytoplasm, and cell nucleus cancer), parasitic infections and diseases such as-Leishmaniasis. Likewise, Liposomes are extensively utilized as an analytical reagent/tool in biophysics, colloidal science, biochemistry, and biology field [33, 34]. Liposomes as a drug delivery system play a remarkable role in the preparation of formulations of potent drugs and multiply the therapeutic efficacy of the drug, distribute the drug at the specific target site, lessening the drug toxicity. The liposome drug delivery system transports the drug to a specific desired site without or with the expression of target recognition molecules on the lipoidal membrane. Liposomes are comprehensively employed to deliver divergent drug molecules such as antifungal, antiviral, antitubercular drugs, antibiotics, anti-inflammatory drugs, anesthetics, vaccines, and genes [35, 36]. Furthermore, liposomes are extensively utilized for the delivery of therapeutic molecules in peripheral airways using different devices such as medical nebulizers, aerosols, and metered-dose inhalers, contributing toward the safe and controlled/sustained release of drugs in the lungs [37]. Liposomes are employed as carriers for the delivery of antimycobacterials to treat *Mycobacterium avium* intracellular infections within alveolar macrophages [38].

Paclitaxel (PTX) was more effectively delivered to the lungs by liposome aerosol formulations than through intravenous ways, according to research by Koshkina et al. in mice via injection [39]. Fritz et al. demonstrated that clodronate loaded with liposomes decreased the number of macrophages by 50% after 4–6 weeks of treatment and dramatically decreased the capacity of tumor cells to proliferate in a mouse model of carbamate-induced lung tumor [40]. Salbutamol sulfate (SBS) aerosol was encapsulated in liposomes by Chen et al. [41] who also showed that the complexes demonstrated longer-lasting impacts on asthma than unrestricted SBS. In addition, Witten et al. [42] conducted a phase I clinical trial to examine the use of cisplatin liposomal preparation in lung cancer. Their findings suggested that this medication delivery technology might improve drug absorption while minimizing systemic adverse effects. Some more applications of liposome formulation in drug delivery are given in Table 7.1.

7.6.2 Microparticles

Microparticles are solid particulates having sizes in dimensions 1–1000 μm, and behave as a multi-unit drug delivery system. Microparticles are membrane vesicles that are liberated from diverse cell types and vary in size, protein as well as in phospholipid composition. **Microspheres** embody a homogenous, uniform mixture of API and polymers, **microcapsules** composed of polymeric coat that encloses drug molecule. Reliant on their size, shape, and surface characteristics [57], they get deposited in disparate body tissues/parts and contribute towards the sustained/controlled and targeted area-specific drug release. Microparticulates pulmonary drug delivery ameliorates/improves.

Table 7.1 Applications of liposome in drug delivery system for the treatment of pulmonary disease

Drug	Disease	Remarks	Ref.
Amphotericin-B (AmB)	Lung infection, ARDS (Acute Respiratory Distress Syndrome)	AmB-loaded liposomes lead to diminished adverse/toxic effects of amphotericin and enhanced encapsulation efficiency by better interaction of AmB with lipids, reported Suitable for use in infants by pulmonary instillation	[43]
Amphotericin-B	Lung infections (Cryptococcosis, aspergillosis)	Dwindled renal toxicity, improved therapeutic efficacy, long circulation time, and better penetration into tissues, declared not for pulmonary route administration, can be injected by IV route with high amphotericin dose safely (1–30 mg/kg)	[44]
Amikacin	Cystic fibrosis Lung infections, *Mycobacterium avium* complex (MAC Bacterial infection)	Nebulized amikacin administration increases drug penetration to alveolar macrophage (a site of infection) available in dry powder form and is administered by inhalation route/or in nebulization form	[45]
Ciprofloxacin	Cystic fibrosis lung infection [8]	Assures improved protection against Gram-negative bacteria Yersinia Pestis, preferred to administer by the inhalation route	[46]
Vincristine	Leukemia	Highly effective for the treatment of blood cancer, prolonged drug retention in blood, the improved therapeutic index of drug	[47]
Prostaglandin analogue (Iloprost)	Pulmonary Arterial Hypertension (PAH)	Used as a potent vasorelaxing agent in the treatment of pulmonary hypertension, peripheral vascular disease and for treating Raynaud's Phenomenon	[48]
Cisplatin	Lung cancer	PARI LC Star jet nebulizer is used for administration, phase I study results in nausea, fatigue, and hoarseness	[49]

(*Continued*)

Table 7.1 (*Continued*)

Drug	Disease	Remarks	Ref.
IL-2	Lung cancer	Inhalation by Puritan Bennett twin jet nebulizer causes mild cough immediately after inhalation during *in vivo* studies	[50]
Insulin	Diabetes mellitus	Enhancement in drug bioavailability provides sustained/controlled drug release, increased retention in lungs, reduced extra-pulmonary side effects, and better encapsulation of insulin in liposomes used by aerosolization	[51]
N-acetyl cysteine	Mucus hypertension during lung inflammation, ARDS 9	Inhalation results in sustained and controlled release of the drug, and better uptake of chitosan-loaded liposomes by lung epithelial cells	[52]
Cholestryl sulfate + AmB (1:1)	Fungal Lung infection	Miniature size, thin disc-shaped, deliver AmB quickly to phagocytic cells but such liposomal formulations have lesser/short circulation time in comparison to ambisome	[53]
Doxorubicin	Leukemia, Lung & Breast cancer, Ovarian cancer	Ameliorated stability of active ingredient, target site delivery, and improved biodistribution of the drug	[54]
Chemotherapeutic drug-Triptolide	Lung cancer	Enhancement in cellular uptaken efficiency, the efficient killing of tumor cells, provides a sustained effect	[55]
Ciprofloxacin (CPFX)	Respiratory intracellular Parasite infection	Ameliorated antibacterial effect without inducing any cytotoxic effect on lung tissues	[56]

The bioavailability and effectiveness of API in comparability to other routes of drug administration. Techniques that are comprehensively employed for the development of inhalation microparticulate systems are [58] spray drying, supercritical fluid technique, micronization, bottom-up, and spray freezing techniques. Microparticles are broadly used for drug delivery as they certify the target site-specific drug distribution, dwindle the pitfall of dose dumping and burst impact, ameliorate the stability and compatibility, and lessened the intra and inter-subject variations [59]. Microparticles provide appropriate protection/shield to the enclosed active agent from deterioration and assure sustained/controlled drug release and effortless administration [60]. Polymeric microspheres, as well as Solid lipid microparticles, are employed as pulmonary route drug carrier systems to provide sustained-release effect of the therapeutic agent. SLM (Solid lipid microparticles) are physicochemically stable, and physiologically compatible, large-scale production at a lesser cost is achievable [61]. Microparticles are an appropriate tool to target site-specific drug delivery in respiratory airways to treat different pulmonary diseases such as cystic fibrosis, asthma, COPD, pulmonary hypertension, Pulmonary tract infections, and lung cancer [62].

Budesonide inhalable microparticles were created by Parsian et al. utilizing a spray freeze-drying technique. They synthesized budesonide micronized porous particles with L-leucine and hydroxypropyl beta-cyclodextrin (HP-b-CD) as excipients. The resultant particles had an enhanced nanoparticle fraction and suitable MMAD (FPF). Additionally, compared to other formulations, their dissolving rate and aerosolization performance were enhanced [63].

Tacrolimus was made into inhalable microparticles and nanoparticles using this method by Wu et al. to target deep lung tissue delivery. Studies using laser diffraction and scanning electron microscopy demonstrated that the respirable micro-particles had an ideal MMAD with a size range of 1.29–1.62 mm, suited for deep lung administration [64].

Polycaprolactone was used by Dimer et al. to create inhalable microparticles containing resveratrol for the diagnosis of pulmonary arterial hypertension. Vibrational atomization spray drying was used to create the particles, and the aerodynamic behavior of the particles was examined. The particles' sustained-release profile demonstrated the potential for the delivery of resveratrol via the pulmonary route for the therapy of arterial hypertension. They had an MMAD of 2.32 mm and an FPF of 50% [65].

Alireza Vatanara and colleagues considered the utilization of spray freeze-drying to create parathyroid hormone-containing porous microparticles for pulmonary administration. They also examined how other excipients, including L-leucine and HP-b-CD, affected the microparticles. When compared to particles made from HPV-CD, L-leucine-prepared particles displayed improved aerodynamic behavior. The bioavailability of parathyroid hormone significantly increased, indicating that the inhalable microparticulate form of hormone therapy was superior to injectable hormone therapy [66]. Some more applications of microparticle formulation in drug delivery are given in Table 7.2.

7.6.3 Carbon Nanotube

Carbon nanotubes (CNTs) are synthetic nanomaterials that resemble fibers and have distinctive electrical, mechanical, and thermal characteristics (Fig. 7.4). The most extensively used carbon nanotubes are single-walled carbon nanotubes (SWCNTs) and multiwalled carbon nanotubes (MWCNTs). They might either be in their natural state or as constructions with altered surfaces [80, 81]. Due to its large surface area and ability to adsorb or conjugate with a range of pharmacological and diagnostic substances and effectively used in the medical field. Recently, scientists have used CNTs to identify and cure the pulmonary disease [82]. Research has shown that using carbon nanotubes for medical diagnostics is an efficient strategy and research has demonstrated that the immunological reaction *in vivo* is not rare and is used in the targeted therapy [83, 84]. Some carbon nanotube-containing drugs for pulmonary disease are given in Table 7.3.

Table 7.2 Applications of microparticle in drug delivery system for the treatment of pulmonary disease

Drug	Disease	Remarks	Ref.
Salbutamol acetonide loaded SLMs	Employed as broncho-dilator agent in treatment of lung conditions such as asthma attacks	Provides sustained release of therapeutic agent, long-term protection	[61]
Doxorubicin-loaded PLGA (polylactic-co-glycolic acid) microparticles	Lung cancer	Ensures sustained/prolonged local delivery by inhalation	[62]
Corticosteroids	Employed to treat allergic conditions like asthma, allergic bronchopulmonary aspergillosis, diminishes the risk of RDS (respiratory distress condition)	Achieves deep lung deposition, no aggregation under effect of shear force	[67]
Chemotherapeutics	Lung cancer	Deep Lung Deposition, exhibits best efficacy with least adverse effects	[68]
Insulin	Diabetes mellitus (Types I and II)	Prolonged residence time of 6–48 h, improved metabolic control	[69]
Budesonide	Allergic conditions like asthma	Dwindles irritation, swelling, provides sustained release of drug and improved respiratory tract functions	[70]
Paclitaxel	Lung cancer	Paclitaxel-loaded alginate microparticles exhibit similar effectiveness as of free paclitaxel, target site-specific drug distribution, ensure slow release of drug and thereby provide sustained therapeutic API effect	[71]
Docetaxel (DTX)	Employed for treatment of locally advanced and metastatic non-small cell lung cancer	DTX-enclosed chitosan microparticles lead to improved Drug encapsulation efficacy (enhanced up to 88%), reduced systemic toxicity, provides sustained release and improved bioavailability	[72]

(Continued)

Table 7.2 (*Continued*)

Drug	Disease	Remarks	Ref.
Polyketal microparticles	Used to treat inflammation that occurs in lungs distal alveolar spaces during interstitial lung disease	Such polyketal-coated microparticles exhibit anti-inflammatory effect, provide sustained release of drug	[73]
Turbutaline sulfate	Utilized to treat allergic conditions such as asthma, COPD	Turbutaline sulfate act as a bronco-dilator Provide sustain drug release, ensures long-term effect of drug, absence of burst drug release, reduction in repetitive drug use, better patient compliance	[74]
Chitosan beads loaded adriamycin	For target delivery of chemo-therapeutic drugs such as adriamycin (for treatment of small cell lung cancer)	Enhanced efficacy of drug, long-term survival of patients,	[75]
Superpara magnetic iron oxide nanoparticles (SPIONs) and doxorubicin-loaded dry powder NIMs (nano-in-microparticles)	Used for treatment of lung cancer	Target site delivery under presence of magnetic field, enhancement in therapeutic cytotoxicity of doxorubicin	[76]
Camptothecin-loaded Ac-DEX (acetalated dextran microparticles)	For treatment of lung diseases such as lung cancer	Ensure targeted pulmonary delivery of drug to specific target site (alveolar region of lungs)	[77]
Micro RNA (mir-146a) encapsulated NCMPs (Nanocomposite Microparticles)	For treatment of COPD (chronic obstructive pulmonary disease)	Inhalation of NCMPs enclosed micro RNA plays a beneficial role in appropriate treatment and management of COPD	[78]
Azithromycin (AZM) encapsulated FDKP microparticles (N-fumaroylated diketo piperazine	Lung infections: pneumonia (caused by *Streptococcus pneumoniae*)	Efficient target site delivery, reduced systemic toxicity, lessens the chances of developing antibiotic resistance by bacteria	[79]

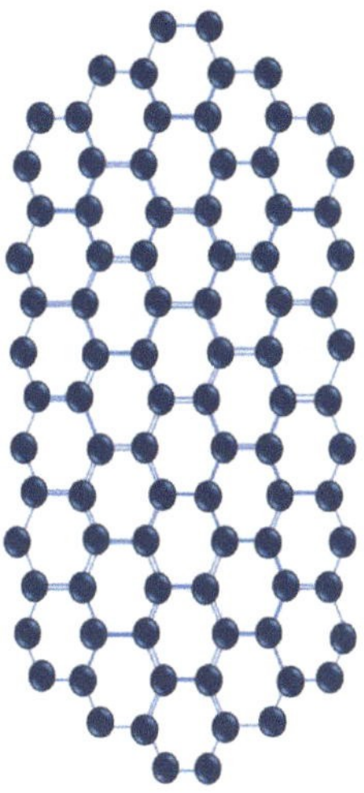

Figure 7.4 Structure of carbon nanotube.

Lodhi et al. developed dexamethasone conjugated multi wall carbon nanotubes (MWCNTs) for controlled delivery of a doxorubicin with reduced toxicity [85]. On cancer cells, the combination of MWCNTs, doxorubicin, and dexamethasone was more toxic, had a less hemolytic impact, and had superior and faster dispersion and diffusion. According to Li et al., the use of MWCNTs in combination with cisplatin as a chemotherapy agent increased treatment efficacy while reducing adverse effects such as liver and renal damage [89]. This effective carrier can raise the concentrations of platinum that accumulate in target organs like the lungs. The research on mice demonstrated that CNTs don't have aberrant immunological or inflammatory reactions. Docetaxel is 136 times more effective when combined with an MWCNT carrier that has been conjugated with the transferrin protein, according to research by Singh et al. and according to reports, A549 cancer cells took the medication in significantly greater amounts. The medication absorption in A549 cancer cells was reportedly considerably greater. A different study from 2016 found that this medication and MWCNT coated with d-alpha-tocopheryl polyethylene glycol 1000 succinate are superior to non-targeted treatment [87]. Some more application of carbon nanotubes formulation in drug delivery is mentioned in following given Table 7.3.

Table 7.3 Applications of carbon nanotubes in drug delivery system for the treatment of pulmonary disease

Type of CNTs	Disease	Drugs/Protein	Remark	Ref.
Multiwall carbon nanotube [MWCNTs]	Lung cancer	Doxorubicin (DOX)	DOX-loaded HA-MWCNTs are targeting the A549 and showed 3.2 times more cytotoxic effects and enhanced apoptotic action was seen	[85]
Multiwall carbon nanotube	Lung cancer	Docetaxel/ Coumarin-6	Multiwalled carbon nanotubes (MWCNT) that were infused with docetaxel and treated with d-alpha-tocopheryl polyethylene glycol 1000 succinate (TPGS)/coumarin-6 are targeting the A549 and showed better Efficacy with safety	[87]
Single-wall carbon nanotube [SWNTs]	Lung cancer	Paclitaxel	SWNT and graphene oxide (GO) are examples of carbon nanostructures (CNs) targeting the NCI-H460 and A549, that can be used to increase the effectiveness of paclitaxel a bioactive chemical that is used to treat lung cancer	[88]
Single-wall carbon nanotube	Lung cancer	Gemcitabine	CNTs were formed by acylation, carboxylation, amination, PEGylation, and formulate GEM conjugation which are targeting the A549 and showing better antitumor effect	[89]
MWCNT	Lung cancer	Methotrexate	A formulation made of chitosan- and multiwalled carbon nanotubes was suggested as a pH-responsive vector for methotrexate targeting the MRC-5 while improving the anticancer efficacy on H1299	[90]
MWCNT	Lung cancer	siRNA	CNT-based siRNA delivery has observed enhanced therapeutic efficacy; the CNT-based siRNA delivery is directly proportional to its enhanced retention in tumor cells	[91]

Type of CNTs	Disease	Drugs/Protein	Remark	Ref.
MWCNT	Lung cancer	Betulinic acid	The MWCNT-BA combination was shown to have an improved antitumor effect against the A549 cell line as compared to the HepG2 cell line	[92]
SWCNT		Curcumin	The study has seen potential of secreted CUR from modified SWCNTs for preventing the spread of cancer cells by causing apoptosis	[93]
MWCNT	Respiratory infection	Amoxicillin	AM-MWNT hybrid material was reported to exhibit increased antibacterial action	[94]
MWCNTs	Tuberculosis	Isoniazid	In combination with its antibacterial activity, MWCNT increases the drug distribution of INZ at lower doses than the medication alone; one of its key antimicrobial mechanisms involves the breakdown of the bacterial cell wall; therefore, a range of *Mycobacterium tuberculosis* strains was more effectively killed by INZ-conjugated MWCNTs	[95]
Multiwall carbon nanotube	Tuberculosis	Pyrazinamide	Creating a compound made of GO and multiwalled carbon nanotubes (MWCNTs) that have been dispersed, which show the better sensitivity of pyrazinamide	[96]
Single-wall carbon nanotube	Lung cancer	Tumor necrosis factor-related apoptosis-inducing ligand (TRAIL)	Through noncovalent 1-pyrenebutanoic acid N-hydrosuccinimide ester (PSE), SWCNT was designed and synthesized with TRAIL, increasing the solubility 20-fold	[97]

7.6.4 Dendrimer

Dendrimers are nanocarrier, which resembles tree-like structurally containing a core in their center and there is a functional group attached to the core. A functional group can be single or repeat itself by being connected (Fig. 7.5). The generation number, which is specified by G, is the repetition of functional groups, or, in other words, the degree of polymerization. It is referred to as the zeroth generation if there is just one functional group that is directly attached to the nucleus, or G-0, in the dendrimer. Whenever functional group 2 or 3 is directly linked to the center, it is referred to as G-2 or G-3 [98]. The biocompatibility of the dendrimer and its flexibility as a nanocarrier are increased by the many functional groups dispersed on its surface [99]. Additionally, by electrostatic contact, their exterior functional groups may be changed by other charged chemicals, and dendrimers with both hydrophilic and hydrophobic group structures can transport a variety of medicinal molecules with various solubilities [100]. The delivered medication may be enveloped in the molecular cavity of the dendrimer or mixed with effective groups on the dendrimer's surface during the distribution process [101]. Researchers studying medication delivery have been interested in dendrimers because of their distinct structural and compositional characteristics (Table 7.4).

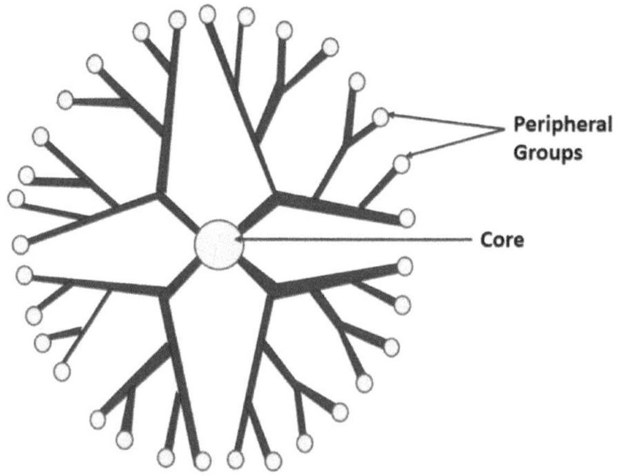

Figure 7.5 Structure of dendrimer.

Table 7.4 Applications of dendrimers in drug delivery system for the treatment of pulmonary disease

Disease	Colloidal system	Drug	Remark	Ref.
Tuberculosis	G-4 PAMAM	Rifampicin	According to current research, PAMAM dendrimers have the potential for pulmonary inhalation, which may be very useful in the case of treating TB and showing high stability and pH-dependent release	[102]
Tuberculosis	G-3 PAMAM	Rifampicin	A combination of rifampicin and G-4 PAMAM showed sustained release, improved absorption, and enhanced bioavailability of drug	[103]
Lung cancer	G-4 PAMAM	siRNA	siRNA-G4NH2 dendriplexes effectively target lung alveolar epithelial A549 cells, silence genes, and have the desired impact	[104]
Lung cancer	G-4 PAMAM	Doxorubicin	According to the research, pulmonary delivery of DOX in conjunction with ligation to PAMAM dendrimer through an intracellular labile bond is a possible tactic to improve therapeutic efficacy and lessen systemic toxicity of DOX	[105]
Asthma	G-4 PAMAM	Methyl-prednisolone	Effectively conjugate methyl-prednisolone to PAMAM-G4 dendrimers, and administering the conjugation intranasally proved successful in lowering the ovalbumin-induced airway inflammation	[106]
Lung cancer	G-3 PAMAM	Cisplatin	Dendrimer delivered the medication at the target spot with minimal loss and controlled rates; synthesized dendrimer was cytocompatible and significantly inhibited cancer cell proliferation, with release rate being greater in tumor pH compared to physiological pH	[107]
Lung cancer	G-5 PAMAM	Paclitaxel	Dendrimers loaded with PTX had a better encapsulation efficiency (95%) and a 25% loading efficiency; the antiproliferative impact of loaded dendrimers on 293T and L132 cells was found to be stronger than that of free PTX; PTX-entrapped dendrimers demonstrated sustained-release phenomena	[108]
Lung cancer	G-5 polylysine dendrimer	Doxorubicin	Intratracheal instillation of dendrimer-conjugated DOX twice weekly led to a >95% decrease in lung tumor burden, whereas intravenous injection of DOX solution reduced tumor burden by around 50%	[109]

For instance, a prior *in vitro* study conducted by Bellini et al. revealed that anti-tuberculosis drug rifampicin embedded in fourth-generation polyamidoamide (G4-PAMAM) dendrimers exhibited high stability under physiological pH conditions [102].

Similar to this, Rajabnezhad et al. formulated inhalable nanodrugs for the treatment of tuberculosis by using several generations of PAMAM dendrimer-loaded rifampicin. Their findings demonstrated that third-generation PAMAM dendrimers provided prolonged drug release and greatly enhanced medication solubility and bioavailability as compared to standard intravenous delivery [103].

Conti et al. used an amine-terminated G4PAMAM dendrimer (G4NH2) embedded with siRNA to reduce the expression of enhanced green fluorescent protein in an A549 epithelial cancer cell model. The demonstrated G4NH2 siRNA profoundly targets the alveolar epithelial cells and successfully silences the target gene [104].

Zhong et al. formulated a complex containing DOX and carboxyl-terminated G4-PAMAM dendrimers for the treatment of pulmonary metastasis. They found that on intravenous administration the dendrimer complex increased the drug's formation and retention time in the lung. Also, it has decreased systemic toxicity and improved DOX's effectiveness on carcinoma [105]. Some more applications of dendrimer formulation in drug delivery are given in Table 7.4.

7.6.5 Solid Lipid Nanoparticles

Solid lipid nanoparticles can be described as colloidal drug carriers with specified diameters ranging from 50 nm to 1 μm. They are composed of solid lipids or a combination of solid lipids and different liquids that are stabilized with the help of an emulsifier (Fig. 7.6). Lipids are generally utilized in the preparation of SLNs that includes physiological lipids like triglycerides, fatty acids, waxes, and steroids which can be well absorbed by the body and are biocompatible. SLNs are preferred over liposomes because of the enhanced stability of drug-encapsulated nanoparticles due to emulsion-based stabilization. SLNs offer specialized properties like a target-based release, easy manufacturing, controllable particle size, controlled release, incorporation of a lipophilic and hydrophilic drug, simple scale-up, and reduced toxicity. SLNs prevent drug molecules' interaction with physical, chemical, and enzymatic degradation [110].

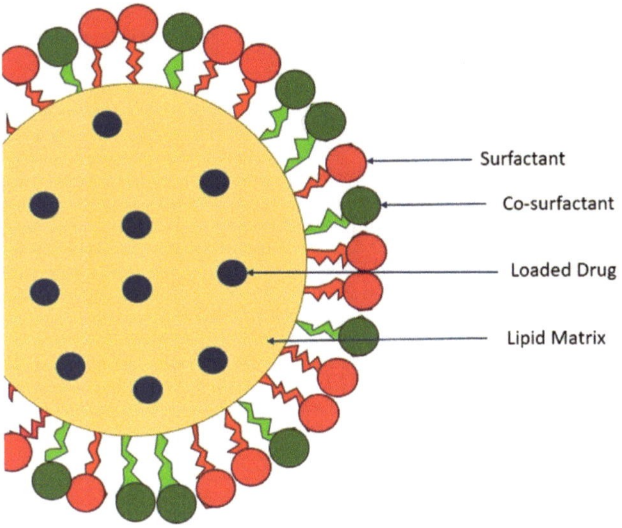

Figure 7.6 Structure of solid lipid nanoparticles.

Rosiere et al. evaluated the efficiency of paclitaxel-loaded solid lipid nanoparticles for enhanced delivery to lung tumors. It was concluded that prolonged exposure to paclitaxel was exhibited by *in vivo* pulmonary delivery of coated solid lipid nanoparticles [111]. According to the research by Ji et al. conducted a study in which the hydrophobic drug naringenin was encapsulated into solid lipid nanoparticles using the low-temperature solidification method and emulsification. The study found that when the drug-loaded SLNs were administered via pulmonary instillation, their bioavailability was significantly improved compared to that of the containing drug suspension, confirming that SLNs can be utilized for delivery and improving the bioavailability of poorly water-soluble drugs [112]. In contrast to traditional oral delivery, Makled et al. investigated the potential of sildenafil citrate-loaded SLNs for the management of pulmonary hypertension using targeted inhalational delivery. The drug-loaded SLNs showed good colloidal stability, a sustained-release profile, and high encapsulation efficiency for a duration of over 24 h. The stability was unaffected when inhaled using a jet nebulizer [113]. Some more applications of SLP formulation in drug delivery are given in Table 7.5.

Table 7.5 Applications of solid lipid nanoparticles in drug delivery system for the treatment of pulmonary disease

Disease	Drug	Remarks	Ref.
Lung cancer	Paclitaxel	Evaluated efficiency of paclitaxel-loaded solid lipid nanoparticles for enhanced delivery to pulmonary metastasis	[111]
	Epirubicin	*In vitro* studies proposed that SLNs are stabilized during nebulization with enhanced respirable fraction; *in vivo* studies showed that drug concentration of EPI-SLNs (Epirubicin loaded solid lipid nanoparticles) was significantly higher than the drug concentration in plasma	[116]
Pulmonary hypertension	Sildenafil	Drug-loaded SLNs shown good colloidal stability, a sustained-release profile, and high encapsulation efficiency for a duration of over 24 h; the stability was unaffected when inhaled using a jet nebulizer	[113]
Thrombosis	Bromelain	Bromelain encapsulated hybrid SLNs (Br-HNPs) were formulated and characterized; results indicated that Br-HNPs can be a substitute to commercial therapies for thrombosis treatment	[114]
Cystic fibrosis	Amikacin	Pulmonary delivery of SLNs enhances patient compliance by reducing side effects in kidneys and increased drug dosing intervals	[115]
Asthma	Curcumin	Curcumin solid lipid nanoparticles enhance its therapeutic efficacy; curcumin concentrations in plasma concentrations are higher than curcumin; this formulation can be an option for asthma therapy	[117]

Disease	Drug	Remarks	Ref.
Tuberculosis	Isoniazid	Isoniazid-solid lipid nanoparticles were prepared to achieve prolonged effect and enhanced bioavailability by reducing pulsatile plasma concentrations	[118]
	Cisplatin	Cisplatin aimed to improve the efficacy, therapeutic index and reduced toxicity; SLNs of cisplatin preferably target lungs, liver, and brain	[119]
Lung cancer	Methotrexate (MTX)	MTX SLNs are formulated by melt emulsification method; MTX SLNs are an adequate oral delivery system to improve the bioavailability according to invitro and *in vivo* studies	[120]
Lung inflammation and pulmonary dysfunction	Dimethyl fumarate	According to a study, breathing in DMF-encapsulated SLN protects against inflammatory conditions and pulmonary dysfunction, also reduces the CNS inflammatory process	[121]

7.6.6 Polymeric Nanoparticles

Polymeric nanoparticles (NPs) are the formulations that entrap active compounds within the polymeric core (Fig. 7.7). The particle size ranges from 1 to 1000 nm. Nanocapsules and nanospheres are the forms of nanoparticles that are differentiated based on their structure. Polymeric nanoparticles can be used to target drug delivery for various diseases [122, 123]. For the creation of nanocarriers to carry therapeutic and diagnostic medicines, polymers with specific physicochemical and biological benefits are utilized.

Different substances that are introduced into the polymer surface or disseminated in the polymeric matrix can be delivered using polymer-based nanocarriers [124]. Polymers used in polymeric nanoparticles are such as polyanhydrides, polyethyleneimine (PEI), poly-lactic-co-glycolic acid (PLGA), polyacrylates, polyethyleneimine (PEI), and PEG. As a pulmonary delivery method, PLGA offers several benefits but also some drawbacks. For instance, the slow rate of PLGA breakdown may cause an excessive build-up of PLGA in the respiratory tract [125]. The release duration ranges from several weeks to several months, and the drug's rate of degradation is dependent on the molecular weight and composition of the polymeric nanocarriers. Additionally, ongoing PLGA hydrolysis may result in an acidic core being created inside the delivery system. The hydrolysis also lowers the pH of the microenvironment and harms pH-sensitive proteins that are encapsulated, like proteins and peptides [126].

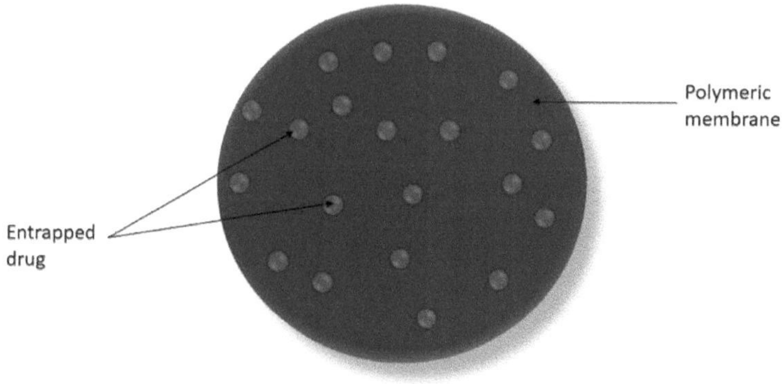

Figure 7.7 Structure of polymeric nanoparticle.

To evaluate whether ciprofloxacin-loaded PLGA NPs might treat cystic fibrosis brought on by bacterial infection in Calu-3 cells and CFBE41o cells, Türeli et al. [127] synthesized the NPs. The findings demonstrated that the nanoparticles had high drug loading efficiency and better permeability, enabling them to attain high and sustained local drug concentrations while also allowing for a reduction in medication dosage to lessen adverse effects.

Kim et al. formulated a sustained-release inhalation system of DOX using PLGA. It has shown high drug loading efficiency and had better nebulization. According to the results, the DOX nanoparticles have been effective in inhibition of tumor cell growth inhibition. It can be indicated for the treatment of metastatic lung cancer [128].

An earlier investigation in guinea pigs by Pandey et al. [129] showed that the embedding of PLGA increased the bioavailability and decreased the frequency of administration of anti-tuberculosis medications by extending their average residence duration and elimination half-life.

Tomoda et al.'s [130] research showed that TAS-103-loaded PLGA NPs boosted drug toxicity to A549 lung cancer cells and raised drug concentrations in rats' lungs. PLGA is also thought to be a suitable option for the transfer of genes for the treatment of pulmonary diseases. Some more applications of polymeric nanoparticle formulation in drug delivery are given in Table 7.6.

7.7 Patents

From the above discussion, we can understand that novel technology has the potential to deliver drugs to the pulmonary target site. Researchers have been working on developing and improving delivery systems for the target delivery of drugs. With new advancements in delivery systems, toxicity and efficacy should be acknowledged by researchers. A diverse range of nanotechnology-based delivery has been developed and studied for pulmonary disease/disorder. Some of the patents related to nanotechnology for pulmonary delivery such as liposomes, microparticles, nanoparticles, powders, and microemulsions for pulmonary diseases are listed in Table 7.7.

7.8 Clinical Case Report

Waldrep et al. evaluated the safety and tolerability of the liposome aerosol formulation of beclomethasone dipropionate (Bec)-dilauroyl phosphatidylcholine (DLPC) in patients. Ten healthy subjects received a single dosage of Bec-DLPC liposome aerosol to be inhaled. The tolerability and safety of the formulation were assessed by spirometry and hematological investigations. Through the study, it was concluded that the Bec-DLPC liposome aerosol formulation can be an alternative for an MDI or dry powder inhalers (DPI) devices [171]. Inspired by this study, Saari et al. further continued the work on Bec-DLPC liposome aerosol formulation. They studied the difference in distribution and clearance of Bec-DLPC in patients suffering from mild (n = 10) and severe asthma (n = 10). The open, parallel-group study was carried out by using radioactive Bec-DLPC liposome formulation. After administration, the mucociliary clearance was evaluated. According to the results, it was observed that

Table 7.6 Applications of polymeric nanoparticles in drug delivery system for the treatment of pulmonary disease

Disease	Drug	Remark	Ref.
Cystic fibrosis	Ciprofloxacin	Ciprofloxacin complex-loaded PLGA [poly-lactic-co-glycolic acid] NPs penetrate the bacteria-into, into negatively charged, thick Cystic Fibrosis mucus and show antibacterial activity.	[127]
Metastatic lung cancer	Doxorubicin	Doxorubicin PLGA [poly-lactic-co-glycolic acid] formulation showed excellent aerosolization properties, was very porous and had great encapsulation efficiency. After pulmonary administration, Doxorubicin PLGA MPs were deposited in the lungs and stayed there for up to 14 days. Doxorubicin was progressively released from DOX PLGA for 2 weeks.	[128]
Tuberculosis	Rifampicin, Isoniazid and Pyrazinamide	PLGA loaded with Isoniazid, Rifampicin, Pyrazinamide Increase the bioavailability, extend the elimination half-life, and mean residence duration, and decrease the rate of administration.	[129]
Lung cancer	TAS-103	PLGA nanoparticles with the anticancer drug 6-{[2-(dimethylamino) ethyl] amino}-3-hydroxyl-*7H*-indeno [2, 1-*c*] quinolin-7-one dihydrochloride (TAS-103) prepared are used in the treatment of pulmonary metastasis.	[130]
Cystic fibrosis	Tobramycin	Alginate/chitosan nanoparticles enhance the Drug penetration for the effectiveness of pulmonary infection treatment.	[131]

Disease	Drug	Remark	Ref.
Respiratory disease	Salbutamol	In respiratory treatment, poly (D,L-lactide-co-glycolide) (VS (72)-10) nanoparticles loaded with salbutamol that exhibit sustained release are employed.	[132]
Lung cancer	Paclitaxel	Nanoparticles made of poly (lactic-co-glycolic acid) and poly ethylenimine coated with paclitaxel and cyanine-5 are known as PLGA-PEI-TAX-Cy5-S3SI, which are used in lung cancer treatment.	[133]
Lung cancer	Curcumin	In this work, we essentially created polymeric nanoparticles of curcumin loaded with poly (lactic-co-glycolic acid) and compared their cytotoxicity to that of their unloaded counterparts. When compared to free curcumin, the cytotoxicity of nanoparticles was shown to be higher after 24, 48, and 72 h. Therefore, it may be inferred that curcumin polymeric nanoparticles could function as a possible delivery mechanism for lung cancer treatment.	[134]
Chronic obstructive pulmonary disease	Azithromycin	PLGA nanoparticles that have been AZI-loaded are intended to enhance antibacterial effects and promote medication delivery to cells. These nanoparticles will be used to create an inhalable AZI formulation for the treatment of respiratory infections.	[135]

Table 7.7 List of patents related to novel formulation applied for pulmonary disease

Dosage form	Patent no.	Title	Remarks	Ref.
Liposomes	US20150110855 A1	Inhaled surfactant-modified liposomal formulations providing both an immediate and sustained-release profile	While preparing the liposomal formulation the addition of surfactant is modified; formulation contains anti-infectives such as ciprofloxacin indicated for treatment of respiratory tract infection	[136]
	US9549939B2	Lipid-based compositions of anti-infectives for treating pulmonary infections and methods of use thereof	Aerosolized lipid-based formulation for respiratory infections; anti-infectives are available in free form for immediate antimicrobial activity, and lipid-based compositions were in responsible to maintain anti-infective levels in the lungs	[137]
	US9545401B2	Concentrated, inhalable ciprofloxacin formulation	Ciprofloxacin liposomal composition for treating a range of respiratory tract illnesses	[138]
	CN103784403A	Long-acting liposome preparation for pulmonary drug delivery and preparation method thereof	For delivery of polypeptide drugs used in treatment of pulmonary diseases carrier such as polyethylene glycol was modified	[139]
	CN110559280A	Paclitaxel-loaded liposome bacterium inhalation preparation for treating lung cancer	High efficacy and safety paclitaxel-loaded liposome bacterial inhalation preparation for lung tumor targeting	[140]
	CN107260678B	Anti-lung cancer Docetaxel active targeting liposome	Docetaxel-loaded liposomes for active targeting in the treatment of lung cancer	[141]

Dosage form	Patent no.	Title	Remarks	Ref.
	RU2493874C2	Transpulmonary liposomes for controlling drug delivery	Gene delivery through liposomes modified with terminal hydrophobic polyvinyl alcohol for Pulmonary disease treatment	[142]
	JP2003504321A	Pulmonary delivery of liposome-encapsulated cannabinoid	Cannabinoid mimetic drug encapsulated in Liposomes hypothesized for possessing psychoactive effect in mammalian lung tissue	[143]
	KR20060123341A	Stable liposome compositions comprising lipophilic amine-containing pharmaceutical agents	Drugs solely having amines in a stable liposome composition for pulmonary administration	[144]
Microparticles	US8697653B2	Microparticle formulation for pulmonary drug delivery of anti-infective molecule for treatment of infectious diseases	Microparticles made of lipid and drug are biodegradable and inhalable and are used to treat pulmonary tuberculosis and multidrug-resistant tuberculosis	[145]
	CN109674773A	A kind of Xiduofeng drug microparticles of pulmonary administration and the preparation method and application thereof	Drug microparticles of Xiduofeng for pulmonary administration demonstrated improved systemic efficacy and bioavailability	[146]
	EP1204409A1	Microparticles for pulmonary administration	Supercritical fluid technology used to synthesize biodegradable microparticles (1–30 μm) for greater pulmonary deposition and improved effectiveness	[147]

(*Continued*)

Table 7.7 *(Continued)*

Dosage form	Patent no.	Title	Remarks	Ref.
	WO2006124446A2	Sustained-release microparticles for pulmonary delivery	Multilamellar lipid bilayer-encapsulated in sustained-release microparticles for pulmonary distribution that contain the therapeutic agent	[148]
	WO2010007604A2	Inhalable microparticles and methods for the production thereof	Drug delivery via the lungs using a three-dimensional interpenetrating network of microparticles made of cross-linked polysaccharide and polymeric protein with a mass median aerodynamic diameter of 1 to 5 μm	[149]
	JP2008507585A	Treatment with iloprost inhalation using a microparticle formulation for pulmonary hypertension	Carbohydrates derived hydrophobic iloprost microparticles for the management and treatment of pulmonary hypertension	[150]
	PT1259228E	Therapeutic compositions for pulmonary delivery	Micronized insulin combined with lactose carrier particles is contained in a drug powder inhaler for pulmonary administration	[151]
Nanoparticles	US20110190245	Nanosuspension with antifungal medication to be administered via inhalation with improved impurity profile and safety	Antifungal azole derivative nanosuspension for the successful treatment of respiratory tract fungal infection	[152]
	CN110384681A	A kind of nanometer formulation and preparation method thereof for pulmonary fibrosis	In order to treat pulmonary fibrosis effectively, a nanometer formulation for deep alveolar drug delivery was formulated which inhibits the release of inhibitory factor	[153]

Dosage form	Patent no.	Title	Remarks	Ref.
	CN110090307A	A kind of load medicine black phosphorus chitosan composite Nano ball and its preparation method and application	Surface-modified chitosan composite nanoballs for improved pulmonary diseases therapy effectiveness	[154]
	CN 110251689A	A kind of chitosan nanomaterial and preparation method thereof for lung cancer therapy	Chitosan nanomaterial shows how molecular thermal therapy and synergistic effects work together to effectively treat and manage lung cancer	[155]
	WO2009/121631 A2	Nanoparticles for targeted delivery of active agents to the lungs	For the diagnosis and therapy of lung cancer or bronchial dysplasia, monoclonal antibody encapsulated in polymeric nanoparticles linked cytotoxic drugs have advantages such as prolonged residence duration, target delivery, and increased efficacy	[156]
	WO2016199146A1	A controlled release system for pulmonary delivery of surfactant protein D	Controlled release of surface protein D loaded with PLGA (polylactic-co-glycolic acid) nanoparticles for treatment of various pulmonary disease	[157]
	AU2013271392B2	Pulmonary delivery of mRNA to non-lung targeting	mRNA for cytosolic proteins is delivered through the lungs to treat or prevent diseases linked to non-lung cells	[158]
Powder	US20120247462A1	Antibiotic formulations, unit doses, kits, and methods	Improved unit concentration dose and antibiotic formulation kits for aerosolized composition with longer lung residence time	[159]

(*Continued*)

Table 7.7 (*Continued*)

Dosage form	Patent no.	Title	Remarks	Ref.
	US9433576	Cationic dry powder	For the treatment, prophylaxis, or diagnosis of respiratory illnesses, a respirable dry powder containing cations (such as calcium, magnesium, strontium, etc.) and the active pharmaceutical ingredient	[160]
	US20150283069	Inhalable vaccine compositions and methods	For oral or nasal inhalation, a stable dry powder vaccine formulation; the vaccine comes in monovalent or multivalent forms, both of which can be kept at room temperature for a long time	[161]
	US9802012B2	Dry powder drug delivery system and methods	For the development of drug delivery formulations of diketopiperazine and the active ingredient for the treatment of respiratory diseases/disorders, inhalers and cartridges were used	[162]
	WO2019204583A1	Antifungal formulations for pulmonary administration comprising itraconazole	Itraconazole inhalable drug powders are crystalline particulate with less toxicity and improved effectiveness against pulmonary infections	[163]
	WO2001093837A2	Protein powder for pulmonary delivery	Surfactant-coated therapeutic protein core for treatment of a variety of pulmonary diseases	[164]
	AU753014B2	Dry powder active agent pulmonary delivery	Micronized food supplements, vitamins, nutrient delivery through the lungs combined with a lactose carrier	[165]

Dosage form	Patent no.	Title	Remarks	Ref.
	RU2571331C1	Systems and methods for dry powder drug delivery	For the treatment of endocrine disorders, a dry powder inhalation mixture containing diketopiperazine and micro-organic molecules, proteins, and peptides is used	[166]
Microemulsion	WO1999024016A1	Emulsions for aerosolization and drug delivery	Aerosolized emulsion compositions comprising fluorocarbons and therapeutic agent solutions for drug delivery to the lungs	[167]
	WO2015009776A1	Low-dose corticosteroid microemulsion compositions and methods of treatment thereof	Treatment of diseases affecting the lower and upper respiratory airways with mometasone furoate microemulsions	[168]
	WO2019110099A1	Inhalable clofazimine formulation	Clofazimine pharmaceutical emulsion formulation for the treatment of lung infection	[169]
	JP2001517692A	Stabilizing preparations for use in the nebulizer	For pulmonary drug administration of medication, a stabilized dispersion of colloidal preparation of antihistamine, anticholinergic, anti-inflammatory, antitumor agent, and anti-tuberculosis with reduced molecular attraction for better stability was proposed	[170]

patients dealing with severe asthma have a higher clearance rate in comparison with mild asthmatic patients. The distribution of Bec-DLPC liposomes was more in the central part of lower airways in severe asthmatic patients [172]. This study on Bec-DLPC liposome was further investigated and this time it was compared with Bec. Containing dipalmitoylphosphatidylcholine (DPPC) liposomes. A total of 11 healthy volunteers were taken for the comparison study. After the study, it was concluded that clearance of both forms of liposome formulation is slow. The aerosol clouds were efficiently made in DLPC containing liposome suspension. Hereafter we can conclude that liposomes are a good choice for the sustained release of drugs at a local site for pulmonary disease [173].

Jakobsson et al. investigated the difference in the deposition of the nanoparticle in distal lungs in healthy volunteers and patients suffering from respiratory disease. A total of 48 subjects were taken and were divided into three groups: healthy non-smoker subjects, smoker subjects, and subjects dealing with chronic obstructive pulmonary disease. The deposition fraction (DF) of nanoparticles was examined and it was shown that patient group with the respiratory disease the DF was lower in comparison with the other two groups. The lower DF value of emphysematous subjects indicates enlargement of airspaces in the lungs, which increases the deposition of nanoparticles in the lungs [174].

Haworth et al. conducted a randomized, double-blind, placebo-controlled phase 3 trial to examine the effectiveness of liposomal ciprofloxacin (ARD-3150) in patients with non-cystic fibrosis bronchiectasis and lung infection with *Pseudomonas aeruginosa* are associated with frequent pulmonary exacerbations. A total of 1047 patients were examined for pulmonary exacerbations after receiving the ARD-3150. According to the findings, it was concluded that ARD-3150 significantly increases the median time to first pulmonary Exacerbation and reduces the frequency of pulmonary exacerbations [175].

Tsuji et al. examined the efficiency of a combination of carboplatin and nanoparticle albumin-bound paclitaxel (nab-PTX) in a 65-year-old male patient. The research showed that nab-PTX is more effective at reaching the tumor microenvironment than solvent-based paclitaxel (sb-PTX) [176].

In a study, it was revealed that severely affected COVID-19 patients are suffering from a decrease in albumin level and an increase in inflammatory response. Park et al. studied the effect of PEGylated nanoparticle albumin-bound (PNAB) in COVID-19 patients. The efficacy of PNAB was evaluated in the animal model. The study suggested that PNAB steroidal ginsenoside drugs can treat symptoms of COVID-19 [177].

Winthrop et al. studied the safety, efficacy, and tolerance of amikacin liposome inhalation suspension with the guideline-based therapy. The study was expanded for over 12 months with a total of 163 patients. Of the 163 patients, 56 were withdrawn from the study. They further continued with 107 patients and completed the study. It was a 12-month open-label convert clinical study. The patients were divided into two groups: one assigned with GBT alone and the other with amikacin liposome formulation and GBT. At the end of the investigation, it was observed that in patients with amikacin lipoma therapy, the efficacy and tolerance are the same as those of the patients receiving GBT alone. There were no differences with respect to the respiratory adverse events [178].

References

1. Cazzola, M., Cavalli, F., Usmani, O. S., and Rogliani, P. (2020). Advances in pulmonary drug delivery devices for the treatment of chronic obstructive pulmonary disease. *Expert Opinion on Drug Delivery*, **17**(5), 635–646.
2. Patil, J. S., and Sarasija, S. (2012). Pulmonary drug delivery strategies: A concise, systematic review. *Lung India: Official Organ of Indian Chest Society*, **29**(1), 44.
3. Ahookhosh, K., Pourmehran, O., Aminfar, H., Mohammad pourfard, M., Sarafraz, M. M., and Hamishehkar, H. (2020). Development of human respiratory airway models: a review. *European Journal of Pharmaceutical Sciences*, **145**, 105233.
4. Person, A., and Mintz, M. L. (2006). Anatomy and physiology of the respiratory tract. In *Disorders of the Respiratory Tract*, Humana Press, pp. 11–15.
5. Thakur, A. K., Chellappan, D. K., Dua, K., Mehta, M., Satija, S., and Singh, I. (2020). Patented therapeutic drug delivery strategies for

targeting pulmonary diseases. *Expert Opinion on Therapeutic Patents*, **30**(5), 375–387.

6. Mangal, S., Gao, W., Li, T., and Zhou, Q. T. (2017). Pulmonary delivery of nanoparticle chemotherapy for the treatment of lung cancers: challenges and opportunities. *Acta Pharmacologica Sinica*, **38**(6), 782–797.
7. Fröhlich, E., Mercuri, A., Wu, S., and Salar-Behzadi, S. (2016). Measurements of deposition, lung surface area and lung fluid for simulation of inhaled compounds. *Frontiers in Pharmacology*, **7**, 181.
8. Knudsen, L., and Ochs, M. (2018). The micromechanics of lung alveoli: structure and function of surfactant and tissue components. *Histochemistry and Cell Biology*, **150**(6), 661–676.
9. Man, W. H., de Steenhuijsen Piters, W. A., and Bogaert, D. (2017). The microbiota of the respiratory tract: gatekeeper to respiratory health. *Nature Reviews Microbiology*, **15**(5), 259–270.
10. Gehr, P. (1994). Annexe A. Anatomy and morphology of the respiratory tract. *Annals of the International Commission on Radiological Protection*, 24(1–3), 121–166.
11. Girod, S., Zahm, J.M., Plotkowski, C., Beck, G., and Puchelle, E. (1992). Role of the physiochemical properties of mucus in the protection of the respiratory epithelium. *European Respiratory Journal*, **5**(4), 477–487.
12. Kaialy, W., and Nokhodchi, A. (2015). Particle engineering for improved pulmonary drug delivery through dry powder inhalers. *Pulmonary Drug Delivery: Advances and Challenges*. eds., Nokhodchi, A., Martin, G. P., pp. 171–198.
13. Martini, A., Muggetti, L., and Warchol, M. P. (2000). Nasal and pulmonary drug delivery systems. *Expert Opinion on Therapeutic Patents*, **10**(3), 315–323.
14. Patil, J. S., and Sarasija, S. (2012). Pulmonary drug delivery strategies: a concise, systematic review. *Lung India: Official Organ of Indian Chest Society*, **29**(1), p. 44.
15. Di Sant'Agnese, P. A., and Davis, P. B. (1976). Research in Cystic Fibrosis: (Third of Three Parts). *New England Journal of Medicine*, **295**(11), 597–602.
16. Subramanian, J., and Govindan, R. (2007). Lung cancer in never smokers: a review. *Journal of Clinical Oncology*, **25**(5), 561–570.
17. Sharma, R., Saxena, D., Dwivedi, A. K., and Misra, A. (2001). Inhalable microparticles containing drug combinations to target alveolar

macrophages for treatment of pulmonary tuberculosis. *Pharmaceutical Research*, **18**(10), 1405–1410.

18. Siafakas, N. M., Vermeire, P., Pride, N. A., Paoletti, P., Gibson, J., Howard, P., Yernault, J. C., Decramer, M., Higenbottam, T., and Postma, D. S. (1995). Optimal assessment and management of chronic obstructive pulmonary disease (COPD). The European Respiratory Society Task Force. *European Respiratory Journal*, **8**(8), 1398–1420.
19. Mishra, B., and Singh, J. (2020). Novel drug delivery systems and significance in respiratory diseases. In *Targeting Chronic Inflammatory Lung Diseases Using Advanced Drug Delivery Systems*, Academic Press, pp. 57–95.
20. Javadzadeh, Y., and Yaqoubi, S. (2017). Therapeutic nanostructures for pulmonary drug delivery. In *Nanostructures for Drug Delivery*, pp. 619–638.
21. Gangurde, H. H., Chordiya, M. A., Baste, N. T. S., and Upasani, C. (2012). Approaches and devices used in pulmonary drug delivery system: a review. *Asian Journal of Pharmaceutical Research and Health Care*, **4**(1), 11–27.
22. Yu, C. P., and Xu, G. B. (1987). Predicted deposition of diesel particles in young humans. *Journal of Aerosol Science*, **18**(4), 419–429.
23. Yu, C. P. (1978). Exact analysis of aerosol deposition during steady breathing. *Powder Technology*, **21**(1), 55–62.
24. Chandel, A., Goyal, A. K., Ghosh, G., and Rath, G. (2019). Recent advances in aerosolised drug delivery. *Biomedicine & Pharmacotherapy*, **112**, 108601.
25. Newman, S. P. (2017). Drug delivery to the lungs: challenges and opportunities. *Therapeutic Delivery*, **8**(8), 647–661.
26. Patton, J. S., Brain, J. D., Davies, L. A., Fiegel, J., Gumbleton, M., Kim, K. J., Sakagami, M., Vanbever, R., and Ehrhardt, C. (2010). The particle has landed—characterizing the fate of inhaled pharmaceuticals. *Journal of Aerosol Medicine and Pulmonary Drug Delivery*, **23**(S2), 71.
27. Cipolla, D. (2016). Will pulmonary drug delivery for systemic application ever fulfill its rich promise? *Expert Opinion on Drug Delivery*, **13**(10), 1337–1340.
28. Sanchis, J., Gich, I., Pedersen, S., and Team, A. D. M. I. (2016). Systematic review of errors in inhaler use: has patient technique improved over time? *Chest*, **150**(2), 394–406.
29. Groneberg, D. A., Witt, C., Wagner, U., Chung, K. F., and Fischer, A. (2003). Fundamentals of pulmonary drug delivery. *Respiratory Medicine*, **97**(4), 382–387.

30. Singh, A., Malviya, R., and Sharma, K. P. (2011). Pulmonary drug delivery system: a novel approach for drug delivery. *Current Drug Therapy*, **6**(2), 137–151.

31. Paranjpe, M., and Müller-Goymann, C. C. (2014). Nanoparticle-mediated pulmonary drug delivery: a review. *International Journal of Molecular Sciences*, **15**(4), 5852–5873.

32. Kaur, G., Narang, R. K., Rath, G., and Goyal, A. K. (2012). Advances in pulmonary delivery of nanoparticles. *Artificial Cells, Blood Substitutes, and Biotechnology*, **40**(1–2), 75–96.

33. Bozzuto, G., and Molinari, A. (2015). Liposomes as nanomedical devices. *International Journal of Nanomedicine*, **10**, 975.

34. Akbarzadeh, A., Rezaei-Sadabady, R., Davaran, S., Joo, S. W., Zarghami, N., Hanifehpour, Y., Samiei, M., Kouhi, M., and Nejati-Koshki, K. (2013). Liposome: classification, preparation, and applications. *Nanoscale Research Letters*, **8**(1), 1–9.

35. Samad, A., Sultana, Y., and Aqil, M. (2007). Liposomal drug delivery systems: an update review. *Current Drug Delivery*, **4**(4), 297–305.

36. Allen, T. M., and Cullis, P. R. (2013). Liposomal drug delivery systems: from concept to clinical applications. *Advanced Drug Delivery Reviews*, **65**(1), 36–48.

37. Elhissi, A. (2017). Liposomes for pulmonary drug delivery: the role of formulation and inhalation device design. *Current Pharmaceutical Design*, **23**(3), 362–372.

38. Ali, M. E., McConville, J. T., and Lamprecht, A. (2015). Pulmonary delivery of anti-inflammatory agents. *Expert Opinion on Drug Delivery*, **12**(6), 929–945.

39. Koshkina, N. V., Waldrep, J. C., Roberts, L. E., Golunski, E., Melton, S., and Knight, V. (2001). Paclitaxel liposome aerosol treatment induces inhibition of pulmonary metastases in murine renal carcinoma model. *Clinical Cancer Research*, **7**(10), 3258–3262.

40. Fritz, J. M., Tennis, M. A., Orlicky, D. J., Yin, H., Ju, C., Redente, E. F., Choo, K. S., Staab, T. A., Bouchard, R. J., Merrick, D. T., and Malkinson, A. M. (2014). Depletion of tumor-associated macrophages slows the growth of chemically induced mouse lung adenocarcinomas. *Frontiers in Immunology*, **5**, 587.

41. Chen, X., Huang, W., Wong, B. C., Yin, L., Wong, Y. F., Xu, M., and Yang, Z. (2012). Liposomes prolong the therapeutic effect of anti-asthmatic medication via pulmonary delivery. *International Journal of Nanomedicine*, **7**, 1139.

42. Wittgen, B. P., Kunst, P. W., Van Der Born, K., Van Wijk, A. W., Perkins, W., Pilkiewicz, F. G., Perez-Soler, R., Nicholson, S., Peters, G. J., and Postmus, P. E. (2007). Phase I study of aerosolized SLIT cisplatin in the treatment of patients with carcinoma of the lung. *Clinical Cancer Research*, **13**(8), 2414–2421.

43. Faustino, C., and Pinheiro, L. (2020). Lipid systems for the delivery of amphotericin B in antifungal therapy. *Pharmaceutics*, **12**(1), 29.

44. Barratt, G., and Bretagne, S. (2007). Optimizing efficacy of amphotericin B through nanomodification. *International Journal of Nanomedicine*, **2**(3), 301.

45. Griffith, D. E., Thomson, R., Flume, P. A., Aksamit, T. R., Field, S. K., Addrizzo-Harris, D. J., Morimoto, K., Hoefsloot, W., Mange, K. C., Yuen, D. W., and Ciesielska, M. (2021). Amikacin liposome inhalation suspension for refractory Mycobacterium avium complex lung disease: sustainability and durability of culture conversion and safety of long-term exposure. *Chest*, **160**(3), 831–842.

46. Hamblin, K. A., Armstrong, S. J., Barnes, K. B., Davies, C., Laws, T., Blanchard, J. D., Harding, S. V., and Atkins, H. S. (2017). Inhaled liposomal ciprofloxacin protects against a lethal infection in a murine model of pneumonic plague. *Frontiers in Microbiology*, **8**, 91.

47. Douer, D. (2016). Efficacy and safety of vincristine sulfate liposome injection in the treatment of adult acute lymphocytic leukemia. *The Oncologist*, **21**(7), 840–847.

48. Jain, P. P., Leber, R., Nagaraj, C., Leitinger, G., Lehofer, B., Olschewski, H., Olschewski, A., Prassl, R., and Marsh, L. M. (2014). Liposomal nanoparticles encapsulating iloprost exhibit enhanced vasodilation in pulmonary arteries. *International Journal of Nanomedicine*, **9**, 3249.

49. Wittgen, B. P., Kunst, P. W., Van Der Born, K., Van Wijk, A. W., Perkins, W., Pilkiewicz, F. G., Perez-Soler, R., Nicholson, S., Peters, G. J., and Postmus, P. E. (2007). Phase I study of aerosolized SLIT cisplatin in the treatment of patients with carcinoma of the lung. *Clinical Cancer Research*, **13**(8), 2414–2421.

50. Khanna, C., Hasz, D. E., Klausner, J. S., and Anderson, P. M. (1996). Aerosol delivery of interleukin 2 liposomes is nontoxic and biologically effective: canine studies. *Clinical Cancer Research: An Official Journal of the American Association for Cancer Research*, **2**(4), 721–734.

51. Bi, R., Shao, W., Wang, Q., and Zhang, N. (2008). Spray-freeze-dried dry powder inhalation of insulin-loaded liposomes for enhanced pulmonary delivery. *Journal of Drug Targeting*, **16**(9), 639–648.

52. Raviv, S. A., Alyan, M., Egorov, E., Zano, A., Harush, M. Y., Pieters, C., Korach-Rechtman, H., Saadya, A., Kaneti, G., Nudelman, I., and Farkash, S. (2022). Lung targeted liposomes for treating ARDS. *Journal of Controlled Release*, **346**, 421–433.

53. Guo, L. S., Fielding, R. M., Lasic, D. D., Hamilton, R. L., and Mufson, D. (1991). Novel antifungal drug delivery: stable amphotericin B-cholesteryl sulfate discs. *International Journal of Pharmaceutics*, **75**(1), 45–54.

54. Sercombe, L., Veerati, T., Moheimani, F., Wu, S. Y., Sood, A. K., and Hua, S. (2015). Advances and challenges of liposome assisted drug delivery. *Frontiers in Pharmacology*, **6**, 286.

55. Lin, C., Wong, B. C. K., Chen, H., Bian, Z., Zhang, G., Zhang, X., KashifRiaz, M., Tyagi, D., Lin, G., Zhang, Y., and Wang, J. (2017). Pulmonary delivery of triptolide-loaded liposomes decorated with anti-carbonic anhydrase IX antibody for lung cancer therapy. *Scientific Reports*, **7**(1), 1–12.

56. Chono, S., Tanino, T., Seki, T., and Morimoto, K. (2006). Influence of particle size on drug delivery to rat alveolar macrophages following pulmonary administration of ciprofloxacin incorporated into liposomes. *Journal of Drug Targeting*, **14**(8), 557–566.

57. VanWijk, M. J., VanBavel, E., Sturk, A., and Nieuwland, R. (2003). Microparticles in cardiovascular diseases. *Cardiovascular Research*, **59**(2), 277–287.

58. He, S., Gui, J., Xiong, K., Chen, M., Gao, H., and Fu, Y. (2022). A roadmap to pulmonary delivery strategies for the treatment of infectious lung diseases. *Journal of Nanobiotechnology*, **20**(1), 1–22.

59. Lengyel, M., Kállai-Szabó, N., Antal, V., Laki, A. J., and Antal, I. (2019). Microparticles, microspheres, and microcapsules for advanced drug delivery. *Scientia Pharmaceutica*, **87**(3), 20.

60. Siepmann, J., and Siepmann, F. (2006). Microparticles used as drug delivery systems. In *Smart Colloidal Materials*. Springer, Berlin, Heidelberg, pp. 15–21.

61. Jaspart, S., Bertholet, P., Piel, G., Dogné, J. M., Delattre, L., and Evrard, B. (2007). Solid lipid microparticles as a sustained release system for pulmonary drug delivery. *European ournal of Pharmaceutics and Biopharmaceutics*, **65**(1), 47–56.

62. Yang, Y., Bajaj, N., Xu, P., Ohn, K., Tsifansky, M. D., and Yeo, Y. (2009). Development of highly porous large PLGA microparticles for pulmonary drug delivery. *Biomaterials*, **30**(10), 1947–1953.

63. Parsian, A. R., Vatanara, A., Rahmati, M. R., Gilani, K., Khosravi, K. M., and Najafabadi, A. R. (2014). Inhalable budesonide porous microparticles tailored by spray freeze drying technique. *Powder Technology*, **260**, 36–41.

64. Wu, X., Hayes Jr, D., Zwischenberger, J. B., Kuhn, R. J., and Mansour, H. M. (2013). Design and physicochemical characterization of advanced spray-dried tacrolimus multifunctional particles for inhalation. *Drug Design, Development and Therapy*, **7**, 59.

65. Dimer, F. A., Ortiz, M., Pohlmann, A. R., and Guterres, S. S. (2015). Inhalable resveratrol microparticles produced by vibrational atomization spray drying for treating pulmonary arterial hypertension. *Journal of Drug Delivery Science and Technology*, **29**, 152–158.

66. Poursina, N., Vatanara, A., Rouini, M. R., Gilani, K., and RouholaminiNajafabadi, A. (2017). Systemic delivery of parathyroid hormone (1–34) using spray freeze-dried inhalable particles. *Pharmaceutical Development and Technology*, **22**(6), 733–739.

67. Sethi, G. R., and Singhal, K. K. (2008). Pulmonary diseases and corticosteroids. *The Indian Journal of Pediatrics*, **75**(10), 1045–1056.

68. Feng, S. S., and Chien, S. (2003). Chemotherapeutic engineering: application and further development of chemical engineering principles for chemotherapy of cancer and other diseases. *Chemical Engineering Science*, **58**(18), 4087–4114.

69. Fuso, L., Pitocco, D., and AntonelliIncalzi, R. (2007). Inhaled insulin and the lung. *Current Medicinal Chemistry*, **14**(12), 1335–1347.

70. Naikwade, S. R., Bajaj, A. N., Gurav, P., Gatne, M. M., and Singh Soni, P. (2009). Development of budesonide microparticles using spray-drying technology for pulmonary administration: design, characterization, *in vitro* evaluation, and *in vivo* efficacy study. *American Association of Pharmaceutical Scientists PharmSciTech*, **10**(3), 993–1012.

71. Alipour, S., Montaseri, H., and Tafaghodi, M. (2010). Preparation and characterization of biodegradable paclitaxel loaded alginate microparticles for pulmonary delivery. *Colloids and Surfaces B: Biointerfaces*, **81**(2), 521–529.

72. Comer, A. M., and Goa, K. L. (2000). Docetaxel. *Drugs & Aging*, **17**(1), 53–80.

73. Fiore, V. F., Lofton, M. C., Roser-Page, S., Yang, S. C., Roman, J., Murthy, N., and Barker, T. H. (2010). Polyketal microparticles for therapeutic delivery to the lung. *Biomaterials*, **31**(5), 810–817.

74. Sahin, S., Selek, H., Ponchel, G., Ercan, M. T., Sargon, M., Hincal, A. A., and Kas, H. S. (2002). Preparation, characterization and *in vivo* distribution of terbutaline sulfate loaded albumin microspheres. *Journal of Controlled Release*, **82**(2–3), 345–358.
75. Perevodchikova, N. I., Bychkov, M. B., and Ausekar, B. V. (1983). Adriamycin in the combined chemotherapy of small-cell lung cancer. *Antibiotiki*, **28**(8), 628–632.
76. Price, D. N., Stromberg, L. R., Kunda, N. K., and Muttil, P. (2017). *In vivo* pulmonary delivery and magnetic-targeting of dry powder nano-in-microparticles. *Molecular Pharmaceutics*, **14**(12), 4741–4750.
77. Meenach, S. A., Kim, Y. J., Kauffman, K. J., Kanthamneni, N., Bachelder, E. M., and Ainslie, K. M. (2012). Synthesis, optimization, and characterization of camptothecin-loaded acetalated dextran porous microparticles for pulmonary delivery. *Molecular Pharmaceutics*, **9**(2), 290–298.
78. Mohamed, A., Pekoz, A. Y., Ross, K., Hutcheon, G. A., and Saleem, I. Y. (2019). Pulmonary delivery of Nanocomposite Microparticles (NCMPs) incorporating miR-146a for treatment of COPD. *International Journal of Pharmaceutics*, **569**, 118524.
79. Wang, Q., Mi, G., Hickey, D., Li, Y., Tu, J., Webster, T. J., and Shen, Y. (2018). Azithromycin-loaded respirable microparticles for targeted pulmonary delivery for the treatment of pneumonia. *Biomaterials*, **160**, 107–123.
80. Sharma, A., Hong, S., Singh, R., and Jang, J. (2015). Single-walled carbon nanotube based transparent immunosensor for detection of a prostate cancer biomarker osteopontin. *Analytica Chimica Acta*, **869**, 68–73.
81. Yamada, K., Kim, C. T., Kim, J. H., Chung, J. H., Lee, H. G., and Jun, S. (2014). Single walled carbon nanotube-based junction biosensor for detection of Escherichia coli. *PLoS One*, **9**(9), e105767.
82. Sheikhpour, M., Golbabaie, A., and Kasaeian, A. (2017). Carbon nanotubes: a review of novel strategies for cancer diagnosis and treatment. *Materials Science and Engineering: C*, **76**, 1289–1304.
83. Shaikhpoor, M., Ahangari, G., Sadeghizadeh, M., Khosravi, A., and Derakhshani Deilami, G. (2012). Significant changes in D2-like dopamine gene receptors expression associated with non-small-cell lung cancer: could it be of potential use in the design of future therapeutic strategies? *Current Cancer Therapy Reviews*, **8**(4), 304–310.

84. Sheikhpour, M., Ahangari, G., Sadeghizadeh, M., and Deezagi, A. (2013). A novel report of apoptosis in human lung carcinoma cells using selective agonist of D2-like dopamine receptors: a new approach for the treatment of human non-small cell lung cancer. *International Journal of Immunopathology and Pharmacology*, **26**(2), 393–402.

85. Datir, S. R., Das, M., Singh, R. P., and Jain, S. (2012). Hyaluronate tethered,"smart" multiwalled carbon nanotubes for tumor-targeted delivery of doxorubicin. *Bioconjugate Chemistry*, **23**(11), 2201–2213.

86. Li, J., Pant, A., Chin, C. F., Ang, W. H., Ménard-Moyon, C., Nayak, T. R., Gibson, D., Ramaprabhu, S., Panczyk, T., Bianco, A., and Pastorin, G. (2014). *In vivo* biodistribution of platinum-based drugs encapsulated into multi-walled carbon nanotubes. *Nanomedicine: Nanotechnology, Biology and Medicine*, **10**(7), 1465–1475.

87. Singh, R. P., Sharma, G., Singh, S., Kumar, M., Pandey, B. L., Koch, B., and Muthu, M. S. (2016). Vitamin E TPGS conjugated carbon nanotubes improved efficacy of docetaxel with safety for lung cancer treatment. *Colloids and Surfaces B: Biointerfaces*, **141**, 429–442.

88. Arya, N., Arora, A., Vasu, K. S., Sood, A. K., and Katti, D. S. (2013). Combination of single walled carbon nanotubes/graphene oxide with paclitaxel: a reactive oxygen species mediated synergism for treatment of lung cancer. *Nanoscale*, **5**(7), 2818–2829.

89. Razzazan, A., Atyabi, F., Kazemi, B., and Dinarvand, R. (2016). *In vivo* drug delivery of gemcitabine with PEGylated single-walled carbon nanotubes. *Materials Science and Engineering C*, **62**, 614–625.

90. Cirillo, G., Vittorio, O., Kunhardt, D., Valli, E., Voli, F., Farfalla, A., Curcio, M., Spizzirri, U. G., and Hampel, S. (2019). Combining carbon nanotubes and chitosan for the vectorization of methotrexate to lung cancer cells. *Materials*, **12**(18), 2889.

91. Guo, C., Al-Jamal, W. T., Toma, F. M., Bianco, A., Prato, M., Al-Jamal, K. T., and Kostarelos, K. (2015). Design of cationic multiwalled carbon nanotubes as efficient siRNA vectors for lung cancer xenograft eradication. *Bioconjugate Chemistry*, **26**(7), 1370–1379.

92. Tan, J. M., Karthivashan, G., Arulselvan, P., Fakurazi, S., and Hussein, M. Z. (2014). Characterization and *in vitro* studies of the anticancer effect of oxidized carbon nanotubes functionalized with betulinic acid. *Drug Design, Development and Therapy*, **8**, 2333.

93. Singh, N., Sachdev, A., and Gopinath, P. (2018). Polysaccharide functionalized single walled carbon nanotubes as nanocarriers for delivery of curcumin in lung cancer cells. *Journal of Nanoscience and Nanotechnology*, **18**(3), 1534–1541.

94. Kumar, A. S., Sornambikai, S., Deepika, L., and Zen, J. M. (2010). Highly selective immobilization of amoxicillin antibiotic on carbon nanotube modified electrodes and its antibacterial activity. *Journal of Materials Chemistry*, **20**(45), 10152–10158.

95. Zomorodbakhsh, S., Abbasian, Y., Naghinejad, M., and Sheikhpour, M. (2020). The effects study of isoniazid conjugated multi-wall carbon nanotubes nanofluid on Mycobacterium tuberculosis. *International Journal of Nanomedicine*, **15**, 5901.

96. Mani, S., Cheemalapati, S., Chen, S. M., and Devadas, B. (2015). Anti-tuberculosis drug pyrazinamide determination at multiwalled carbon nanotubes/graphene oxide hybrid composite fabricated electrode. *International Journal of Electrochem. Sci*, **10**, 7049–7062.

97. Zakaria, A. B., Picaud, F., Rattier, T., Pudlo, M., Saviot, L., Chassagnon, R., Lherminier, J., Gharbi, T., Micheau, O., and Herlem, G. (2015). Nanovectorization of TRAIL with single wall carbon nanotubes enhances tumor cell killing. *Nano Letters*, **15**(2), 891–895.

98. Medina, S. H., and El-Sayed, M. E. (2009). Dendrimers as carriers for delivery of chemotherapeutic agents. *Chemical Reviews*, **109**(7), 3141–3157.

99. Mehta, M., Tewari, D., Gupta, G., Awasthi, R., Singh, H., Pandey, P., Chellappan, D. K., Wadhwa, R., Collet, T., Hansbro, P. M., and Kumar, S. R. (2019). Oligonucleotide therapy: an emerging focus area for drug delivery in chronic inflammatory respiratory diseases. *Chemico-Biological Interactions*, **308**, 206–215.

100. Ahmad, J., Akhter, S., Rizwanullah, M., Amin, S., Rahman, M., Ahmad, M. Z., Rizvi, M. A., Kamal, M. A., and Ahmad, F. J. (2015). Nanotechnology-based inhalation treatments for lung cancer: state of the art. *Nanotechnology, Science and Applications*, **8**, 55.

101. Palmerston Mendes, L., Pan, J., and Torchilin, V. P. (2017). Dendrimers as nanocarriers for nucleic acid and drug delivery in cancer therapy. *Molecules*, **22**(9), 1401.

102. Bellini, R. G., Guimarães, A. P., Pacheco, M. A., Dias, D. M., Furtado, V. R., de Alencastro, R. B., and Horta, B. A. (2015). Association of the anti-tuberculosis drug rifampicin with a PAMAM dendrimer. *Journal of Molecular Graphics and Modelling*, **60**, 34–42.

103. Rajabnezhad, S., Casettari, L., Lam, J. K., Nomani, A., Torkamani, M. R., Palmieri, G. F., Rajabnejad, M. R., and Darbandi, M. A. (2016). Pulmonary delivery of rifampicin microspheres using lower generation polyamidoamine dendrimers as a carrier. *Powder Technology*, **291**, 366–374.

104. Conti, D. S., Brewer, D., Grashik, J., Avasarala, S., and da Rocha, S. R. (2014). Poly (amidoamine) dendrimer nanocarriers and their aerosol formulations for siRNA delivery to the lung epithelium. *Molecular Pharmaceutics*, **11**(6), 1808–1822.

105. Zhong, Q., Bielski, E. R., Rodrigues, L. S., Brown, M. R., Reineke, J. J., and da Rocha, S. R. (2016). Conjugation to poly (amidoamine) dendrimers and pulmonary delivery reduce cardiac accumulation and enhance antitumor activity of doxorubicin in lung metastasis. *Molecular Pharmaceutics*, **13**(7), 2363–2375.

106. Inapagolla, R., Guru, B. R., Kurtoglu, Y. E., Gao, X., Lieh-Lai, M., Bassett, D. J. P., and Kannan, R. M. (2010). *In vivo* efficacy of dendrimer–methylprednisolone conjugate formulation for the treatment of lung inflammation. *International Journal of Pharmaceutics*, **399**(1–2), 140–147.

107. Nguyen, H., Nguyen, N. H., Tran, N. Q., and Nguyen, C. K. (2015). Improved method for preparing cisplatin-dendrimer nanocomplex and its behavior against NCI-H460 lung cancer cell. *Journal of Nanoscience and Nanotechnology*, **15**(6), 4106–4110.

108. Zhang, W. W., Wang, Y. C., Kan, X. M., Wang, X. M., and Geng, D. M. (2017). Preparation and evaluation of peptide-dendrimer-paclitaxel conjugates for treatment of heterogeneous stage 1 nonsmall cell lung cancer in 293T and L132 cell lines. *Tropical Journal of Pharmaceutical Research*, **16**(4), 737–742.

109. Kaminskas, L. M., McLeod, V. M., Ryan, G. M., Kelly, B. D., Haynes, J. M., Williamson, M., Thienthong, N., Owen, D. J., and Porter, C. J. (2014). Pulmonary administration of a doxorubicin-conjugated dendrimer enhances drug exposure to lung metastases and improves cancer therapy. *Journal of Controlled Release*, **183**, 18–26.

110. Nafee, N., Makled, S., and Boraie, N. (2018). Nanostructured lipid carriers versus solid lipid nanoparticles for the potential treatment of pulmonary hypertension via nebulization. *European Journal of Pharmaceutical Sciences*, **125**, 151–162.

111. Rosiere, R., Van Woensel, M., Gelbcke, M., Mathieu, V., Hecq, J., Mathivet, T., Vermeersch, M., Van Antwerpen, P., Amighi, K., and Wauthoz, N. (2018). New folate-grafted chitosan derivative to improve delivery of paclitaxel-loaded solid lipid nanoparticles for lung tumor therapy by inhalation. *Molecular Pharmaceutics*, **15**(3), 899–910.

112. Ji, P., Yu, T., Liu, Y., Jiang, J., Xu, J., Zhao, Y., Hao, Y., Qiu, Y., Zhao, W., and Wu, C. (2016). Naringenin-loaded solid lipid nanoparticles:

preparation, controlled delivery, cellular uptake, and ulmonary pharmacokinetics. *Drug Design, Development and Therapy*, **10**, 911.

113. Makled, S., Nafee, N., and Boraie, N. (2017). Nebulized solid lipid nanoparticles for the potential treatment of pulmonary hypertension via targeted delivery of phosphodiesterase-5-inhibitor. *International Journal of Pharmaceutics*, **517**(1–2), 312–321.

114. Sharma, M., and Chaudhary, D. (2022). *In vitro* and *in vivo* implications of rationally designed bromelain laden core-shell hybrid solid lipid nanoparticles for oral administration in thrombosis management. *Nanomedicine: Nanotechnology, Biology and Medicine*, **42**, 102543.

115. Varshosaz, J., Ghaffari, S., Mirshojaei, S. F., Jafarian, A., Atyabi, F., Kobarfard, F., and Azarmi, S. (2013). Biodistribution of amikacin solid lipid nanoparticles after pulmonary delivery. *BioMed Research International*, 2013.

116. Hu, L., and Jia, Y. (2010). Preparation and characterization of solid lipid nanoparticles loaded with epirubicin for pulmonary delivery. *Die Pharmazie-An International Journal of Pharmaceutical Sciences*, **65**(8), 585–587.

117. Wang, W., Zhu, R., Xie, Q., Li, A., Xiao, Y., Li, K., Liu, H., Cui, D., Chen, Y., and Wang, S. (2012). Enhanced bioavailability and efficiency of curcumin for the treatment of asthma by its formulation in solid lipid nanoparticles. *International Journal of Nanomedicine*, **7**, 3667.

118. Bhandari, R., and Kaur, I. P. (2013). Pharmacokinetics, tissue distribution and relative bioavailability of isoniazid-solid lipid nanoparticles. *International Journal of Pharmaceutics*, **441**(1–2), 202–212.

119. Doijad, R. C., Manvi, F. V., Godhwani, D. M., Joseph, R., and Deshmukh, N. V. (2008). Formulation and targeting efficiency of cisplatin engineered solid lipid nanoparticles. *Indian Journal of Pharmaceutical Sciences*, **70**(2), 203.

120. Surve, C. H. A. I. T. A. L. I., Singh, R. U. C. H. I., Banerjee, A. N. A. N. Y. A., Patnaik, S. R. I. N. I. V. A. S., and Shidhaye, S. U. P. R. I. Y. A. (2021). Formulation and QBD based optimization of methotrexate-loaded solid lipid nanoparticles for an effective anti-cancer treatment. *International Journal of Applied Pharmaceutics*, **13**(5), 132–143.

121. Pinto, B. F., Ribeiro, L. N. B., Da Silva, G. B. R. F., Freitas, C. S., Kraemer, L., Oliveira, F. M. S., Clímaco, M. C., Mourão, F. A. G., Santos, G. S. P. D., Béla, S. R., and Gurgel, I. L. D. S. (2022). Inhalation of

dimethyl fumarate-encapsulated solid lipid nanoparticles attenuate clinical signs of experimental autoimmune encephalomyelitis and pulmonary inflammatory dysfunction in mice. *Clinical Science*, **136**(1), 81–101.

122. Soppimath, K. S., Aminabhavi, T. M., Kulkarni, A. R., and Rudzinski, W. E. (2001). Biodegradable polymeric nanoparticles as drug delivery devices. *Journal of Controlled Release*, **70**(1–2), 1–20.

123. d'Angelo, I., Conte, C., Miro, A., Quaglia, F., and Ungaro, F. (2015). Pulmonary drug delivery: a role for polymeric nanoparticles? *Current Topics in Medicinal Chemistry*, **15**(4), 386–400.

124. Marasini, N., Haque, S., and Kaminskas, L. M. (2017). Polymer-drug conjugates as inhalable drug delivery systems: a review. *Current Opinion in Colloid & Interface Science*, **31**, 18–29.

125. Dailey, L. A., and Kissel, T. (2005). New poly (lactic-co-glycolic acid) derivatives: modular polymers with tailored properties. *Drug Discovery Today: Technologies*, **2**(1), 7–13.

126. Xu, Y., Kim, C. S., Saylor, D. M., and Koo, D. (2017). Polymer degradation and drug delivery in PLGA-based drug–polymer applications: a review of experiments and theories. *Journal of Biomedical Materials Research Part B: Applied Biomaterials*, **105**(6), 1692–1716.

127. Türeli, N. G., Torge, A., Juntke, J., Schwarz, B. C., Schneider-Daum, N., Türeli, A. E., Lehr, C. M., and Schneider, M. (2017). Ciprofloxacin-loaded PLGA nanoparticles against cystic fibrosis P. aeruginosa lung infections. *European Journal of Pharmaceutics and Biopharmaceutics*, **117**, 363–371.

128. Kim, I., Byeon, H. J., Kim, T. H., Lee, E. S., Oh, K. T., Shin, B. S., Lee, K. C., and Youn, Y. S. (2012). Doxorubicin-loaded highly porous large PLGA microparticles as a sustained-release inhalation system for the treatment of metastatic lung cancer. *Biomaterials*, **33**(22), 5574–5583.

129. Pandey, R., Sharma, A., Zahoor, A., Sharma, S., Khuller, G. K., and Prasad, B. (2003). Poly (D,L-lactide-co-glycolide) nanoparticle-based inhalable sustained drug delivery system for experimental tuberculosis. *Journal of Antimicrobial Chemotherapy*, **52**(6), 981–986.

130. Tomoda, K., Ohkoshi, T., Hirota, K., Sonavane, G. S., Nakajima, T., Terada, H., Komuro, M., Kitazato, K., and Makino, K. (2009). Preparation and properties of inhalable nanocomposite particles for treatment of lung cancer. *Colloids and Surfaces B: Biointerfaces*, **71**(2), 177–182.

131. Deacon, J., Abdelghany, S. M., Quinn, D. J., Schmid, D., Megaw, J., Donnelly, R. F., Jones, D. S., Kissenpfennig, A., Elborn, J. S., Gilmore, B. F., and Taggart, C. C. (2015). Antimicrobial efficacy of tobramycin polymeric nanoparticles for Pseudomonas aeruginosa infections in cystic fibrosis: formulation, characterisation and functionalisation with dornasealfa (DNase). *Journal of Controlled Release*, **198**, 55–61.

132. Beck-Broichsitter, M., Gauss, J., Gessler, T., Seeger, W., Kissel, T., and Schmehl, T. (2010). Pulmonary targeting with biodegradable salbutamol-loaded nanoparticles. *Journal of Aerosol Medicine and Pulmonary Drug Delivery*, **23**(1), 47–57.

133. Su, W. P., Cheng, F. Y., Shieh, D. B., Yeh, C. S., and Su, W. C. (2012). PLGA nanoparticles codeliver paclitaxel and Stat3 siRNA to overcome cellular resistance in lung cancer cells. *International Journal of Nanomedicine*, **7**, 4269.

134. Saikia, T. R. I. D. E. E. P., Lalhlenmawia, H. A. U. Z. E. L., Laldinchhana, R. P., and Thanzami, K. A. W. L. (2020). Effect of polymeric nanoparticles of curcumin on a549 cell line. *International Journal of Current Pharmaceutical Research*, 2020, 50–3.

135. Ghari, T., Mortazavi, S. A., Khoshayand, M. R., Kobarfard, F., and Gilani, K. (2014). Preparation, optimization, and *in vitro* evaluation of azithromycin encapsulated nanoparticles by using response surface methodology. *Journal of Drug Delivery Science and Technology*, **24**(4), 352–360.

136. Cipolla, D. C., Gonda, I., Aradigm, Corp. Inhaled surfactant-modified liposomal formulations providing both an immediate and sustained release profile. US20150110855A1.2015.

137. Weers, J. Insmed Inc., Lipid-based compositions of antiinfectives for treating pulmonary infections and methods of use there of.US9549939B2.2017.

138. Cipolla, D. C., Blanchard, J., Aradigm, Corp., Concentrated, inhalable ciprofloxacin formulation. US9545401B2.2017.

139. Zhiyong, Y., Xinyu, L., Zhiqin, et al. Long-acting liposome preparation for pulmonary drug delivery and preparation method thereof. CN103784403A.2014.

140. Yiguang, J., Mengmeng, Z., Lina, D. Military Mediccal Research Institute, Chinese Academy of Military Sciences. Paclitaxel-loaded liposome bacterium inhalation preparation for treating lung cancer. CN110559280A.2019.

141. Kaihua, L., Qian, W., Meiling, Z. Anti-lung cancer Docetaxel active targeting liposome. CN107260678B.2019.

142. Takeuti, H., Hakaho, K., Toyobuku, H. Otsuka Pharmaceutical Co. Ltd., Transpulmonary liposome for controlling drug delivery. RU2493874C2.2013.

143. Han, O., Zameknik, J., Schek, P. N., et al. Orlando Han., Pulmonary delivery of liposome encapsulated cannabinoid. JP2003504321A.2003.

144. Lee, H., Listevsky, B., Boylan, J. C., et al. Derek Ceraputix Corp., Stableliposome compositions comprising lipophilic amine containing pharmaceutical agents. KR20060123341A.2006.

145. Chimote, G. C., Mahajan, G. B., Vasudevan, A., et al. Priamal Enterprises Ltd., Microparticle formulation for pulmonary drug delivery of anti-infective molecule for treatmen to finfectious diseases. US8697653B2.2014.

146. Tingming, F., Wenqiang, S., Nanjing University of Chinese Medicine. Akind of 'Xiduofeng' drug microparticles of pulmonary administra tion and the preparation method and application thereof. CN109674773A.2019.

147. Benoit, J. P., Dulieu, C., Meurlay, D. L., et al. Microparticles for pulmonary administration. EP1204409A1.2002.

148. Tzannis, S. T., Sadrzadeh, N., Schiavone, H. Therapeutics. Sustained release micro particles for pulmonary delivery. WO2006124446A2.2006.

149. Cryan, S. A., Sivadas, N. Royal College of Surgeons In Ireland. Inhalable microparticles and methods for the production thereof. WO2010007604A2.2010.

150. Curtis, L. Coselix Ink Cotherix Inc., Treatment with iloprost inhaled using a microparticle formulation of pulmonary hypertension. JP2008507585A.2008.

151. Martyn, G. P. Quadrant Drug Delivery Ltd., Therapeutic compositions for pulmonary distribution. PT1259228E.2010.

152. Rundfeldt, C., Steckel, H., Rainer Schlichthaar, S. H. Nanosuspension with antifungal medication to be administered via inhalation with improved impurity profile and safety. US20110190245A1.2011.

153. Hulin, J., Xin, C., Lei, X., et al. China Pharmaceutical University. A kind of nanometer formulation and preparation method thereof for pulmonary fibrosis. CN110384681A.2019.

154. Zhibin, L., Xuefeng, Y. Shenzhen Institute of Advanced Technology, Chinese Academy of Sciences. A kind of load medicine black phosphorus chitosan composite nano ball and its preparation method and application. CN110090307A.2019.

155. Yu, G., Ziying, L., Lisheng, Z., et al. Fuzhou University. A kind of chitosan nano-material and preparation method thereof for lung cancer therapy. CN110251689A.2019.

156. Borlak, J., Benita, S., Debotton, N., et al. The Hebrew University of Jerusalem. Nanoparticles for targeted delivery of active agents to the lung. WO2009121631A2.2009.

157. Kost, J., Traitel, T., Goldbart, R., et al. Children's Hospital Medical Center. A controlled release system for pulmonary delivery of surfactant protein D. WO2016199146A1.2016.

158. Derosa, F., Guild, B. C., Heartlein, M., et al. Shire Human Genetics Therapies Inc., Pulmonary delivery of mRNA to non-lung target cells. AU2013271392B2.2018.

159. Charan, C., Dwivedi, S. Bayer Health Care AG. Antibiotic formulations, unit doses, kits, and methods. US20120247462A1.2012.

160. Lipp, M. M., Sung, J. C., Pulmatrix Inc., Cationic dry powder. US9433576B2.2016.

161. Smutney, C. C., Leone-Bay, A., Galarza, J. M., et al. Techno Vax Inc., Inhalable vaccine compositions and methods. 20150283069A1.2015.

162. Smutney, C. C., Adamo, B., Laurenzi, B. F., et al. Dry powder drug delivery system and methods. US9802012B2.2017.

163. Perry, J. M., Hava, D. L., Saunders, R. C., et al. Pulmatrix Operating Company. Antifungal formulations for pulmonary administration comprising it raconazole. WO2019204583A1.2019.

164. Bhat, M. G., Cuff, G. W., Wolff, R. K., Eli Lilly and Co., Protein powder for pulmonary delivery. WO2001093837.2001.

165. Aldous, B. J., Clark, A., Kuo, M.-C., et al. Nektar Therapeutics. Dry powder active agent pulmonary delivery. AU753014B2.2002.

166. Smatni, C. S., Adamo, B., Polidoro, J. M., et al. Mannkind Corporation. Systems and methods for dry powder drug delivery. RU2571331C1.2015.

167. Lai, J., Kessler, D. R., Quay, S. C. Sonus Pharmaceuticals Inc., Emulsions for aerosolization and drug delivery. WO1999024016A1.1999.

168. Shah, S. A., Sandidge, J. A., Sharp, M., et al. Low dose corticosteroid microemulsion compositions and methods of treatments thereof. WO2015009776A1.2015.

169. Ufer, S., Hofmann, T., Qrumpharma Inc., Inhalable clofazimine formulation. WO2019110099A1.2019.

170. Weirs, J. G., Knob, C. A., Sut, E. G., et al. Inhal Therapeutic Systems Inc., Stabilizing preparations for use in the nebulizer. JP2001517692A.2001.

171. Waldrep, J. C., Gilbert, B. E., Knight, C. M., Black, M. B., Scherer, P. W., Knight, V., and Eschenbacher, W. (1997). Pulmonary delivery of beclomethasone liposome aerosol in volunteers: tolerance and safety. *Chest*, **111**(2), 316–323.

172. Saari, S. M., Vidgren, M. T., Koskinen, M. O., Turjanmaa, V. M., Waldrep, J. C., and Nieminen, M. M. (1998). Regional lung deposition and clearance of ^{99m}Tc-labeled beclomethasone-DLPC liposomes in mild and severe asthma. *Chest*, **113**(6), 1573–1579.

173. Saari, M., Vidgren, M. T., Koskinen, M. O., Turjanmaa, V. M., and Nieminen, M. M. (1999). Pulmonary distribution and clearance of two beclomethasone liposome formulations in healthy volunteers. *International Journal of Pharmaceutics*, **181**(1), 1–9.

174. Jakobsson, J. K., Aaltonen, H. L., Nicklasson, H., Gudmundsson, A., Rissler, J., Wollmer, P., and Löndahl, J. (2018). Altered deposition of inhaled nanoparticles in subjects with chronic obstructive pulmonary disease. *BMC Pulmonary Medicine*, **18**(1), 1–11.

175. Haworth, C. S., Bilton, D., Chalmers, J. D., Davis, A. M., Froehlich, J., Gonda, I., Thompson, B., Wanner, A., and O'Donnell, A. E. (2019). Inhaled liposomal ciprofloxacin in patients with non-cystic fibrosis bronchiectasis and chronic lung infection with Pseudomonas aeruginosa (ORBIT-3 and ORBIT-4): two phase 3, randomised controlled trials. *The Lancet Respiratory Medicine*, **7**(3), 213–226.

176. Tsuji, T., Kim, Y. H., Ozasa, H., Sakamori, Y., Nagai, H., Ajimizu, H., Yagi, Y., Furukawa, A., Haga, H., and Mishima, M. (2015). Successful treatment with carboplatin and nanoparticle albumin-bound paclitaxel in a patient with pulmonary spindle cell carcinoma. *Respiratory Medicine Case Reports*, **15**, 48–50.

177. Park, H. H., Kim, H., Lee, H. S., Seo, E. U., Kim, J. E., Lee, J. H., Mun, Y. H., Yoo, S. Y., An, J., Yun, M. Y., and Kang, N. W. (2021). PEGylated nanoparticle albumin-bound steroidal ginsenoside derivatives ameliorate SARS-CoV-2-mediated hyper-inflammatory responses. *Biomaterials*, **273**, 120827.

178. Winthrop, K. L., Flume, P. A., Thomson, R., Mange, K. C., Yuen, D. W., Ciesielska, M., Morimoto, K., Ruoss, S. J., Codecasa, L. R., Yim, J. J., and Marras, T. K. (2021). Amikacin liposome inhalation suspension for Mycobacterium avium complex lung disease: a 12 month open-label extension clinical trial. *Annals of the American Thoracic Society*, **18**(7), 1147–1157.

Chapter 8

The Potential of Nanotechnology in Transdermal Drug Delivery Systems

Arvind Sharma,[a] Sumitra Singh,[b] Sunny Dhiman,[c] and Rakesh K. Sindhu[d]

[a]*School of Pharmaceutical and Health Sciences, Career Point University, Hamirpur, Himachal Pradesh, India*
[b]*Department of Pharmaceutical Sciences, Guru Jambheshwar University of Science and Technology, Hisar, Haryana, India*
[c]*Chandigarh College of Pharmacy, SAS Nagar, Mohali, Punjab, India*
[d]*School of Pharmacy, Sharda University, Greater Noida, Uttar Pradesh, India*

rakeshsindhu16@gmail.com

The stratum corneum presents a tough barrier for the delivery of drugs through the skin. There is interest in the use of nanoparticles as drug delivery carrier systems because these systems are potentially superior to other carrier systems in terms of controlled release, targeting, and stability. In recent years, a great deal of attention has been given to polymeric nanoparticles for delivering drugs to the skin. A detailed explanation of the interaction of the skin and nanoparticles will enhance the reader's understanding of new concepts and the use of drug delivery carriers in transdermal delivery. The mechanism of penetration/permeation of drug from different nanocarriers plays an important role not only in targeting drugs within the skin but also in the development strategies of nanocarriers. This chapter provides an overview

Nanotechnology and Drug Delivery: Principles and Applications
Edited by Rakesh K. Sindhu

ISBN 978-981-4968-83-6 (Hardcover), 978-1-003-43040-7 (eBook)
www.jennystanford.com

of the design of nanodrug delivery systems for transdermal drug delivery. The potential of nanotechnology in transdermal drug delivery is highlighted. The influence of the physicochemical properties of nanocarriers on transdermal drug delivery has also been given attention. Finally, the chapter concludes with future perspectives on nanotechnology in transdermal drug delivery.

8.1 Introduction

The word "nanoscale" describes to particle size within 100 to 1 nm [1]; however, depending on the mode of administration, nanoparticles between 50 and 500 nm are acceptable for drug delivery. The way a drug is administered can significantly affect how efficiently it is delivered to the desired site. Some medicaments have a range of optimal concentrations where the most effectiveness is obtained; dosages outside or inside of this range might be harmful or have no therapeutic potential. A diversified strategy for the delivery of therapies to targeted tissues is becoming more necessary as a result of the gradual improvement in the efficacy of treating a number of diseases [2]. After topical application to the skin's surface, transdermal drug delivery systems (TDDS) or patches are acceptable pharmaceutical delivery systems that contain the drug candidate for targeted management of disease conditions either administered topically or transdermally [3]. Even though the formulation matrix of various delivery systems varies, TDDS are suitable for a variety of drugs under investigation. The following ways set them apart from traditional topical formulations:

The formulation matrix of the patch maintains the drug concentration gradient within the device after application so that drug delivery to the interface between the patch and the skin is sustained [4]. They also have an impermeable occlusive backing film that prevents intense water loss from the skin beneath the patch. Finally, TDDS are kept in place on the skin surface by an adhesive layer, ensuring drug contact with the skin and ongoing drug delivery.

Drug administration through the skin, whether topical/transdermal, is difficult as the skin serves as a natural protective barrier. The US market for TDDS was first opened up in the middle of the 1970s [5], but transdermal (TD) drug had been used for a very long period. Previous studies have mentioned the use of belladonna plasters as an analgesic and mustard plasters to relieve chest congestion. The mustard plasters could be created at home or bought professionally. They were made by combining water and powdered mustard seeds to form a paste, which was then used to create a dispersion-style delivery method. The use of a nanoparticulate delivery system is one strategy that has been investigated to boost the penetration of bioactive substances into and through the skin.

When systemic, localized, or topical effects are indicated, the skin has traditionally been a key channel for drug administration. The skin stratum corneum (SC) serves as an effective restriction, but it also poses challenges for the TD administration of therapeutic agents since few compounds have the properties required to penetrate it sufficiently to achieve a therapeutic concentration within the blood [6]. Diverse approaches have been researched, created, and patented in an attempt to improve medicine transdermal absorption. Transdermal medication delivery is once again receiving attention as a result of advancements in physical permeation-enhancement technology. ultrasound, microneedles, iontophoresis and electroporation to open the skin, and more significantly, transdermal nanodrug delivery systems are a few of these cutting-edge technologies that improve transdermal penetration.

8.2 Structure of Skin

With a surface area of between 1.8 and 2.0 m^2, the human skin is the largest organ in the body.

The epidermis, dermis, and hypodermis (subcutaneous layer) make up its three primary layers (Fig. 8.1). The skin is a strong barrier that guards the body against outside threats and controls heat and loss of water in the body.

8.3 Mechanism of Drug Permeation through the Skin

Diffusion of therapeutics via the intact epidermis and skin appendages is crucial for drug penetration into the skin (hair

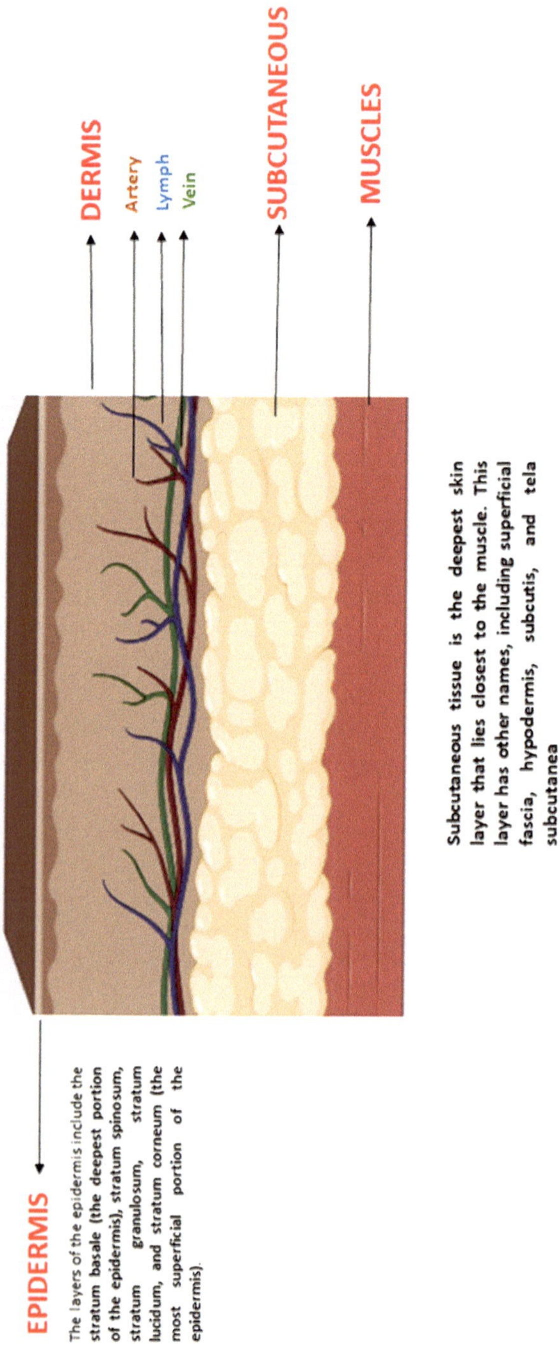

Figure 8.1 The basic structure of the skin.

follicles and sweat glands). These skin appendages, which account for approximately 0.1% of total human skin, establish shunt channels across the intact epidermis. The stratum corneum is recognized to provide a barrier to medication penetration through the skin. Interlamellar areas, particularly linker regions, have less ordered hydrophobic chains and lipids. Nonplanar spaces result from this between crystalline lipid lamellae and cell membranes. Skin fats transepidermal diffusion of lipidic and amphiphilic insertion and movement of molecules via intercellular lipid layers [7]. Hydrophilic compounds disperse "laterally" through or through water-filled interlamellar gaps; Polar molecules can utilize the gap between lamella and corneocyte membranes as shown in (Fig. 8.2).

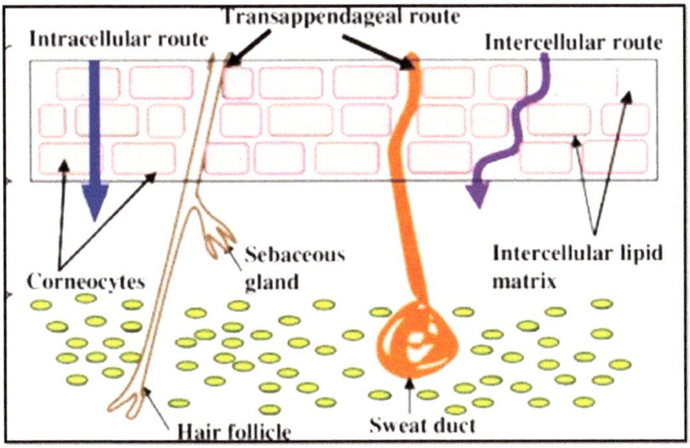

Figure 8.2 Mechanism of skin penetration.

Keratin is abundant in the stratum corneum's intracellular macromolecular matrix, which does not contribute directly to the skin diffusive barrier but maintains mechanical stability and intactness. Transcellular diffusion isn't crucial for transdermal medication delivery [8]. Confocal laser scanning microscopy reveals transepidermal aqueous channels. Poor cellular and intercellular lipid packing coincides with wrinkles on the skin surface and lowers the skin barrier to hydrophilic transport. This low-resistance route connects corneocyte clusters without lateral overlap. TD drug transport can enhance with route broadening or multiplication, e.g., by exposing the stratum corneum to a high electrical, mechanical, thermal, or skin penetrant stimulation.

8.4 Physicochemical Properties of Nanocarriers for Transdermal Drug Delivery

8.4.1 Particle Size Distribution (PSD), Zeta Potential and Particle Size

Size and shape impact nanoparticle cellular absorption, stability and drug release. Operations in-process and parameters such as rate of stirring, temperature, type and quantity of dispersion agent, and organic and aqueous phase viscosity alter yield and size distribution [9, 10]. Dispersion stability demands zeta potential [11].

8.4.2 Properties of Surface

Nanoparticle surface charge influences cell membrane adhesion. Variation of particle surface charge may regulate tissue binding and nanoparticle delivery in vitro and in vivo. Negatively charged sulfated proteoglycans have a key influence on the proliferation of cells, motility and migration [12]. Proteoglycans present on the cell surface are made up of a core protein attached to a membrane and connected to multiple glycosaminoglycan side chain (chondroitin sulfates, heparan, dermatan and keratin).

8.4.3 Nanoparticulate Drug Delivery Systems

Dermatological applications have been explored for a variety of nanodrug delivery systems, such as solid lipid nanoparticles, polymer-based nanoparticles, nanostructured lipid carriers as well as magnetic nanoparticles. These have overcome the shortcomings of classic TDDS such as ointments, gels, and so on in some way. Various delivery systems have been developed to promote drug transport via the skin, allowing for drug retention and in minor cases controlled release [6].

Skin penetration is critical for a variety of contemporary problems, including microbial and chemical contamination, medicine distribution to and via the skin (dermatological and transdermal therapies), and skincare and protection (cosmetics) [6]. Nanocarriers' small size, high surface energy, composition, architecture, and associated molecules are all merits and disadvantages of employing them for TDDS in general. Table 8.1 lists the benefits and drawbacks of typical transdermal nanocarriers.

8.4.3.1 Vesicular systems

8.4.3.1.1 *Liposomes*

Liposomes are colloidal dispersions having spherical vesicles that comprise a bilayer composed of phospholipid sequesters a portion of solvent where they easily disperse within the core [13]. Their benefit in pharmaceutical applications as drug carriers is the large range of molecules that may be added as well as the inherent biocompatibility of natural phospholipids. It is currently being debated whether liposomes can enter intact skin in terms of penetration behavior [14–17]. Liposomes have become a popular pharmaceutical nanotechnology-based drug delivery system for a variety of uses. Many vesicular system-based pharmaceuticals and biomedical formulations have recently been authorized for clinical use. Membrane processes and membrane-bound polypeptides were studied using them. Liposomes have also been considered as medication carriers with the potential to lower toxicity while increasing effectiveness. Liposomes are one of the greatest medication delivery options since they are nontoxic and stay in the bloodstream for an extended period of time. They've had good results for cancer treatment and skin melanoma [6]. Currently, the structural stability of many molten nanocosmetic carriers, including such as liposomes, is unstable. They stick to the interior walls of skin cells when passing through the skin, triggering the collapse of phospholipid-association bodies and the leakage of their contained components. As a result, they are unlikely to be able to deliver active substances deep into the skin. As a result, the use of flexible liposomes (elastic liposomes or transferosomes) is a promising technique for achieving the goal of transdermal medication administration. Examples of APIs delivered through the skin using a liposomal drug delivery system include melatonin, ketoprofen, methotrexate, estradiol, ketoprofen, lignocaine and amphotericin B, in comparison to diclofenac, insulin, tetanus toxoid, corticosteroids, DNA, clindamycin hydrochloride, triamcinolone-acetonide, and indinavir administered parentally.

8.4.3.1.2 *Niosomes (non-ionic surfactant-based vesicular systems)*

The drug molecule is enclosed in a vesicle in these non-ionic surfactant vesicular new drug delivery systems. Niosomes are vesicles that could entrap both hydrophilic and hydrophobic solutes. They can be unilamellar or multilamellar. Practically saying, niosomes are potential drug delivery systems as they are more stable and do not possess many of the drawbacks of liposomes, such as their expensive price and difficulties with changeable phospholipid purity [18]. Another benefit is the simplest procedure for producing niosomes on a continuous basis and in large quantities without the use of incompatible solvents. The hydrated composition of cholesterol and non-ionic surfactants such alkyl ethers, alkyl esters, or alkyl amides is one substitute for phospholipids [18, 19]. The vesicles developed by the above-mentioned combination are referred to as niosomes or non-ionic surfactant vesicles. Biocompatible, non-immunogenic, and biodegradable noisome surfactants are provided. Niosomes are adaptive delivery devices that may be applied transdermal, among many other ways [20, 21].

The use of niosomes as effective cutaneous and transdermal medicament delivery methods has received special attention [22, 23]. Niosomes, in particular, are thought to be promising medication delivery mechanisms for dermatological conditions.

Minoxidil and ellagic acid are two examples of transdermal medication delivery using niosomes. It has been demonstrated that niosomes can prolong the time that drugs remain in the stratum corneum and epidermis while reducing systemic absorption and enhancing the penetration of trapped molecules via the skin. Furthermore, these devices have been shown to reduce side effects and provide a significant medication release [24].

Table 8.1 Summary of typical components, structure, and transdermal mechanisms of transdermal nanocarriers [50]

Nanocarriers	Classification	Mechanism (TDDS)	Composition	Shape
Vesicular systems	Liposomes	The SC's lipids interact well with the phospholipid component	Phospholipid, cholesterol	Spherical vesicles with an aqueous inner core and one or maybe more lipid bilayers
	Elastic liposomes	For passing through the narrow pores, the edge activators boost flexibility and deformability	Phospholipid and edge activators	
	Ethosomes	The fluidity of lipid bilayers is enhanced by ethanol, which disrupts the SC membrane barrier	20–50% additional Ethanol	
	Invasomes	The lipid structure of the SC is disrupted by ethanol and terpenes, which increases membrane flexibility	Terpenes, phospholipids, and ethanol (low concentrations as low as 3% w/w)	
	Niosomes	Non-ionic surfactants improve the effectiveness of drug encapsulation	Non-ionic surfactants in addition to cholesterol	
	Glycerosomes	Comparable to transferosome; glycerol promotes deformability and elasticity	Cholesterol, glycerol, and phospholipid	
Inorganic nanoparticles	CuS nanoparticles	Near-infrared absorption triggers localized thermal ablation of SC, making penetration easier	Copper sulfide	Rigid as well as spherical particle

(Continued)

Table 8.1 (*Continued*)

Nanocarriers	Classification	Mechanism (TDDS)	Composition	Shape
	Gold nanoparticles	Some nanoscale nanoparticles can permeate the skin via the stratum corneum's lipidic matrix and hair follicle orifices	Gold	
	Fe_3O_4 nanoparticles	Transfollicular penetration allows them to reach the deeper dermis	Ferric oxide	
Lipid-based nanoparticles	Solid lipid nanoparticles	To broaden the inter-keratinocyte gap, the lipid nanoparticles produce a mono-layer lipid film	Lipid is solid	
	Nanostructured lipid carriers	The lipid components and associated surfactant may cause skin structure to be disrupted and the intercellular space to enlarge	Solid as well as liquid lipids	
Nanoemulsions		Improving the solubility of both lipid-soluble and water-soluble medicament by disrupting the skin's lipid bilayers	Surfactants, oil, water	Dispersions of oil and water
Nanogel		The nanocarrier dispersions boost localized medicament concentration and extend topical contact time; nanogels that are cationically charged interact with the epidermis	Polymers	Cross-linked network structure

During treating hair loss, niosomes synthesized from sorbitan monoesters (Spans) with a cholesterol molar ratio of 1:1 are an effective method for administering minoxidil to the scalp [25]. The Span 60 and Tween 60 niosomes have been shown to be promising carriers for cutaneous administration of ellagic acid [26].

8.4.3.1.3 *Elastic liposomes (transferosome)*

A lipid bilayer with characteristics that are deliberately constructed encapsulates at least one inner aqueous compartment in transferosomes, which are characterized as precisely engineered vesicular particles. Due to this, transferosomes, resemble lipid vesicles, or liposomes, in structure, but they are functionally flexible enough to pass through apertures that are much smaller than their own size [27]. They are metastable, which provides the vesicle membrane and the vesicles great mutability. The very great membrane adaptability of transferosomes, vesicles permits them to adjust to a restricting pore and so trespass through it. In contrast to conventional lipid vesicles like liposomes, typical transferosomes, have a membrane that is at least one order of magnitude more elastic. To convert liposomes into transferosomes, the vesicular membrane can include one or more edge-active substance(s); surfactants have been suggested as potential examples of such edge activators [28–30]. The enhanced hydrophilicity of transferosomes, which allows the membrane to enlarge more than the bilayers of ordinary lipid vesicles, is another difference between them and liposomes.

8.4.3.1.4 *Ethosomes*

Ethosomes are lipid vesicular systems that contain relatively high amounts of ethanol for improved medicament penetration through the skin [31]. Phospholipids, ethanol, and water make up the majority of them. The high ethanol content, which distinguishes ethosomes from other vesicular carriers, aids skin permeability, allowing encapsulated medication particles to be released into deeper layers and systemic circulation. Touitou created ethosomes in 1996 while researching the use of a lipid bilayer drug delivery system in drug delivery systems for skin therapy [32].

An ethosomal vesicle is composed of an aqueous inner core with the entrapped active component and a phospholipid bilayer. They are flexible and supple. An ethosome vesicle is in the nanometer range in size [33]. Furthermore, because of the high alcohol concentration, the ethosome vesicle is smaller than a liposome when generated under the same conditions. As the percentage of alcohol consumed grew from 20% to 45% [34], the size dropped. The ethanol conferred a net negative charge on the vesicle surface, which caused the size to decrease. Other excipients commonly used in the formulation of ethosomes include phospholipids such as cholesterol, soya lecithin (vesicle membrane stability), Span 60, 80 and Ethanol (permeation enhancers), and marker dyes (6-carboxy fluorescein and rhodamine) for characterization studies. Cholesterol has a stabilizing effect because it prevents vesicle aggregation and expansion during storage [35]. Because of their tiny size and malleability, ethosomes can pass past the skin or membrane barrier and impact transdermal permeability. The higher the amount of penetration, the smaller the size [31]. Unlike traditional liposomes, ethosomes penetrate the stratum corneum barrier and have a substantially higher transdermal flow. Deeper distribution and penetration in skin lipid bilayers are thought to be triggered by these interactions between linked phospholipids and high ethanol concentrations in vesicular formulations [33]. Technical ease, non-invasive administration (topical), enhanced TD distribution, and bypassing first-pass metabolism impact are just a few advantages of using ethosomes in drug delivery [36–38]. Improved patient compliance as a result of non-invasiveness leads to better treatment outcomes. High entrapment efficiency for a wide variety of substances, including lipophilic pharmaceuticals, has been established for ethosomes [34, 39], due to the multilamellar property of the vesicular systems and the presence of C_2H_5OH. Ethosomes are reported to have improved drug distribution unlike liposomes and elastic liposomes to the skin in both occlusive [40] and non-occlusive [35, 41, 42] situations.

The use of transformable liposomes lipid bilayer of the SC, which are able to squeeze and permeate throughout the skin when the gradient is developed, has grown. Tacrolimus-loaded ethosomes, for example, might be effective as a treatment for dermatitis especially atopic [43]. Skin permeability related to drugs formulated as ethosomes was measured using confocal laser scanning microscopy (CSLM), and the Rhodamine 123 loaded formulation had higher permeation than the ethanolic solution. Another Ketoprofen encapsulated ethosomal formulation has been shown as potentially promising vehicle for transdermal administration [44]. A psoriasis therapeutic approach which provides long-term therapeutic advantages, such as being nontoxic, and improves patient compliance is transferosomal carrier (phosphati-dylethanolamine). When 5-aminolevulinic acid (ALA)-containing ethosomal carriers are administered to hyperproliferative murine skin, ALA penetration and proto-porphyrin IX synthesis are enhanced, and tumor necrosis factor is significantly decreased in this disordered skin [45]. Ammonium glycyrrhizinate's ability to reduce inflammation was shown to be enhanced by ethanolosomes more so than by ethanolic or aqueous solutions [46].

Furthermore, the transferosomal system considerably increased skin permeability in vitro as compared to ethanolic, hydroethanolic, or phospholipid–ethanolic-micellar formulations of minoxidil. Moreover, TD testosterone distribution from an transferosomal patch was higher than that from commercially available patches both in vitro and in vivo [47]. Tacrolimus [43], clotrimazole [48], trihexyphenidyl HCl [49], ketoprofen [44], and testosterone are examples of transdermal drug delivery utilizing ethosomes.

The various commercially available transdermal formulations present in the market are discussed in Table 8.2.

8.4.3.2 Lipid nanoparticles

Lipid nanoparticles, unlike lipid nanocarriers, are solid entities that encapsulate pharmacological molecules in a lipid core. Solid lipid nanoparticles (SLN) are made up entirely of lipids that are solid in nature, while NLC or nanostructured lipid carriers comprise both solid as well as lipids. In comparison to SLNs, NLCs (Liquid lipids) prevent solid lipid recrystallization, increasing stability. Surfactants are employed to promote stability in formulations by reducing the tension between the hydrophobic-lipid structure and the aqueous phase [50]. Lipid nanoparticles' transdermal distribution method is unknown. The proposed causes are as follows: lipid nanoparticles have skin adhesion properties and create a mono-layer lipid film, resulting in the "occlusion effect," which prevents water evaporation, widens the inter-keratinocyte gap, and so improves drug penetration [51]. By interacting with the skin lipid layer, the lipid components and included surfactant have been shown to disturb skin structure and broadening of intercellular space, notably in SC. Gu et al., after treating the skin with triptolide-loaded lipid nanoparticles, observed skin structure [11] and SC as loose texture and dilated epidermis were visible in SEM pictures and histological examination, indicating a lipid nanoparticle-skin interaction.

8.4.3.3 Inorganic nanoparticles

With their potential for bio-imaging and phototherapy, inorganic nanostructures are frequently used for drug delivery for cancer management. By passively entering SC, certain nanoparticles with + charge, high surface lipophilicity, and tiny size exhibit TD capacity [2].

Various research has examined the transdermal drug delivery efficacy of some inorganic nanoparticles due to their excellent stability and potential for functionalization of the surface. Because of their minimum cell toxicity and controlled size of particles, gold nanoparticles have been extensively studied as TDDS [52]. According to reports, the volume and rate of skin penetration increase as particle size decreases; also, 15 nm size range entity accumulate in the deep dermis [53]. Furthermore, the surface ligands form an Au–S bond with the gold nanoparticles, allowing diverse ligands to be easily conjugated to the surface of particles by pre-thiolation [12]. This unique property of gold nanoparticles makes them suitable for gene transfer. Zheng et al. used Au–S bonding to combine GPs with EGFR-thiolated epidermal growth factor receptor, siRNA duplexes. In a mouse model, SNA-NCs penetrated the whole skin layer and efficiently suppressed EGFR expression. Other metallic particles for transdermal administration have also been discovered. Trans-follicular Fe_3O_4 nanoparticles with a pH-sensitive amide link effectively enter deeper dermis [54]. Light as well heat sensitive CuS nanoparticles irrigated with near-infrared cause localized thermal dissipation of SC and promote particle penetration [55].

Table 8.2 Marketed formulations for transdermal route of administration [59]

API/Drug	Manufacturer	Trade name	Transdermal patch	Indication
Nitroglycerine	Schwarz Pharma	Deponit	Drug in adhesive	Angina Pectoris
	3M Pharmaceuticals	Minitran	Drug in adhesive	
	Alza/Novartis	TransdermNitro	Reservoir	
	Schering-Plough	Diafusor	Matrix	
	Nitroderm TTS	Novartis	Face	
	Nitrodur	Key Pharmaceuticals	Matrix	
	NTS	Bolar, Major, Bio-Line, Goldline, Warner-Chilcott Laboratory Geneva, Rug	RIM	
Isosorbide-dinitrate	Frandol (Tape)	Yamanouchi, Toaeiyo, Pharmaceutical	Matrix	
Nicotine	Pro-step	Lederie/ElanCorp/Laboratory	Reservoir	Cessation of Smoking
	Habitraol	Novartis	Drug in adhesive	
	Nicotinell	Novartis	Matrix	
	Nicotrol	McNeil Consumer-Cygnus Inc-Products Ltd	Drug in adhesive	
	Nikofrenon	Novartis	Matrix	

(*Continued*)

Table 8.2 (*Continued*)

API/Drug	Manufacturer	Trade name	Transdermal patch	Indication
Testosterone	Androderm	GlaxoSmithKline/ Thera Tech	Reservoir	Male hypogonadism
	Testoderm TTS	Alza	Reservoir	
Lidocaine	Lidoderm	Cerner Multum, Inc.	Drug in adhesive	Anesthetic
Clonidine	Catapres-TTS	Alza/Boehinger Ingelheim	Membrane matrix hybrid type	Hypertension
Minoxidil 4%	Nanominox	Sinere, Germany		Promotion of hair growth
Sco-polamine	Transderm-(Scop)	Alza/Novarti	Matrix-membrane hybrid type	Motion-sickness
Hyoscine	Kimite-patch	Myun Moon Pharm. Co	Matrix	
Estradiol	Climara	3M Pharmaceuticals/Berlex Labs	Drug in adhesive	Postmenstrual syndrome
Acyclovir	Supravir cream	Trima, Israel		Herpes infection
Ethinyl-Estradiol	Ortho Evra		Drug in adhesive	Postmenstrual Syndrome

8.4.3.4 Additional nanocarriers

Dendrimers are high-branched polymeric nanocarriers that are utilized as TDDS to transport hydrophobic chemicals and macromolecules like photosensitizers and chemotherapeutics. Traditional poly (amidoamine) dendrimers demonstrated penetration enhancer potential, but they were unable to successfully penetrate the skin barrier due to their interaction with the lipid bilayers that make up the skin [56]. Some recent investigations have focused on dendrimer size and surface charge, leading to the development of second-generation dendrimers with reduced sizes and skin-penetrating capabilities [57]. Micelles are polymeric nanocarriers that are made up of amphiphilic polymers or surfactants that clump together in an aqueous solution [58]. Micelles have the capacity to co-deliver drugs due to their variable composition. Lipophilic medications are usually found in the core, whereas hydrophilic drugs are mostly found in the shell [30]. Micelles, like TDDS, can improve medication water solubility and hence boost skin penetration. Because intact SC blocks the polymer components, low-permeability medicines have less improvement [59].

8.5 Future Prospects of Nanodrug Delivery Systems

Physicochemical features use, and transport mechanisms of several transdermal nanocarriers are explored in this paper. According to the findings, the lipophilic part can interfere with the skin's lipid layer, disturb structure, increase space within cells, and therefore make skin penetration easier. TDDS can be made from nanovesicles or solid nanoparticles. The bilayer membrane structure gives nanovesicles a lot of flexibility and elastic nature, while the lipoidal core gives solid nanoparticles more stability. Hydrophilic pharmaceuticals are encapsulated in aqueous internal cores, whereas hydrophobic medications are loaded in exterior lipid bilayers. Solid nanoparticles, on the other hand, protect hydrophobic pharmaceuticals in the lipid core while absorbing hydrophilic medications in the outside aqueous phase. Furthermore, smaller sizes are indicated for increased

SA, which promotes non-specific cell absorption and enables transcellular penetration. However, there is no absolute relationship between size and penetration effectiveness, and drug encapsulation efficiency is dependent on nanoparticle size. Furthermore, the impact of surface charge is still debatable. Although + surface charge is thought to facilitate penetration through the skin by increasing electrostatic contact with the cell membrane, several studies have found that negatively charged nanoparticles have better transdermal efficiency. Excessive cell internalization and skin retention will result in decreased skin penetration. As a result, the optimal particle size and surface charge range must be investigated. In addition, their surface modification tactics are examined in order to address the issues of limited penetration, uncontrolled release, and lack of targeting. As previously stated, we categorized the surface modifications based on their purposes. The use of a penetration enhancer boosts transdermal penetrability, allowing therapeutic medicines to pass through thick skin tissue in dermatitis and dense fibrous tissue in scars. The ability to build the TD nanocarrier according to the ideal tissue drug concentration is made feasible by the implementation of both sustained and triggered regulated drug release. Furthermore, transdermal nanocarriers achieve active drug targeting delivery capacity within selected particular ligands for target receptors, which is critical for skin cancer treatment.

References

1. Hatto, P (2011). ISO consensus definitions relevant to nanomaterials and nanotechnologies. 4th Annual Nano Safety for Success Dialogue. ISO TC 229 and BSI NTI/1 Nano-Nanoparticles for Dermal and Transdermal Drug Delivery. http://dx.doi.org/10.5772/586722-23.
2. Devi, VK, Saisivam, S, Maria, GR, Deepti PU (2003). Design and evaluation of matrix diffusion controlled transdermal patches of verapamil hydrochloride. *Drug Dev Ind Pharm*. 29: 495–503.
3. Valenta, C, Auner, BG (2004). The use of polymers for dermal and transdermal delivery. *Eur J Pharm Biopharm*. 58: 279–289.
4. Block, HL (2010). Biopharmaceutics and drug delivery systems. In: *Comprehensive Pharmacy Review*. eds. Shargel, L, Mutnick, AH,

Souney, PF, Swanson, LN, Lippincott Williams and Wilkins, USA. pp. 83–96.

5. Prausnitz, MR, Langer, R (2008). Transdermal drug delivery. *Nat Biotech.* 26(11): 1261–1268.
6. Escobar-Chávez, JJ, Díaz-Torres, R, Rodríguez-Cruz, IM, Domínguez-Delgado, CL, Morales, RS, Ángeles-Anguiano, E, Melgoza-Contreras, LM (2012). Nanocarriers for transdermaldrug delivery. *Res Rep Transdermal Drug Deliv.* 1: 3–17.
7. Geinoz, S, Guy, RH, Testa, B, Carrupt, PA (2004). Quantitative structure–permeation relationships (QSPeRs) to predict skin permeation: a critical evaluation. *Pharm Res.* 21: 83–92.
8. Cevc, G, Vier IU (2010). Nanotechnology and the transdermal route. A state of the art review and critical appraisal. *J Control Rel.* 141: 277–299.
9. Pinto Reis, C, Nuefel, RJ, Ribeiro, AJ (2006). Nanoencapsulation 1. Methods for preparation of drug-loaded polymeric nanoparticles. *Nanomedicine.* 2: 8–21.
10. Maestrelli, F, Capasso, G, Gonzalez-Rodriguez, M, et al. (2009). Effect of preparation technique on the properties and in vivo efficacy of benzocaine-loaded ethosomes. *J Liposome Res.* 19(4): 253–60.
11. Attama, AA, Schicke, BC, Paepenmüller, T, Müller-Goymann, CC (2007). Solid lipid nano-dispersions containing mixed lipid core and a polar heterolipid: Characterization. *Eur J Pharm Biopharm.* 67: 48–57.
12. Bernfild, M, Gotte, M, Park, PW, Reizes, O, Fitzgerald, ML, Lincecum, J, Zako, M (1999). Functions of cell surface heparan sulphate proteoglycans. *Annu Rev Biochem.* 68: 729–777.
13. Kumar, VS, Asha, K (2011). Herbosome a Novel carrier for herbal drug delivery. *Int J Curr Pharm Res.* 3(3): 36–41.
14. Jung, S, Otberg N, Thiede, G, Richter, H, Sterry, W, Panzner, S, Lademann, J (2006). Innovative liposomes as a transfollicular drug delivery system: penetration into porcine hair follicles. *J Invest Dermatol.* 126: 1728–1732.
15. Honeywell-Nguyen, PL, Wouter Groenink, HW, de Graaff, AM, Bouwstra, JA (2003). The in vivo transport of elastic vesicles into human skin: effects of occlusion, volume and duration of application. *J Control Rel.* 90: 243–255.
16. Honeywell-Nguyen, PL, de Graaff, AM, Groenink, HW, Bouwstra, JA (2002). The in vivo and in vitro interactions of elastic and rigid vesicles with human skin. *Biochim Biophys Acta.* 1573: 130–140.

17. Verma, DD, Verma, S, Blume, G, Fahr, A (2003). Liposomes increase skin penetration of entrapped and non-entrapped hydrophilic substances into human skin: a skin penetration and confocal laser scanning microscopy study. *Eur J Pharm Biopharm.* 55: 271–277.
18. Uchegbu, IF, Florence, AT (1995). Non-ionic surfactant vesicles (niosomes): physical and pharmaceutical chemistry. *Adv Colloid Interface Sci.* 58: 1–55.
19. Vora, B, Khopade, AJ, Jain, NK (1998). Proniosome based transdermal delivery of levonorgestrel for effective contraception. *J Control Rel.* 54: 149–165.
20. Alsarra, IA, Bosela, AA, Ahmed, SM, Mahrous, GM (2005). Proniosomes as a drug carrierfor transdermal delivery of ketorolac. *Eur J Pharm Biopharm.* 59: 485–490.
21. Muzzalupo, R, Tavano, L, Cassano, R, Trombino, S, Ferrarelli, T, Picci, N (2011). A new approach for the evaluation of niosomes as effective transdermal drug delivery systems. *Eur J Pharm Biopharm.* 79: 28–35.
22. Manconi, M, Caddeo, C, Sinico (2011). Ex vivo skin delivery of diclofenac by transcutol containing liposomes and suggested mechanism of vesicle–skin interaction. *Eur J Pharm Biopharm.* 78: 27–35.
23. Mura S, Manconi, M, Sinico, C, Valenti D, Fadda, AM (2009). Penetration enhancer containingvesicles (PEVs) as carriers for cutaneous delivery of minoxidil. *Int J Pharm.* 380: 72–79.
24. Guinedi, AS, Mortada, ND, Mansour, S, Hathout, RM (2005). Preparation and evaluation of reverse-phase evaporation and multilamellar niosomes as ophthalmic carriers of acetazolamide. *Int J Pharm.* 306: 71–82.
25. Balakrishnana, P, Shanmugama, S, Lee, WS (2009). Formulation and in vitro assessmen to fminoxidil niosomes for enhanced skin delivery. *Int J Pharm.* 377: 1–8.
26. Junyaprasert, VB, Singhsa, P, Suksiriworapong, J, Chantasart, D (2012). Physicochemical properties and skin permeation of Span 60/Tween 60 niosomes of ellagic acid. *Int J Pharm.* 423: 303–311.
27. Jain, S, Jain, P, Umamaheshwari, RB, Jain, NK (2003). Transfersomes a novel vesicular carrier for enhanced transdermal delivery: development, characterization, and performance evaluation. *Drug Dev Ind Pharm.* 29 (9): 1013–1026.

28. Planas, ME, Gonzalez, P, Rodriguez, S, Sanchez, G, Cevc, G (1992). Non-invasive percutaneous induction of topical analgesia by a new type of drug carrier and prolongation of the local pain intensity by liposomes. *Anesth Analge.* 95: 615–621.

29. Cevc, G, Schatzlein, A, Blume, G (1995). Transdermal drug carrier basic properties, optimization and transfer efficiency in the case of epicutaneously applied peptides. *J Control Rel.* 36: 3–16.

30. Paul, A, Cevc, G, Bachhawat, BK (1998). Transdermal immunization with an integral membrane component gap junction protein, by means of ultradeformable drug carriers, transfersomes. *Vaccine.* 16: 188–195.

31. Mbah, CC, Builders PF, Attama, AA (2014). Nanovesicular carriers as alternative drug delivery systems: ethosomes in focus. *Expert Opin Drug Deliv.* 11(1): 1–15.

32. Touitou, E (1996). Composition of applying active substances to or through the skin. US5716638.

33. Jain, S, Tiwary, AK, Sapra, B, Jain, NK (2007). Formulaion and evaluation of thosomes for transdermal delivery of lamivudine. *AAPS PharmSciTech.* 8(4): Article 111.

34. Touitou, E, Dayan N, Bergelson, L (2000). Ethosomes–novel vesicular carriers for enhanced delivery: characterization and skin penetration properties. *J Control Rel.* 65: 403–18.

35. Coderch, L, Fonollosa, J, De Pera, M (2000). Influence of cholesterol on liposome fluidity by EPR: relationship with percutaneous absorption. *J Control Rel.* 68: 85–95.

36. Serikawa, T, Kikuchi, A, Sugaya, S (2006). *In vitro* and *in vivo* evaluation of novel cationic liposomes utilized for cancer gene therapy. *J Control Rel.* 113(3): 255–260.

37. Barry, BW (2004). Breaching the skin' barrier to drugs. *Nat Biotechnol.* 22: 165–167.

38. Honeywell-Nguyen, PL, Bouwstra, JA (2005). Vesicles as a tool for transdermal and dermal delivery. *Drug Discov Today.* 2: 67–74.

39. Elsayed, MMA, Abdallah, OY, Naggar, VF (2007a). Lipid vesicles for skin delivery of drugs: reviewing three decades of research. *Int J Pharm.* 332: 1–16.

40. Paolino, D, Lucania, G, Mardente, D, et al. (2005). Ethosomes for skin delivery of ammonium glycyrrhizinate: in vitro percutaneous

permeation through human skin and in vivo anti-inflammatory activity on human volunteers. *J Control Rel.* 106: 99–110.

41. Dayan, N, Touitou, E (2000). Carriers for skin delivery of tri-hexyphenidyl HCl: ethosomes vs. liposomes. *Biomaterials.* 21: 1879–85.
42. Elsayed, MM, Abdallah, OY, Naggar, VF (2007b). Deformable liposomes and ethosomes as carriers for skin delivery of ketotifen. *Pharmazie.* 62: 133–137.
43. Li G, Fan Y, Fan C, Li X, Wang X, Li M, Liu Y (2012). Tacrolimus-loaded ethosomes: physicochemical characterization and in vivo evaluation. *Eur J Pharm Biopharm.* 82(1): 49–57.
44. Chourasia, MK, Kang, L, Chan, SY (2011). Nanosized ethosomes bearing ketoprofen for improved transdermal delivery. *Results Pharm Sci.* 1: 60–67.
45. Fang, YP, Huang YB, Wua, PC, Tsai, YH (2009). Topical delivery of 5-aminolevulinic acid-encapsulated ethosomes in a hyper-proliferative skin animal model using the CLSM technique to evaluate the penetration behavior. *Eur J Pharm Biopharm.* 73: 391–398.
46. Paolino, D, Lucania, G, Mardente, D, Alhaique, F, Fresta, M (2005). Ethosomes for skin delivery of ammonium glycyrrhizinate: in vitro percutaneous permeation through human skin and in vivo anti-inflammatory activity on human volunteers. *J Control Rel.* 106: 99–110.
47. Touitou, E, Dayan, N, Bergelson, L, Godina, B, Eliaz, M (2000). Ethosomes–novel vesicular carriers for enhanced delivery: characterization and skin penetration properties. *J Control Rel.* 65: 403–418.
48. Maheshwari, RGS, Tekade, RK, Sharma, PA (2012). Ethosomes and ultra-deformable liposomes for transdermal delivery of clotrimazole: a comparative assessment. *Saudi Pharm J.* 20: 161–170.
49. Dayan, N, Touitou, E (2000). Carriers for skin delivery of trihexy-phenidyl HCl: ethosomes vs liposomes. *Biomaterials.* 21: 1879–1885.
50. Ranade, VV, Cannon, JB (2011). *Drug Delivery Systems*, 3rd ed, Taylor and Francis, Boca Raton.
51. Schaefer, H, and Redelmeir, TE (1996). *Skin Barrier, Principles of Percutaneous Absorption*, eds, Karger Publishers.
52. Chikazawa, M, Takei, T (1997). *Specific Surface Area in Powder Technology Handbook* (eds Gotoh, K, Masuda, H, and Higashitani, K), 2nd edn, Marcel Dekker, Inc., New York, NY, Ch. III. 8, pp. 337–349.

53. Hueber, F, Schaefer, H, Wepierre, J (1994). Role of trans-epiderma and trans-follicular routes in percutaneous absorption of steroids: *in vitro* studies on human skin. *Skin Pharmacol.* 7: 237–244.

54. Rougier, A, Rallis, M, Kiren, P, Lotte, C (1990). "*In vivo* percutaneous absorption: A key role for stratum corneum/vehicle partitioning." *Arch Dermatol Res.* 282: 498–505.

55. Kalpana, SP, Mikolaj, M, Courtney, LS, Nicole, KB, Priyanka, G, Audra, LS (2010). Challenges and opportunities in dermal/transdermal delivery. *Ther Deliv.* 1(1): 109–131.

56. Bos, JD, Meinardi, MMHM (2000). The 500 Dalton rule for the skin penetration of chemical compounds and drugs. *Ex Dermatol.* 9(3): 165–169.

57. Ishida-Yamamoto, A, Simon, M, Kishibe, M, Miyauchi, Y, Takahashi, H, Yoshida, S, O'Brien, TJ, Serre, G, Iizuka, H (2004). 'Epidermal lamellar granules transport different cargoes as distinct aggregates. *J Invest Dermatol.* 122(5): 1137–1144.

58. Tsutomu, I, Tohru, M (2010). Techniques for efficient entrapment of pharmaceuticals in biodegradable solid micro/nanoparticle. *Expert Opinion Drug Deliv.* 7(6): 1–11.

59. Marcato, PD, Duran, N (2008). New aspects of nano-pharmaceutical delivery systems. *J Nanosci Nanotechnol.* 6: 2216–2229.

Multiple-Choice Questions

1. Physicochemical factor that affect TDDS:
   (a) Sunlight
   (b) Partition coefficient
   (c) Air pollution
   (d) Cold season

2. The characteristic that is suitable for transdermal drug:
   (a) Large drug dose
   (b) Large molecular size
   (c) Drug with narrow therapeutic index
   (d) Drugs which are metabolized in the skin

3. The primary barrier to transdermal drug delivery:
   (a) Dermis
   (b) Epidermis (stratum corneum)

(c) Hypodermis
(d) All of the above

4. Transdermal drug delivery system is related to

(a) Dosage form applied to the skin
(b) Dosage forms administered in the colon
(c) Dosage form administered systemically

5. The ideal molecular weight for the drug for transdermal drug delivery system:

(a) Not more than 800 Dalton
(b) Not more than 1000 Dalton
(c) Not more than 400 Dalton
(d) Not more than 1200 Dalton

6. Liposomes consists of a bilayer of

(a) Hydrophilic molecules
(b) Hydrophobic molecules
(c) Both a and b
(d) None

7. Which of the following is not an advantage of liposomes?

(a) Tissue targeting
(b) Increased therapeutic index
(c) Reduction in drug toxicity
(d) Faster dissolution

8. Liposome phospholipid undergoes

(a) Oxidation
(b) Hydrolysis
(c) Acetylation
(d) Both a and b

9. Liposomes are spherical structures, usually between _____ and ________ in diameter.

(a) 80 nm and 100 nm
(b) 60 nm and 100 nm
(c) 55 nm and 1000 nm
(d) 15 nm and 1000 nm

10. Liposomes are made up of
    (a) Phospholipids
    (b) Glycoproteins
    (c) Polysaccharides
    (d) Monosaccharides

11. Niosomes are formulated by using ____ surface-active agents.
    (a) Cationic
    (b) Non-ionic
    (c) Anionic
    (d) Zwitter-ionic

12. Advantages of niosomes:
    (a) They are osmotically active and stable.
    (b) They increase the stability of the entrapped drug.
    (c) They are biodegradable, non-immunogenic and biocompatible.
    (d) All the above.

13. Non-ionic surfactants used to formulate niosomes:
    (a) Tween-80
    (b) Cetrimide
    (c) Alkyl sulfates
    (d) All of the above

14. In niosomes, phospholipids are:
    (a) Present
    (b) Absent
    (c) Both a and b
    (d) None

15. Which of the following is false regarding the merits of the TDDS?
    (a) Avoidance of the first-pass effect
    (b) A stable and controlled blood level
    (c) Termination at any time is conceivable
    (d) Skin irritation and allergic response

16. The innermost layer of the skin is
    (a) Hypodermis
    (b) Stratum lucidum
    (c) Dermis
    (d) Epidermis
17. The stratum corneum is composed of
    (a) Melanin
    (b) Granules
    (c) Keratin cells
    (d) Squamous cells
18. The primary barriers for the TDDS is
    (a) Dermis
    (b) Hypodermis
    (c) Subcutaneous tissue
    (d) Epidermis
19. Which of the following statement is true with regard to the effect of "skin thickness" on the rate of permeation?
    (a) The rate of permeation is not dependent on the thickness of the skin.
    (b) The rate of permeation increases with an increase in skin thickness.
    (c) The rate of permeation decreases with an increase in skin thickness.
    (d) The rate of permeation increases skin thickness.
20. Which of the following molecular weight is considered ideal for a TDDS candidate?
    (a) Not more than 400 Dalton
    (b) Not more than 600 Dalton
    (c) Not more than 800 Dalton
    (d) Not more than 1000 Dalton
21. The following characteristic is/are true for noisome:
    (a) Biocompatible
    (b) Non-immunogenic
    (c) Biodegradable
    (d) All of the above

22. Advantages of solid lipid nanoparticles:
    (a) Easy to scale up and sterilize
    (b) Water-based technology
    (c) More affordable
    (d) All the above
23. The range of the size of the colloidal particles used as nanoparticle is
    (a) 10–1000 nm
    (b) 1–100 nm
    (c) 100–10,000 nm
    (d) All the above
24. Which route is the most common way of drug penetration into the skin?
    (a) Transcellular route
    (b) Intercellular route
    (c) Appendageal route
    (d) Both a and b
25. Liposomes have ___________ water solubility.
    (a) Lower
    (b) Higher
    (c) Intermediate
    (d) Both a and b
26. The nanoparticles that are used as a " novel drug delivery systems" are
    (a) Nanotubes
    (b) Nanocapsules
    (c) Nanoarrays
    (d) Nanocarriers

Answer Key

1.	(b)	**2.**	(c)	**3.**	(b)	**4.**	(b)	**5.**	(c)	**6.**	(c)	**7.**	(d)
8.	(d)	**9.**	(d)	**10.**	(a)	**11.**	(b)	**12.**	(d)	**13.**	(a)	**14.**	(a)
15.	(d)	**16.**	(a)	**17.**	(c)	**18.**	(d)	**19.**	(c)	**20.**	(a)	**21.**	(d)
22.	(d)	**23.**	(a)	**24.**	(d)	**25.**	(a)	**26.**	(d)				

Chapter 9

Novel Drug Delivery Systems for Infection Treatment

Shashi Kiran Mishra,[a] **Anupriya Kapoor,**[a] **and Kamla Pathak**[b]

[a]*School of Pharmaceutical Sciences,*
CSJM University Kanpur, Uttar Pradesh, India
[b]*Faculty of Pharmacy, Uttar Pradesh University of Medical Sciences,*
Saifai, Etawah, India

kamlapathak5@gmail.com

Approximately, 60% of the infectious diseases in developing countries are transmitted through animal sources (zoonotic) which silently affect vital organs and result in life-threatening diseases. The size, shape and mode of transmission of these pathogens are highly compatible with host biological tissues and compartments. Although enormous antibiotics and antivirals have been discovered and clinically approved, their systemic toxicity and drug resistance are major hurdles to effective therapy. Furthermore, the emergence of new variants of infectious agents poses new challenges to therapy. Advanced technologies in delivery systems are stipulated that can control and eradicate pathogens and alleviate infection. Novel drug delivery systems (NDDS) are sought as an effective and specific tool for targeting pathogens and imparting better patient compliance. Reduced dosing frequency, diminished adverse effects, high biocompatibility, short treatment

Nanotechnology and Drug Delivery: Principles and Applications
Edited by Rakesh K. Sindhu

ISBN 978-981-4968-83-6 (Hardcover), 978-1-003-43040-7 (eBook)
www.jennystanford.com

time and cost-effective parameters of NDDS always remain the prominent area. The chapter focuses on different NDDS including micro/nanospheres, vesicular, polymeric, particulate and their applications in the management of myriad infectious diseases.

9.1 Introduction

In developing countries, the emergence and re-emergence of contagious infections are proving a community health threat. Infections may occur via bacteria, viruses, fungi, parasites (protozoa, helminths) and worms that transmit diseases through intake of infected food, insect bite, sexual intercourse, droplet dispersion and skin contact. These invaders easily attack the immuno-compromised, diseased state and post-operated patients where these microorganisms flourish according to their growth requirements [1].

Today's world faces infectious diseases as a leading cause of death, particularly among young children in middle-income countries. Respiratory tract infections (COVID-19, coronary obstructive pulmonary disease and pneumonia), diarrhea, tuberculosis, dengue, malaria, human immunodeficiency virus (HIV)/acquired immunodeficiency syndrome (AIDS), hepatitis B and influenza are ranked in the top 10 infections [2]. The co-evolution of infectious agents (pathogens) with living beings including the environment creates critical challenges. A list containing human pathogenic organisms (1000 bacteria, 270 viruses, 450 fungi, 80 protozoans and 300 helminths) was compiled in the year 2008 in which most of the infections were transmitted through animal sources (zoonotic) [3]. Rapid urbanization, climate change, poor nutritional choice and modern living style lead to the risk of infections day by day. Poverty, deficient infrastructure (poor water quality, unhygienic hospitals, and open sewage system) and malnutrition intensify severity of infection in a community [4]. Drastic climate changes and shifted geographical distribution significantly contribute emergence and transmission of infectious pathogens in a community. According to a WHO report (2018), more than 17 million people are sufferers of bacterial infections in a year. Further, antibiotics-resistant bacteria are harder to manage and require higher medical costs and prolonged hospital stays [5].

A survey demonstrated that amid 9.7% universal infectious disease, tuberculosis ranked first (2.3%) in global death, followed by 2% diarrhea and 0.5% meningitis, 0.2% gonorrhea, syphilis, Chlamydia (sexually transmitted) and 0.19% encephalitis. Moreover, bacterial infection resistant to a particular medicine can be transmitted to others in a community, which would lead to serious health issues or even death. In the year 2019, WHO declared antimicrobial resistance associated deaths from six leading bacteria, i.e., *Escherichia coli* (cephalosporins and fluoroquinolones resistant), *Klebsiella pneumonia (*cephalosporin and carbapenem resistant), *Staphylococcus aureus* (methicillin resistant), *Pseudomonas aeruginosa* (tetracycline and erythromycin resistant), *Streptococcus pneumonia* (fluoroquinolones) *and Acinetobacter baumannii* (carbapenem resistant). Inappropriate and irrational usages of antimicrobials (antibiotics) are major issues which should be resolved to achieve efficient action against bacteria-resistant infections [6]. Misuse of antibiotics lets the exposure of bacteria in a sub-minimum inhibitory concentration environment for an extended time. That leads to drug-resistant mutation, produces antibiotic-resistant genes and sharply increases the MIC level of antibiotics [7]. In the USA, more than USD 55 billion per year is invested in the management of infections caused by antibiotic-resistant bacteria [8]. Traditional remedies, i.e., cream, lotion, gel and powders, may inhibit the growth of pathogens at the prelim stage and work as prophylactic. Figure 9.1 displays various novel drug delivery approaches designed for the alleviation of diverse infections caused by bacteria, viruses and fungi. But, at severe and advanced stages of infection, these preparations seem to be ineffective due to issues such as poor drug release, frequent administration, reduced half-life, peak valley plasma concentration, side effects and patient incompliance. Sometimes, the conventional preparations may trigger the immune system of the host and exhibit hypersensitivity or allergic reactions also. Irrational, increased and nonspecific use of antibiotics against bacterial infection often leads to the risk of super infection in case of surgery and organ transplantation. Moreover, patients receiving substantial doses of steroids, chemotherapeutic agents,

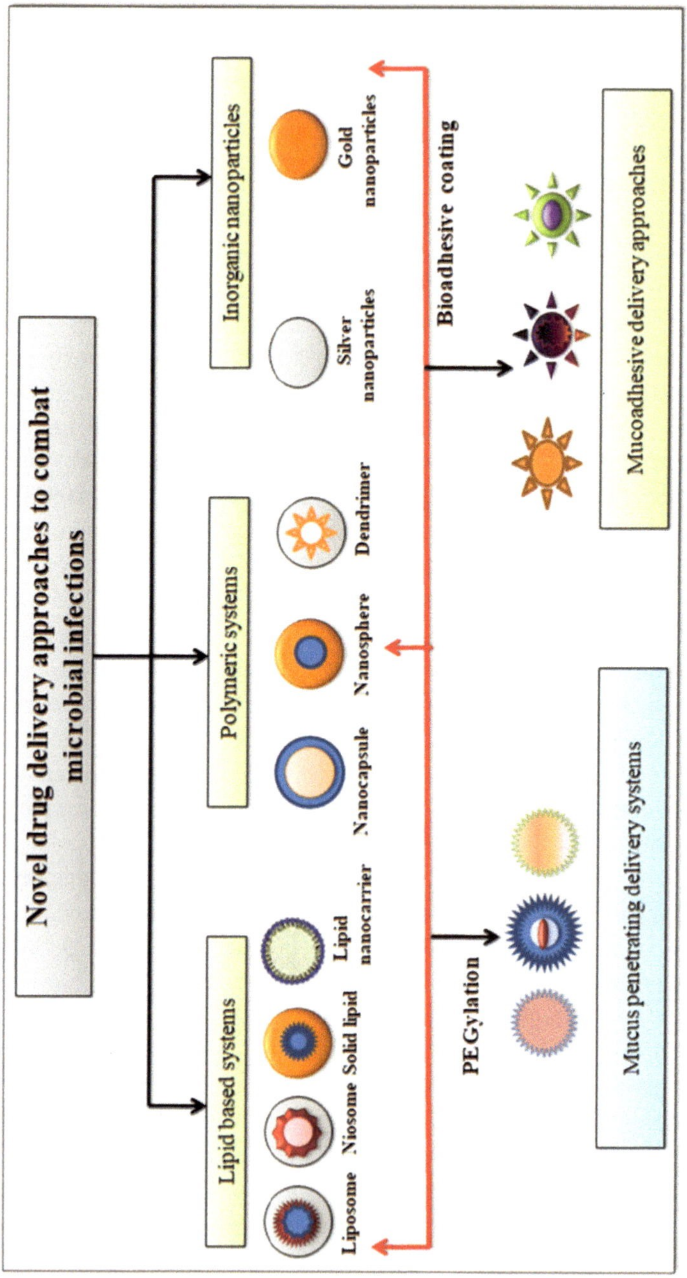

Figure 9.1 Various novel drug delivery approaches for the management of infections.

dependent on parenterals, are more susceptible to infections. So, an understanding of the emergence and speed of resistance for antibiotic treatment is required [9]. Development of newer antibiotics has been restricted by more rigorous legislations and poor economic incentives in developing countries. The US FDA, the principal drug regulator, approved only six antibiotics against Gram-positive bacteria between 2015 and 2018 [10].

Several approaches, including proteins, peptides, genes, nucleic acids, antibodies, aptamers, etc., are proven to mitigate infections and are suggested to co-administer with other bioactive agents to treat multiple diseases. The conventional delivery systems fail to deliver them due to oscillation in plasma concentration, poor bioavailability, enzymatic degradation and insufficient penetration of intestinal mucosa. Further, altered microenvironment at the infection site (low pH, overexpressive enzymes, release of hydrogen peroxide and toxins) and bacterial surface properties are major concerns for designing efficient and responsive drug delivery systems [11].

NDDS have been extensively utilized to completely eradicate pathogens and their infection from the site. Improved pharmacokinetics decreased dosing frequency, high therapeutic action, controlled release, minimum adverse effects and improved patient compliance can be achieved through designing novel technology and innovation in methodology. The past decade witnesses extensive research on innumerable innovative strategies for the management of infections. Polymeric particles, vesicular (liposomes, niosomes, aquasomes), lipid carriers and inorganic-based materials have been developed to combat infections caused by myriad microorganisms.

9.2 NDDS for the Management of Bacterial Infections

Bacteria, the most widespread pathogens, have the potential to affect body functional units, including facial, neural, respiratory, gastric, genital and urinary systems. Antibiotics are advised in most of the infections that target the cell wall, protein synthesis, metabolism, nucleic acid synthesis (DNA and RNA) of bacteria [12].

In the past decade, antibiotic-embedded novel drug delivery strategies that exhibit desirable bactericidal action with improved patient compliance have been frequently designed. Abiotic drug carriers (vesicle, conjugated, polymeric, lipid-based systems) and biological carriers (lysozyme and attenuated vectors) specifically target the pathogens and infected cells [13]. Figure 9.2 compiles several diseases caused by different strains of bacteria.

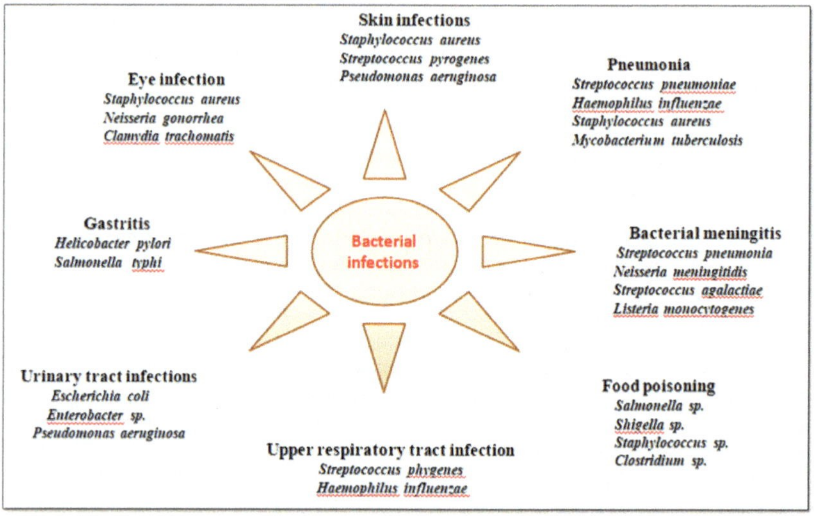

Figure 9.2 Different novel strategies are discussed to alleviate bacterial infections.

9.2.1 Neuroinfection and Bacterial Meningitis

It is a major detrimental condition of nervous tissues and cells, caused by bacterial pathogens which progressively lead to neurological disorders [14]. Few antibiotics or antimicrobial therapeutics are hydrophilic and poorly permeate the bacterial cells. Further, the internalized antimicrobial agent was readily destroyed by the lysozyme action thus reducing the therapeutic action achieved. Hence, the passive action of novel delivery systems on directly infected cells targeting through phagocytosis is preferred that ensures better therapeutic action. Meningitis is an infection around the membrane covering the brain and the spinal cord. It may result in life-threatening issues quickly, such as brain damage, stroke and paralysis. Bacteria, including *Streptococcus, Listeria* and *Escherichia*, are the prime causes of meningitis in neonates, whereas *Neisseria* and *Haemophilus* are more common in children [15]. Polymeric-based drug delivery approaches present potential advantages in the treatment of meningitis owing to the direct delivery of therapeutic agents at the infection site and circumventing obstacles of the blood-brain barrier [16]. Moreover, polymers with inherited antimicrobial action and biocide polymers exhibit enhanced effect after conjugating with antimicrobials and can be implanted on the delivery system and medical devices to alleviate infection. Apart from their exclusive effects, these polymers get adhered on the cell surface of bacteria and lead to the destruction of the bacterial cell [17]. Polymeric nanoparticles from amphiphilic lipopolysaccharides (*N,N′*-methylene bisacrylamide and acrylamide) are derived that had an affinity towards *Pseudomonas aeruginosa*. Small-scale (40 nm) developed polymeric particles exhibited selective targeting efficiencies for meningitis and keratitis models at a dose of 5 mg/kg after intra-cerebroventricular administration [18]. Another meningococcal nanoparticle-containing vaccine was developed via containing meningococcal capsular polysaccharide (the main virulence factor in bacterial meningitis) that slowly delivered antigen at the infection site. The system was biocompatible, biodegradable and stable and could be stored as dry powder. 250 µg of developed polymeric nanoparticles were evaluated against DC2.4 dendritic cell line to analyze antigenicity and cell maturation. Enhanced antigenicity for MHCI, MHC II and CD40,80, 86 in dendritic cells was achieved [19].

Cationic peptide-based antibiotics have the potential to combat multidrug-resistant bacteria, i.e., *Streptococcus aureus*, causative agent of meningitis. Positively charged peptides containing alpha or beta helices-like architectures show an affinity for negatively surfaced bacterial cells. These peptides can be modulated in self-assembled micelle form that can readily cross the blood-brain barrier (BBB) and efficiently suppress bacterial growth at the infection site [20]. Polymeric micelles are potentially active and successful approach for the management of meningitis, cerebritis and other cerebral inflammations in the brain and the spinal cord. Self-assembled cholesterol-linked polyethylene glycol micelles were fabricated and anchored with transcriptional activator peptide (TAT) to facilitate the efficient delivery of ciprofloxacin across the BBB. Ultra-small spherical micelles (180 nm) exhibited sustained release of ciprofloxacin for 6 h in saline phosphate buffer, pH 7.4. Augmented uptake of formulated micelles via human astrocytes was reported through confocal laser scanning microscopy that suggested rapid permeation of polymeric micelles across BBB for the alleviation of meningitis caused by bacterial species of *Escherichia* and *Neisseria* [21]. Pegylated self-assembled micelles embedded with bacitracin A were designed for the potential action against penicillin-sensitive and penicillin-resistant pneumococcal meningitis caused by *S. pneumonia*. Rabies virus glycopeptides-29 (RVG, brain targeting peptide) and Pluronic P85 unimers (a p-glycoprotein inhibitor) were used to design self-assembled micelles. Superb cellular uptake and enhanced BBB permeation through brain capillary endothelial cells were by virtue of synergistic action of RVG and Pluronic P85 unimers. The developed micelles sufficiently accumulated in the brain parenchyma, suppressed bacterial growth, performed receptor-mediated transcytosis and deducted membrane microviscosity, thus showing potential antibacterial application for the effective management of pneumococcal meningitis [22]. Lipoid liposomes are a favorable drug carrier for antimicrobial drug delivery in multidrug-resistant conditions. These vesicular systems can be conjugated easily with targeting templates including proteins, antibodies, enzymes and other bioactive agents. Liposomes not only facilitate localized delivery of the antimicrobial agent but also their superb stability ensures the safety of antibiotics from the adverse environment of the infection site. Prolonged distribution of antibiotics in the bloodstream, specific targeting and improved pharmacokinetic and pharmacodynamic parameters favor liposomes for the treatment of meningitis via different routes of administration [23]. The functional ability of liposomes can be amplified through the conjugation of cell-penetrating peptides (TAT_{47-57}). Bartomeu et al. (2016) designed spherical, small-scale TAT_{47-57} functionalized fusogenic liposomes (100 nm) encapsulated with different antibiotics such as methicillin, vancomycin and ampicillin to combat meningitis-causing bacterial pathogens (*Staphylococcus aureus* and *Escherichia coli*). Significant decrement in antibiotic MICs and total eradication of bacteria were observed when treated with functionalized methicillin liposomes. A cytotoxic study against BBB cellular components (astrocytes and endothelial cells) revealed promising effects by developed functionalized liposomes that suggested clinical applications in meningitis [24]. Dendrimers are another effective drug delivery strategy against bacterial meningitis. The star-shaped three-dimensional branched architecture of dendrimers offers conjugation of numerous antibiotics and bioactive therapeutics. Biocompatibility, low polydispersity index, high water solubility and exclusive outer and inner layers attract researchers for the functionalization and encapsulation of dendrimers for the management of neuro-infectious diseases [25].

Numerous studies on gold nanoparticles exhibited their high potential against the treatment of neurological disorders and central nervous system infections owing to their surface morphology, biocompatibility, surface affinity for several functional moieties and ability to cross layers of the BBB [26]. Sub-colloidal gold particles have shown high surface modification alternatives by the virtues of their tunable physicochemical properties. A variety of proteins can be adorned over their surface via electrostatic interactions and perform antipathogenic or antimicrobial functions [27]. Anwar et al. (2019) synthesized gold and silver nanoparticles embedded with novel bioactive agents such as hesperidin (flavonoid) and naringin (antimicrobial). The system was targeted against brain cells eating neuropathogens, i.e., methicillin-resistant *Staphylococcus aureus* and *E. coli*. Green-synthesized silver and gold nanoparticles were stabilized with plant gums acacia and tragacanth, respectively. Spherical and nanodimensional particles (100–250 nm) were cytocompatible and exhibited preeminent bactericidal action while analyzed through anti-microbial assays [28, 29].

9.2.2 Urinary Tract Infection

Both Gram-negative (*E.* and *K. pneumonia*) and Gram-positive (*Enterococcus faecalis* and *S. saprophyticus*) bacteria are associated with urinary tract infections (UTIs). They enter through the gastrointestinal tract into the region of the urinary bladder and urethra and start to multiply there, resulting in full-blown infection. Anatomically, the female urethra is close to the vagina, hence sexually transmitted diseases (gonorrhea and herpes) may also lead to bacterial urethritis [30]. Globally, UTIs are the most common infections distressing more than 150 million patients annually. Frequent reoccurrences result in painful and critical conditions that may need bacteria-resistant antimicrobial medications. Particularly, lower UTI is prevalent in elderly patients and ignorance of this disease leads to serious complications such as septicemia and pyelonephritis [31]. Polymeric microspheres were designed by Labbaf et al. (2013) by encapsulating a high dose of gentamycin sulfate antibiotic. Nontoxic polymethylsilsesquioxane was selected as a polymer owing to its high stability, compatibility, biodegradability and superior physicochemical properties. The formulation was prepared using the coaxial electrohydrodynamic method and has the potential to target *Enterococcus faecalis* after being delivered through a routine urinary catheter. The developed microcapsules contained fluorescent tracer dye and confirmed the release of antibiotic into the cells of uropathogen at the site of the human bladder [32].

Kristian et al. (2021) developed a unique antimicrobial catheter from a silicon-derived interpenetrating polymer network (IPN). It worked like balloon material and aimed for the slow release of antibiotic at the site of the urinary bladder. The developed system targeted local urinary infections that were associated with frequent use of catheters in patients, developing biofilm and other nosocomial infections. Antimicrobials, i.e., nitrofurazone and nitrofurantoin were loaded into the IPN worked as a reservoir and exhibited zero-order drug kinetics that significantly diminished bacterial growth around the urinary bladder and destroyed the biofilm formed over the urinary catheter [33]. In an alternate approach, trimethoprim-embedded microparticles were designed to target uropathogen *E. coli*. Low-molecular-weight PLGA 2300 (poly-D,L-lactic-co-glycolic acid) was used as a matrix material to depict a slow drug release pattern from the developed microparticles. An initial burst release (30%) within 24 h followed by sustained effect for 2 days was observed that was desirable to eradicate colonies of bacteria at the bladder region [34]. Unusual ultrasound-activated lipid-based microbubbles were fabricated using a urothelial organoid model to release the antimicrobial agent into the apical cell cytoplasm. Initially, non-cell permeant gentamicin and fluorescent dye were loaded in the liposomes. The formulated liposomes were adhered on to the gas-filled microbubbles and subjected to buffer simulation with the apical surface of bladder. The ultrasound-activated intracellular-containing microbubbles were more efficient than traditional oral antibiotic regimens and thus have the potential for the safe delivery of high amounts of antibiotics into urothelial cells [35]. A nanoemulsion containing polyphenon 60 and curcumin was prepared to provide a combined effect against uropathogens, i.e., *E. coli*. To achieve efficient antibacterial effects and prevention of gastrointestinal enzyme degradation, the vaginal route was preferred to administer the medicament. The nanoemulsion system was developed by the ultrasonication method and optimized through the Box-Behnken drug design model. The nanoemulsion revealed an average globule size of 211 nm, minimum poly-dispersity index (0.343), optimum stability (–32.7 mV) at 4°C and sustained permeation for 12 h. An *in vivo* study on Sprague-Dawley rats exhibited distribution of drugs, i.e., polyphenon 60 (3.07% per g) and curcumin (3.35% per gram) after 3 h and was found effective for 12 h in the affected areas [36].

9.2.3 Gastrointestinal Tract Infection

Various bacterial species such as *Salmonella, Escherichia, Listeria, Staphylococcus,* and *Clostridium* frequently cause food-borne infections, including food poisoning. Other risk factors for gastric infections are undercooked meat (*E. coli*), contaminated water/juice (Vibrio, Salmonella), unpasteurized dairy (*Staphylococcus* and *Salmonella*), unwashed raw vegetables and fruits (*Shigella* spp.) [37]. *Helicobacter pylori* is the most common bacterial pathogen causing gastritis, gastrointestinal ulcer and cancer. Enormous research and projects containing microspheres, microbeads and gels are under way for the eradication of *H. pylori* [38]. Although Gram-negative *H. pylori* pathogens are highly sensitive to any single antibiotic, clinically their complete eradication rate is very slow. There are several explanations for this. The first one is the degradation or instability of various antimicrobials in the acidic pH of the stomach. The second reason is the attainment of low concentration or low bioavailability of therapeutic to the bacteria. The third possibility is the low residence time of the dosage form in the pathogen-affected area of the gastrointestinal tract. Although multidrug therapy is advised, different adverse effects, poor patient compliance and high level of drug resistance are a few serious issues. Thus, drug delivery systems that are stable in the gastric region and extend the residence time of the drug with minimum side effects are appropriate to overcome gastritis and gastric ulcer. Myriad formulations, including mucoadhesive, floating, expendable, high-density and magnetic systems, are well suited for the management of bacterial infection in the stomach [39].

Gastroretentive floating gel beads are the most suitable drug delivery system for the complete elimination of pathogens from the gastric region. This dosage form offers a controlled-release pattern with sufficient residence time [40]. Various natural polymers, including sodium alginate, pectin, agar/agarose, chitosan and casein, are widely explored for the preparation of gel beads owing to their biocompatibility, nontoxicity and biodegradability features [41]. Salmonellosis, another gastric infection, occurs through food-borne enteropathogen *Salmonella enterica*. It is a Gram-negative facultative anaerobe and frequently causes gastrointestinal diseases. Annually, more than 150 million cases of gastroenteritis are reported worldwide with symptoms of stomach cramps and acute diarrhea [42]. Oral rehydration therapy is advised in mild cases of salmonellosis, but antimicrobials and probiotics are recommended for severely ill, infants and immune-compromised patients [43].

Antimicrobials, including sulfonamides and quinolones, are systemically absorbed readily; hence, their insufficient concentration is retained at the enteric sites if given orally. Additionally, poorly absorbed oral antimicrobials (beta lactam antibiotics and aminoglycosides) provide prolonged localized action but may alter the balance of gut flora (microbiome) and allow the overgrowth of other opportunistic bacteria [44]. To sort out these issues Mu et al. (2019) have introduced pathogen-targeting glycovesicles for the alleviation of gastroenteritis caused by *Salmonella enterica serovar typhimurium* (active in both humans and animals). They conjugated xylo-oligosaccharides with long-chain fatty acid through bridging with disulfide bonds. The resultant conjugate was an amphiphilic, self-assembled molecule that has a tendency to generate H_2S-triggered antimicrobial (ciprofloxacin) at the infected site. The system was biocompatible, stable and safe for oral administration. The disulfide bond is important while developing reduction-responsive dosage forms as the bond can easily degrade by H_2S produced by sulfate-reducing pathogens including *H. pylori, S. enterica, Fusobacterium* and *Enterobacter*. Thus, the developed H_2S-responsive glycovesicles worked both as cargo to release antimicrobial and prebiotic xylo-oligosaccharides at the infection site [45]. Polymeric nanoplexes have been synthesized via admixing polycationic gentamicin with macromolecular block copolymers through electrostatic interaction. Polyethylene oxide-b-sodium acrylate and polyethylene oxide-b-sodium methacrylate were individually mixed with PAA before complexing with gentamicin. The resulting nanoplexes were nanodimensional (90–120 nm) and stable (zeta potential –11 to –17 mV). An *in vivo* study revealed a reduced number of viable salmonella pathogens at the infection site [46]. Ciprofloxacin-embedded lipid-coated mesoporous silica nanoparticles have been developed for the management of intracellular eradication of enteritis-causing *Salmonella* bacteria. The average particle size of lipid-coated mesoporous silica particles was in the nano range (50–100 nm) with 5 nm thickness. Developed lipid-coated nanoparticles exhibited lesser cytotoxicity and enhanced antibacterial activity compared to non-lipid-coated mesoporous silica particles. After oral administration, the data obtained from confocal microscopy suggested improvement in intravacuolar targeting owing to the lipoidal surface and augmented eradication of viable cells of pathogens at a lower dose of antibiotic ciprofloxacin [47]. Salmonella serotypes are accountable for food-borne infections and are associated with meat products and pet foods [48]. Kumar et al. (2020) explored the antimicrobial use of pelargonic acid present in tomatoes. Pelargonic acid-loaded microemulsion was prepared with different surfactants such as TritonX100, Tween 80, Quillaja and sodium dodecyl sulfate. Thereafter, formed micelles were evaluated for antimicrobial action against three pathogens, i.e., *Salmonella, Typhimurium* and *Oranienburg. In vitro* study reflected that microemulsion containing sodium dodecyl sulfate exhibited the lowest MIC for *Salmonella* Newport (7.82 mM) [49]. Enterotoxigenic *E. coli* is a proven fatal cause of diarrhea that leads to morbidity and mortality in socioeconomic communities. Intestinal gut barrier dysfunction and inflammation are mostly associated with *E. coli* [50]. Poor oral bioavailability, systemic toxicity and developed multidrug resistance create issues for antibiotic administration. To overcome these shortcomings nanocarrier-based drug delivery approaches are recommended. Paudel et al. (2021) investigated enrofloxacin-embedded polymeric nanoparticles of PLGA (poly(lactide-co-glycolide)) and lignin-grafted PLGA. Synthesized spherical particles of each polymer were nanodimensional (approximately 111–117 nm) and biocompatible. The polymeric nanoparticles have the potential to prevent more than 50% bacterial infection than bare antibiotic (enrofloxacin) while tested against IPEC-J2 cells. Additionally, a 25% higher inhibition of bacterial growth was observed owing to particle uptake through endocytosis. Further, sustained release of drug from polymeric nanoparticles suggested the prevention of rapid *E. coli* growth inside the cells [51]. Nuria et al. (2021) developed pH-responsive targeted and controlled delivery of narrow-spectrum bacteriocins (protein) to alleviate *E. coli* from the lower gastrointestinal tract. Colicin E9/Ia or plasmid-encoded bacteriocin is very toxic to strains of *E. coli* and other related pathogens. To protect from the degradation in the upper gastric region and enable the controlled release of colicin E9/Ia, pH-responsive hydrogel microcapsules with nontoxic alginic acid were designed via the membrane emulsification method. Encapsulation ensured the safe delivery of bioactive colicin in the lower tract of the gastrointestinal tract in the murine *E. coli* colonization model. The microencapsulation of antibiotic colicin has the potential to decolonize gut microbiota particularly multidrug-resistant dominant Enterobacteriaceae pathogens [52].

9.2.4 Vaginal Infection

Vaginal infection or bacterial vaginosis is a common health issue, often reported in females at their reproductive age. It occurs due to vaginal microflora dysbiosis where one or more microorganisms are dominant to the others in that region [53, 54]. Women at the age of 40 or higher are vulnerable to vaginosis due to less release of estrogen, which affects the living environment of the bacteria *Lactobacillus*. Off-white discharge, itching and a burning sensation with a fishy smell are prominent symptoms of bacterial vaginosis [55]. A healthy vagina preserves the bacteria *Lactobacillus*, which is accountable for the production of lactic acid and maintains acidity there. The acidic environment protects from other invaders in the region of the vagina. The overgrowth of pathogenic microflora including species of *Staphylococcus*, *Mycoplasma*, *Gardnerella* and *Peptostreptococcus* leads to the imbalance of the acidic milieu of the vagina, resulting in vaginal infection [56]. Topically administered metronidazole has been the preferred antibacterial agent against bacterial vaginosis over the last decade. Although its gel, cream, suppositories and lavages are widely accepted, the prolonged drug release pattern is not established. To modify the local efficiency of metronidazole, mucoadhesive tablets were prepared with a blend of bioadhesive polymers such as chitosan FG90C, polycarbophil PCPAA1 and polyvinylpyrrolidone (PVPK90). The developed mucoadhesive tablets displayed a controlled release of metronidazole at the infection site [57].

Alqahtami et al. (2020) developed chitosan nanoparticles to explore their antimicrobial action against the bacterial pathogen *Neisseria gonorrhea*, a Gram-negative bacteria causing sexually transmitted infections. Globally, more than 106 million new cases of this pathogen are reported annually; the pathogen colonizes the mucosal tissues of the urethra, rectum and upper genital regions in women [58]. Chitosan nanoparticles were prepared via the emulsion gelation method and evaluated for the average particle size and zeta potential on varying the chitosan concentration from 1 to 5 mg/ml. The data obtained showed that on increasing the chitosan concentration, the average particle diameter and the zeta potential increased from 193 to 530 nm and 14 to 20 mV, respectively. Additionally, mucoadhesive chitosan particles were effective not only against various multidrug-resistant species of *Neisseria* but also were cytocompatible for HeLa cells at lower a concentration (less than 2.5 mg/ml) [59].

Further, silver nanoparticles were developed that significantly reduced the colony of antibiotic-resistant *N. gonorrhea* itself. Thereafter, silver nanoparticles (120 nm) were combined with cefmetazole to provide an additive effect at the infection site. Both silver nanoparticles and their amalgamation with antibiotic exhibited potent action on bacterial cell integrity (MIC 12.5 μg/ml) and did not produce adverse effects or cytotoxicity for human epithelial and fibroblast cells [60]. Tugcu-Demiroz et al. (2020) very first studied the efficacy of metronidazole-embedded PVP (Polyvinyl pyrrolidone) nanofibers for the management of infection at the site of the female genital organ. The prime features of these nanofibers including mucoadhesion, biocompatibility and high drug permeability offered potential usage for efficient metronidazole activity compared to bare gel or solution [61]. Thereafter, benzydamine (antiseptic and anti-inflammatory therapeutic) and chitosan nanoparticles were loaded in the polymeric PVP nanofibers and compared its efficiency with their hydroxy propylmethyl cellulose (HPMC) gels and evaluated against different pathogens causing vaginal infections. Controlled and prolonged drug delivery, sufficient mechanical strength, hydrophilicity and mucoadhesive property displayed superiority of fabricated nanofibers compared to conventional remedies [62].

9.2.5 Skin Infection

Topical infections such as leprosy, cellulitis, boils and impetigo are the most common infections caused by bacterial pathogens. Among them, leprosy, or Hansen's disease, covers considerable percentage of the world's population [63]. Instead of advanced socioeconomic status of developing countries, it is still considered as endemic in many areas of America and South Asia. In 2019, India, Indonesia, and Brazil reported more than a thousand new cases of leprosy [64]. Leprosy is caused by the bacterial pathogen *Mycobacterium leprae* and is characterized as chronic granulomatous on the skin and peripheral nerves. Multi-drug therapy (MDT) has been widely recommended worldwide as an efficient treatment against leprosy. However, several adverse effects and drug resistance are significant issues with MDT.

Frequently prescribed conventional antileprotic dosages containing dopamine and clofazimine display slow dissolution in the gastrointestinal tract and poor or limited bioavailability hence novel dosages including nanocarriers are required [65]. A liposomal drug delivery system containing clofazimine cholesterol and phosphotidyl choline was prepared to modify residence time at the site of infection and reduced the treatment time for leprosy. The system was aimed for local delivery and hence avoided systemic absorption. Both liposomal gel and its suspension were stable at body, refrigerator and room temperatures [66]. Polymeric nanoparticles containing PLGA-clofazimine were developed as a promising tool to manage leprosy. The system improved solubility and bioavailability and minimized associated adverse effects. PLGA–clofazimine nanoparticles were spherical, nanodimensional and exhibited a controlled-release pattern. Cell viability study of developed nanoparticles did not expose intrinsic clofazimine toxicity performed against Caco-2 and HT29-MTX cells. After oral administration, these PLGA-clofazimine nanoparticles represented a potential platform to alleviate stubborn bacterial pathogens with improved bioavailability and patient compliance [67]. Solid dispersion containing clofazimine and hypromellose phthalate was prepared to modify solubility and drug loading capacity. Formulated solid dispersion exhibited proton transfer between clofazimine and polymer hypromellose phthalate that mediated the amorphous form and augmented solubility of the preparation [68]. Alike clofazimine, dapsone also shows poor bioavailability and nonspecific distribution in the vital organs including skin, kidney and liver. That leads to serious undesirable effects. Enormous dosage forms including niosomes, bilosomes, polymeric nanocapsules, lipid nanocarriers embedded with dapsones have been reported in the past decade [69]. In this series, covalently bonded polymer-dapsone conjugate was developed that exhibited controlled pharmacokinetics with efficient therapeutic value. Acrylic functional groups of macromolecular chains of hydroxyethyl methacrylate, HEMA polymer offer covalent functionalization with dapsone molecule. The formed stable conjugate showed superior anti-inflammatory activity against bacterial pathogens and was hence suggested for clinical application in leprosy [70].

El-Nabarawi et al. (2018) discussed potential applications of novel vesicles invasomes that have enhanced percutaneous permeation. Dapsone-loaded invasomes with phosphatidylcholine, terpenes and ethanol were formulated through the thin-film hydration technique. Several terpenes including cineol, citral, limonene and fenchone were explored for improving dapsone retention on the skin. Pharmacokinetic parameters such as drug deposition and area under the curve (AUC) of dapsone-loaded invasomes and dapsone solution were compared. Both drug deposition and AUC of dapsone-loaded invasomes were high approximately 2.5 and 2 times compared to conventional dapsone solution respectively [71]. Chen et al. (2018) utilized mesoporous silica as a nanocarrier the for delivery of poorly soluble clofazimine to treat multidrug-resistant tuberculosis and leprosy. FDA-approved food additive acetophenone was added that modified the loading of poorly soluble antibiotic (clofazimine) into the mesoporous silica nanocarrier and facilitated the release from pores also. Developed nanocarrier-based drug delivery systems exhibited dose-dependent anti-bacterial action against bacterial pathogen-infected macrophages [72].

Cellulitis is a deep skin infection often caused by *Streptococcus pneumonia* and *Staphylococcus aureus*. Skin breakage, trauma or surgeries invite pathogens for infection [73]. For the management of deep skin infection or cellulitis, elastic liposomes and their gels have been formulated using hydrophilic neomycin sulfate, Phospholipon® 90G, Tween 80/Span 80 and carbopol. The stability of elastic liposomes and elastic liposome-containing gels was reported for 14 days and 2 months, respectively. Outcomes of confocal laser scanning microscopy suggested deep penetration (180 μm) and enhanced deposition (~26%) of neomycin sulfate in the rat skin on 24 h. Histological findings described efficient eradication of *Staphylococcus aureus* localized in stratum corneum through elastic liposomes within 7 days [74]. Nitric oxide-releasing nanoparticles have been developed for the mitigation of methicillin-resistant *Staphylococcus aureus* (MSRA) colonized in the wounded area. MSRA is a common threat for both invasive and superficial infections primarily associated with hospital settings. Prepared nanoparticles displayed accelerated antibacterial action against the MSRA-affected wound model. Histological studies revealed minimum MSRA pathogen burden, minimum inflammation and less collagen degradation after treatment with nitric oxide-releasing nanoparticles [75]. Electrospun nanofibers are versatile drug delivery scaffolds owing to their superior architecture that mimics the extracellular matrix of the cell. These scaffolds are promising therapy for wound healing, potentiate absorption of released exudates, allow transportation of gaseous exchange and proficiently diminish bacterial load at the site of infection. Biocompatible and biodegradable polymeric (Polycaprolactone/collagen) nanofibers containing gentamicin or clindamycin have been fabricated for the effective differentiation of human dermal fibroblast at the site of the wound. The novel fabricated antibiotic scaffolds have great utility for cell proliferation, infection mitigation and skin grafting for wound healing and tissue engineering [76].

9.2.6 Oral Cavity Infection

The human oral cavity is an integral part of the digestive system with multifaceted anatomical structures. Complexed bacterial colonies exist all around teeth, mucosal layer, bones (maxillary/mandibular) and periodontal tissues that account for oral health. This ecological niche prevents pathogenic growth and maintains the balance of microecology in the oral cavity [77]. The composition of microbiota present in the oral cavity may be altered due to poor or ignored oral hygiene, imbalanced diet and diseased state that create oral infectious ailments such as dental caries, periodontitis and peri-implantitis [78]. Dong et al. (2017) explored pH-dependent silver nanoparticles releasing titanium implant for the effective eradication of pathogenic Gram-positive and Gram-negative causing peri-implant infections. Antimicrobial strategies are far from satisfactory as control delivery cannot be maintained. At the time of peri-implant infection, the pH decreases below 5.5 hence pH-dependent controlled drug delivery from the surface of the implant is required. Silver nanoparticles grafted titania nanotube structured implants were designed with low pH sensitive acetal linker for the management of oral infection. The system was efficacious at pH 5.5 and released a high dose of silver nanoparticles (broad spectrum) hence, robust antimicrobial and osteoinductive actions were displayed [79]. Table 9.1 compiles different novel drug delivery approaches for the management of oral infections caused by bacteria.

Table 9.1 Novel drug delivery systems and their potential applications to combat oral infections

Drug delivery system	Therapeutics	Oral infections	Applications	Ref.
Hydrogel	Human fibroblast growth factor type 2 with hyaluronic acid	Periodontitis	Periodontal wound healing and intrabony defects	[80]
Nanocapsules	Indomethacin encapsulated on adhesive resin	Inflammation in pulp tissues	Adhesive resin disk to treat deep cavities	[81]
Micelles	Triclosan, alendronate	Dental caries	Tooth binding micelles, inhibitor of biofilm developed by *Streptococcus mutans*	[82]
Dendrimers	Triclosan, carboxyl terminated polyamidoamine	Dental caries and damaged dentine	Remineralization	[83]
Silica nanoparticles	Titanium-based mesoporous silica and silver nanoparticles	Peri-implantitis	Dental implant rehabilitation	[84]
Nanofibrous dental implant	Tetracycline, titanium disk	Periodontal infection	Antimicrobial and osteogenic	[85]

Maurya et al. 2019 designed a localized drug delivery system containing Eudragit RS 100-coated pectin microspheres of moxifloxacin for the management of periodontal diseases caused by Gram-negative bacteria. Periodontal diseases are identified by degradation of teeth, bones, periodontal ligaments, dental cementum followed by severe inflammation of subgingival plaque. Moxifloxacin microspheres were formulated via the emulsion dehydration method. Superb drug entrapment efficiency (80%) and drug release (90%) in phosphate buffer pH 6.8 suggested prolonged localized antimicrobial action with high patient compliance [86]. Periodontitis, an inflammatory condition around teeth supporting tissues can be alleviated by the removal of plaque and stayed microorganisms there. Localized antimicrobial therapy is recommended for effective antimicrobial action. A competent and safe locally administered minocycline microspheres have been prepared that were clinically trialed on 748 periodontitis sufferers. The antimicrobial action was dependent on smoking status, gender, age and diseased condition. Outcomes suggested the potential usage of minocyclin microspheres along scaling and root planing in periodontitis patients [87].

9.2.7 Pulmonary Infections

Bacteria such as *S. pneumonia, S. aureus, K. pneumonia, H. influenza* and *P. aeruginosa* get adhered to the pulmonary mucous layer and have strong efficiency to form biofilm there that creates resistance to antimicrobial agents [88]. Few of them are extracellular and primarily adhere in the extracellular fluid, tissue fluid and blood lymphocytic fluid and ingest nutrients for their growth and multiplication [89]. Localized inhalation preparations administered through the pulmonary route effectively manage pulmonary infections caused by bacteria. Several nebulizers, pulmonary metered dose inhalers (pMDIs), dry powdered inhalers (DPIs) and soft mist inhalers are recommended for the eradication of stubborn mucosal adhered pathogens. Delivered smaller droplets from an inhaler device cover the maximum infected affected surface and kill bacterial pathogens [90]. pMDI and DPI are most frequently prescribed to people with pulmonary infection. pMDIs are a pressurized system where antimicrobial drugs are dissolved or dispersed in single or mixed propellants. On the other hand, DPIs are in the dry form and do not necessitate the addition of propellants and cold chain storage conditions. Physicochemical (particle size, shape, mechanism of drug release, flow behavior, solubility, pH and osmolarity), pharmacokinetic (absorbance, clearance and bioavailability) and device-based parameters (type of device, flow rate and breath pattern) are prominent factors that affect therapeutic efficacy of antimicrobial agent at the infected site [91]. Srichana et al. (2016) compared the drug delivery performance of Aeronide inhaler (pressurized metered dose inhaler) and Pulmicort Turbuhaler (dry powder inhaler) against mild to moderate pulmonary infections and asthma. Budesonide was used as a model drug and aerodynamic particle size and spirometer parameters including forced vital capacity, forced expiratory volume and peak expiratory flow rate were analyzed. Both the device systems provided uniform performances and no significant differences in the frequency of bronchodilation, urinary cortisol and other spirometric parameters were observed [92]. Different drug delivery systems including polymeric nanoparticles, liposomes, micelles, solid lipid nanocarriers, dendrimers and gene therapies are well established for the controlled and targeted release of antimicrobial agents to cure pulmonary bacterial infections. Polymeric nanoparticles loaded with tobramycin-alginate/chitosan were developed for the treatment and prevention of mucosa adhered *P. aeruginosa* in the case of cystic fibrosis. To enhance penetration of developed polymeric nanoparticles, functionalization with dornase alfa was carried out which exhibited dose-dependent efficacy against *P. aeruginosa* PA01. The novel system demonstrated the development of clinically effective antimicrobial nanoparticles that have the potential for mucus penetration, localized action with minimum adverse effects [93]. Solid lipid nanoparticles (SLNs) containing rifabutin, mannitol and trehalose have been designed for effective eradication of *M. tuberculosis* via pulmonary administration. Prepared aerodynamic SLNs were capable of reaching the alveolar region and targeting adhered pathogens there. The formulation was delivered in dry form into the deep lung where rifabutin encapsulated SLNs reached the target site within 15–30 min. The enhanced antimycobacterial activity in the murine model suggested a potential clinical application of developed SLNs for the treatment of pathogen *M. tuberculosis* [94]. Isoniazid-loaded microparticles and polymeric (poly-ε-caprolactone) microparticles were synthesized and evaluated against drug-resistant

M. tuberculosis bacterium. Histological examination revealed a significantly higher accumulation of released isoniazid from both dosage forms into the alveolar macrophages. Nitric acid was also produced, which was not toxic to healthy cells. Further, hepatotoxicity was determined via SGOT (serum glutamate transferase) and SGPT (serum glutamate pyruvate transferase) which indicated safe drug delivery from microparticles. Thus, both systems exhibited potential for the management of tuberculosis [95]. Table 9.2 outlines the utility of NDDS for the alleviation of myriad pulmonary bacterial infections.

Table 9.2 Various novel drug delivery approaches for the eradication and inhibition of bacterial pathogens in the pulmonary region

Advanced drug delivery approaches	Therapeutic agent	Applications	Ref.
Polymeric nanoparticles	Alginate-capped iron oxide nanoparticles	Inhibition of *P. aeruginosa* and formed biofilm	[96]
Liposomal suspension	Amikacin	Management of *P. aeruginosa* in cystic fibrosis-affected lungs	[97]
Solid lipid nanoparticles	Levofloxacin	Antimicrobial against *P. aeruginosa* and *S. aureus* and inhibit biofilm formation	[98]
Microparticles	Rifampicin	Management of tuberculosis and multidrug-resistant tuberculosis	[99]
Micelles	Curcumin acetate and Nile red	Pulmonary infections	[100]

9.3 Novel Drug Delivery for the Management of Viral Infections

The major concern associated with the viral infection is fast replication in the host cell, which can have a deleterious effect on any part of the host cell. Figure 9.3 compiles different viral pathogens and their devastating infections in humans.

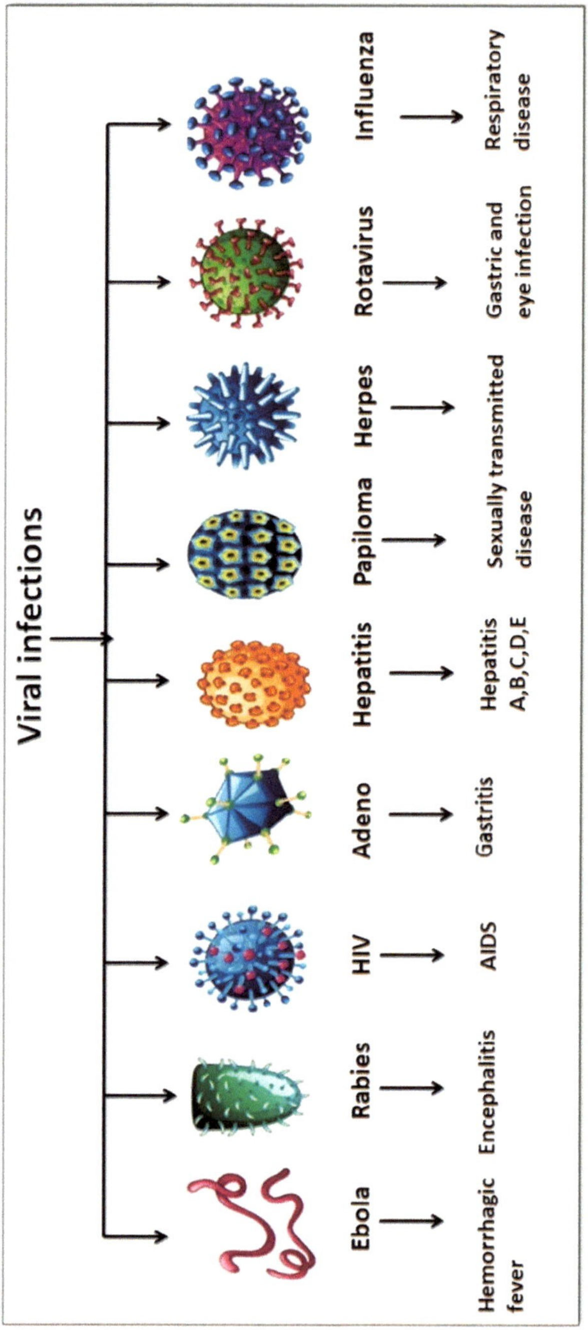

Figure 9.3 Different viral infections and their causative agents.

Although oral and parental formulations have been utilized for the management of viral infections several shortcomings associated with them like first-pass metabolism, reduced clinical efficacy and bioavailability of antiviral drugs have paved the way for the usage of novel drug delivery approaches to minimize the adverse effects and enhance the therapeutic efficacy of antiviral drugs [101].

9.3.1 Respiratory Infections

Respiratory viruses are the most common causative agents that are responsible for diseases in humans which have a significant effect on the health of an individual. Several virus families are responsible for human transmission at the global level. Respiratory tract infecting viruses include influenza virus, rhinovirus, and the most recent pandemic that has brought the entire world to a halt; coronavirus [102]. The majority of viruses can cause potential damage to the lungs; so pulmonary drug delivery is the first choice of the treatment regimen. Although the pulmonary route offers benefits like avoidance of first-pass metabolism and high bioavailability structural characteristics of lungs and the presence of biological barriers resist the utilization of conventional dosage forms and have subsequently led to the usage of novel delivery systems like nanoparticles, niosomes, liposomes, etc. Influenza, commonly referred to as "the flu", may vary from mild to severe and often include fever, runny nose, sore throat, muscle pain, headache, coughing, and fatigue. It may lead to pneumonia, supported by subsequent bacterial infection. Other complications are acute respiratory diseases, asthma and associated cardio-vascular ailments. Various drugs and vaccines have been used for the management of influenza, but still, the drugs have failed to show ideal efficacy. There are several factors responsible for decreased drug effect, like the emergence of the resistant viral strain, poor drug solubility, and poor permeability of the drug across biological barriers. The development of novel formulations for the management of influenza can be of aid in reducing unfavorable public health and social impact [103]. Virus-like particles (VLPs) are spherical supramolecular assemblies produced by the expression of the viral envelope or capsid proteins. VLPs show resemblance to the natural assemblies of the antigenic epitopes of their corresponding viruses, but may lack any infectious genetic material. This characteristic property of VLPs allows the immune system to recognize VLPs similar to the original virus to promote phagocytosis by antigen-presenting cells, thereby, offering protection against multiple influenza virus serotypes via induction of humoral and cellular immune responses [104]. Microcapsules have been widely demonstrated as a useful tool for the management of influenza infection. Layer-by-layer assembled hollow polyelectrolyte microcapsules possess biomimetic properties and features like shape, size, thickness, and ability to incorporate several types of biomolecules that allow their utilization in the management of influenza [105]. Microparticles are novel formulations that can help deliver vaccines through the oral route. Owing to their small size (1 to 1000 μm), microparticles can have the potential for delivering the drug through the pulmonary route [106]. Dendrimers are another type of nano-drug delivery system that has been explored for their ability to deliver antigenic molecules for the management of influenza. Dendrimers are three-dimensional, branched, and star-shaped delivery systems that have unique features such as good water solubility, good biocompatibility, and low polydispersity index [107]. Dendrimer encapsulating various antigens has been found to elicit powerful antibody and T-cell responses against the influenza H1N1 virus [108]. Polymeric nanoparticles are often utilized in the delivery of anti-influenza drugs and vaccines. These are beneficial due to their biodegradability and biocompatibility, as well as, the ability to incorporate various drugs and antigens.

Another, rhinovirus affects the human population and is associated with the common cold. The virus possesses the ability to proliferate at 33–35°C; which corresponds to the temperature of the nose. The infection is transmitted either as aerosols or in the form of fomites, direct person-to-person contact can also be a cause of transmission of the virus [109]. Organic nanoparticles are the most extensively researched type of nanoparticle for the delivery of antiviral drugs. Polymeric nanoparticles exhibit colloidal properties with sizes ranging from 10 to 1000 nm. The small particle size facilitates capillary penetration and uptake by cells resulting in increased concentrations of drug at target sites [110]. Incorporation of antiviral drugs in micelles for the treatment of viral infection is one of the appealing nano-technologies that impart the dual property of enhancing the water solubility of the poorly soluble drug and also improving the stability of same. An additional positive attribute associated with micelles is that they demonstrate a slow dissociation rate and thus result in longer retention time and accumulation of drug at target sites [111].

COVID-19 is caused by a novel coronavirus SARS-CoV-2, earlier referred as 2019-nCoV. Currently, there is no standard drug or vaccine available for the treatment; therefore, repurposing existing drugs using NDDS is the only solution [112]. Although the usage of strategies like repurposing drugs, providing symptomatic treatments, and adopting alternative systems have been of help in management to a lesser extent; there is an urgent need of designing an effective option that incorporates the combined properties of both diagnostic as well as a therapeutic agent. Such an approach is likely to be mentioned as theranostics could be a potential approach to resist the spread of coronavirus [113]. Recent studies have revealed that theranostic drug therapies of chloroquine have resulted in effective *in vitro* inhibition of novel coronavirus [114]. Chen et al. (2020) formulated Lanthanide-doped polystyrene nanoparticles that proved to be effective in detecting anti-SRV-CoV-2 IgG in human serum, which could be of help in tracking COVID-19 progression [115]. Vesicular drug delivery systems like liposomes, polymersomes, gold nanoparticles, and peptide-based vesicles exhibit desired properties that make them suitable carriers for delivering drugs. These vesicular drug delivery systems control the fate of drug molecules by controlling the release kinetics, increasing bioavailability, and reducing the side effects of the drug [116].

9.3.2 Hepatitis

Viral hepatitis is one of the common causes of chronic liver infection. The liver is an essential part of the body that performs several functions like detoxification, and protein synthesis, and serves as a site for several biochemical reactions. A patient suffering from chronic liver disease requires immediate treatment and that too for a prolonged duration to sustain life. Prolonged exposure to drugs and nonspecificity of conventional dosage forms for hepatocytes/nonparenchymal cells are often accomplished with off-target interactions that limit the use of the same for the fabrication of novel targeted delivery systems that could specifically deliver the drug at the target site [117]. A lot of progress has been done in designing new and safe vaccines for the treatment of hepatitis; however, the major setback with the currently available vaccines is the induction of humoral immune response, three-dose schedule, storage issues, and economic constraints related to pilot plant scale-up. To overcome the flaws nanotechnology-based formulations are explored as a new platform. The development of nano-based formulations can display good patient compliance [118]. Nanoparticles, owing to their small size of < 1000 nm are easily taken up by the phagocytic cells, antigen-presenting cells, and mucosa-associated lymphoid tissues; the nanoparticles facilitate antigen recognition and presentation. The generally used vaccine delivery systems are liposomes, nanoemulsions, nanospheres, and polymer-based nanoparticles, several nano-/microparticles formulations have been approved by FDA (Decapeptyl®, Lupron Depot®, Nutropin Depot®, Zoladex®, etc.). Jaganathan and Vyas formulated surface-modified DL-lactide/glycolide copolymer (PLGA) microspheres employing chitosan for nasal immunization using recombinant HBsAg. These modified PLGA microspheres exhibited humoral and cellular immune responses upon nasal administration [119]. A novel version of the liposome/niosome system is the evolution of bilosomes, which are nonionic surfactant vesicles with bile salts. The nanoformulation offered stability after oral administration of an immunogen, and also prompted antibody titers. These formulations are so stable, that the requirement for a "cold chain" supply is also not mandatory [120].

9.3.3 Sexually Transmitted Viral Infections

Sexually transmitted viral infections have reached the stage where they are considered an epidemic and are responsible for global health concerns. Infections caused by herpes simplex virus (HSV), papillomaviruses (HPV), and HIV are the predominant virally transmitted venereal diseases that are generally incurable [121]. In the case of sexually transmitted viral infections, the causative pathogen displays a diverse mode of transmission, symptoms, and treatment.

Multiple reasons hinder the development of antiviral agents; the fact that viruses are obligate parasites, i.e., they require a host cell for replication; therefore only a few virus-specific metabolic functions are targeted by antiviral agents without hampering the host cell. Another challenge with antiviral molecules is the physicochemical and biopharmaceutical aspects of the drug. The novel formulations of the nano range display characteristic properties like small size, high surface-to-volume ratio, and modifiable surfaces which make them a potential carrier for antiviral drugs in the treatment of sexually transmitted diseases.

Herpes simplex virus infection, globally known as herpes, is primarily caused by HSV-1 and HSV-2 types. HSV-1 is responsible for oral infection, while HSV-2 is a cause of genital herpes. HSV-2 infection can be asymptomatic or have mild symptoms, however, in severe cases; the herpes infection shows the occurrence of blisters or ulcers in genital areas [122]. Seth et al. (2004) formulated idoxuridine-loaded liposomal gel by the reverse-phase evaporation method. The findings of the study revealed increased efficiency of topical liposomal gel in comparison to the plain liposome. The enhanced drug retention and permeation through the skin resulted in the effective treatment of HSV-2 infection [123]. Acyclovir is pharmacologically active against HSV-2. The conventional formulation like cream of acyclovir confers the problem of poor penetration of the drug via stratum corneum and thereby increases the frequency of application of the cream. The issue was overcome by developing microemulsions of acyclovir that can improve the stability of active molecules as well as increment in flux and permeation coefficient [124]. Microspheres of Acyclovir formulated by cross-linking method with acrylamide, dextran, chitosan, and glutaraldehyde demonstrated prolonged release of the drug, which proved its better efficacy in comparison to the conventional formulation [125].

Another, human papillomavirus (HPV) is a DNA virus belonging to the *Papillomaviridae* family. The virus is responsible for the cause of human papillomavirus infection. About 90% of the cases tend to show no symptoms and the situation resolves within two years of infection. In severe cases, warts and precancerous lesions are observed that can cause cancer in affected areas like the cervix, vulva, vagina, anus, mouth, and throat [126]. Concerning the treatment of HPV infection two strategies are mainly employed: drug-based and non-drug-based. The drug-based treatment involves the employment of drugs like 5-fluorouracil, bleomycin, acyclovir, and immunomodulators while the non-drug-based treatment is based on the use of cryotherapy, laser techniques, and CO_2. Problems like a reoccurrence of infection and scar hyperplasia are associated with the above-described treatment strategies, as the solution to the above-mentioned problem novel formulations came into existence for the treatment of HPV infection. Nanotechnology has played a key role in the diagnosis of cervical cancer caused by HPV, Zehbe et al. (1997) first realized the application of gold nanoparticles in the diagnosis of cervical cancer, and their study also demonstrated that the diagnostic technique involving gold nanoparticles is more accurate in diagnosis when compared with polymerase chain reaction method [127].

Development of hyperbranched copolymers by utilizing poly (amideamine) (PAMAM, G0) and poly (β-amino ester) (PBAE) has been reported. The fabricated hyperbranched copolymer was used to deliver CRISPR/Cas9 to target the HPV16 E7, which subsequently led to enhanced cellular uptake of plasmid and increased frequency of gene editing. Kampel et al. (2021) fabricated cationic lipid nanoparticles with the intent to deliver a gene (small interfering RNA against HPV E6/E7 oncoproteins) for the treatment of HPV infection. Surface modification of lipid nanoparticles with epidermal growth factor receptor antibodies reflected significant suppression of xenograft tumors in mice [128]. A biomimetic dual drug delivery system was designed that encapsulated paclitaxel and siRNS as a target for E7. With the aid of HeLa cell membranes camouflage, the biomimetic system results in the avoidance of immune system activation and leads to enhanced accumulation of drugs in tumor cells that hinder the growth of tumor tissues.

Further, HIV disease is associated with AIDS, one of the major health concerns worldwide in the 21st century. HIV upon invasion in the mucosal membrane weakens the immune system which results in rendering the body more susceptible to the attack of different microbes. Several antiretroviral drugs are available on the market in the present scenario that has the potential to prolong the life span of HIV-infected patients. The prime challenges offered by the antiretroviral drugs include poor solubility, limited controlled release, low permeability, and less bioavailability; to resolve the mentioned issues, nanoscale drug delivery technologies are employed to design therapeutically efficient formulations of active molecules [129]. Various nano-range formulations are utilized in the treatment of HIV infection, including liposomes, dendrimers, nanocrystals, nanoparticles, and polymeric micelles. Oussoren et al. (1999) developed a liposomal drug delivery system for Zalcitabine. The results of the studies performed in the murine acquired immune deficiency model provided evidence of improved chemical stability, enhanced retention, and reduced viral load in both spleen and bone marrow [130]. Clayton et al. (2009) fabricated stealth immunoliposomes of HIV-1 protease inhibitor coated with Fab fragments of HIV-gp120-directed monoclonal antibody F105. The immunoliposomal formulation showed increased and prolonged antiviral activity as compared to the free drug and the drug entrapped in plain liposomes [131]. Nanoparticles have been explored as a delivery system that is used as a promising carrier for drug delivery of drugs capable of improving pre-exposure prophylaxis. Mandal et al. (2017) formulated nanoparticles of emtricitabine and demonstrated improved bioavailability of the drug with significantly low inhibitory concentration [132]. Dendrimers are synthetic macromolecules that are characterized by their highly branched structure; they are also referred to as nanocontainers owing to their small size and ability to entrap drugs inside them. These specifically designed carriers are used as a tool for targeted drug delivery. Poly(propyleneimine) dendrimer-based nanocontainers for targeting efavirenz to Mo/Mac were designed by Dutta et al. (2007). The results of the study indicated that the dendrimers possess the potential as a carrier and can alter the efficacy and toxicity of the drug [133].

9.3.4 Encephalitis

Encephalitis is an acute, diffused inflammatory infection of the brain that is primarily caused by HSV types 1 and 2, varicella-zoster virus, and enteroviruses. In usual instances, the infection with the herpes virus is accomplished with cold sores but under severe circumstances, the inflammation in the brain occurs that is responsible for the mortality ratio associated with herpes infection. Brain disorders are the major quagmire for health and demand the development of strategies that augment the ability to cross the BBB and blood-cerebrospinal fluid barrier (BSCFB) as they protect the central nervous system from exogenous molecules and create obstacles in the treatment of brain disorders, the efflux across the barriers is regulated by P-gp, so it's inhibition is required for penetration of drug across BBB and BSCFB. In recent years, nanoformulations emerged as a pivotal option for altering the delivery of the active molecules to the brain. The advancement in nanotechnology has manifested its applications in diagnosis as well as treatment of brain disorders, by specifically delivering the drug to its site of action. As an attribute of small size nanoparticles are reported to enhance the efficacy of drugs. Graverini et al. (2018) performed a study by incorporating andrographolide (a neuroprotective drug) in SLNs. The results of the study revealed that SLNs potentially improve the penetration of drugs across BBB as compared to free drugs [134]. Micelles are vesicles of size ranging from 10 to 100 nm. The vesicles have drawn the attention of researchers as a suitable carrier for the delivery of drugs to the CNS. Micelles are of two types depending on the composition: nonpolymeric micelles (amphiphilic surfactants) and polymeric micelles (amphiphilic copolymers). The vesicles have a core and shell structure in which the inner core is hydrophobic and the outer shell is hydrophilic. The external shell offers stability to the carrier in an aqueous environment and protection from the reticuloendothelial system, the shell is also responsible for promoting the accumulation of micelles in leaky vasculature. Micelles are associated with the delivery of low molecular mass active pharmaceutical ingredients to the brain by the virtue of improved solubility and stability in plasma [135].

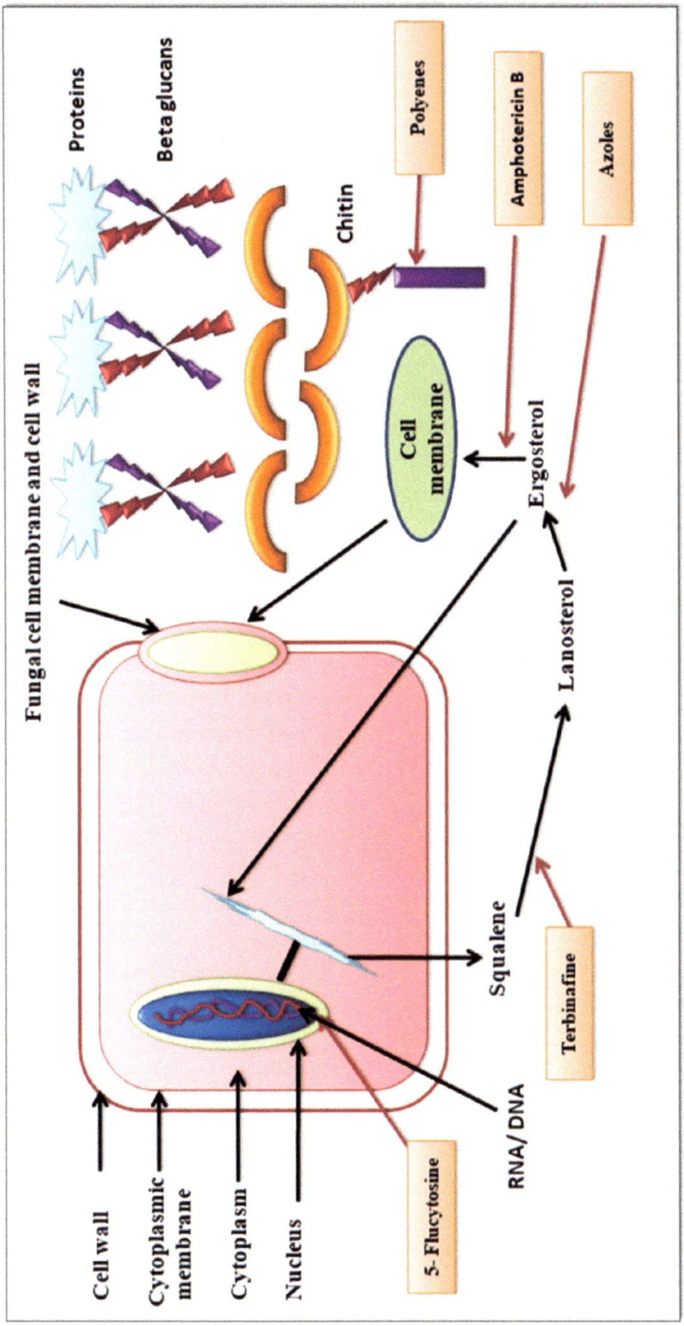

Figure 9.4 Antifungal agents targeting different components of fungal cell.

9.4 NDDS for the Management of Fungal Infections

Globally, fungal infections are growing community health threats which are largely associated with socioeconomic factors (unhealthy food, unhygienic, modern lifestyle) and ignoring primary infection symptoms [136]. Although a wide range of broad-spectrum antibiotics are prescribed to manage fungal diseases, severe adverse effects are associated with the therapy due to their eukaryotic nature. Patients with prolonged medication, diseased state, immune-compromised and surgery/operated persons are highly susceptible to fungal infections [137]. Additionally, the development of antibiotic resistance and undesirable side effects worsen the cases that lead to a high percentage of mortality rate. Figure 9.4 displays fungal cell and target sites of antifungal drugs.

9.4.1 Cutaneous Infection

Globally, fungal infection or mycosis is one of the major treacherous threats that influence approximately 40 million people in developed and developing countries annually. Initially, fungal pathogen attacks the skin surface and later by the process of desquamation it proliferates into the deeper layers of skin. Dermatophytes are fungal pathogens that invade not only the upper stratum corneum but also penetrate the other parts of the skin devastatingly if ignored [138]. Several topical ailments such as *Tinea corporis* (covers the whole body), *Tinea pedis* (legs or feet), *Tinea capitis* (scalp) and *Tinea cruris* (groin area) are highly significant diseases caused by myriad strains of fungi, i.e., *Trichophyton, Microsporum,* and *Epidermophyton* [139, 140]. Topical drug delivery proves the best route for effective healing of major dermatophytosis as it ensures direct reach with a high retention rate at the infected site with minimum adverse effects. Several topical azole and allyamine derivatives are successfully employed for the designing of antifungals. Traditional remedies require a high dose and frequent or repeated applications on the affected skin area that lead to hypersensitivity, itching and poor patient compliance. Advanced or novel drug carrier-embedded delivery systems have been introduced that offer a controlled release of the drug with less local and systemic toxic effects. Although the mechanism of antifungals should be clear for the selection of appropriate dosage that can maintain adequate therapeutic concentration at the target site. Most of the antifungal check synthesis of ergosterol, a desired growth nutrient for fungal pathogens [141].

Candidiasis caused by yeast (Candida genus) is another common superficial skin disease. It affects mostly the immunocompromised individuals and those in intensive care. Approximately 20 species of Candida yeast are reported in which *Candida albicans* and *Candida glabrata* are prominent for causing devastating topical infections (oral, skin and vaginal) to humans [142]. Human skin covers approximately 2 m^2 surface area and is hence considered the largest vital part of the body. Stratum corneum, the outermost layer of the epidermis, is contained keratinized and dead cells. It is also the prime barrier for invading of pathogens and penetration of antifungal therapeutics. Novel preparations such as niosomes, liposomes, micro/nanoemulsions, solid lipid carriers are targeted to kill skin-adhered fungal pathogens [143]. Enormous research is disclosed related to novel and carrier-mediated antifungal drug delivery systems which are discussed in Table 9.3.

Imidazole derivative clotrimazole and ketoconazole-loaded two lipid-based formulations, i.e., SLNs and nanostructured lipid carriers were designed for the management of topical fungal infections. polyacrylic acid and carbopol were selected owing to the formation of in situ gel and mucoadhesiveness. HPLC analysis reported higher antimycotic action by clotrimazole-embedded solid lipid nanoparticles and lipid carriers, 91.7% and 98.7%, respectively, compared to ketoconazole-loaded SLN and NLC, i.e., 62% and 70%, respectively. Hence, these novel delivery systems have the potential to inhibit the growth of fungal pathogens present on the skin [144]. Antifungal fluconazole-embedded nonionic niosomes were developed using various surfactants such as Span 40/60 and Brij 72 via the film hydration method. The formulations were stable and had micron size range (~0.287–0.378 μm) with satisfactory entrapment efficiency (greater than 41%). An *in vitro* skin permeation study revealed sufficient accumulation of released fluconazole and hence exhibited localized antifungal remedy with enhanced skin retention time [145].

Table 9.3 Different antifungal agents containing novel dosages for the management of fungal infections

Drug delivery system	Therapeutics	Objectives	Outcomes	Ref.
Solid lipid nanoparticles and nanostructured lipid carriers	Clotrimazole, climbazole and ketoconazole	Feasibility of sucrose ester stabilized formulations and comparison of gels prepared with SLN and NLC loaded with therapeutics	The drug release rate was climbazole > ketoconazole > clotrimazole from SLN and NLC contained gels; the formulations exhibited sustained delivery of therapeutics	[146]
Solid lipid nanoparticles	Fluconazole	Preparation of fast and effective topical treatment against *Pityriasis versicolor* (*Tinea versicolor*) compared to marketed cream Candistan®	Findings displayed stable formulation with zeta potential-21–31 mV and high entrapment efficiency (~83%); superior antimycotic action by fluconazole-loaded SLN was found compared to marketed preparation	[147]
Liposomes	Fluconazole	Localized vesicular delivery of fluconazole against fatal cutaneous candidiasis	Developed vesicular system exhibited sustained release and high accumulation of drug while performed against cutaneous candidiasis-induced albino rats	[148]
Niosomes	Naftifine hydrochloride	Development of alcohol-free naftifine hydrochloride niosomal gel that would impart improved antifungal results without hazarding skin	The negatively charged niosomes were formulated with HEC (hydroxyethyl cellulose) and exhibited more stability and potency for superficial fungal pathogens	[149]

Drug delivery system	Therapeutics	Objectives	Outcomes	Ref.
Microemulsion	Ketoconazole	Development of ketoconazole-loaded microemulsion with permeation enhancer nigella oil for the effective management of onychomycosis	A thermodynamically stable and sustained released (more than 10 h) antifungal microemulsion was prepared that exhibited greater skin permeation compared to marketed ketoconazole cream	[150]
Nanoemulsion	Amphotericin B	Nanoemulsion containing amphotericin B were designed to mitigate candidiasis and aspergillosis	Developed amphotericin B-embedded nanoemulsion displayed potential against local fungal infections without systemic toxicity	[151]
Micelles	Econazole nitrate, clotrimazole, fluconazole	Formulation of aqueous micelles with block polymers to improve antifungal efficacy against superficial infections	Different antifungal-loaded micelles were developed that exhibited improved bioavailability of antifungal agents	[152]
Microneedle	Voriconazole	Enhanced antifungal efficacy of biodegradable polyglycolic acid microneedle was proposed	Voriconazole contained microneedles worked by the principle of piezoelectric inkjet printing and was helpful for designing of antifungal transdermal drug delivery devices	[153]

Voriconazole is an effective antifungal agent but poor solubility and serious side effects limit its frequent uses in topical drug delivery systems. To overcome voriconazole-related issues, microemulgel has been prepared using Parker neem® oil and carbomer 934P. Improved solubility and prolonged antifungal efficiency suggested potential application of emulgel (microemulsion-based gel) against the treatment of superficial dermatophytes [154]. Further, allylamine-derived butenafine hydrochloride has limited aqueous solubility, which was modified by the addition of surfactant (aerosol OT) and co-surfactant (Sorbitol monooleate) during the formulation of microemulsion. Isopropyl palmitate and carbopol/sodium alginate/HPMC were employed as oil phase (microemulsion) and gelling agent (microgel), respectively. The formulated microgel exhibited superior skin permeation and antimycotic action compared to marketed butenafine hydrochloride cream [155].

9.4.2 Fungal Meningitis

In the year 2012, an outbreak of fungal meningitis appeared due to intrathecal methylprednisolone steroidal injection already contaminated with fungal strain *Exserohilum rostratum* that resulted in more than 50 casualties accompanied by 700 cases of illness in England [156]. Fungal species such as *Cryptococcus neoformans, Histoplasma, Blastomyces* and *Coccidioides* are prevalent pathogens that cause fungal meningitis. This infection spreads through blood to the brain and spinal cord. Commonly, amphotericin B and azole derivatives are prescribed to manage the infection. But poor solubility, high systemic toxicity and poor BBB permeability necessitate the designing of advanced drug delivery strategies. Different types of nanoparticles, nanocrystals, and lipoidal vesicular systems are approached for the preparation of efficient and targeted drug delivery systems. In this context, fusogenic liposomes have been designed that has the potential for effective rapid drug release against fungal meningitis [157].

Febrile neutropenia has been well treated with liposomal amphotericin B and caspofungin (a new echinocandin). These antifungals alter membrane permeability; disturb metabolic process that causes leakage of nutrients and ultimately fungal cell death. Dose-dependent efficacy was achieved in adult patients after the intravenous administration of drug-loaded liposomes. The rapid and extensive biodistribution of amphotericin B displayed no tissue accumulation and hence proved safe for normal cells [158]. Moreover, amphotericin B deoxycholate-polybutylcyanoacrylate nanoparticles were reported to treat cryptococcal meningitis. The developed nanoparticles were modified with polysorbate 80, which could be detected within 30 min after systemic administration in mice. An improved antifungal property was revealed, which was due to the improved transportation capacity of polysorbate-coated amphotericin B nanoparticles across the BBB [159].

9.4.3 Oropharyngeal Infection

Oropharyngeal candidiasis, a Candida infection mainly covers the oral cavity. The clinical features of oral candidiasis are highly prevalent in immunodeficient patients (HIV individuals). *Candida albicans* acts as an opportunistic pathogen that is supposed to be more virulent in humans [160].

Dental hygiene and regular mouthwash prevent most cases of oropharyngeal infections caused by *Candida* sp. Anti-Candida rinses including hexetidine or chlorhexidine antimicrobial agents are recommended [161]. Nystatin-encapsulated polymeric nanoparticles in toothpaste and gels were prepared and compared with unloaded polymeric nanoparticles. The developed system revealed prolonged adhesion of polymeric nystatin-embedded nanoparticles in the buccal mucosa. Moreover, it is alcohol-free, and the reduced frequency of application augmented patient compliance [162]. Ahmad et al. (2020) demonstrated modified PMMA dentures and their effective role in the mitigation of oral candidiasis. They compiled antifungal actions shown by different nanomaterials (copper–titanium dioxide, graphene sheet, zinc oxide, silver, zirconium oxide and curcumin-loaded nanoparticles) entrapped in PMMA dentures to modify cytotoxicity against *Candida albicans*. Versatile mechanisms of action were displayed by these nanoparticles such as disruption of cell wall and membrane, conjugation with the cell wall and by generation on reactive oxygen species due to their exclusive physicochemical properties [163]. Ho et al. (2020) developed itraconazole-loaded nanoparticles through the evaporation emulsion method. The developed nanoparticles were embedded in carbopol 934 polymeric gel and evaluated for efficacy against *Candida albicans*, a primary source of oropharyngeal ailments. Formulated nanosystem was colloidal; the particles were spherical with a nanorange dimension [164]. Recently, bilayered mucoadhesive buccal films containing antibiotics have emerged for the complete eradication of adhered pathogens in the buccal cavity. Gajdosova et al. (2021) explored ciclopirox olamine, which is a broad-spectrum antifungal and preferred for topical dermal infections. Bilayer mucoadhesive buccal films were fabricated with polyacrylate Eudragit®NM 30D and polyethylene oxide. Ex vivo studies highlighted that the mucoadhesive films mediated prolonged release and accumulated in the porcine buccal tissue, which suggested the clinical significance for the alleviation of oral candidiasis [165].

Mady et al. (2018) fabricated miconazole buccal film with and without the addition of urea and evaluated antifungal efficiency (specifically, the role of the penetration enhancer) against *Candida albicans*. Urea-added miconazole patches displayed synergistic antifungal action due to cytoplasmic leakage and necrosis of cells. *In vitro* evaluation of urea-incorporated miconazole buccal films exhibited significantly higher zone of inhibition (30–40 mm) compared to the miconazole-alone film (18 mm) [166]. Buccal films and patches are proven remedies for the management of oromucosal fungal disorders, specifically candidiasis. These are easily fabricated, microbiologically stable and exhibit higher retention on the affected site of buccal mucosa [167].

9.4.4 Vaginal Candidiasis

Vulvovaginal or vaginal candidiasis is a very common female genital infection caused by the yeast species *Candida*. The symptoms such as itching, pruritis, vulvar erythema and dyspareunia are frequently complained by the sufferer. Prolonged use of antibiotics, spermicides, diseased patients (diabetes, AIDS), intra-uterine devices and imbalance of vaginal biota are risk factors of vulvovaginal candidiasis. Conventional vaginal dosages including suppositories, creams and gels exhibit poor residence time. Moreover, the self-cleansing attribute of vagina limits the adherence of therapeutics at site and requires repetitive application of dosage [168]. Frequent applications and limited therapeutic efficacy ultimately lead to inconvenience to the patients. Several mucoadhesive formulations are suggested to overcome limitations associated with conventional drug delivery systems. Biocompatible mucoadhesive natural and semi-synthetic polymers are widely employed for designing NDDS owing to their superb binding efficacy to the mucosal tissues for long periods of time [169]. Novel formulations including microspheres, nanocapsules, mucoadhesive tablets and microemulsions have been proved to be the effective treatments for the eradication of fungal/yeast pathogens around the area of the vagina. Table 9.4 summarizes a few novel strategies designed for the clinical management of vulvovaginal candidiasis. Vaginal formulations containing cyclodextrin have been highlighted owing to their tendency to amplify solubility, absorption, bioavailability and stability. Mucoadhesive in situ gels containing itraconazole, HPMC and poloxamer are reported for combatting vaginal candidiasis. The formulation exhibited pseudoplastic-type flow and thermostability on varying the temperature. Texture analysis displayed that poloxamer polymer provided more bioadhesion and prolonged release of itraconazole from the gel compared to HPMC [170].

Kenechukwu et al. (2018) investigated the potential use of miconazole nitrate microparticles developed using different phytolipids for vulvovaginal candidiasis. Biocompatible phytolipids including hydrogenated palm oil, Softisan® 154 and super refined sunflower seed oil were employed for the preparation of SLNs via melt homogenization. Formulated miconazole nitrate nanoparticles were pegylated with PEG 400 that enhanced physicochemical and pharamacokinetic parameters of the system. Improved antifungal property was observed through analyzing the inhibition zone diameter when compared with the marketed Fungusol® topical solution. Augmented fungicidal rate of miconazole nitrate SLNs (7.1×10^{-3} min^{-1}) than commercial Fungusol® (8.0×10^{-3} min^{-1}) suggested clinical application to combat vaginal infection [178].

Table 9.4 Novel drug approaches for the management of vaginal candidiasis

Drug delivery system	Ingredients	Research highlights	Applications	Ref.
Bioadhesive tablets	Clotrimazole, HPMC, Carbopol, Sodium CMC, Eudragit RL/RS100	Clotrimazole–Eudragit RL/RS 100 microspheres were employed for preparation of bioadhesive tablets	Controlled intravaginal drug delivery	[171]
	Ketoconazole, carbomers (Carbopol 934P and 974P), HPMC and HPC	Bioadhesive effervescent tablets exhibited biocompatibility and retention of dosage for more than 24 h in rat model	Effective against *Candida albicans*	[172]
Acid buffering bioadhesive vaginal gel	Clotrimazole, metronidazole, monosodium citrate, xanthan gum gum, HPMC (K4M) and guar gum	*Lactobacillus* spores were added along with therapeutics for the management of mixed vaginal infections; prolonged retention (12–13 h) was observed	Antimicrobial in vaginal infection	[173]
Microemulsion-based vaginal gel	Fluconazole, Carbopol ETD 2020	Significantly superior antifungal efficacy and bioadhesion were observed when compared to marketed Candid V (clotrimazole gel)	Antifungal vaginal diseases and irritation	[174]
Mucoadhesive thermosensitive gel (MTG)	Clotrimazole, Polaxomers (P407, P188), Polycarbophil,	Prolonged drug release was exhibited by clotrimazole MTG; after 10 h post dose, tenfold colony forming units of *C. albicans* were reported	Vaginal candidiasis	[175]
Coconut oil core vaginal nanocapsule suspension	Clotrimazole, coconut oil, Eudragit RS 100	Clotrimazole nanocapsule-containing suspension was stable in temperature and UV radiations as well; in acidic pH, drug release was higher without the burst effect	Effective against candidiasis caused by *C. albicans* and *C. glabrata*	[176]
Peptide vaccine	Hepcidin (Hep 20)	Human cationic Hep 20, a fungicide peptide displayed susceptibility for *C. glabrata* without harming human healthy cells	Vaginal infections caused by fluconazole-resistant *Candida glabrata*	[177]

9.5 Conclusion

The effective alleviation of pathogenic diseases requires the designing of carrier-mediated delivery systems that not only stabilize therapeutic agents but also improve drug action at the infected site and resolve the issues associated with cell permeation and drug resistance. The chapter highlights myriad research and novel formulations for the management of different infectious agents, i.e., bacteria, viruses and fungi. Polymeric nanoparticles, micelles, vesicular and lipid-based drug delivery approaches are highly entertained for the management of these devastating infections owing to their local and targeted drug release efficiencies. Although a few issues related to clinical trial and approval from registered governing bodies are still in the pipeline.

References

1. Louria, D. B., and Carbon, C. J. (2004). Introduction to infectious diseases. In Armstrong, D., and Cohen, J. (eds.), *Infectious Diseases*, Vol 1, 1st ed. Mosby Publishers, London, U.K., 1999.
2. World Health Organization. The top 10 causes of death. 2020. https://www.who.int/news-room/fact-sheets/detail/the-top-10-causes-of-death.
3. Wardeh, M., Risley, C., McIntyre, M. K., Setzkorn, C., and Baylis, M. (2015). Database of host-pathogen and related species interactions, and their global distribution, *Sci Data*, **2**, 150049.
4. Wang, P., Li, Z., Jones, A., Bodner, M. E., and Dean, E. (2019). Discordance between lifestyle-related health behaviors and beliefs of urban mainland Chinese: a questionnaire study with implications for targeting health education, *AIMS Public Health*, **6**, 49–66.
5. World Health Organization (WHO). Global health estimates 2016: diseases burden by cause, age, sex, by country and by region, 2000–2016.
6. Murray, K. A., Olivero, J., Roche, B., Tiedt, S., and Guégan, J.-F. (2018). Pathogeography: leveraging the biogeography of human infectious diseases for global health management, *Ecography*, **41**, 1411–1427.
7. Zheng, K., Li, K., Chang, T. H., Xie, J., and Chen, P. Y. (2019). Synergistic antimicrobial capability of magnetically oriented graphene oxide conjugated with gold nanoclusters, *Adv. Funct. Mater.*, **29**, 1970320.

8. Wu, Z. L., Zhao, J., and Xu, R. (2020). Recent advances in oral nano-antibiotics for bacterial infection therapy, *Int. J. Nanomed.*, **15**, 9587–9610.
9. Laxminarayan, R., Bhutta, Z., and Duse, A. (2006). Drug resistance. In: Jamison, D. T., Breman, J. G., Measham, A. R, Evans, D. B., Jha, P., Mills, A., and Musgrove, P. (eds.), *Disease Control Priorities in Developing Countries*, 2nd ed., Washington (DC): The International Bank for Reconstruction and Development/The World Bank.
10. Ruddaraju, L. K., Pammi, S. V. N., Guntuku, G. S., Padavala, V. S., and Kolapalli, V. R. M. (2020). A review on anti-bacterials to combat resistance: from ancient era of plants and metals to present and future perspectives of green nano technological combinations, *Asian. J. Pharm. Sci.*, **15**, 42–59.
11. Chen, H., Jin, Y., Wang, J., Wang, Y., Jiang, W., Dai, H., Pang, S., Lei, L., Ji, J., and Wang, B. (2018). Design of smart targeted and responsive drug delivery systems with enhanced antibacterial properties, *Nanoscale*, **10**, 20946–20962.
12. Hooper, C. D. (2001). Mechanisms of action of antimicrobials: focus on fluoroquino-lones, *Clin. Infect. Diseases*, **32**, S9–S15.
13. Zhang, W., Hu, E., Wang, Y., Miao, S., Liu, Y., Hu, Y., Liu, J., Xu, B., Chen, D., and Shen, Y. (2021). Emerging antibacterial strategies with application of targeting drug delivery system and combined treatment, *Int. J. Nanomed.*, **16**, 6141–6156.
14. Thakur, K., and Zunt, J. (2015). Tropical neuroinfectious diseases, *Continuum (Minneap Minn)*, **21**, 1639–1661.
15. Parikh, V., Tucci, V., and Galwankar, S. (2012). Infections of the nervous system, *Int. J. Crit. Illness Injury Sci.*, **2**, 82–97.
16. Halliday, A. J., and Cook, M. J. (2009). Polymer-based drug delivery devices for neurological disorders, *CNS Neurol. Disord. Drug Targets*, **8**, 205–221.
17. Kamaruzzaman, N. F., Tan, L. P., Hamdan, R. H., Choong, S. S., Wong, W. K., Gibson, A. J., Chivu, A., and Pina, M. F. (2019). Antimicrobial polymers: the potential replacement of existing antibiotics? *Int. J. Mol. Sci.*, **20**, 2747.
18. Long, Y., Li, L., Bi, Q., Deng, C., Chen, Z., Bhattachayya, S., and Li, C. (2016). Novel polymeric nanoparticles targeting the lipopolysaccharides of Pseudomonas aeruginosa, *Int. J. Pharm.*, **502**, 232–241.
19. Gala, R. P., D'Souza, M., and Zughaier, S. M. (2016). Evaluation of various adjuvant nanoparticulate formulations for meningococcal capsular polysaccharide-based vaccine, *Vaccine*, **34**, 3260–7.

20. Liu, L., Xu, K., Wang, H., Tan, P. K., Fan, W., Venkatraman, S. S., Li, L., and Yang, Y. Y. (2009). Self-assembled cationic peptide nanoparticles as an efficient antimicrobial agent, *Nat. Nanotechnol.*, **4**, 457–463.

21. Liu, L., Venkatraman, S. S., Yang, Y.-Y., Guo, K., Lu, J., He, B., Moochhala, S., and Kan, L. (2008), Polymeric micelles anchored with TAT for delivery of antibiotics across the blood brain barrier, *Biopolymers*, **90**, 617–623.

22. Hong, W., Zhang, Z., Liu, L., Zhao, Y., Zhang, D., and Liu, M. (2018). Brain-targeted delivery of PEGylated nano-bacitracin A against Penicillin-sensitive and -resistant Pneumococcal meningitis: formulated with RV_{G29} and Pluronic® P85 unimers, *Drug Deliv.*, **25**, 1886–1897.

23. Vieira, D. B., and Gamarra, L. F. (2016). Getting into the brain: liposome-based strategies for effective drug delivery across the blood-brain barrier, *Int. J. Nanomed.*, **18**, 5381–5414.

24. Bartomeu Garcia, C., Shi, D., and Webster, T. J. (2017). Tat-functionalized liposomes for the treatment of meningitis: an *in vitro* study, *Int. J. Nanomed.*, **12**, 3009–3021.

25. Zandile, M., and Blessing, A. (2018). Application of dendrimers for the treatment of infectious diseases, *Molecules*, **23**, 2205.

26. Rizvi, S. M. D., Hussain, T., Ahmed, A. B. F., Alshammari, T. M., Moin, A., Ahmed, M. Q., Barreto, G. E., Kamal, M. A., and Ashraf, G. M. (2018). Gold nanoparticles: a plausible tool to combat neurological bacterial infections in humans, *Biomed. Pharmacother.*, **107**, 7–18.

27. Bucharskaya, A., Maslyakova, G., Terentyuk, G., Yakunin, A., Avetisyan, Y., Bibikova, O., Tuchina, E., Khlebtsov, B., Khlebtsov, N., and Tuchin, V. (2016). Towards effective photothermal/photodynamic treatment using plasmonic gold nanoparticles, *Int. J. Mol. Sci.*, **17**, 1295.

28. Anwar, A., Masri, A., Rao, K., Rajendran, K., Khan, N. A., Shah, M. R., and Siddiqui, R. (2019). Antimicrobial activities of green synthesized gums-stabilized nanoparticles loaded with flavonoids, *Sci. Rep.*, **9**, 3122.

29. Barani, M., Mukhtar, M., Rahdar, A., Sargazi, G., Thysiadou, A., and Kyzas, G. Z. (2021). Progress in the application of nanoparticles and graphene as drug carriers and on the diagnosis of brain infections, *Molecules*, **26**, 186.

30. Flores-Mireles, A. L., Walker, J. N., Caparon, M., and Hultgren, S. J. (2015). Urinary tract infections: epidemiology, mechanisms of infection and treatment options, *Nat. Rev. Microbiol.*, **13**, 269–284.

31. Irwin, D. E., Kopp, Z. S., Agatep, B., Milsom, I., and Abrams, P. (2011). Worldwide prevalence estimates of lower urinary tract symptoms, overactive bladder, urinary incontinence and bladder outlet obstruction, *BJU Int.*, **108**, 1132–8.

32. Labbaf, S., Horsley, H., Chang, M. W., Stride, E., Malone-Lee, J., Edirisinghe, M., and Rohn, J. L. (2013). An encapsulated drug delivery system for recalcitrant urinary tract infection, *J. Royal Soc. Interface*, **10**, 20130747.

33. Kristian, S., Birkholm, G. R., Yaseelan, P., Jørn, K. H., Lars, L., Martin, A., Peter, T., and Emil, A. T. A. (2021). Novel device-integrated drug delivery system for local inhibition of urinary tract infection, *Front. Microbiol.*, **12**, 685698.

34. Brauner, B., Schuster, C., Wirth, M., and Gabor, F. (2020). Trimethoprim-loaded microspheres prepared from low-molecular-weight PLGA as a potential drug delivery system for the treatment of urinary tract infections, *ACS Omega*, **5**, 9013–9022.

35. Horsley, H., Owen, J., Browning, R., Carugo, D., Malone-Lee, J., Stride, E., and Rohn, J. L. (2019). Ultrasound-activated microbubbles as a novel intracellular drug delivery system for urinary tract infection, *J. Control. Release*, **301**, 166–175.

36. Kaur, A., Saxena, Y., Bansal, R., Gupta, S., Tyagi, A., Sharma, R. K., Ali, J., Panda, A. K., Gabrani, R., and Dang, S. (2017). Intravaginal delivery of polyphenon 60 and curcumin nanoemulsion gel, *AAPS PharmSciTech*, **18**, 2188–2202.

37. Zhao, S., Lv, Y., Zhang, J. B., Wang, B., Lv, G. J., and Ma, X. J. (2014). Gastro-retentive drug delivery systems for the treatment of Helicobacter pylori, *World J. Gastroenterol.*, **20**, 9321–9329.

38. Goh, K. L., Chan, W. K., Shiota, S., and Yamaoka, Y. (2011). Epidemiology of Helicobacter pylori infection and public health implications, *Helicobacter*, **1**, 1–9.

39. Khan, S., Misra, S. K., and Sharma, N. (2015). Formulation and evaluation of multiparticulate gel beads containing tinidazole for stomach specific delivery, *Int. J. Pharm. Tech. Res.*, **8**, 196–205.

40. Mishra, S. K., and Pathak, K. (2008). Formulation and evaluation of oil entrapped gastroretentive floating gel beads of loratadine, *Acta Pharm.*, **58**, 187–197.

41. Mishra, S. K., Philip, A. K., and Pathak, K. (2008). Passage-delaying microbeads for controlled delivery of loratadine, *PDA J. Pharm. Sci. Technol.*, **62**, 421–428.

42. Hunter, J. C., and Watkins, L. K. F. (2017). *CDC Yellow Book 2018: Health Information for International Travel.* (ed. Brunette, G. W.), Ch. 3, Oxford University Press, New York, USA, pp. 304–305.

43. Cameron, D., Hock, Q. S., Kadim, M., Mohan, N., Ryoo, E., Sandhu, B., Yamashiro, Y., Jie, C., Hoekstra, H., and Guarino, A. (2017). Probiotics for gastrointestinal disorders: proposed recommendations for children of the Asia-Pacific region, *World J. Gastroenterol.*, **23**, 7952–7964.

44. Bäumler, A. J., and Sperandio, V. (2016). Interactions between the microbiota and pathogenic bacteria in the gut, *Nature*, **535**, 85–93.

45. Mu, H., Bai, H., Sun, F., Liu, Y., Lu, C., Qiu, Y., Chen, P., Yang, Y., Kong, L., and Duan, J. (2019). Pathogen-targeting glycovesicles as a therapy for salmonellosis, *Nat. Commun.*, **10**, 4039.

46. Ranjan, A., Pothayee, N., Seleem, M., Jain, N., Sriranganathan, N., Riffle, J. S., and Kasimanickam, R. (2010). Drug delivery using novel nanoplexes against a Salmonella mouse infection model, *J. Nanoparticle Res.*, **12**, 905–914.

47. Mudakavi, R. J., Raichur, A. M., and Chakravortty, D. (2014). Lipid coated mesoporous silica nanoparticles as an oral delivery system for targeting and treatment of intravacuolar Salmonella infections, *RSC Adv.*, **4**(105), 61160–61166.

48. Seys, S. A., Sampedro, F., and Hedberg, C. W. (2017). Assessment of meat and poultry product recalls due to *Salmonella* contamination: product recovery and illness prevention, *J. Food Prot.*, **80**, 1288–1292.

49. Kumar, D. G., Solval, K. M., Mishra, A., and Macarsin, D. (2020). Antimicrobial efficacy of pelargonic acid micelles against *Salmonella* varies by surfactant, serotype and stress response, *Sci. Rep.*, **10**, 10287.

50. Brubaker, J., Zhang, X., Bourgeois, A. L., Harro, C., Sack, D. A., and Chakraborty, S. (2021). Intestinal and systemic inflammation induced by symptomatic and asymptomatic enterotoxigenic *E. coli* infection and impact on intestinal colonization and ETEC specific immune responses in an experimental human challenge model, *Gut Microbes*, **13**, 1–13.

51. Paudel, S., Peña-Bahamonde, J., Shakiba, S., Astete, C., Louie, S., Sabliov, C. M., and Rodrigues, D. F. (2021). Prevention of infection caused by enteropathogenic *E. coli* O157:H7 in intestinal cells using enrofloxacin entrapped in polymer based nanocarriers, *J. Hazard. Mater.*, **414**, 125454.

52. Carpena, N., Richards, K. B., Gonzalez, T. D. J., Bravo-Blas, A., Housden, N. G., Gerasimidis, K., Milling, S. W. F., Douce, G., Malik, D. J., and Walker, D. (2021). Targeted delivery of narrow-spectrum protein antibiotics to the lower gastrointestinal tract in a murine model of *Escherichia coli* colonization, *Front. Microbiol.,* **12**, 670535.

53. Haahr, T., Zacho, J., Bräuner, M., Shathmigha, K., Skov, Jensen, J., and Humaidan, P. (2019). Reproductive outcome of patients undergoing *in vitro* fertilisation treatment and diagnosed with bacterial vaginosis or abnormal vaginal microbiota: a systematic PRISMA review and meta-analysis, *BJOG Int. J. Obstet. Gynaecol.,* **126**, 200–207.

54. Pandey, M., Choudhury, H., Abdul-Aziz, A., Bhattamisra, S. K., Gorain, B., Carine, T., Wee Toong, T., Yi, N. J., and Win, Yi, L. (2020). Promising drug delivery approaches to treat microbial infections in the vagina: a recent update, *Polymers,* **13**, 26.

55. Balkus, J. E., Srinivasan, S., Anzala, O., Kimani, J., Andac, C., Schwebke, J., Fredricks, D. N., and McClelland, R. S. (2017). Impact of periodic presumptive treatment for bacterial vaginosis on the vaginal microbiome among women participating in the preventing vaginal infections trial, *J. Infect. Dis.,* **215**, 723–731.

56. Ranjit, E., Raghubanshi, B. R., Maskey, S., and Parajuli, P. (2018). Prevalence of bacterial vaginosis and its association with risk factors among non-pregnant women: a hospital based study, *Int. J. Microbiol.,* **8**, 1–10.

57. Perioli, L., Ambrogi, V., Pagano, C., Scuota, S., and Rossi, C. (2009). FG90 chitosan as a new polymer for metronidazole mucoadhesive tablets for vaginal administration, *Int. J. Pharm.,* **377**, 120–127.

58. Burnett, A. M., Anderson, C. P., and Zwank, M. D. (2012). Laboratory-confirmed gonorrhea and/or Chlamydia rates in clinically diagnosed pelvic inflammatory disease and cervicitis, *Am. J. Emerg. Med.,* **30**, 1114–1117.

59. Al-Qahtani, F., Aleanizy, F., El Tahir, E., Alhabib, H., Alsaif, R., Shazly, G., Al-Qahtani, H., Alsarra, I., and Mahdavi, J. (2020). Antibacterial activity of chitosan nanoparticles against pathogenic *N. gonorrhoea, Int. J. Nanomed.,* **15**, 7877–7887.

60. Li, L. H., Yen, M. Y., Ho, C. C., Wu, P., Wang, C. C., Maurya, P. K., Chen, P. S., Chen, W., Hsieh, W. Y., and Chen, H. W. (2013). Non-cytotoxic nanomaterials enhance antimicrobial activities of cefmetazole against multidrug-resistant Neisseria gonorrhoeae, *PLoS One,* **8**, e64794.

61. Tuðcu-Demiröz, F., Saar, S., Tort, S., and Acartürk, F. (2020). Electrospun metronidazole-loaded nanofibers for vaginal drug delivery, *Drug Dev. Ind. Pharm.*, **46**, 1015–1025.

62. Tuðcu-Demiröz, F., Saar, S., Kara, A. A., Yýldýz, A., Tunçel, E., and Acartürk, F. (2021). Development and characterization of chitosan nanoparticles loaded nanofiber hybrid system for vaginal controlled release of benzydamine, *Eur. J. Pharm. Sci.*, **161**, 105801.

63. Virmond, M. D. C. L., Grzybowski, A., and Virmond, L. (2015). Leprosy: a glossary, *Clin. Dermatol.*, **33**, 8–18.

64. Chaves, L. L., Patriota, Y., Soares-Sobrinho, J. L., Vieira, A. C. C., Lima, S. A. C., and Reis, S. (2020). Drug delivery systems on leprosy therapy: moving towards eradication? *Pharmaceutics,* **12**, 1202.

65. Chaves, L. L., Vieira, A. C. C., Reis, S., Sarmento, B., and Ferreira, D. (2014). Quality by design: discussing and assessing the solid dispersions risk, *Curr. Drug Deliv.*, **11**, 253–269.

66. Patel, V. B., and Misra, A. N. (1999). Encapsulation and stability of clofazimine liposomes, *J. Microencapsul.*, **16**, 357–367.

67. Chaves, L. L., Lima, S. A. C., Vieira, A. C. C., Barreiros, L., Segundo, M. A., Ferreira, D., Sarmento, B., and Reis, S. (2018). Development of PLGA nanoparticles loaded with clofazimine for oral delivery: assessment of formulation variables and intestinal permeability, *Eur. J. Pharm. Sci.*, **112**, 28–37.

68. Nie, H., Su, Y., Zhang, M., Song, Y., Leone, A., Taylor, L. S., Marsac, P. J., Li, T., and Byrn, S. R. (2016). Solid-state spectroscopic investigation of molecular interactions between clofazimine and hypromellose phthalate in amorphous solid dispersions, *Mol. Pharm.*, **13**, 3964–3975.

69. Schneider-Rauber, G., Argenta, D. F., and Caon, T. (2020). Emerging technologies to target drug delivery to the skin—the role of crystals and carrier-based systems in the case study of dapsone, *Pharm. Res.*, **37**, 240.

70. Rojo, L., Fernandez-Gutierrez, M., Deb, S., Stevens, M. M., and San, R. J. (2015). Designing dapsone polymer conjugates for controlled drug delivery, *Acta Biomater.*, **27**, 32–41.

71. El-Nabarawi, M. A., Shamma, R. N., Farouk, F., and Nasralla, S. M. (2018). Dapsone-loaded invasomes as a potential treatment of acne: preparation, characterization, and *in vivo* skin deposition assay, *AAPS PharmSciTech,* **19**, 2174–2184.

72. Chen, W., Cheng, C. A., Lee, B. Y., Clemens, D. L., Huang, W. Y., Horwitz, M. A., and Zink, J. I. (2018). Facile strategy enabling both high loading and high release amounts of the water-insoluble drug clofazimine using mesoporous silica nanoparticles, *ACS Appl. Mater. Interfaces*, **10**, 31870–31881.

73. Toleman, M. S., Vipond, I. B., and Brindle, R. (2016). Specific PCR, bacterial culture, serology and pharyngeal sampling to enhance the aetiological diagnosis of cellulitis, *J. Med. Microbiol.*, **65**, 44–47.

74. Darwhekar, G., Jain, D. K., and Choudhary, A. (2012). Elastic liposomes for delivery of neomycin sulphate in deep skin infection, *Asian J. Pharm. Sci.*, **7**, 230–240.

75. Martinez, L. R., Han, G., Chacko, M., Mihu, M. R., Jacobson, M., Gialanella, P., Friedman, A. J., Nosanchuk, J. D., and Friedman, J. M. (2009). Antimicrobial and healing efficacy of sustained release nitric oxide nanoparticles against Staphylococcus aureus skin infection, *J. Invest. Dermatol.*, **129**, 2463–2469.

76. Albright, V., Xu, M., Palanisamy, A., Cheng, J., Stack, M., Zhang, B., Jayaraman, A., Sukhishvili, S. A., and Wang, H. (2018). Micelle-coated, hierarchically structured nanofibers with dual-release capability for accelerated wound healing and infection control, *Adv. Health Mater.*, **7**, e1800132.

77. Scannapieco, F. A. (2013). The oral microbiome: its role in health and in oral and systemic infections, *Clin. Microbiol. Newsl.*, **35**, 163–169.

78. Wade, W. G. (2013). The oral microbiome in health and disease, *Pharm. Res.*, **69**, 137–143.

79. Dong, Y., Ye, H., Liu, Y., Xu, L., Wu, Z., Hu, X., Ma, J., Pathak, J. L., Liu, J., and Wu, G. (2017). pH dependent silver nanoparticles releasing titanium implant: a novel therapeutic approach to control peri-implant infection, *Colloids Surf. B Biointerfaces*, **158**, 127–136.

80. de Santana, R. B., and de Santana, C. M. (2015). Human intrabony defect regeneration with rhFGF-2 and hyaluronic acid—a randomized controlled clinical trial, *J. Clin. Periodontol.*, **42**, 658–665.

81. Genari, B., Leitune, V. C., Jornada, D. S., Camassola, M., Pohlmann, A. R., Guterres, S. S., Samuel, S. M., Collares, F. M. (2017). Effect of indomethacin-loaded nanocapsules incorporation in a dentin adhesive resin, *Clin. Oral Investig.*, **21**, 437–446.

82. Chen, F., Rice, K. C., Liu, X. M., Reinhardt. R. A., Bayles, K. W., Wang, D. (2010). Triclosan-loaded tooth-binding micelles for prevention and treatment of dental biofilm, *Pharm. Res.*, **27**, 2356–2364.

83. Zhou, Y., Yang, J., Lin, Z., Li, J., Liang, K., Yuan, H., Li, S., and Li, J. (2014). Triclosan-loaded poly (amido amine) dendrimer for simultaneous treatment and remineralization of human dentine, *Colloids Surf. B Biointerfaces*, **115**, 237–243.

84. Massa, M. A., Covarrubias, C., Bittner, M., Fuentevilla, I. A., Capetillo, P., Von Marttens, A., Carvajal, J. C. (2014). Synthesis of new antibacterial composite coating for titanium based on highly ordered nanoporous silica and silver nanoparticles, *Mater. Sci. Eng. C Mater. Biol. Appl.*, **45**, 46–53.

85. Bottino, M. C., Münchow, E. A., Albuquerque, M. T. P., Kamocki, K., Shahi, R., Gregory, R. L., Chu, T. G., and Pankajakshan, D. (2017). Tetracycline-incorporated polymer nanofibers as a potential dental implant surface modifier, *J. Biomed. Mater. Res. B Appl. Biomater.*, **105**, 2085–2092.

86. Maurya, R., Singh, M. P., and Kymonil, K. M. (2019). Formulation and evaluation of moxifloxacin microspheres implant for intra-periodontal pockets, *Int. J. Pharm. Sci. Res.*, **10**, 3891–3897.

87. Williams, R. C., Paquette, D. W., Offenbacher, S., Adams, D. F., Armitage, G. C., Bray, K., Caton, J., Cochran, D. L., Drisko, C. H., Fiorellini, J. P., Giannobile, W. V., Grossi, S., Guerrero, D. M., Johnson, G. K., Lamster, I. B., Magnusson, I., Oringer, R. J., Persson, G. R., Van Dyke, T. E., Wolff, L. F., Santucci, E. A., Rodda, B. E., and Lessem, J. (2001). Treatment of periodontitis by local administration of minocycline microspheres: a controlled trial, *J. Periodontol.*, **72**, 1535–1544.

88. Singh, N., Paknikar, K. M., and Rajwade, J. (2019). Gene expression is influenced due to 'nano' and 'ionic' copper in pre-formed Pseudomonas aeruginosa bioflms, *Environ. Res.*, **175**, 367–375.

89. Belon, C., and Blanc-Potard, A.-B. (2016). Intramacrophage survival for extracellular bacterial pathogens: MgtC as a key adaptive factor, *Front. Cell Infect. Microbiol.*, **6**, 52.

90. Muchao, F. P., and da Silva, L. V. R. F. (2010). Advances in inhalation therapy in pediatrics, *J. Pediatr.*, **86**, 367–376.

91. Mishra, B., and Singh, J. (2020). Novel drug delivery systems and significance in respiratory diseases. In: *Targeting Chronic Inflammatory Lung Diseases Using Advanced Drug Delivery Systems*, Elsevier, pp. 57–95.

92. Srichana, T., Juthong, S., Thawithong, E., Supaiboonpipat, S., and Soorapan, S. (2016). Clinical equivalence of budesonide dry powder inhaler and pressurized metered dose inhaler, *Clin. Respir. J.*, **10**, 74–82.

93. Deacon, J., Abdelghany, S. M., Quinn, D. J., Schmid, D., Megaw, J., Donnelly, R. F., Jones, D. S., Kissenpfennig, A., Elborn, J. S., Gilmore, B. F., Taggart, C. C., Scott, C. J. (2014). Antimicrobial efficacy of tobramycin polymeric nanoparticles for Pseudomonas aeruginosa infections in cystic fibrosis: formulation, characterisation and functionalisation with dornase alfa (DNase), *J. Control. Release*, **198**, 55–61.

94. Gaspar, D. P., Gaspar, M. M., Eleutério, C. V., Grenha, A., Blanco, M., Gonçalves, L. M. D., Taboada, P., Almeida, A. J., and Remuñán-López, C. (2017). Microencapsulated solid lipid nanoparticles as a hybrid platform for pulmonary antibiotic delivery, *Mol. Pharm.*, **14**, 2977–2990.

95. Parikh, R., Dalwadi, S., Aboti, P., and Patel, L. (2014). Inhaled microparticles of antitubercular antibiotic for *in vitro* and *in vivo* alveolar macrophage targeting and activation of phagocytosis, *J. Antibiot.*, **67**, 387–394.

96. Armijo, L. M., Wawrzyniec, S. J., Kopciuch, M., Brandt, Y. I., Rivera, A. C., Withers, N. J., Cook, N. C., Huber, D. L., Monson, T. C., Smyth, H. D. C., and Osiński, M. (2020). Antibacterial activity of iron oxide, iron nitride, and tobramycin conjugated nanoparticles against Pseudomonas aeruginosa biofilms, *J. Nanobiotechnol.*, **18**, 35.

97. Ehsan, Z., and Clancy, J. P. (2015). Management of Pseudomonas aeruginosa infection in cystic fibrosis patients using inhaled antibiotics with a focus on nebulized liposomal amikacin, *Fut. Microbiol.*, **10**, 1901–1912.

98. Islan, G. A., Tornello, P. C., Abraham, G. A., Duran, N., and Castro, G. R. (2016). Smart lipid nanoparticles containing levofloxacin and DNase for lung delivery. Design and characterization, *Colloids Surf. B Biointerfaces*, **143**, 168–176.

99. Parikh, R., Patel, L., and Dalwadi, S. (2014). Microparticles of rifampicin: comparison of pulmonary route with oral route for drug uptake by alveolar macrophages, phagocytosis activity and toxicity study in albino rats, *Drug Deliv.*, **21**, 406–411.

100. Hu, X., Yang, F. F., Quan, L. H., Liu, C. Y., Liu, X. M., Ehrhardt, C., and Liao, Y. H. (2014). Pulmonary delivered polymeric micelles-pharmacokinetic evaluation and biodistribution studies, *Eur. J. Pharm. Biopharm.*, **88**, 1064–1075.

101. Sharma, P., Chawla, A., Arora, S., and Pawar, P. (2012). Novel drug delivery approaches on antiviral and antiretroviral agents, *J. Adv. Pharm. Technol. Res.*, **3** 147–159.

102. Bartlett, N. W., Walton, R. P., Edwards, M. R. (2008). Mouse models of rhinovirus-induced disease and exacerbation of allergic airway inflammation, *Nat. Med.*, **14**, 199–204.

103. Gansukh, E., Anthonydhason, V., Jung, S., Kim, D. H., Muthu, M., Gopal, J., and Chun, S. (2018). Nanotherapeutic anti-influenza solutions: current knowledge and future challenges, *J. Clust. Sci.*, **29**, 933–941.

104. KhalajHedayati, A., Chua, C. L. L., Smooker, P., and Lee, K. W. (2020). Nanoparticles in influenza subunit vaccine development: immunogenicity enhancement, *Influenza Other Respi. Viruses*, **14**, 92–101.

105. He, Q., Cui, Y., and Li, J. (2009). Molecular assembly and application of biomimetic microcapsules, *Chem. Soc. Rev.*, **38**, 292–303.

106. Shastri, P. N., Kim, M. C., Quan, F. S., D'Souza, M. J., and Kang, S. M. (2012). Immunogenicity and protection of oral influenza vaccines formulated into microparticles, *J. Pharm. Sci.*, **101**, 623–635.

107. Mhlwatika, Z., and Aderibigbe, B. A. (2018). Application of dendrimers for the treatment of infectious diseases. *Molecules*, **23**, 2025.

108. Pati, R., Shevtsov, M., and Sonawane, A. (2018). Nanoparticle vaccines against infectious diseases, *Front. Immunol.*, **9**, 2224.

109. Kolinski, John, M., Schneider, and Tobias, M. (2021). Superspreading events suggest aerosol transmission of SARS-CoV-2 by accumulation in enclosed spaces, *Phys. Rev. E*, **103**, 033109.

110. Ochekpe, N. A., Olorunfemi, P. O., Ngwuluka, N. C. (2009). Nanotechnology and drug delivery part 2: nanostructures for drug delivery. *Trop. J. Pharm. Res.*, **8**, 275–287.

111. Mahajan, S. D., Aalinkeel, R., Law, W. C. (2012). Anti-HIV-1 nanotherapeutics: promises and challenges for the future, *Int. J. Nanomed.*, **7**, 5301–5314.

112. Shashi, K. M., Kapoor, A., Kumar, A., aand Katiyar, A. (2021). An overview on SARS-CoV-2 variants, *IJARESM*, **9**, 962–966.

113. Singh, Y., Gupta, G., Satija, S., Negi, P., Chellappan, D. K., and Dua, K. (2020). RAAS blockers in hypertension posing a higher risk towards the COVID-19, *Dermatol. Ther.*, 33, 13501.

114. Wang, M., Cao, R., and Zhang, L. (2020). Remdesivir and chloroquine effectively inhibit the recently emerged novel coronavirus (2019-nCoV) *in vitro*, *Cell Res.*, 30, 269–271.

115. Chen, Z., Zhang, Z., and Zhai, X. (2020). Rapid and sensitive detection of anti-SARS-CoV-2 IgG using lanthanide-doped nanoparticles-based lateral flow immunoassay, *Anal. Chem.*, **92**, 7226–7231.

116. Mehta, M., and Tewari, D. (2019). Oligonucleotide therapy: an emerging focus area for drug delivery in chronic inflammatory respiratory diseases, *Chem. Biol. Interact.*, 308, 206–215.

117. Virovic, L., Wu, C. H., Konishi, M., and Wu, G, Y. (2005). Novel delivery methods for treatment of viral hepatitis: an update, *Expert Opin. Drug Deliv.*, **2**, 707–717.

118. Perazzo, P., Valle, N. R. D., Sordelli, A., Gonzalez, R. H., and Cuestas, M. L. (2015). Nanotechnology, drug delivery systems and their potential applications in hepatitis B vaccines, *Int. J. Vaccines Vaccin.*, **1**, 00007.

119. Jaganathan, K. S, and Vyas, S. P (2006). Strong systemic and mucosal immune responses to surface-modified PLGA microspheres containing recombinant hepatitis B antigen administered intranasally, *Vaccine*, **24**, 4201–4211.

120. Wilkhu, J., McNeil, S. E., Kirby, D. J., and Perrie, Y. (2011). Formulation design considerations for oral vaccines, *Ther. Deliv.*, **2**, 1141–1164.

121. World Health Organization. *Report on Global Sexually Transmitted Infection Surveillance.* (2018).

122. Roizman, B., and Whitley, R. J. (2001). The nine ages of herpes simplex virus. *Herpes*, **8**(1), 23–27.

123. Seth, A. K., Misra, A., and Umrigar, D. (2004). Topical liposomal gel of idoxuridine for the treatment of herpes simplex: pharmaceutical and clinical implications, *Pharm. Dev. Technol.*, **9**, 277–289.

124. Shishu, Rajan, S., and Kamalpreet. (2009). Development of novel microemulsion-based topical formulations of acyclovir for the treatment of cutaneous herpetic infections, *AAPS PharmSciTech*, **10**, 559–565.

125. Rokhade, A. P., Patil, S. A., and Aminabhavi, T. M. (2007). Synthesis and characterization of semi-interpenetrating polymer network microspheres of acrylamide grafted dextran and chitosan for controlled release of acyclovir, *Carbohydr. Polym.*, **67**, 605–613.

126. Suzana, L., and Mihael, S. (2014). HPV-associated diseases, *Clin. Dermatol.*, **32**, 227–234.

127. Zehbe, I., Hacker, G. W., Su, H., Hauser, K. C., Hainfeld, J. F., and Tubbs, R. (1997). Sensitive in situ hybridization with catalyzed reporter deposition, streptavidin-nanogold, and silver acetate autometallography: detection of single-copy human papillomavirus, *Am. J. Pathol.*, **150**, 1553–1561.

128. Kampel, L., Goldsmith, M., Ramishetti, S., Veiga, N., Rosenblum, D., and Gutkin, A. (2021). Therapeutic inhibitory RNA in head and neck cancer via functional targeted lipid nanoparticles, *J. Control. Release*, **337**, 378–389.

129. McArthur, J. C., Brew, B. J., and Nath, A. (2005). Neurological complications of HIV infection. *Lancet Neurol.*, **4**, 543–555.

130. Oussoren, C., Magnani, M., Fraternale, A., Casabianca, A., Chiarantini, L., Ingebrigsten, R., Underberg, W. J., and Storm, G. (1999). Liposomes as carriers of the antiretroviral agent dideoxycytidine-5′-triphosphate, *Int. J. Pharm.*, **180**, 261–270.

131. Clayton, R., Ohagen, A., Nicol, F., Del Vecchio, A. M., Jonckers, T. H., Goethals, O., Van Loock, M., Michiels, L., Grigsby, J., Xu, Z., Zhang, Y. P., Gutshall, L. L., Cunningham, M., Jiang, H., Bola, S., Sarisky, R. T., and Hertogs, K. (2009). Sustained and specific *in vitro* inhibition of HIV-1 replication by a protease inhibitor encapsulated in gp120-targeted liposomes, *Antiviral. Res.*, **84**, 142–149.

132. Mandal, S., Khandalavala, K., Pham, R., Bruck, P., Varghese, M., and Kochvar, A. (2017). Cellulose acetate phthalate and antiretroviral nanoparticle fabrications for HIV pre-exposure prophylaxis, *Polymers Basel.*, **9**, 423–440.

133. Dutta, T., Agashe, H. B., Garg, M., Balakrishnan, P., Kabra, M., and Jain, N. K. (2007). Poly (propyleneimine) dendrimer-based nano-containers for targeting of efavirenz to human monocytes/macrophages *in vitro*, *J. Drug Target.*, **15**, 89–98.

134. Graverini, G., Piazzini, V., Landucci, E., Pantano, D., Nardiello, P., and Casamenti, F. (2018). Solid lipid nanoparticles for delivery of andrographolide across the blood-brain barrier: *in vitro* and *in vivo* evaluation, *Coll. Surf. B Biointerf.*, **161**, 302–313.

135. Aliabadi, H. M., and Lavasanifar, A. (2006). Polymeric micelles for drug delivery, *Expert. Opin. Drug Deliv.*, **3**,139–162.

136. Alangaden, G. J. (2011). Nosocomial fungal infections: epidemiology, infection control, and prevention, *Infect. Dis. Clin. North Am.*, **25**, 201–225.

137. Misra, S. K., Pandey, H., Pathak, K., and Patil, S. (2021). Biocompatible antidermatophytic Scaffolds (TfG-Nf) for controlled and impressive management of topical tinea diseases, *ASPS*, **5**, 8–11.

138. Pandey, S., Misra, S. K., and Sharma, N. (2020). Development of usnic acid embedded eudragit microspheres for alleviation of nosocomial infections, *Anti-Infective Agents*, **18**, 79–87.

139. Ameen, M. (2010). Epidemiology of superficial fungal infections, *Clin. Dermatol.*, **28**, 197–201.

140. Sharma, N., and Misra, S, K. (2019). Smart Gn-keto nanohybrid embedded topical system for effective management of dermatophytosis, *Drug Deliv. Lett.*, **9**, 21–28.

141. Gungor, S., Erdal, M., and Aksu, B. (2013). New formulation strategies in topical antifungal therapy, *J. Chem. Dermatol. Sci. Appl.*, **3**, 56–65.

142. Sharma, R., Sharma, S., and Rana, V. (2020). Nanostructure drug delivery system: an inimitable approach for candidiasis therapy. In: Talegaonkar, S., Rai, M. (eds.), *Nanoformulations in Human Health*, Springer, Cham. https://doi.org/10.1007/978-3-030-41858-8_15.

143. Williams, A. (2003). *Transdermal and Topical Drug Delivery: from Theory to Clinical Practice,* Pharmaceutical Press, London.

144. Souto, E. B., and Müller, R. H. (2006). The use of SLN and NLC as topical particulate carriers for imidazole antifungal agents, *Pharmazie*, **61**, 431–437.

145. Gupta, M., Vaidya, B., Mishra, N., and Vyas, S. P. (2011). Effect of surfactants on the characteristics of fluconazole niosomes for enhanced cutaneous delivery, *Artif. Cells Blood Substit. Immobil. Biotechnol.*, **39**, 376–384.

146. Das, S., Ng, W. K., and Tan, R. B. (2014). Sucrose ester stabilized solid lipid nanoparticles and nanostructured lipid carriers. II. Evaluation of the imidazole antifungal drug-loaded nanoparticle dispersions and their gel formulations, *Nanotechnology*, **25**, 105102.

147. El-Housiny, S., Shams, E. M. A., El-Attar, Y, A., Salem, H. A., Attia, D., Bendas, E. R., and El-Nabarawi, M. A. (2018). Fluconazole-loaded solid lipid nanoparticles topical gel for treatment of pityriasis versicolor: formulation and clinical study, *Drug Deliv.*, **25**, 78–90.

148. Gupta, M., Goyal, A. K., Paliwal, S. R., Paliwal, R., Mishra, N., Vaidya, B., Dube, D., Jain, S. K., and Vyas, S. P. (2010). Development and characterization of effective topical liposomal system for localized treatment of cutaneous candidiasis, *J. Liposome Res.*, **20**, 341–350.

149. Barakat, H. S., Darwish, I. A., El-Khordagui, L. K., and Khalafallah, N. M. (2009). Development of naftifine hydrochloride alcohol-free niosome gel, *Drug Dev. Ind. Pharm.*, **35**, 631–637.

150. Amra, K., and Momin, M. (2019). Formulation evaluation of ketoconazole microemulsion-loaded hydrogel with Nigella oil as a penetration enhancer, *J. Cosmet. Dermatol.*, **18**, 1742–1750.

151. Sosa, L., Clares, B., Alvarado, H. L., Bozal, N., Domenech, O., and Calpena, A. C. (2017). Amphotericin B releasing topical nanoemulsion for the treatment of candidiasis and aspergillosis, *Nanomedicine*, **13**, 2303–2312.

152. Bachhav, Y. G., Mondon, K., Kalia, Y. N., Gurny, R., and Möller, M. (2011). Novel micelle formulations to increase cutaneous bioavailability of azole antifungals, *J. Control. Release*, **153**, 126–132.

153. Boehm, R. D., Daniels, J., Stafslien, S., Nasir, A., Lefebvre, J., and Narayan, R. J. (2015). Polyglycolic acid microneedles modified with inkjet-deposited antifungal coatings, *Biointerphases*, **10**, 011004.

154. Ashara, K. C., Paun, J. S., Soniwala, M. M., and Chavda, J. R. (2017). Micro-emulgel of voriconazole: an unfathomable protection to counter fungal contagiousness, *Folia Med. (Plovdiv)*, **59**, 461–471.

155. Pillai, A. B., Nair, J. V., Gupta, N. K., and Gupta, S. (2015). Microemulsion-loaded hydrogel formulation of butenafine hydrochloride for improved topical delivery, *Arch. Dermatol. Res.*, **307**, 625–633.

156. Lovato, L. M. (2013). Update on emerging infections: news from the Centers for Disease Control and Prevention. Commentary, *Ann. Emerg. Med.*, **61**, 366–367.

157. Alex, I., Jose, J., Rahul, R., Gopal, A., and Priya, A. (2018). Fusogenic liposome for the treatment of fungal meningitis: an overview, *Asian. J. Pharm. Clin. Res.*, **11**, 95–101.

158. Moen, M. D., Lyseng-Williamson, K. A., and Scott, L. J. (2009). Liposomal amphotericin B: a review of its use as empirical therapy in febrile neutropenia and in the treatment of invasive fungal infections, *Drugs*, **69**, 361–392.

159. Xu, N., Gu, J., Zhu, Y., Wen, H., Ren, Q., and Chen, J. (2011). Efficacy of intravenous amphotericin B-polybutylcyanoacrylate nanoparticles against cryptococcal meningitis in mice, *Int. J. Nanomed.*, **6**, 905–913.

160. Thompson, G. R., Patel, P. K., Kirkpatrick, W. R., Westbrook, S. D., Berg, D., Erlandsen, J., Redding, S. W., and Patterson, T. F. (2010). Oropharyngeal candidiasis in the era of antiretroviral therapy, *Oral Surg. Oral Med. Oral Pathol. Oral Radiol. Endod.*, **109**, 488–495.

161. Akpan, A., and Morgan, R. (2002). Oral candidiasis, *Postgrad. Med. J.*, **78**, 455–459.

162. Roque, L., Castro, P., Molpeceres, J., Viana, A. S., Roberto, A., Reis, C., Rijo, P., Tho, I., Sarmento, B., and Reis, C. (2018). Bioadhesive polymeric nanoparticles as strategy to improve the treatment of

yeast infections in oral cavity: *in vitro* and ex vivo studies, *Eur. Polymer J.*, **104**, 19–31.

163. Ahmad, N., Jafri, Z., and Khan, Z. H. (2020). Evaluation of nanomaterials to prevent oral Candidiasis in PMMA based denture wearing patients, A systematic analysis, *J. Oral Biol. Craniofac. Res.*, **10**, 189–193.

164. Ho, H. N., Le, T. G., Dao, T. T. T., Le, T. H., Dinh, T. T. H., Dang, H., Nguyen, D. H., Tran, T. C., and Nguyen, C. N. (2020). Development of itraconazole-loaded polymeric nanoparticle dermal gel for enhanced antifungal efficacy, *J. Nanomater.*, **2020**, 1–11.

165. Gajdošová, M., Vetchý, D., Muselík, J., Gajdziok, J., Juřica, J., Vetchá, M., Hauptman, K., and Jekl, V. (2021). Bilayer mucoadhesive buccal films with prolonged release of ciclopirox olamine for the treatment of oral candidiasis: *in vitro* development, ex vivo permeation testing, pharmacokinetic and efficacy study in rabbits, *Int. J. Pharm.*, **592**, 120086.

166. Mady, O. Y., Donia, A. M., and Al-Madboly, L. A. (2018). Miconazole-urea in a buccal film as a new trend for treatment of resistant mouth fungal white patches, *Front. Microbiol.*, **9**, 837.

167. Potaś, J., Szymańska, E., Wróblewska, M., Kurowska, I., Maciejczyk, M., Basa, A., Wolska, E., Wilczewska, A. Z., Winnicka, K. (2021). Multilayer films based on chitosan/pectin polyelectrolyte complexes as novel platforms for buccal administration of clotrimazole, *Pharmaceutics*, **13**, 1588. https://doi.org/10.3390/pharmaceutics13101588.

168. Johal, H. S., Garg, T., Rath, G., and Goyal, A. K. (2016). Advanced topical drug delivery system for the management of vaginal candidiasis, *Drug Deliv.*, **23**, 550–563.

169. Kataria, K., Garg, T., Goyal, A. K., and Rath, G. (2014). Novel technology to improve drug loading in polymeric nanofibers, *Drug Deliv. Lett.*, **4**, 79–86.

170. Karavana, S. V., Rençbe, S., Þenyiðit, S. A., and Baloðlu, E. (2012). A new in situ gel formulation of itraconazole for vaginal administration, *J. Pharm. Pharmacol.*, **3**, 417–426.

171. Natasha, S., Getyala, A., and Bhat, R. S. (2013). Bioadhesive vaginal tablets containing spray dried microspheres loaded with clotrimazole for treatment of vaginal Candidiasis, *Acta Pharm.*, **63**, 359–372.

172. Wang, L., and Tang, X. (2008). A novel ketoconazole bioadhesive effervescent tablet for vaginal delivery: design, *in vitro* and '*in vivo*' evaluation, *Int. J. Pharm.*, **350**, 181–187.

173. Ahmad, F. J., Alam, M. A., Khan, Z. I., Khar, R. K., and Ali, M. Development and *in vitro* evaluation of an acid buffering bioadhesive vaginal gel for mixed vaginal infections, *Acta Pharm.*, **58**, 407–419.

174. Bachhav, Y. G., and Patravale, V. B. (2008). Microemulsion based vaginal gel of fluconazole: formulation, *in vitro* and *in vivo* evaluation, *Int. J. Pharm.*, **365**, 175–179.

175. Chang, J. Y., Oh, Y. K., Kong, H. S., Kim, E. J., Jang, D. D., Nam, K. T., and Kim, C. K. (2002). Prolonged antifungal effects of clotrimazole-containing mucoadhesive thermosensitive gels on vaginitis, *J. Control. Release*, **82**, 39–50.

176. Santos, S. S., Lorenzoni, A., Pegoraro, N. S., Denardi, L. B., Alves, S. H., Schaffazick, S. R., and Cruz, L. (2014). Formulation and *in vitro* evaluation of coconut oil-core cationic nanocapsules intended for vaginal delivery of clotrimazole, *Colloids Surf. B Biointerfaces*, **116**, 270–276.

177. Del Gaudio, G., Lombardi, L., Maisetta, G., Esin, S., Batoni, G., Sanguinetti, M., Senesi, S., and Tavanti, A. (2013). Antifungal activity of the noncytotoxic human peptide hepcidin 20 against fluconazole-resistant *Candida glabrata* in human vaginal fluid, *Antimicrobial. Agents Chemotherapy*, **57**, 4314–4321.

178. Kenechukwu, F. C., Ibezim EC, Nnamani, P. O., Umeyor, C. E., Uronnachi, E. M., Momoh, M. A., Akpa, P. A., and Ozioko, A. C. (2018). Novel intravaginal drug delivery system based on molecularly PEGylated lipid matrices for improved antifungal activity of miconazole nitrate, *BioMed Res. Int.*, **2018**, 3714329.

Multiple Choice Questions

1. Identify the factors responsible for poor management of viral infections by conventional dosage forms.
   a. Viral resistance
   b. Poor solubility of drug
   c. Poor stability of drug
   d. All of the above
2. Three-dimensional, highly branched drug delivery systems are referred as
   a. Dendrimers
   b. Nanocrystals

c. Nanoparticles
d. Microparticles

3. Theranostics is the term used to describe the combination of
   a. Diagnostic and therapeutic drug
   b. Diagnostic agent
   c. Either a or b
   d. Both a and b
4. The vesicular drug delivery systems control the fate of drug molecules
   a. By controlling the release kinetics
   b. Increasing bioavailability
   c. Reducing side effects of the drug
   d. All of the above
5. Novel formulations of the nano range display characteristic properties like
   a. Small size
   b. High surface to volume ratio
   c. Both of the above
   d. None of the above
6. Micelles are vesicles of size ranging
   a. 10 to 100 nm
   b. 100 to 1000 nm
   c. 1000 to 10000 nm
   d. 10000 to 100000 nm
7. Barriers for delivery of drug to brain are
   a. BBB
   b. BSCFB
   c. Both
   d. None of the above
8. The micelles have a core and shell structure in which the inner core is
   a. Hydrophobic
   b. Hydrophilic
   c. Amphiphilic
   d. None of above

9. Biomimetic system results in
    a. Avoidance of immune system activation
    b. Immune system activation
    c. Either a or b
    d. None of the above
10. Novel drug delivery includes
    a. Powder
    b. Solution
    c. Microspheres
    d. None
11. Which one is related to peptic ulcer
    a. Virus
    b. Fungi
    c. Bacteria
    d. All
12. Drawback associated with conventional preparations for treatment of infection
    a. Poor efficacy
    b. Poor penetration
    c. Nonspecific cell targeting
    d. All
13. Causes of drug resistance
    a. Prolonged antimicrobial therapy
    b. Poor immunity
    c. Diseased state
    d. All
14. Development of newer antibiotics are restricted due to
    a. Deficiency of antimicrobial agents
    b. Strict legislations
    c. Require high capital
    d. Both b and c
15. The major factors for designing novel dosages to combat infection is/are
    a. Altered microenvironment
    b. Microbial surface properties

c. Both
d. Not related

16. Which one is not included in vesicular drug delivery system
    a. Liposomes
    b. Niosomes
    c. Metallic particles
    d. Phytosomes
17. Meningitis cover area of
    a. Brain and spinal cord
    b. Myocardial tissues
    c. Pleural membrane
    d. Nephran cells
18. Urinary tract infection (UTI) is/are caused by
    a. *E. coli*
    b. Klebsilla
    c. Enterobacters
    d. All
19. For the management of antibiotic resistant bacteria
    a. Anionic peptide-based antibiotic is required
    b. Cationic peptide-based antibiotic is required
    c. Any antibiotic irrespective to charge
    d. Nonrelated
20. Penicillin sensitive and penicillin resistant pneumococcal meningitis are cured by
    a. Bacitracin A
    b. Nimesulide
    c. Ranitidine
    d. Beta blocker
21. Liposomes successfully mitigate neurological bacterial infection via
    a. Prolong distribution of antibiotic in blood stream
    b. Specific targeting
    c. Improve pharmacokinetic and pharmacodynamic parameters of antibiotic
    d. All

22. Poorly absorbed antimicrobials are
    a. Sulfonamide
    b. Quinolones
    c. Aminoglycosides
    d. All
23. Sulfate reducing pathogens are
    a. *H. pylori*
    b. *S. enterica*
    c. *Fusobacterium*
    d. All of them
24. Polio virus multiplies in
    a. Nerve cells
    b. Brain cells
    c. Intestine cells
    d. Blood cells
25. Which one of fungi is not associated with dermatophytosis
    a. Microsporum
    b. Macrosporum
    c. Tryptophyton
    d. Epidermophyton
26. Bacterial vaginosis is characterized through
    a. Less level of estrogen
    b. Imbalance in acidic milieu
    c. Both a and b
    d. Either a or b
27. Which factors amplify the spread of fungal disease
    a. Cold and dry
    b. Heat and moist
    c. Cold and humid
    d. All
28. Which fungal disease does not spread through fomite transmission
    a. Ring worm
    b. Common cold

c. AIDS
d. Influenza

29. In humans, topical fungal infection is known as
    a. Mucorsis
    b. Dermatophytosis
    c. Fungosis
    d. Micromia

30. Recently, which virus infected millions worldwide
    a. MERS
    b. SARS
    c. HKU1
    d. OC43

Answer Key

1.	d	**2.**	a	**3.**	a	**4.**	d	**5.**	c	**6.**	a
7.	c	**8.**	a	**9.**	a	**10.**	c	**11.**	d	**12.**	d
13.	d	**14.**	d	**15.**	c	**16.**	c	**17.**	a	**18.**	d
19.	b	**20.**	d	**21.**	d	**22.**	c	**23.**	d	**24.**	c
25.	b	**26.**	c	**27.**	b	**28.**	a	**29.**	b	**30.**	b

Short Answer Questions

1. What are the constraints observed with brain targeted drug delivery for the management of meningitis?
2. Describe the applications of novel drug delivery in treatment of viral infections.
3. What are the challenges in treatment of viral infections?
4. What are the major sexually transmitted diseases, how nanotechnology has proved as an asset in treatment of HIV?
5. Elaborate the role of dendrimers in management of microbial infections.
6. Why treatment of fungal infection is more critical than bacterial infection.
7. What is dermatophytosis? How it is caused?

8. Write different bacterial infections and their causative agents.

Long Answer Questions

1. What is infection? Give an account on different infection causing agents.
2. Why do conventional preparations fail to control pathogenic infections? What are advantages of novel drug delivery systems over conventional preparations?
3. Discuss in detail on bacterial diseases in different parts of body.
4. What are micelles? How they enhance the solubility and stability of drugs?
5. Discuss different novel drug delivery approaches employed for the management of bacterial, viral and fungal infections.

Chapter 10

Novel Drug Delivery System Approach in Cancer Treatment

Renu Saharan,[a] Shikha Sachdeva,[a] Inderjeet Verma,[a] and Suresh Kumar[b]

[a]*M. M. College of Pharmacy, M. M. Deemed to be University, Mullana, Haryana, India*
[b]*Bharat Institute of Pharmacy, Pehladpur, Babain, Kurukshetra, Haryana, India*

indupup@gmail.com

Cancer is the abnormal growth of body cells in an uncontrolled manner. It is the leading cause of death worldwide. However, today there are several strategies and technologies for the treatment of cancer, such as chemotherapy, radiation, surgery, and chemoimmunotherapy, a combination of chemotherapeutics and immunotherapeutic drugs. Despite all these strategies, the survival rate is very poor and the treatment is quite challenging and unsatisfactory. To address the limitations associated with the present strategies, nanodrug delivery systems (NDDS) have been introduced in this field and it has been seen that the progression of nanotechnology and a delve into tumor biology have brought several achievements and success in cancer treatment. The approaches based on NDDS have developed rapidly as they impart several advantages over conventional approaches for cancer therapy. In addition, NDDS such as nanocomposites,

Nanotechnology and Drug Delivery: Principles and Applications
Edited by Rakesh K. Sindhu

ISBN 978-981-4968-83-6 (Hardcover), 978-1-003-43040-7 (eBook)
www.jennystanford.com

nanoparticles, dendrimers, liposomes, microspheres, and hydrogels have the potential to improve the bioavailability, stability, and solubility of the therapeutical agent and to effectively deliver it in a controlled manner at the target site with an appropriate route in sufficient concentration. Hence, with all such qualities, NDDS could be a remarkable approach for future cancer treatment. This chapter discusses various NDDS their development, and applications in cancer therapy by addressing the cancer background.

10.1 Introduction

Cancer is the deadliest disease worldwide. In 2019, the WHO estimated that cancer is the major cause of death and in 2020 nearly 10 million deaths were accounted for worldwide, and in the future, the figure could cross ~13.1 million by 2030 [1, 2]. Several strategies have been implemented for the treatment of this fatal disease like chemotherapy, radiation, surgery, chemoimmunotherapy, combining chemotherapeutics and immunotherapeutic drugs. Among these, chemotherapy is the most commonly used technology. In chemotherapy, the anticancer drug is systemically delivered to the patient to control the abnormal proliferation of cancerous cells, but the frequency of survival of patients is very poor, because of nonspecific targeting and lack of proper drug delivery in sufficient amounts [3]. In the treatment of cancer, there are two major concerns: The first one is the early detection of the tumor and the second is the targeted drug delivery [4]. Here, nonspecificity and toxicity are the major challenges associated with traditional approaches. The researchers are doing regular efforts in developing and improving cancer treatment strategies to overcome the observed challenges; however, ideas like improving the pharmacological activity of drugs and preventing negative side effects are still in progress [5, 6]. Therefore, to address the limitations and challenges with the currently practiced strategies, the concept of nanotechnology has been introduced in this sector. Nanotechnology enables researchers to develop novel, versatile targeted drug delivery systems aimed to deliver the therapeutics agent at the right time at the right sight in the right amount for the treatment of cancer [7, 8].

In pharmaceutical sciences, drug delivery approaches are basically utilized for administrating pharmaceutical products in a controlled manner to increase therapeutic efficacy, and they have received much attention in the past two-three decades for cancer treatment [9]. Earlier, DDS were generally of two types on the basis of their size: macro- and micro-scale DDS [10].

10.1.1 Causes of Cancer

There are numerous factors that can cause cancer in different parts of the body, including tobacco use (22% of deaths), malnutrition (10% of deaths), obesity (10% of deaths), physical inactivity (10% of deaths), increased consumption of alcohol (10% of deaths), excessive exposure to ionizing radiation, infection, and environmental pollution. Cancer-causing infections like human papillomavirus and hepatitis B, C, and Epstein-Barr virus cause about 15% of cancer worldwide. These variables are partially responsible for gene changes. Cancer is also caused by aging. The most common cause of cancer is advanced age. Genetics is the most common factor in cancer and tumour development, including skin, ovarian, colorectal, breast, and prostate cancer. Consumption of large amounts of cooked meat can further raise the risk due to chemicals formed at high temperatures [11, 12].

10.1.2 Prevalence of Cancer

The number of people in a defined group who have been diagnosed with a specific type of cancer at a specific time in the past and are still living at the end of a given year. Usually expressed as a figure and a percentage per 100,000 people. At the end of 2008, about 29 million people who had been diagnosed with cancer within the previous 5 years were still alive. Following colon cancer, which impacted both men and women (3.3 million), prostate cancer, which affected men most frequently (3.2 million), and breast cancer, which affected women (5.2 million), were the most prevalent [13, 14].

Types of cancer [12, 15]

Various types of cancer are shown in Table 10.1 [12, 15].

Table 10.1 Types of cancer

Type of cancer	Description
Carcinomas	Begins in the tissue or skin that covers the glands and the surface of internal organs. Prostate cancer, lung cancer, colorectal cancer, and breast cancer are examples of carcinomas.
Sarcomas	Begins in the connective and supportive tissues of the body. Joints Nerves, tendons, lymph vessels, blood vessels, bone, fat, cartilage, and muscles can all create it.
Leukemia's	It starts when healthy blood cells expand and alter uncontrolled. Acute myeloid leukemia, chronic myeloid leukemia, acute lymphocytic leukemia, and chronic lymphocytic leukemia are the four types of leukemia.
Lymphomas	It starts in the lymphatic system. Non-Hodgkin lymphoma (NHL) and Hodgkin lymphoma (HL) are the two main types of lymphomas.
Central nervous system cancers	Cancers of the central nervous system include primary CNS lymphomas, meningiomas, gliomas, pituitary adenomas, vestibular schwannomas, vestibular schwannomas, and primitive neuro-ectodermal tumors which start in the brain tissues and spinal cord.
Multiple Myeloma	It starts in plasma cells. It accumulates in the bone marrow and causes malignancies. Plasma cell myeloma is also known as Kahler disease.
Melanoma	It begins in cells that develop into melanocytes. These are specialized cells that produce melanin, the pigment that gives the skin its color.

Table 10.2 Types of cancer treatment with their limitations

S. No.	Type of cancer treatment	Description	Limitations
1	Surgery	The surgeon may remove lymph nodes to prevent or slow the spread of the disease and to remove cancer from the body. During surgery, surgeons utilize scalpels, small thin knives, and other sharp tools to cut through muscle, skin, and occasionally bones. These wounds are uncomfortable after surgery, so the patient is given an anesthetic to ease the discomfort [16]. The common problems associated with surgery are pain and infection. After surgery on the colon, mouth, throat, or stomach, the patient's food intake will vary.	The major limitation of surgery is a lack of improvement in survival rate and tumor cells may remain in the patient after surgery.
2	Radiotherapy	This therapy uses high doses of radiation to reduce tumors, kill cancer cells, and inhibit the growth of cancer cells by damaging their DNA. Damaged DNA does not repair, and the cell dies, and the body removes it. The treatment takes weeks or months to complete and prevents the condition from recurring. The external beam is used to treat pain, loss of bowel and bladder control, and problems breathing caused by the shrinking tumor, whereas radiopharmaceuticals are medications used in systemic radiation treatment to treat pain that has spread to the bones [17–20].	The limitation of radiotherapy is that it will damage the surrounding tissues of the tumor and inability to kill tumor cells that cannot be seen on imaging scans [21].
3	Chemotherapy	It is a type of cancer treatment in which chemicals are used to block or reduce the growth of cancer cells, kill cancer cells, or decrease tumors that cause pain and other issues but have serious adverse effects. Chemotherapy is used alone or in combination with other cancer treatments, depending on the type of cancer [23–25].	Chemotherapeutic medicines have a number of limitations including the development of resistance, interference with normal cell metabolism, and nonspecific targeting [22].

(*Continued*)

Table 10.2 (*Continued*)

S. No.	Type of cancer treatment	Description	Limitations
4	Immunotherapy	Medication or other therapies are used to enhance the immune system. WBC and lymph node tissues make up the immune system, which gives the body the strength it needs to fight sickness and infection. It is also known as biological therapy, which refers to the compounds utilized in cancer treatment that are derived from living organisms. The most prevalent side effects are skin responses at the needle site along this pain, soreness, rash, chills, redness, swelling, joint pain, diarrhea, weakness, and fatigue [23–27].	The availability of known targetable tumor-specific antigens (TSAs), also known as "neoantigens," that are primarily expressed by tumor cells, is a fundamental limitation of cancer immunotherapy [23].
5	Precision/ Personalized Medicine	This is a recent technique in which genetic testing is used to determine the optimal treatment for a patient. Nowadays, cancer treatments are the same for patients with the same cancer and stage of cancer, although some patients' reactions differ. Scientists have discovered that tumors have genetic alterations that cause cancer cells to develop and spread after extensive investigation. Precision medicine, according to scientists, has a bright future because it aids in receiving the best cancer therapy. Many medications are utilized as treatments known as target therapies in order to try treating patients with treatments that target the cancer-causing genetic alterations in the tumor. Precision medicine assists clinicians in determining the best treatment options because it contains all of the information on the tumor's genetic changes, size, kind, and spread [28].	The limitation of precision medicine is the understudy of a mutation may or may not be important to the malignancy and the actual tumor may respond to the same therapy in a different way due to sampling mistake.

10.1.3 Current Strategies and Their Limitations

There are a variety of cancer therapies available with their limitations as shown in Table 10.2, depending on the type of cancer and how far it has progressed. Some cancer patients have only one treatment, but the majority receive a mix of treatments, such as surgery and radiation therapy.

Despite the fact that cancer nanomedicine has been around for 30 years and has made significant progress in the field of cancer treatment, it still has significant drawbacks that must be addressed as shown in Fig. 10.1.

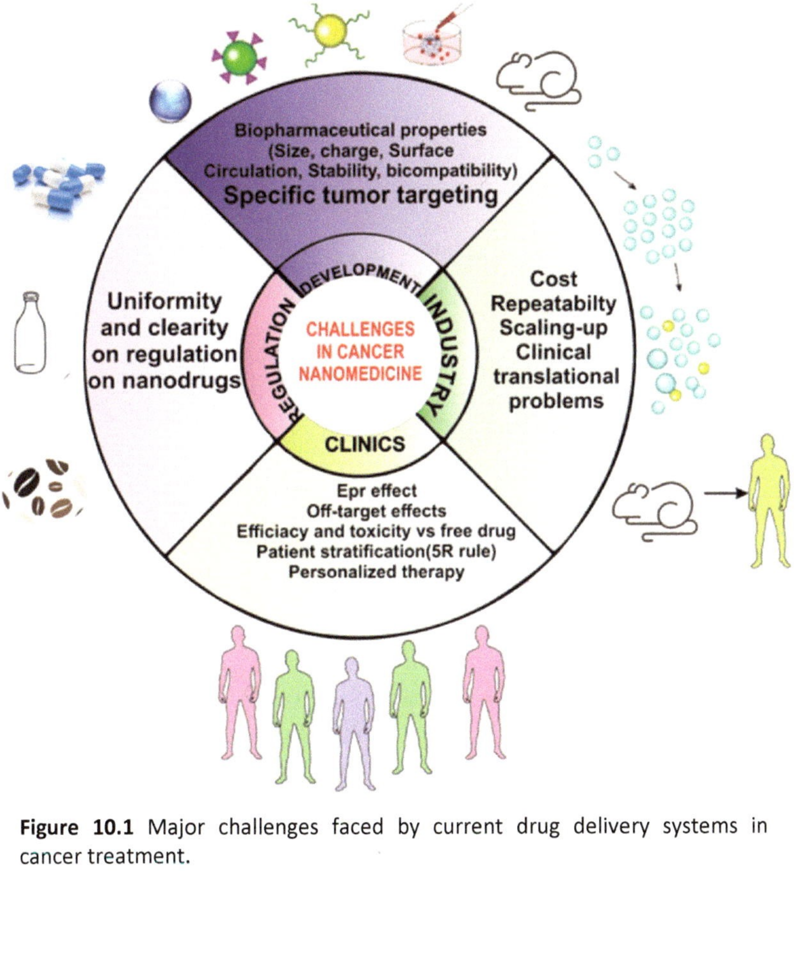

Figure 10.1 Major challenges faced by current drug delivery systems in cancer treatment.

10.2 Use of Nanotechnology in the Treatment of Cancer

In the last few years, multiple versatile NDDS have been developed such as liposomes, microspheres, polymeric nanoparticles, micelles, dendrimers, carbon-based materials like carbon nanotubes (CNT), graphene to deliver chemotherapeutic agents to tumor sites with improved therapeutic efficacy [2, 29–31]. A nanocarrier-based drug delivery system possessing remarkable features is shown in Fig. 10.2.

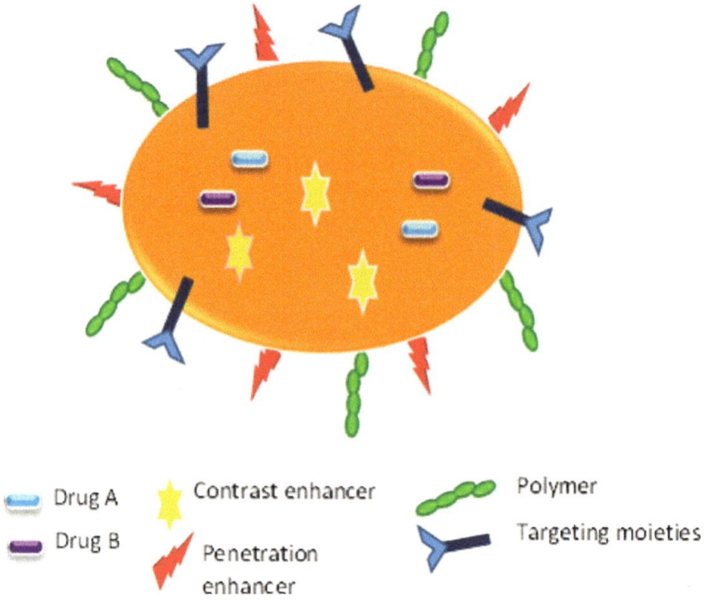

Figure 10.2 Multifunctional nanocarrier system-based drug delivery [9, 31].

Some of the features of NDDS through which the cancer treatment efficacy could be improved are as follows [22, 32]:

- Site-specific targeting, that can be achieved by conjugating the nanocarriers consisting of a chemotherapeutic agent.
- Minimizing the toxicity by accumulating in the infected site via enhanced permeability and retention (EPR) effect and active cellular uptake

- Sustained release of the chemotherapeutic agent for a couple of days or months
- Stimuli-responsive drug release for effective delivery of anticancer drug

Nowadays more than twenty NDDS are available commercially to treat different diseases including cancer, infections, and hormonal disorders, some clinically approved or under clinical trial nanomedicines are given in Table 10.3 [33]. The advantages of FDA-approved nanomedicines mainly include:

- improved stability
- enhanced site-specific targeted drug delivery in tumor
- increased drug loading and bioavailability, which results in lower toxicity and higher efficacy
- increase distribution of anticancer agents at the targeted site (tumor) may be through passive targeting, active targeting, or triggered drug release [34, 35]

Table 10.3 Clinically approved or under clinical trial nanomedicines [9–25]

Product	Drug	Carrier components	Stage
Apealea	PTX	Micelle: two isoforms of N-retinoyl-1 cysteic acid	EMA approved
Vyxeos	Cytarabine and daunorubicin	Liposome: DSPC, DSPG, cholesterol	FDA and EMA approved
Mepact	Mifamurtide	Liposome: OOPS, POPC	EMA approved
Doxil	DOX	Liposome: cholesterol, HSPC, mPEG-DSPE	FDA and EMA approved
Nab-Paclitaxel (Abraxane)	PTX	Human serum albumin	FDA and EMA approved
Onivyde	Irinotecan	Liposome: cholesterol, DSPC, mPEG-DSPE	Phase II/III
NC-6004	Cisplatin	Micelle: PEG-P(Glu)	Phase I/II
NKTR-102	Irinotecan	PEG (Four-arm) conjugation	Phase II
Lipoplatin	Cisplatin	Liposome: SPC/cholesterol/DPPG/mPEG-DSPE	Phase II/III

Product	Drug	Carrier components	Stage
Genexol-PM	PTX	Micelle: mPEG-PDLLA	Approved in Korea
Lipusu	PTX	Liposome: lecithin/ cholesterol	Phase IV
Myocet	DOX	Liposome: phosphatidylcholine, cholesterol	EMA approved
Nanoparticle generator	DOX	Porous silicon microparticle with polymeric doxorubicin	Planning of Phase I
CRLX101	CPT	PEG-modified beta-cyclodextrin	Phase II
ThermoDox	DOX	Thermosensitive liposomal doxorubicin	Phase III completed
Marqibo	Vincristine sulfate	Liposome: sphingomyelin, cholesterol	FDA approved
DOTAP-Chol-TUSC2	TUSC2	DOTAP: Chol	Phase I/II

10.2.1 Role of Nanotechnology-Based Approaches in Cancer Treatment

The applications of nanotechnology for anticancer therapy are rapidly growing and have made a remarkable contribution to treatment approaches by enabling the site-specific release of chemotherapeutic agents, depending on their physicochemical characteristics and biological attributes [3, 36]. The role of nanotechnology approaches has been described by the following postulates [37]:

- Several studies carried out with nanoparticle (NP) formulations have shown that they offer high loading capacity and more stability and both hydrophilic and lipophilic substances can be administered by using NP through various routes.
- NDDS are also capable of utilizing the unique patho-physiology of cancer cells to selectively carry the loaded chemotherapeutic drug to the target site.

- NDDS based on the nanotechnology for cancer targeting generally have a longer shelf-life and better distribution of chemotherapeutic drugs at the effective site.
- Use of nanotechnology enables the delivery of biomacromolecules like DNA, small interfering RNA (siRNA), mRNA, and protein) to intracellular sites of action.
- It made the codelivery of multiple drugs possible to improve therapeutic efficacy and overcome drug resistance, by providing more precise control of exposure to stimuli to each drug and the delivery of appropriate drug ratio to the target of interest.
- By combining therapeutic agents with imaging moiety visualization of sites of drug delivery is possible and hence diagnosis and imaging of cancer become more sensitive and sophisticated.
- It led to the miniaturized medical devices for cancer diagnosis, drug screening, and drug delivery.

Figure 10.3 depicts some disadvantages of the current drug delivery systems and the advantages of the novel drug delivery systems [38].

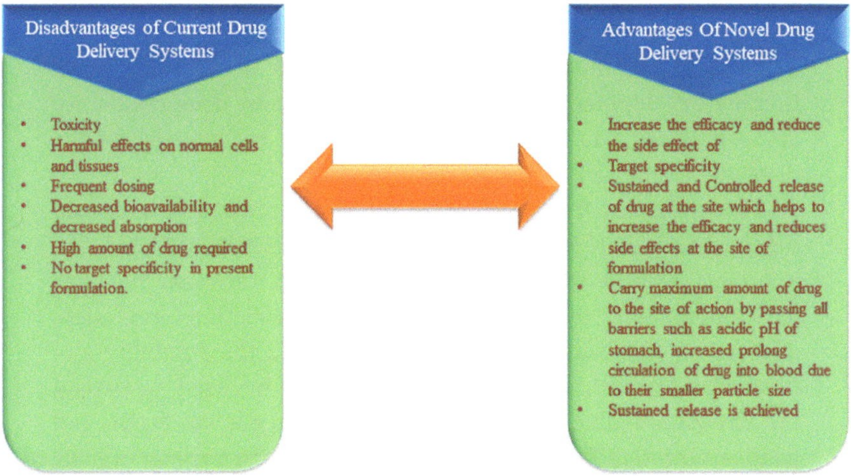

Figure 10.3 Disadvantages of the current drug delivery systems and the advantages of the novel drug delivery systems.

According to the FDA's criteria, nanotechnological products are those containing materials whose size ranges from 1 to 100 nm [39]. Size is one of the main parameters which determines the behavior of transport of nanoparticles through the bloodstream and their accumulation in tumor cells. It has been observed that smaller nanomedicines are able to deliver the drug to the tumor cells better than the large molecules, but with the possibility of getting distributed to the healthy cells too. The size of NDDS is usually in the range of 10–100 nm, which is necessary for the accumulation of the drug at the target site or tissue [40]. Apart from size, the charge can also affect the biopharmaceutical properties of nanomedicines. Neutral-charged NDDS diffused faster at the tumor as compared to the positively charged and negatively charged, while positively charged NDDS diffuse better [41]. The variability in the charge can be achieved by attaching ligands and it could improve blood circulation time and cellular uptake of these nanoparticles [42]. Moreover, the surface modification of NDDS can increase the adsorption of circulating proteins which modifies the targeting properties of nanoparticles [22, 43].

The growing interest in novel and efficient drug delivery systems with minimum toxicity and adverse effect has created a demand for developing NDDS in cancer therapy. Further, the increase in healthcare spending, investments in R&D for novel therapy development, and new drug approvals by drug regulatory authorities are also the major factors that are responsible for the development of NDDS.

The results from studies conducted around the world demonstrate that NDDS applications in the medical field are a promising and innovative approach. They can also be used in combination therapy to improve penetration, retention, and therapeutic action as well as to increase the solubility and bioavailability of the agents. They can also be used to extend the circulation time of a chemotherapeutic agent via active and passive targeting [44]. NDDS are developed using various organic and inorganic materials by loading natural or synthetic drugs onto these nanocarrier materials. Before 1995 several nanodrug carriers were developed by researchers, which included liposomes, polymeric systems, dendrimers, and PEGylated liposomes [45]. Moreover, the potential of NDDS is better depicted earlier in Fig. 10.1 which showed a multifunctional nanoparticle illustrating the ability to carry one or more drugs, a targeting bimolecular moiety in conjugation with one or more antibodies or some recognition agent, a contrast-enhancing agent which assists the amplification of the imaging signal, a permeation enhancer for the smooth crossing of the bio barriers and a selective polymer for the avoidance of macrophage uptake by macrophages [31, 46].

10.2.1.1 Polymer–drug conjugates

The covalent binding between a polymer and a drug results in a polymer–drug conjugate as shown in Fig. 10.4, which leads to high solubility, and stability with reduced immunogenicity for peptide drugs or proteins along with an increase in clearance time [47, 48]. Among polymers, PEG is the first choice for polymer–drug conjugation due to its simple structure and biodegradability.

Formulations: Oncaspar® is a commercialized FDA-approved cancer treatment. L-asparagine is an amino acid of natural origin whose decomposition is catalyzed by enzyme asparaginase into aspartic acid and ammonia. Decreased concentration of L-asparagine in the systemic circulation results in decreased synthesis of protein, DNA, and RNA. However, the use of naked asparaginases has been limited by a high rate of hypersensitivity reactions and the development of anti-asparaginase antibodies, which neutralize its activity. But PEGylated asparaginase under clinical trials (I and II) suggested that its mean half-life time is 357 h as compared to the naked drug, which is 20 h; hence, this demonstrated that a single dose of PEG-asparaginase can replace 6–9 doses of native *E. coli* asparaginase injections. So here, PEG-asparaginase with a longer half-life and reduced number of doses is a good example of a polymer–drug conjugate [33, 46, 49, 50].

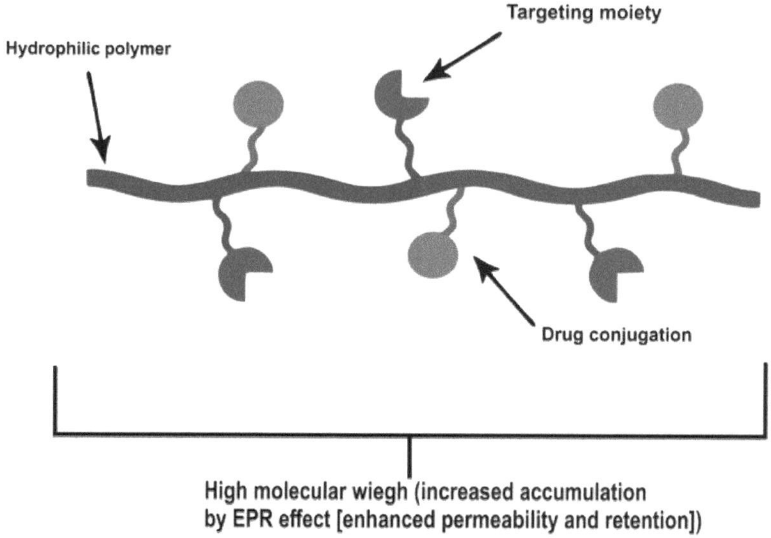

Figure 10.4 Polymer–drug conjugate.

10.2.1.2 Polymeric micelles

Micelles are about 5–100 nm-sized colloidal particles basically proposed to carry hydrophobic drugs in anticancer therapy and the polymeric micelles are nanostructures made up of amphiphilic copolymer that assembled themselves in an aqueous solution. Its structure can be easily tailored and its hydrophobic core can be made to load hydrophobic drugs such as camptothecin, docetaxel, paclitaxel, and simultaneously. The hydrophilic shell makes the whole system soluble in an aqueous medium and stabilizes the core. With a size less than 100 nm, polymeric micelles have a narrow distribution and show delayed renal excretion; hence, they get accumulated at the tumor site through the EPR effect. In addition, their polymeric shell restrains non-specific interactions with biological components. Thus these structures permit stability and bioavailability to chemotherapeutic molecules. A typical structure of polymeric micelles is shown in Fig. 10.5.

In recent years, polymeric micelles have been extensively utilized in pre-clinical studies for delivering poorly soluble chemotherapeutic agents in cancer. Polymeric micelles are formed via the self-assembly of amphiphilic polymers in facile manners. The wide availability of hydrophobic and, to some extent, hydrophilic polymeric blocks allow researchers to explore various polymeric combinations for optimum loading, stability, systemic circulation, and delivery to the target cancer tissues. Moreover, polymeric micelles could easily be tailor-made by increasing and decreasing the number of monomers in each polymeric chain. Some of the widely accepted hydrophobic polymers are poly (lactide) (PLA), poly (caprolactone) (PCL), poly (lactide-co-glycolide) (PLGA), polyesters, poly (amino acids), and lipids. The hydrophilic polymers used to wrap the hydrophobic core are poly (ethylene glycol), poly (oxazolines), chitosan, dextran, and hyaluronic acids. Drugs could be conjugated to polymers at the distal ends to prepare pharmacologically active polymeric systems that impart enhanced solubility and stability of the conjugates and provide an opportunity for combination drug delivery. Their nano-size enables them to accumulate in the tumor microenvironment via the EPR effect. Moreover, the stimuli-sensitive breakdown provides the micelles with an effective means to deliver the therapeutic cargo effectively. The tumor micro-environmental stimuli are pH, hypoxia, and upregulated enzymes. Externally applied stimuli to destroy micellar disassembly to release the payload include light, ultrasound, and temperature [22, 51, 52]. Polymeric micelles under clinical trials are shown in Table 10.4.

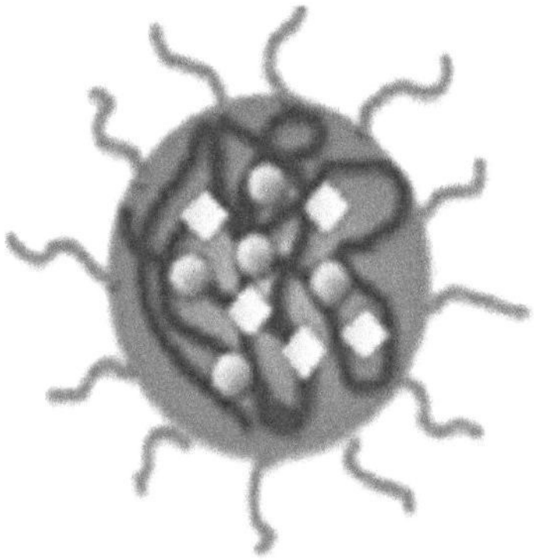

Figure 10.5 Polymeric micelles.

Table 10.4 Polymeric micelles in clinical trials

Polymeric micelle	Block copolymer	Drug	Clinical phase	Indication
NK105	PEG-P (aspartate)	Paclitaxel	II	Advanced stomach cancer
Genoxol-PM	PEG-P (D,L-lactide)	Paclitaxel	IV	Breast cancer, pancreatic cancer
NK012	PEG-PGlu (SN-38)	SN-38	II	Breast cancer
SP1049C	Pluronic L61 and F127	Doxorubicin	III	Adenocarcinoma of esophagus, gastroesophageal junction, and stomach
NC-6004	PEG-PGlu(cisplatin)	Cisplatin	I/II	Solid tumors

10.2.1.3 Microspheres

Microspheres are solid spherical porous particles with a diameter range of 1 to 1000 μm and allow a uniform distribution of the drug in the polymer matrix. They could be biodegradable or nonbiodegradable depending on the material chosen [53]. These are one of the approaching NDDSs that are widely integrated and tailored so that the carcinogenic drugs can be delivered with site-specific targeting with improved therapeutic activity with minimal adverse effects further microspheres can be injected and ingested to due ease of modification as per the need hence with such properties, microspheres play an essential role in the treatment of cancer [54]. A wide range of polymeric materials can be considered for the formulation of microspheres, such as lipids, proteins, polysaccharides, and polyesters. Also, there are several techniques which can be adopted for their development such as phase inversion technology, emulsification and heat stabilization, and coacervation. Anticancer drugs such as doxorubicin, mitomycin C, cisplatin, and 5-fluorouracil have been subjected to various studies by using microspheres. Nevertheless, with all such applications, these persistent instability problems so need more optimization and characterization [44, 53, 55, 56].

Figure 10.6 shows the modes of drug release from different types of microspheres: (a) bulk-eroding polymer and (b) surface-eroding polymer.

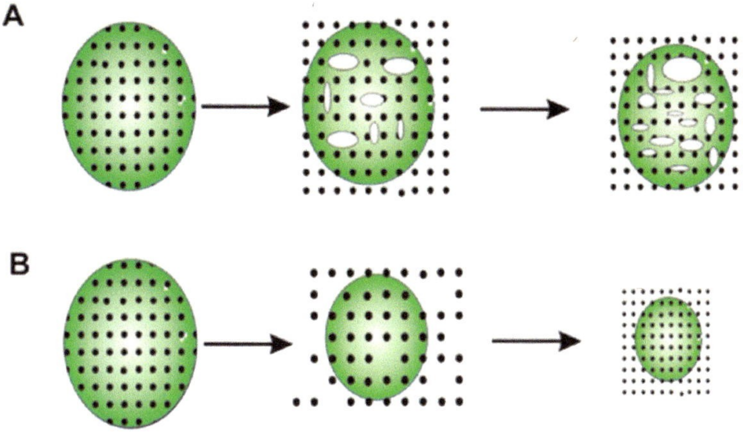

Figure 10.6 Modes of drug release from different types of microspheres: (A) bulk-eroding polymer and (B) surface-eroding polymer.

10.2.1.4 Hydrogels

Hydrogels are quite flexible three-dimensional networks of water-soluble cross-linked polymer. They are highly biocompatible and have a wide range of applications in many fields, especially in biomedical and commonly used in clinical studies. Their porous, flexible structure can be easily tailored by governing the density of cross-links in the gel matrix, and their porous structure along with the gel-sol phenomenon permits the loading and release rate of therapeutic molecules through these three-dimensional networks. Hydrogel formulations showed a significant impact on the pharmacokinetics of drugs by creating a depot which keeps a high concentration of the drug at the local site and in the surroundings for an extended period. Using hydrogels two or more drugs can be delivered concurrently hence this approach can be used to avoid drug resistance and adverse effect of a potent drug. The design of a hydrogel for controlled release is shown in Fig. 10.7.

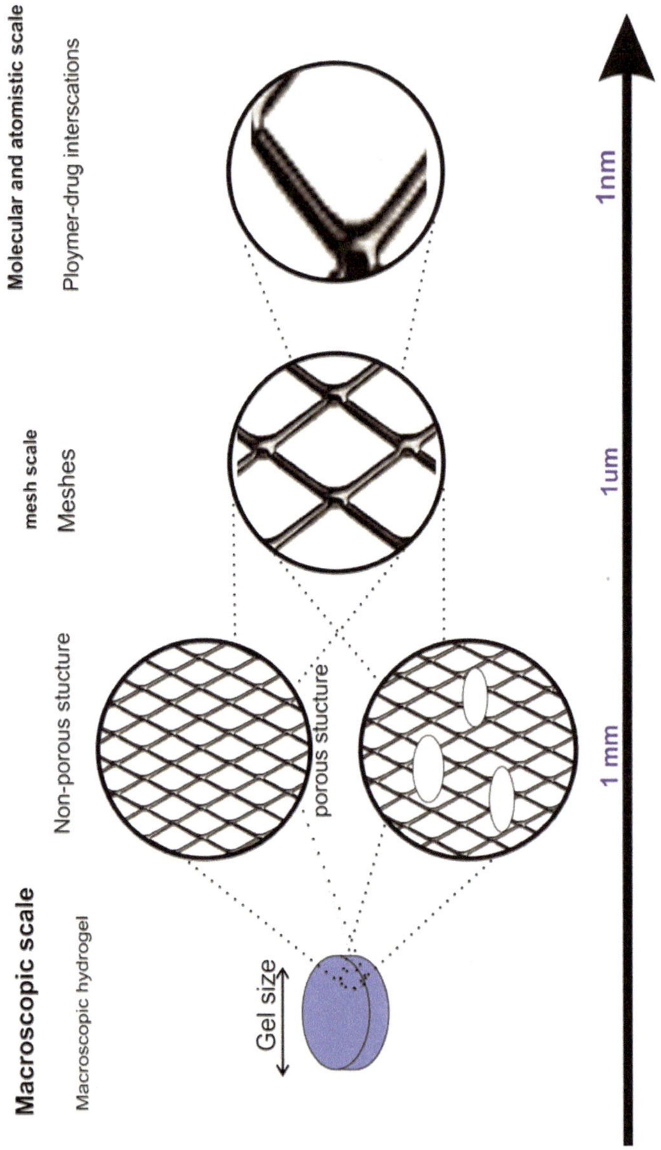

Figure 10.7 Design of hydrogel for controlled release.

Studies have shown synergistic administration of lapatinib and paclitaxel results in the accumulation of lapatinib at the cancerous site in an acceptable safe concentration, and the codelivery of microparticles of lapatinib and nanoparticles of paclitaxel were incorporated into a thermosensitive hydrogel was conducted to achieve a localized delivery. In another study, a poly(N-isopropylacrylamide-co-acrylamide) hydrogel with near-infrared absorbing silica–gold nanoshells successfully carried concurrent doxorubicin and DNA.

Besides several applications, hydrogels also impart some limitations such as the initial burst release of the drug due to the poor mechanical strength of polymers and less load-bearing capacity. Hence, it demands efforts in this direction so that the remarkable properties of such nanocarriers can be utilized in targeted delivery [10, 44, 55, 57].

10.2.1.5 Nanoparticles

Nanoparticles (NPs) are particles that have dimensions not more than 100 nm, and at such size, they show different properties and behavior compared with the bulk sample of the same substance. Nanoparticles may be 0D, 1D, 2D, or 3D depending on their shape. They possess some extraordinary properties such as high surface-to-volume ratio, sub-micron size, and enhanced targeting system, they showed deep tissue penetration hence increasing the EPR effect. The special features offered by the optimal size of NPs allow the therapeutic molecule to be encapsulated/loaded/or conjugated to the surface and distributed to the target site directly. The rate of therapeutic molecules can be easily controlled by activating or changing the external and internal stimuli such as environmental pH, temperature, chemicals, and radiations [36, 58, 59].

For example, PEGylation of nanoparticles increased the stability, minimized the opsonization, and circumvented the immune system clearance. Also, the optimization of the release rate of drugs or active moiety by manipulating particle polymer characteristics could be possible [48, 60]. Different nanomaterials are used in drug delivery for cancer treatment as shown in Fig. 10.8.

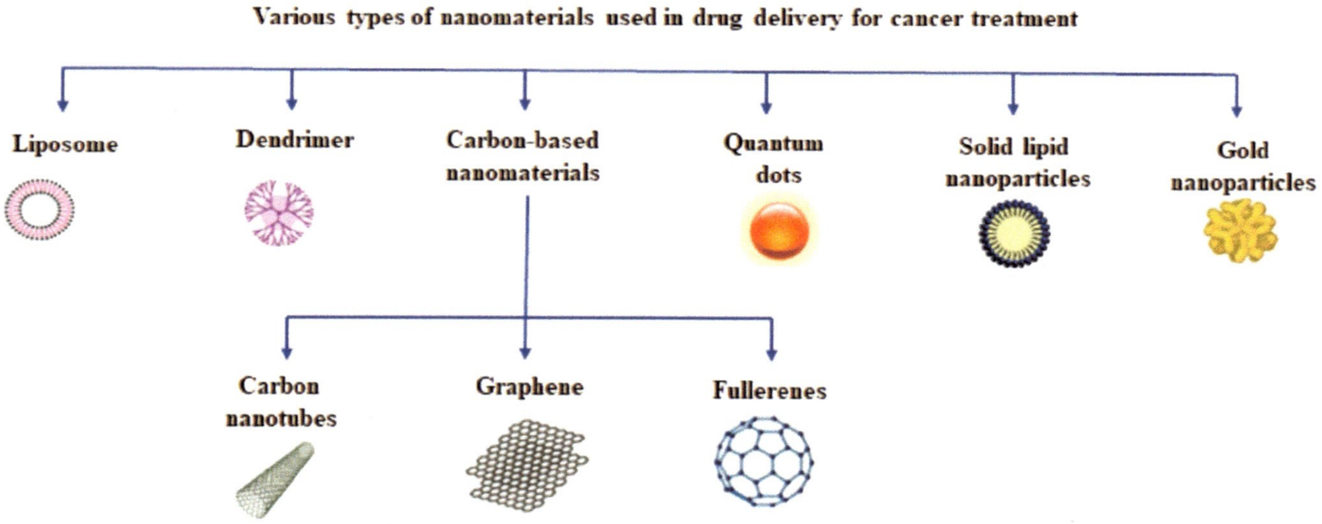

Figure 10.8 Various types of nanomaterials used in drug delivery for cancer treatment.

10.2.1.6 Liposomes

The discovery of liposomes in 1960 by Alec Bangham brought a significant revolution to the drug discovery systems, liposomes are basically concentric bi-layered vesicles composed of either natural or synthetic phospholipids and cholesterol enclosing aqueous volume inside them and are usually spherical in shape [5]. Generally, they are manufactured in size less than 20 μm in diameter and interact with the membrane components in a predicted way. Both hydrophobic and hydrophilic chemotherapeutic molecules can be delivered by using liposomes as a DDS, like the hydrophobic molecules can be encapsulated inside into lipid bilayer, or the hydrophilic molecules can be enclosed in an aqueous core or can be adsorbed onto the surface via charge interaction or through chemical linkers. They have created a wide interest as they are very flexible nontoxic, highly biocompatible, improve the therapeutic efficacy, reduce peak-valley fluctuations, and provide sustained release at the target site. Till now more than 20 liposome formulations are commercialized and several are under pre-clinical and clinical trials. It has been observed that liposomes due to hydrophobicity show early clearance time so sometimes they are conjugated with polymers like polyethylene glycol (PEG), such liposomes are known as Stealth® liposomes with increased blood circulation time.

Formulations: Doxil® and Myocet® are commercialized liposomes that encapsulate the broad-spectrum anticancer drug doxorubicin. It was observed that the side effects have been reduced but the clearance time was rapid hence the drug was loaded through an "active loading" approach via potential gradients and pH on Doxil® and Myocet,® respectively. The results were significant and Doxil® showed more remarkable improvement in its pharmacokinetic profile than Myocet® which was due to PEG coating. Overall, the results demonstrated both Doxil® and Myocet® proved quite significant in reducing the toxicity of doxorubicin [44, 45, 53, 55, 61].

10.2.1.7 Dendrimers

Dendrimers are globular-shaped 3-D structures and they can be easily modified through surface functionalization in a controlled manner apart from the structural benefits dendrimers possessed some special features which lend them as a promising nanocarrier for oncological approaches. Following are their features:

a. They show biocompatibility due to the presence of negative charge or no charge but the presence of positive charge results in toxicity.
b. The architecture and design of dendrimers can affect pharmacokinetics to a great extent.
c. The PEGylation of dendrimers leads to an increase in its aqueous solubility and retention time with improved biodistribution characteristics.
d. The surface of dendrimers offers easy functionalization due to which the chemotherapeutic agents can be attached to the functionalized groups via covalent bonding, electrostatic interaction, or can be trapped into the void surface available.
e. To improve the specificity and efficacy, some other moieties can be attached to the surface of dendrimers like targeting moiety, imaging moiety, etc.

Hence, these properties generated the interest of researchers to develop dendrimer-based anticancer therapies.

For example, Jain et al. developed doxorubicin-folate-conjugated poly-l-lysine dendrimers which showed pH-dependent drug release with 121.5-fold increased concentration of doxorubicin in tumor area in comparison to free drug after 24 h. Further, Kaur et al. described folate-conjugated polypropylene imine pH-sensitive dendrimer to carry methotrexate to cancer cells, the results of *in vitro* studies showed a sustained release with increased drug concentration and low toxicity on MCF-7 cell lines as compared to free drug delivery [3, 46, 49, 50].

10.2.1.8 Carbon nanoparticles

Because of their amazing optical, mechanical, and electronic properties, carbon NPs are widely utilized in the medicinal field [62–65]. Drugs are basically encapsulated in such structures via π–π stacking due to their hydrophobic nature [66, 67]. Carbon NPs are further categorized into

- **Graphene:** is a 2D sp2-hybridized honeycomb structure with extraordinary physicochemical properties and it can be further modified as graphene oxide (GO) and reduced graphene oxide (rGO) which possess more desired characteristics, biocompatibility, and oxygenated groups for functionalization, for example, doxorubicin conjugated with GO exhibits better anticancer activities in a cellular model of breast cancer as compared to the free drug [67–70].
- **Carbon nanotubes:** are 1D cylindrically shaped tube-like structures obtained by folding a graphene sheet and depending upon the number of sheets of graphene it is classified as single-walled carbon nanotube (SWNT) and multi-walled carbon nanotube (MWNT). They are capable of producing immune responses by interacting with immune cells and therefore can be used to suppress tumor growth. For example, encapsulating doxorubicin to a fluorescent SWNT with mAb was used to target colon cancer cells and it was found that the complex was effectively engulfed by the cancer cells and released doxorubicin intracellularly, whereas the CNTs were retained in the cytoplasm [62, 65, 71, 72].
- **Fullerenes:** are 3D carbon cage-like structures generally spherical in shape and are widely used nanocarriers due to amazing physical, chemical, and electrical properties. Fullerenes modified with PEG brought significant photo-dynamic effects on cancer cells [38, 65].

10.2.1.9 Quantum dots

Quantum dots (QDs) are semiconductor nanocrystals that have a size of a few nanometers (2 to 10 nm). Quantum dots have been vigorously studied as bioimaging, sensors, and targeted drug delivery in the medical field. However, it has been also investigated in the management of cancer. The most widely used of this technique is graphene quantum dots due to their inherent biocompatibility and rapid excretion. For example, quantum dots aptamer—doxorubicin conjugate targets prostate cancer cells. However, the deficiency of optimized processes in producing quantum dots is the major obstacle [73–76].

Table 10.5 Nanoparticle formulations currently available in the market

Product	Drug	Formulations	Applications	Status
Rexin-G	Dominant negative cyclin GI-construct	Pathotropic nanoparticles/IV	Recurrent or metastatic breast cancer	Phase I/II
Abraxane	Paclitaxel	Albumin-bound nanoparticles/IV	Metastatic breast cancer	Marketed
BikDD Nanoparticle	Pro-apoptotic Bik gene (BikDD)	Liposome/IV	Pancreatic cancer	Phase I
Docetaxel-PNP	Docetaxel	Polymeric nanoparticles/IV	Advanced solid malignancies	Phase I
Caelyx	Doxorubicin	Pegylated liposome/IM	Metastatic breast and ovarian cancer; Kaposi sarcoma	Marketed
Doxil	Doxorubicin	Liposome/IV	Kaposi sarcoma	Marketed
Genexol-PM	Paclitaxel	Methoxy PEG-PLA/IV	Breast and lung cancer	Phase II
CALAA-01	Anti-R2 SiRNA	Cyclodextrin-containing polymer (CAL-101) and targeting agent (AD-PEG-Tf)/IV	Solid tumors that are refractory to standard-of-care	Phase I
Myocet	Doxorubicin	Liposome/IV	Metastatic breast cancer	Marketed
L-Annamycin	Annamycin	Liposome/IV	Children and young adults with refractory or relapsed ALL or AML	Phase I/II

10.2.1.10 Solid lipid nanoparticles

Solid lipid nanoparticles (SLN) are generally used for the delivery of hydrophobic substances. They are colloidal with a size range of 50 to 1000 nm consisting of a lipid matrix that remains solid at room temperature and body temperature. The main advantage of SLNs is that they can be produced at a large scale easily and a controlled release with site-specific targeting can be achieved for both hydrophilic and hydrophobic drugs. For example, tryptanthin and oridonin are herbal drugs used for anticancer therapy and have been developed in the form of solid lipid nanoparticles [46, 77].

10.2.1.11 Gold nanoparticles

Gold nanoparticles represent a novel technology in the field of particle-based tumor-targeted drug delivery. Paciotti et al. have reported an application of these carriers for the targeted delivery of tumor necrosis factor-alfa (TNF-α) to solid tumors [5, 36, 78, 79].

Day by day the market of formulations based on nanoparticles is going on expanding and to address the limitations of conventional formulations, some nanoparticle formulations commercially available in the market for the treatment of cancer have been summarized in Table 10.5.

10.3 Conclusion

Every year various authentic organizations present data reports on the cancer status, and the analysis revealed that the current strategies available for the treatment of cancer are limited and are associated with various drawbacks due to which the survival rate of cancer patients is quite unsatisfactory. Most of the conventional methods for cancer therapy are proving toxic and are not able to specifically target the infected region. For researchers, among various fatal diseases, cancer is one of the most challenging life-threatening ailments and continuous efforts are going on to find a suitable strategy. However, the use of nanotechnology revolutionized this field and some remarkable inventions have been made with which researchers got success to some extent in this direction. The current studies have concluded that the use of nanotechnology-based NDDS is proving to be a promising approach for anticancer therapy. NDDS can address the drawbacks associated with conventional therapies and also show suitable results in clinical studies. FDA has also given approval to several NDDS-based systems for the delivery of therapeutic substances, and currently a number of NDDS-based products, such as Abraxane and Doxil, are available on the market and imparting the potential of nanotechnology. In this chapter, we discussed various types of NDDS and their significance in cancer therapy. In addition, cancer background and its treatment with conventional approaches have also been summarized. It is concluded that the unique attribute of NDDS allows and offers researchers to develop new treatments or to use them in combination therapy as an adjunct. Although NDDS are being used as a potential drug delivery carrier, some of them have not been successful during clinical trials. Moreover, several new and existing materials are currently under development and optimization and thereby providing hope for new promising cancer treatments in the near future.

References

1. Sung H, Ferlay J, Siegel RL, Laversanne M, Soerjomataram I, Jemal A, et al. Global cancer statistics 2020: GLOBOCAN estimates of incidence and mortality worldwide for 36 cancers in 185 countries. *CA Cancer J Clin* 2021; 71(3): 209–49.
2. Senapati S, Mahanta AK, Kumar S, Maiti P. Controlled drug delivery vehicles for cancer treatment and their performance. *Signal Transduction Target Ther* 2018; 3(1): 1–19.
3. Mousa SA, Bharali DJ. Nanotechnology-based detection and targeted therapy in cancer: nano-bio paradigms and applications. *Cancers* 2011; 3(3): 2888–903.
4. Zhang Y, Khan AR, Yang X, Fu M, Wang R, Chi L, et al. Current advances in versatile metal-organic frameworks for cancer therapy. *J Drug Deliv Sci Technol.* 2021; 61: 102266.
5. Ho BN, Pfeffer CM, Singh AT. Update on nanotechnology-based drug delivery systems in cancer treatment. *Anticancer Res.* 2017; 37(11): 5975–81.

6. Sikora K. The impact of future technology on cancer care. *Clin Med.* 2002; 2(6): 560.
7. Koushik O, Rao Y, Kumar P, Karthikeyan R. Nano drug delivery systems to overcome cancer drug resistance—a review. *J Nanomed Nanotechnol* 2016; 7(378): 2.
8. Malik P, Gupta R, Malik V, Ameta RK. Emerging nanomaterials for improved biosensing. *Measurement: Sensors* 2021; 16: 100050.
9. Folkman J. How the field of controlled-release technology began, and its central role in the development of angiogenesis research. *Biomaterials* 1990; 11(9): 615–8.
10. Huang P, Wang X, Liang X, Yang J, Zhang C, Kong D, et al. Nano-, micro-, and macroscale drug delivery systems for cancer immunotherapy. *Acta Biomater* 2019; 85: 1–26.
11. Blackadar CB. Historical review of the causes of cancer. *World J Clin Oncol* 2016; 7(1): 54.
12. Saini A, Kumar M, Bhatt S, Saini V, Malik A. Cancer causes and treatments. *Int J Pharm Sci Res.* 2020; 11(7): 3121–4.
13. Ferlay J. GLOBOCAN 2008 v1. 2, Cancer incidence and mortality world-wide: IARC Cancer Base No. 10. http://globocan iarc. 2010.
14. Bray F, Ren JS, Masuyer E, Ferlay J. Global estimates of cancer prevalence for 27 sites in the adult population in 2008. *Int J Cancer.* 2013; 132(5): 1133–45.
15. Siegel R, Naishadham D, Jemal A. Global cancer statistics. *CA Cancer J Clin* 2013; 63(1): 11–30.
16. Delaney G, Jacob S, Featherstone C, Barton M. The role of radiotherapy in cancer treatment: estimating optimal utilization from a review of evidence-based clinical guidelines. *Cancer: Interdisciplinary Int J Am Cancer Soc* 2005; 104(6): 1129–37.
17. Formenti SC, Demaria S. Combining radiotherapy and cancer immunotherapy: a paradigm shift. *J Natl Cancer Inst* 2013; 105(4): 256–65.
18. Boeckman HJ, Trego KS, Turchi JJ. Cisplatin sensitizes cancer cells to ionizing radiation via inhibition of nonhomologous end joining. *Mol Cancer Res* 2005; 3(5): 277–85.
19. Harrison L, Hatahet Z, Wallace SS. *In vitro* repair of synthetic ionizing radiation-induced multiply damaged DNA sites. *J Mol Biol* 1999; 290(3): 667–84.
20. Luqmani Y. Mechanisms of drug resistance in cancer chemotherapy. *Med Principles Pract* 2005; 14(Suppl. 1): 35–48.

21. Care P. Radiation therapy. *Quality Assurance* 2019; 10: 4.
22. Hafeez MN, Celia C, Petrikaite V. Challenges towards targeted drug delivery in cancer nanomedicines. *Processes* 2021; 9(9): 1527.
23. Ventola CL. Cancer immunotherapy, part 3: challenges and future trends. *Pharm Ther* 2017; 42(8): 514.
24. Ventola CL. Cancer immunotherapy, part 1: current strategies and agents. *Pharm Ther* 2017; 42(6): 375.
25. Pardoll D, ed, *Cancer and the Immune System: Basic Concepts and Targets for Intervention. Seminars in Oncology*, 2015; Elsevier.
26. He Q, Liu Z, Liu Z, Lai Y, Zhou X, Weng J. TCR-like antibodies in cancer immunotherapy. *J Hematol Oncol* 2019; 12(1): 1–13.
27. Michel L, Rassaf T, Totzeck M. Cardiotoxicity from immune checkpoint inhibitors. *IJC Heart Vasculature* 2019; 25: 100420.
28. Walko CM, McLeod HL. Personalizing medicine in geriatric oncology. *J Clin Oncol* 2014; 32(24): 2581–6.
29. Shi J, Kantoff PW, Wooster R, Farokhzad OC. Cancer nanomedicine: progress, challenges and opportunities. *Nat Rev Cancer.* 2017; 17(1): 20–37.
30. Chow EK-H, Ho D. Cancer nanomedicine: from drug delivery to imaging. *Sci Trans Med* 2013; 5(216): 216rv4–rv4.
31. Ferrari M. Cancer nanotechnology: opportunities and challenges. *Nat Rev Cancer* 2005; 5(3): 161–71.
32. Maeda H, Wu J, Sawa T, Matsumura Y, Hori K. Tumor vascular permeability and the EPR effect in macromolecular therapeutics: a review. *J Control Release.* 2000; 65(1–2): 271–84.
33. Felice B, Prabhakaran MP, Rodriguez AP, Ramakrishna S. Drug delivery vehicles on a nano-engineering perspective. *Mater Sci Eng C* 2014; 41: 178–95.
34. Primo FL, Rodrigues MM, Simioni AR, Bentley MV, Morais PC, Tedesco AC. *In vitro* studies of cutaneous retention of magnetic nanoemulsion loaded with zinc phthalocyanine for synergic use in skin cancer treatment. *J Magn Magn Mater* 2008; 320(14): e211–e4.
35. Agrawal M, Saraf S, Saraf S, Dubey SK, Puri A, Patel RJ, et al. Recent strategies and advances in the fabrication of nano lipid carriers and their application towards brain targeting. *J Control Release* 2020; 321: 372–415.
36. McNamara K, Tofail SA. Nanosystems: the use of nanoalloys, metallic, bimetallic, and magnetic nanoparticles in biomedical applications. *Phys Chem Chem Phys* 2015; 17(42): 27981–95.

37. Wang Q-S, Gao L-N, Zhu X-N, Zhang Y, Zhang C-N, Xu D, et al. Co-delivery of glycyrrhizin and doxorubicin by alginate nanogel particles attenuates the activation of macrophage and enhances the therapeutic efficacy for hepatocellular carcinoma. *Theranostics* 2019; 9(21): 6239.

38. Sutradhar KB, Amin M. Nanotechnology in cancer drug delivery and selective targeting. *Int Scholarly Res Notices.* 2014; 2014: Article ID 939378 | https://doi.org/10.1155/2014/939378.

39. Guidance D. Guidance for industry considering whether an FDA-regulated product involves the application of nanotechnology. *Biotechnol Law Rep* 2011; 30(5): 613–6.

40. Ma Q, Cao J, Gao Y, Han S, Liang Y, Zhang T, et al. Microfluidic-mediated nano-drug delivery systems: from fundamentals to fabrication for advanced therapeutic applications. *Nanoscale* 2020; 12(29): 15512–27.

41. Stylianopoulos T, Poh M-Z, Insin N, Bawendi MG, Fukumura D, Munn LL, et al. Diffusion of particles in the extracellular matrix: the effect of repulsive electrostatic interactions. *Biophys J* 2010; 99(5): 1342–9.

42. Yue Z-G, Wei W, Lv P-P, Yue H, Wang L-Y, Su Z-G, et al. Surface charge affects cellular uptake and intracellular trafficking of chitosan-based nanoparticles. *Biomacromolecules* 2011; 12(7): 2440–6.

43. Hadjidemetriou M, Al-Ahmady Z, Mazza M, Collins RF, Dawson K, Kostarelos K. *In vivo* biomolecule corona around blood-circulating, clinically used and antibody-targeted lipid bilayer nanoscale vesicles. *ACS Nano* 2015; 9(8): 8142–56.

44. Kushwaha SK, Rastogl A, Rai A, Singh S. Novel drug delivery system for anticancer drug: a review. *Int J PharmTech Res* 2012; 4(2): 542–53.

45. Mu W, Chu Q, Liu Y, Zhang N. A review on nano-based drug delivery system for cancer chemoimmunotherapy. *Nano-Micro Lett* 2020; 12(1): 1–24.

46. Ahmad MZ, Rizwanullah M, Ahmad J, Alasmary MY, Akhter MH, Abdel-Wahab BA, et al. Progress in nanomedicine-based drug delivery in designing of chitosan nanoparticles for cancer therapy. *Intl J Polymeric Mater Polymeric Biomater* 2022; 71(8): 602–23.

47. Pechar M, Ulbrich K, Šubr V, Seymour LW, Schacht EH. Poly (ethylene glycol) multiblock copolymer as a carrier of anti-cancer drug doxorubicin. *Bioconjug Chem.* 2000; 11(2): 131–9.

48. Sinha R, Kim GJ, Nie S, Shin DM. Nanotechnology in cancer therapeutics: bioconjugated nanoparticles for drug delivery. *Mol Cancer Ther* 2006; 5(8): 1909–17.
49. Jain V, Jain S, Mahajan S. Nanomedicines based drug delivery systems for anti-cancer targeting and treatment. *Curr Drug Deliv* 2015; 12(2): 177–91.
50. Wolinsky JB, Grinstaff MW. Therapeutic and diagnostic applications of dendrimers for cancer treatment. *Adv Drug Deliv Rev* 2008; 60(9): 1037–55.
51. Oerlemans C, Bult W, Bos M, Storm G, Nijsen JFW, Hennink WE. Polymeric micelles in anticancer therapy: targeting, imaging and triggered release. *Pharm Res* 2010; 27(12): 2569–89.
52. Ghosh B, Biswas S. Polymeric micelles in cancer therapy: state of the art. *J Control Release.* 2021; 332: 127–47.
53. Zahedi P, Yoganathan R, Piquette-Miller M, Allen C. Recent advances in drug delivery strategies for treatment of ovarian cancer. *Exp Opin Drug Deliv* 2012; 9(5): 567–83.
54. Jose B, Jesy E, Nedumpara RJ. Evaluation of the DPPH free radical scavenging activity of Wrightia tinctoria R. Br. leaf, bark and seed extracts. *World J Pharm Res* 2014; 3(3): 5041–8.
55. Saxena S, Yadav N. Research and Reviews: *J Pharm Pharm Sci* 2017; 6(1): 25–37.
56. More RK, Sonawane DS, Patil MP, Kshirsagar SJ. An overview: use of polymer microspheres in controlled drug delivery. *Res J Pharm Dosage Forms Technol* 2018; 10(3): 193–9.
57. Vinatier C, Mrugala D, Jorgensen C, Guicheux J, Noël D. Cartilage engineering: a crucial combination of cells, biomaterials and biofactors. *Trends Biotechnol* 2009; 27(5): 307–14.
58. Aghebati-Maleki A, Dolati S, Ahmadi M, Baghbanzhadeh A, Asadi M, Fotouhi A, et al. Nanoparticles and cancer therapy: perspectives for application of nanoparticles in the treatment of cancers. *J Cellular Physiol* 2020; 235(3): 1962–72.
59. Chandrakala V, Aruna V, Angajala G. Review on metal nanoparticles as nanocarriers: Current challenges and perspectives in drug delivery systems. *Emergent Mater* 2022; 5(6):1593–615.
60. Mohtar N, Parumasivam T, Gazzali AM, Tan CS, Tan ML, Othman R, et al. Advanced nanoparticle-based drug delivery systems and their cellular evaluation for non-small cell lung cancer treatment. *Cancers* 2021; 13(14): 3539.

61. Li Z, Tan S, Li S, Shen Q, Wang K. Cancer drug delivery in the nano era: an overview and perspectives. *Oncol Rep* 2017; 38(2): 611–24.

62. Maiti D, Tong X, Mou X, Yang K. Carbon-based nanomaterials for biomedical applications: a recent study. *Front Pharmacol* 2019; 9: 1401.

63. Dai L, Chang DW, Baek JB, Lu W. Carbon nanomaterials for advanced energy conversion and storage. *Small* 2012; 8(8): 1130–66.

64. Debnath SK, Srivastava R. Drug delivery with carbon-based nanomaterials as versatile nanocarriers: progress and prospects. *Front Nanotechnol* 2021; 3: 15.

65. Tripathi AC, Saraf SA, Saraf SK. Carbon nanotropes: a contemporary paradigm in drug delivery. *Materials* 2015; 8(6): 3068–100.

66. Lu T, Nong Z, Wei L, Wei M, Li G, Wu N, et al. Preparation and anti-cancer activity of transferrin/folic acid double-targeted graphene oxide drug delivery system. *J Biomater Appl* 2020; 35(1): 15–27.

67. Patra JK, Das G, Fraceto LF, Campos EVR, Rodriguez-Torres MdP, Acosta-Torres LS, et al. Nano based drug delivery systems: recent developments and future prospects. *J Nanobiotechnol* 2018; 16(1): 1–33.

68. Orecchioni M, Cabizza R, Bianco A, Delogu LG. Graphene as cancer theranostic tool: progress and future challenges. *Theranostics* 2015; 5(7): 710.

69. Lakshmanan R, Maulik N. Graphene-based drug delivery systems in tissue engineering and nanomedicine. *Canadian J Physiol Pharmacol* 2018; 96(9): 869–78.

70. Liu L, Ma Q, Cao J, Gao Y, Han S, Liang Y, et al. Recent progress of graphene oxide-based multifunctional nanomaterials for cancer treatment. *Cancer Nanotechnol* 2021; 12(1): 1–31.

71. Zhang W, Zhang Z, Zhang Y. The application of carbon nanotubes in target drug delivery systems for cancer therapies. *Nanoscale Res Lett* 2011; 6(1): 1–22.

72. Tonelli FM, Santos AK, Gomes KN, Lorencon E, Guatimosim S, Ladeira LO, et al. Carbon nanotube interaction with extracellular matrix proteins producing scaffolds for tissue engineering. *Int J Nanomed* 2012; 7: 4511.

73. Kościk I, Jankowski D, Jagusiak A. Carbon nanomaterials for theranostic use. *C J Carbon Res* 2021; 8(1): 3.

74. Pleskova S, Mikheeva E, Gornostaeva E. Using of quantum dots in biology and medicine. *Cellular Mol Toxicol Nanoparticles* 2018: 323–34.

75. Li Z, Fan J, Tong C, Zhou H, Wang W, Li B, et al. A smart drug-delivery nanosystem based on carboxylated graphene quantum dots for tumor-targeted chemotherapy. *Nanomedicine* 2019; 14(15): 2011–25.

76. Jampilek J, Kralova K. Advances in drug delivery nanosystems using graphene-based materials and carbon nanotubes. *Materials* 2021; 14(5): 1059.

77. Chidambaram M, Manavalan R, Kathiresan K. Nanotherapeutics to overcome conventional cancer chemotherapy limitations. *J Pharm Pharm Sci* 2011; 14(1): 67–77.

78. Calixto G, Bernegossi J, Fonseca-Santos B, Chorilli M. Nanotechnology-based drug delivery systems for treatment of oral cancer: a review. *Intl J Nanomed* 2014; 9: 3719.

79. Lee C-S, Kim TW, Oh DE, Bae SO, Ryu J, Kong H, et al. *In vivo* and *in vitro* anticancer activity of doxorubicin-loaded DNA-AuNP nanocarrier for the ovarian cancer treatment. *Cancers* 2020; 12(3): 634.

Multiple Choice Questions

1. From which language is the term 'cancer' is derived?
   a. Sanskrit
   b. French
   c. German
   d. Latin
2. The term cancer means:
   a. Cell division
   b. Out of control
   c. Crab
   d. Lobster
3. In stage 2, the cancer cells:
   a. Have spread to other parts of the body
   b. May or may not have spread to the lymph nodes
   c. Are not spreading and are in situ
   d. Have spread to lymph nodes above the collarbone

4. Which of the following is not a characteristic of cancer cells?
    a. Loss of cell cycle control
    b. Transplantability
    c. Loss of contact inhibition
    d. All are characteristic
5. Cancer is caused by
    a. Uncontrolled mitosis
    b. Uncontrolled meiosis
    c. Rupturing of cell
    d. Loss of immunity of cells
6. To which type of cancer may the exposure to UV radiation lead?
    a. Brain cancer
    b. Oral cavity cancer
    c. Skin cancer
    d. Uterine cancer
7. The most common site for cancer in males in India is:
    a. Oral cancer
    b. Lung cancer
    c. Cervical cancer
    d. Liver cancer
8. The most common site of cancer in males in the world is:
    a. Breast cancer
    b. Lung cancer
    c. Cervical cancer
    d. Liver cancer
9. Cancer cells can be easily destroyed by radiations than normal cells due to:
    a. Fast mutation
    b. Rapid cell mutation
    c. Lack of mutation
    d. Lack of oxygen
10. Which of the following may contribute to causing cancer?
    a. A mutation in a gene that slows the cell cycle

b. Faulty DNA repair
c. Loss of control over telomere length
d. All of the above

11. A lipid bilayer structure that encloses an internal aqueous volume
    a. Niosome
    b. Liposome
    c. Solid lipid nanoparticle
    d. Nanoparticle
12. A spherical solid lipid particle prepared from physiological lipid, dispersed in water or in an aqueous surfactant solution.
    a. Solid lipid nanoparticle
    b. Liposome
    c. Niosome
    d. Nanoparticle
13. A nonionic surfactant based multilamellar or unilamellar vesicular structure
    a. Microspheres
    b. Liposome
    c. Niosome
    d. Nanoparticle
14. Use of monoclonal antibodies for drug delivery to tumor is
    a. Active targeting
    b. Passive targeting
    c. Triggered drug targeting
    d. Vector targeting
15. Which among following is an example of a synthetic biodegradable polymer?
    a. Acrolein
    b. Polyethylene glycol
    c. LDPE
    d. Polystyrene
16. An example of polymer incorporated into dendrimers is
    a. Polyethylene glycol
    b. Polyethyleneimine

c. Polyurethane
d. Styrene copolymer

17. An advantage of novel drug delivery systems is
    a. It causes fluctuation of blood levels
    b. It cannot be target specific
    c. It increases toxicity of the drug
    d. It reduces side effects of the drug
18. One method to prepare nanoparticles is
    a. Pan coating
    b. Filtration
    c. Solubilization
    d. Precipitation
19. Microspheres are prepared by coacervation using
    a. Nonsolvent
    b. Trituration
    c. pH
    d. Pressure
20. Chitosan is a ____________ mucoadhesive polymer.
    a. cationic
    b. anionic
    c. synthetic
    d. nonionic
21. The size of polymeric nanoparticle nanosystems is around?
    a. 1–300 nm
    b. 1–500 mm
    c. 5–100 nm
    d. None of the above
22. Which one of the following is an example of a zero-dimensional nanostructure?
    a. Fullerene
    b. Nanorods
    c. Nanotubes
    d. Graphene sheets

23. Which one of the following is an advantage of nano-technology?
    a. Increased stability
    b. Leakage of drug
    c. Low solubility
    d. All of the above
24. Who defined the term nanotechnology?
    a. Gerd Binning
    b. Alex Zettl
    c. PM Ajayan
    d. Norio Taniguchi
25. Which one of the following are used in cancer therapeutics?
    a. Quantum dots
    b. Hydrogels
    c. Polymeric nanoparticles
    d. All of above

Answer Key

1.	d	**2.**	c	**3.**	b	**4.**	c	**5.**	a	**6.**	c	**7.**	a
8.	b	**9.**	b	**10.**	d	**11.**	b	**12.**	a	**13.**	c	**14.**	a
15.	b	**16.**	b	**17.**	d	**18.**	d	**19.**	a	**20.**	a	**21.**	c
22.	c	**23.**	d	**24.**	d	**25.**	d						

Long-Answer Questions

1. Define and classify cancer. Discuss the various treatment options with their limitations of cancer.
2. Why is nanotechnology so special in the biomedical field? Discuss the role of nanotechnology-based approaches in cancer treatment.
3. What are nanoparticles? Describe various kinds of nano-particles in anticancer therapy.
4. Why are current strategies approaching NDDS for cancer treatment.

Short-Answer Questions

1. Define cancer and its causes.
2. Explain different types of cancer.
3. Write a brief note on chemotherapy and its limitations.
4. What are hydrogels? Why are they important in drug delivery?
5. What are the various types of nanomaterials used in cancer treatment?
6. How are NDDS more important than conventional approaches?
7. Write a short note on the following:
   a. Polymer–drug conjugate
   b. Polymeric micelles
8. Write the role of carbon-based nanomaterials in anticancer therapy.

Chapter 11

Nano-Drug Delivery Systems in the Treatment of Wound Healing

Anjali Saharan,[a] Inderjeet Verma,[b] Meenakshi Dhanawat,[b] and Chander Parkash[c]

[a]*MM School of Pharmacy, Maharishi Markandeshwar University, Sadopur, Ambala, Haryana, India*
[b]*Amity Institute of Pharmacy, Amity University Haryana, Gurugram, Haryana, India*
[c]*Chitkara College of Pharmacy, Chitkara University, Punjab, India*

indupup@gmail.com

To overcome the main limitations of the traditional wound healing and dressing procedure, a new technology with a conjugated form had emerged, leading to several advantages by taking into account nano. The new era of biocompatible agent drug delivery is opened up by nanoparticles. The use of nanomaterials in the treatment and prevention of wound infections has numerous benefits. Numerous research had reported various nanomaterials and nanoproducts for wound healing. They act as a revolving wheel with dynamic properties when combined with other drugs and herbs. They had been utilized commercially in a variety of nanomaterial forms, including hydrogels, metallic nanoparticles, nanofibers, nanocomposites, and nanofibers made of polymers.

Nanotechnology and Drug Delivery: Principles and Applications
Edited by Rakesh K. Sindhu

ISBN 978-981-4968-83-6 (Hardcover), 978-1-003-43040-7 (eBook)
www.jennystanford.com

11.1 Introduction

Wounds are the "hidden epidemic" which reduce the quality of life. In many cases of injury and diseased condition, wound dressings do not meet the standards and fail to integrate properly [1, 2]. These properties in turn resulted in poor bioavailability, systematic delivery of hydrophobic drugs, and high level of reacted oxygen species [3, 4]. A recent analysis conducted in 2018 on acute and chronic wounds revealed that 8 million beneficiaries experienced one or more types of wounds or associated infections [5, 6]. On the other hand, in typical wound care, herbal remedies such as honey, bandages, and dressings leave scars regardless of the possible functional and aesthetic changes [7, 8].

Honey a natural derivative product shows numerous benefits such as immunostimulatory, antibacterial, antioxidant, and anti-inflammatory, actions and it is used in rapid wound healing [9]. However, when used topically for wounds, honey shows some drawbacks or negative effects. For instance, it might be difficult to prepare honey-impregnated dressings [10]. With the rise in temperatures, honey becomes more fluid. Sometimes it might temporarily sting and also increase blood glucose concentration in diabetes mellitus patients at large wound sites [11, 12]. The excessive application of it causes the dehydration of tissues and it can also cause hypersensitivity reactions due to the presence of pollen and bee proteins [13, 14].

In addition to tissue restoration to its original form (i.e., the delay in restoring tissue integrity), these conventional materials have their limitations that make wounds worse. Potential materials for wound healing might thereby improve therapeutic outcomes.

The effective and safe wound dressings include good water vapor transmission rate, exudate-absorbents with high swelling capacity and porosity, and antibacterial and anti-inflammatory characteristics. Exceptionally they have elasticity, flexibility, the ability to load drugs, tensile strength, and spreadability. As the above factors help in the healing process by maintaining a moist environment around the wound [15].

11.1.1 Pathogenesis of Wounds

The cascade of the healing process is divided into four steps, which are depicted below [16]:

Step 1: Hemostasis Phase
Step 2: Defensive/Inflammatory Phase
Step 3: Proliferative Phase
Step 4: Maturation Phase

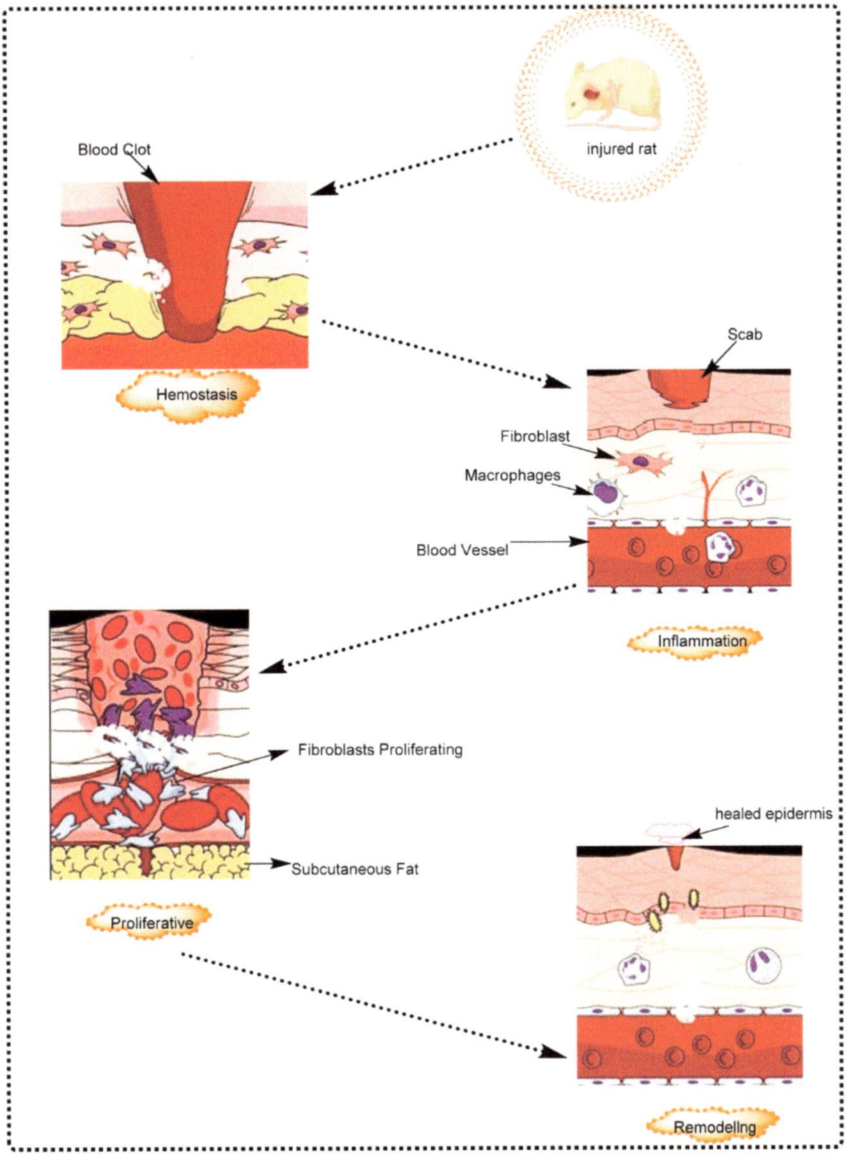

Figure 11.1 Different phases of Wound Healing.

Blood-borne cells including neutrophils control the initial stage of inflammation, and macrophages help in the repairing of tissue damage. Neutrophils and macrophages offer the temporary matrices and platelet-derived growth factor essential for drawing dermal/epidermal cells into the wound bed. In response to autocrine, paracrine, and juxtacrine growth hormones, after three days of injury, the proliferative phase will start which increased the levels of the above growth factors like keratinocyte-fibroblast, migration, and extracellular matrix (ECM) formation [17]. During this stage, angiogenesis and neovascularization also take place. After two weeks of injury, myofibroblasts present in the granulation tissue will start to rebuild the ECM.

An acellular scar is produced as a result of extracellular matrix modification and resident cell death [18, 19]. The phases of wound healing are described in Fig. 11.1.

11.1.2 Role of Nanotechnology in the Wound Healing

Recent advancements in the development of wound dressing materials have improved the understanding of the pathogenesis of chronic wounds. Various novel strategies have been used, such as nanotechnology, which accelerates the healing of both acute and chronic wounds via the movement of various healing phases. The use of various topical nanotechnology formulations such as nanoscaffolds, nanofibers, various small-sized nanomaterials, and biomaterials are used in wound healing [20]. Nanomaterials (10-9 nm) have been increasingly popular in recent years for use in biological and pharmaceutical applications which were used for the dressings of wounds, administration of the drug, and medical procedures [21].

Polymeric nanoscaffolds and innovative polymeric nanofibers have become popular in the treatment of wound healing due to their penetrability and target drug delivery at the site of the wound [22]. The use of nanomaterials in the modern era is rapidly growing in the management of various diseases [23, 24]. When the size of a molecule is converted to nanoscale, it will drastically change the physiological properties such as an increase in volume and surface area [25, 26].

Two principal types of nanoparticles (NPs) are frequently employed in wound healing:

1. NPs possess intrinsic nature which helps in wound closure [27]. They can be further divided into metallic/metal oxide nanomaterials and nonmetallic nanomaterials.
2. NPs used as delivery vectors for therapeutic agents [28].

11.2 Nanoparticles Used in Wound Healing

Wound healing is an important issue today for which wound management is necessary [29]. Nanotechnology plays an intense role in curing and managing this disease by using various biomaterials and various medicines embedded in nanoparticles which act as a good aid in wound dressings by enhancing regeneration, accelerating delayed wound healing, and use in burn treatment [30]. The different types of nanoderivatives used in wound healing are summarized in Fig. 11.2.

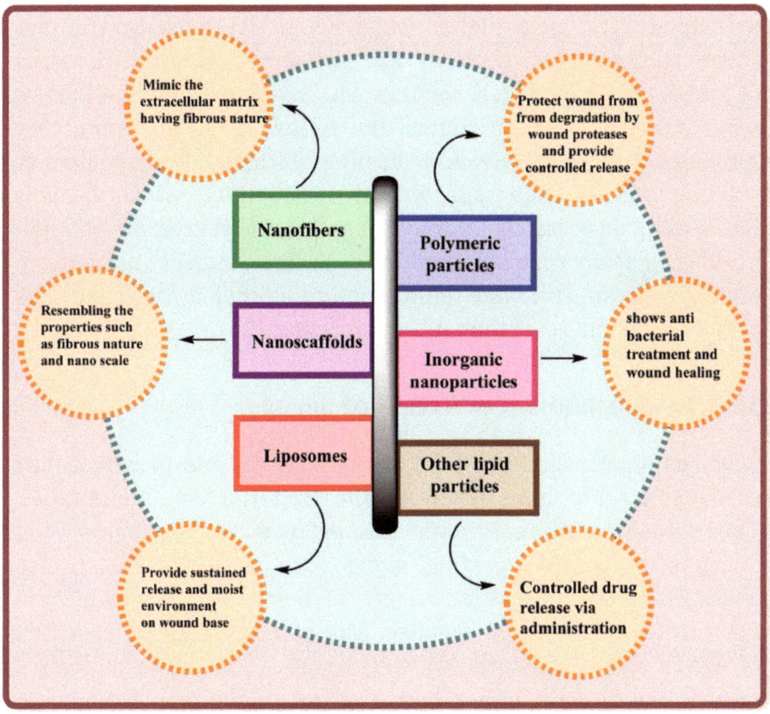

Figure 11.2 The different types and roles of nanoparticles used in wound healing.

11.2.1 Metallic Nanoparticles (Organic/Inorganic)

It has been demonstrated that metal nanostructures in single conjugates may have the ability to heal wounds [31]. They were combined with other dressing materials resulting in the suppression of germs from the wound area. Among various metallic nanoparticles, metals such as silver, gold, and zinc were blended with nanoparticles and exhibited remarkable antimicrobial activities and low *in vivo* toxicity [32].

11.2.1.1 Silver

Due to their unique qualities, silver nanoparticles have been widely used to create burn-specific ointments, pressure ulcer wound dressings, and other medical devices. They must stop the growth of bacteria, fungi, viruses, and protozoa [33]. The silver-coated dressings are frequently used for wound treatment because they can distribute medications effectively. Due to their higher surface-to-volume ratio and higher potency at lower concentrations, silver nanoparticles (AgNPs) are frequently utilized in place of silver material, which reduces the toxicity profile [34]. Pure silver nanoparticles can control the release of anti-inflammatory cytokines to hasten wound healing without causing further scarring. AgNPs encourage wound contractility, which hastens the healing process by encouraging the differentiation of myo-fibroblasts from regular fibroblasts. Besides, AgNPs' mechanism of action is to stimulate epidermal re-epithelialization via the proliferation and relocation of keratinocytes [35].

11.2.2 Mechanism of Action of Silver

Silver nanoparticles have a large surface area due to which they easily adhere to and penetrate the bacterial cell membranes. They cause interaction with the proteins having sulfur and phosphorus groups residing along with the DNA. They also transformed the molecular weight of bacteria to low which in turn protects DNA from damage. The primary method of action of AgNPs against bacteria, causing apoptosis, is the formation of sulfuric bonds with either bacterial cell membrane proteins or thiol groups of different enzymes, especially those included in the respiratory chain. AgNPs may also disrupt DNA synthesis during cell division, which in turn prevents the bacterial proliferation of DNA having sulfurous and phosphorous linkages [36]. AgNPs prevent the production of biofilms and effectively remove bacterial toxins by effectively disrupting quorum sensing. AgNPs are devoid of any biological functions of their own; however, the generated silver ions are only responsible for the said action. Inhibiting the production of adenosine triphosphate (ATP) results in the generation of reactive oxygen species (ROS) and some nonspecific mechanisms. It also delays and interrupts the normal phases of healing [37, 38]. The mechanism of action of silver nanoparticles is illustrated in Fig. 11.3.

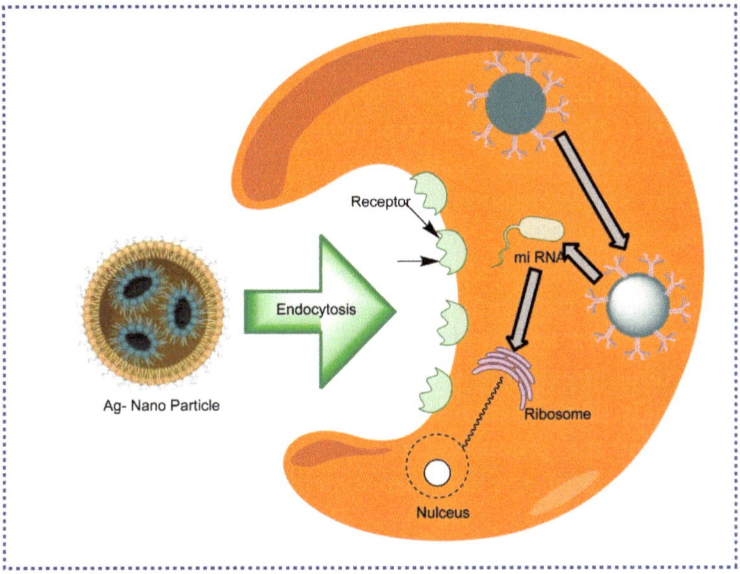

Figure 11.3 Mechanism of action of Ag nanoparticle in invading the bacterial cell.

Some of the reported research findings support the potential role of AgNPs in microbial clearance and enhancing wound healing. Lu et al. integrated AgNPs into mesoporous silica nanoparticles through the aid of disulfide bonds (Ag-MSNs), after their observation in animal trials that inorganic particles such as silica firmly adhere to open wounds. The new compound demonstrated excellent antibacterial activities, with little cellular toxicity [39].

11.2.2.1 Gold

Due to their chemical stability and near-infrared-light–absorbing properties, gold nanoparticles (AuNPs) are useful tools with lengthy chemical stability and the potential to absorb Infrared rays in wound healing therapy. Gold nanoparticles (AuNPs) are connected to the cell surface without changing the collagen's structural integrity through cross-linking with collagen and a number of biomolecules, including polysaccharides, growth factors, and peptides [40, 41]. These particles are widely utilized for wound healing and targeted drug delivery, and they are also biocompatible and aid in tissue regeneration. According to a study on vancomycin-conjugated gold nanoparticles, gold nanoparticles can be complexed with already available antimicrobial medicines or with other nanoparticles to increase their ability to kill bacteria [42]. As it was reported that vancomycin's shown more potent activity against vancomycin-resistant enterococci (VRE) by 50-fold, against E. coli. which earlier remain unaffected by vancomycin [43].

Arafa et al. demonstrated that AuNPs have shown *in vivo* and *in vitro* models their antibacterial and healing properties.

They work by specifically attacking the DNA and cell wall of bacteria, preventing the DNA's double helix from uncoiling, which aids in replication or transcription. They are also known to prevent the production of ROS and inhibit infections like *Staphylococcus aureus* and *Pseudomonas aeruginosa* by acting as antioxidants [44].

AuNP conjugates have been shown by Sherwani et al. to be beneficial in treating mouse wounds that are infected with *Candida albicans*. When the conjugate is administered topically to the lesion site, the wound healing capabilities and improved wound healing are seen [45].

11.2.3 Gold Nanoparticles of Mechanism of Action

AuNPs exert their mechanism of action via two pathways:

1. Alteration of membrane potential and inhibition of the ATP synthase, which in turn results in a depletion of ATP levels

leading to a collapse in energy metabolism and bacterial cell death [46].

2. Cell death induction in multiple drug-resistant bacteria by ROS-independent mechanisms.

11.3 Zinc Oxide

Zinc oxide nanoparticles (ZnONPs) proliferate the cell membrane and act as an antibacterial agent. They show the prolonged site of action when incorporated in hydrogel wound dressings ZnONPs also enhance wound healing by promoting keratinocyte migration, and re-epithelialization [47]. For example, a microporous chitosan hydrogel/ZnONPs dressing was available having a high capacity for wound exudates and enabling the formation of hemostatic blood clots [48].

ZnO nanoparticles are commonly utilized in the formulation of cosmetics, skin creams, and ointments because they have antibacterial, anti-inflammatory, and antiseptic qualities. Zn ions are released from the nanomaterial via a biphasic mechanism. As Zn ions first come into contact with biological fluids, they get hydrated to form hydrated ZnO, which functions as a bactericidal agent [49].

Bellaire et al. performed a study to evaluate the drugs incorporated in ZnONPs with the matrix composed of collagen and essential oil. The nanodressings accelerated the wound closure and prevent fungal growth showing excellent biocompatibility and reduced cytotoxicity [50].

11.4 Polymeric Nanostructures (Hydrogels and Gelatin)

Polymers are long-chain organic molecules, having several repeating monomer units. To overcome the drawbacks of natural polymers such as DNA, hyaluronic acid, gelatin, and collagen. The functional properties of polymers are tailored via the mode of synthesis and made variable with the specific requirements and biological applications. They had a low cost of production and were very adaptable when it came to dressing materials [51]. These polymers are presently utilized in the production of surgical instruments, medical equipment, implanted devices, and vascular grafts. Polyethylene (PE), polypropylene (PP), polystyrene (PS), polyvinyl chloride (PVC), polytetrafluoroethylene (PTFE), polymethyl methacrylate (PMMA), polyamides (nylon), and polysiloxanes (silicone) are some examples of synthetic polymers that are often utilized, whereas natural polymers include [52]. Using synthetic polymeric nanostructures, scaffolds, vascular grafts, biological carriers, and surgical sutures that have a long shelf life and low cost of manufacturing. Some of the commonly used polymeric nanomaterials were discussed below such as polymeric hydrogels, and gelatin [53].

Polymeric hydrogel is a type of polymer having a positive response to enhanced tissue restoration. At the preliminary stage of tissue restoration, the hydrogel scaffold can stimulate the infiltration of inflammatory cells and enhances the activity of angiogenic cells which aids in an improved healing process. The cytokines or growth factors act as an adjuvant to the polymeric hydrogel and enhance the blood vessel formation, neo-vascularization, and microenvironment around the wound area which promotes healing at a rapid rate [54].

Gelatin, a naturally occurring polymer made from collagen, has mostly been used to make biodegradable and biocompatible materials for wound dressings [55].

Bilgic et al. reported in a study about the topical application of gelatin-based scaffolds to rat wounds result in improved and faster-wound healing. Fibrin is a natural polymer, created when the enzyme thrombin reacts with fibrinogen to form fibrin. Fibrin has distinctive qualities that include reducing inflammation, boosting the immune system's response, and enhancing cell adhesion which employs its benefits in tissue engineering and wound healing [56].

11.5 Nanocomposites or Composite Nanoparticles

Polymeric nanoparticles (like chitosan) are used in polymeric nanomaterial therapy as wound dressings or as delivery vehicles because they have antibacterial and re-epithelializing capabilities [57].

Chitosan is a hydrophilic biopolymer having high bioavailability, low toxicity, and antibacterial properties. Chitosan is a biopolymer having chains of linear polysaccharides containing D-glucosamine and N-acetyl glucosamine units [58]. Chitosan's cationic nature causes it to form complexes with anions like sulfate and phosphate as well as with metals, proteins, and dyes. Hydrogels, membranes, films, sponges, and scaffolds are just a few of the different ways that chitosan has been studied for wound-healing treatments. Chitosan nanoparticles possess superior permeability, antibacterial properties, and immune modulation properties [59].

Chen et al. reported in a study that using the chitosan oligosaccharide a novel acellular porcine dermal matrix was developed. To maintain acceptable physicochemical characteristics, the oxidized chitosan oligosaccharide was cross-linked with the acellular network. To create AgNPs in situ, the newly produced compound Ag ions were further treated with the free remaining aldehyde groups (redox reaction). The resulting scaffolds have good biocompatibility, wide spectrum antibacterial activity against *Staphylococcus aureus* and Escherichia coli, and expedited wound healing [60].

Hajji et al. reported in a study that silver nanoparticles increased antioxidant and antibacterial activity against both Gram-positive (*Staphylococcus aureus*) and Gram-negative (Escherichia coli and Klebsiella pneumonia) bacteria when coupled with polyvinyl alcohol and chitosan. This combination enhanced wounds by promoting granulation and re-epithelialization with reducing cytotoxicity *in vivo* models [61].

Mihai et al. observed that coatings containing nanospheres of polylactic acid, chitosan, magnetite, and eugenol reduced the growth of *Staphylococcus aureus* and *Pseudomonas aeruginosa* biofilms while promoting endothelium proliferation [62].

Gao et al. reported In response to activation by near-infrared light, a thermosensitive hydrogel-based drug reservoir was created that can release active ingredients as needed. To integrate complementing antibacterial defense mechanisms, they used ciprofloxacin, glycol chitosan, and polydopamine nanoparticles.

Bacteria were drawn to and trapped on the surface of the gel by the glycol chitosan's positive charge. Near-infrared light can activate polydopamine nanoparticles, causing a photothermal reaction that produced local hyperthermia and caused bacterial annihilation. By being exposed to near-infrared light, polydopamine nanoparticles can be made active. This photothermal response causes local hyperthermia, which kills bacteria. Additionally, ciprofloxacin was loaded into polydopamine nanoparticles and released on demand after stimulation with near-infrared light, despite the hydrogel complex showing less leakage under physiological settings [63].

Hernandez et al. reported that the nanocomposites of AuNPs, chitosan, and calreticulin are used for the treatment of diabetic lesions. The calcium-binding protein called calreticulin controls the amounts of calcium in the cytosol and endoplasmic reticulum. Calreticulin also functions as a molecular chaperone, ensuring that proteins are folded correctly. *In vitro* and *in vivo*, the gold nanoparticles-chitosan-calreticulin composite boosted keratinocytes, fibroblasts, and endothelial cell proliferation, migration, and differentiation without affecting cell survival. The histological analysis also revealed enhanced collagen synthesis, granulation, and re-epithelization [64].

Sun et al. described in a study that cathelicidin, an antibacterial peptide obtained from king cobras, was encapsulated. Bacterial cellulose is a biopolymer produced by a variety of bacteria, including Acetobacter, Pseudomonas, and Salmonella, during the fermentation of carbohydrates. Due to its physicochemical characteristics, such as its extremely large surface area per unit, enhanced biocompatibility, hydrophilicity, and nontoxicity, bacterial cellulose represents a good skin substitute. Bacterial nanocellulose is differentiated by three-dimensional porous networks with a high ability to retain water, ensuring a moist environment ideal for wound healing. ZnONPs were found to have antibacterial characteristics and studied the therapeutic effects of bacterial cellulose mixed with them [65].

Moniri et al. mixed silver nanoparticles with bacterial nanocellulose produced by the fermentation of the Gram-negative *Gluconacetobacter xylinus* (BNC-Ag). The nanocomposite inhibited *Staphylococcus aureus in vitro* colonization and accelerated wound healing [66].

11.6 Nanocarriers for Wound Healing (Nitric Oxide, Curcumin)

Nanomaterials can also act as carriers for therapeutic agents by controlling their release. Nitric oxide plays a key role in inflammatory pathways, cellular proliferation, angiogenesis, and the deposition and remodeling of extracellular matrix. Nitric oxide also inhibits the formation of biofilms and possesses broad-spectrum antibacterial effects. The development of a delivery method with a high loading capacity, regulated release, and low cytotoxicity has thus been the subject of numerous investigations. To have prolonged nitric oxide release, antibacterial action against methicillin-resistant *Staphylococcus aureus* and *Pseudomonas aeruginosa*, and speed up wound healing *in vivo*, poly(lactic-co-glycolic acid)-polyethyleneimine nanoparticles were developed [67].

Nitric oxide: Inflammatory pathways, cell proliferation, angiogenesis, and the deposition and remodeling of an extracellular matrix all demonstrate important roles for nitric oxide. Nitric oxide also hinders the formation of biofilms while exhibiting broad-spectrum antibacterial capabilities. Numerous studies have therefore attempted to develop a delivery method with high loading capacity, regulated release, and little cytotoxicity. To increase the pace of wound healing *in vivo*, methicillin-resistant *Staphylococcus aureus* and *Pseudomonas aeruginosa* antibacterial efficacy, and prolonged nitric oxide release, methicillin-releasing poly(lactic-co-glycolic acid)-polyethyleneimine nanoparticles were developed [68, 69].

Wang et al. for wound treatment developed a novel pH-responsive calcium alginate hydrogel that contains hyaluronan oligosaccharide and protamine nanoparticles. The hydrogel would absorb wound exudates, causing the alkaline fluids to diminish. As a result of the pH change, the calcium alginate released active protamine nanoparticles that killed both Gram-positive and Gram-negative bacteria. Hyaluronan oligosaccharides also increased endothelial cell motility and proliferation, vascular endothelial growth factor expression, and angiogenesis [70].

Curcumin is a natural moiety, that helps in the production of granulation of tissues with antiseptic, antibiotic, and antioxidant properties. In a recent study, the methicillin-resistant *Staphylococcus aureus* and improved wound closure activity of curcumin were demonstrated *in vitro*. The researchers attempted to augment curcumin's poor solubility by encapsulating it inside a saline-hydrogel nanoparticle vector [71].

Moradi et al. Curcumin-loaded super-paramagnetic iron oxide nanoparticles were used to research and analyze pulse photo-biomodulation. They demonstrated a significant reduction in *Staphylococcus aureus* colonies and accelerated wound healing [72].

11.7 Coatings and Scaffolds

The creation of scaffolds with similar qualities is another use for nanomaterials a matrix outside cells. They are made via a variety of processes, including electrospinning, self-assembly, and phase separation. The method most frequently used, electrospinning, produces porous polymeric nanofibers that can act as hybrid scaffolds to help fibroblasts adhere to and grow in wounds. Scaffolds offer strong mechanical support and make it easier to transfer growth factors to the desired areas, which are crucial elements needed for tissue regeneration. However, one significant drawback of scaffolds is that they must be implanted at the desired spot, which restricts their application [73]. An additional class of nano-polymer is called a dendrimer, and it has anti-inflammatory properties as well as the capacity to form networks with antibacterial drugs (e.g., silver).

Another application for nanoparticles is the construction of scaffolds with properties similar to the extracellular matrix. Phase separation, self-assembly, and electrospinning are only a few of the techniques used to make them. Porous polymeric nanofibers produced can be utilized as hybrid scaffolds to promote fibroblast adhesion and growth in wounds. Another type of nano-polymer is dendrimers, which have both anti-inflammatory properties and the capacity to form networks with antibacterial compounds (e.g., silver) [74].

Haik et al. analyzed the healing potential of a polymer nanofiber dressing applied by a portable handheld electrospinning device using a pig model of superficial partial thickness wounds. The outcomes were comparable to the conventional dressing in terms of safety (risk of infection, delayed healing). The benefits of this therapeutic approach include the nontouch method and convenience of use [75].

Chitosan: It was evident from a study that chitosan was used to treat models of diabetic wounds in rats by applying electrospun chitosan-poly-vinyl alcohol nanofibrous blend scaffolds, which shows increased healing rates compared with controls [76].

Hydrogels are versatile materials that can be used to create bandages and dressings for burns, acute/chronic wounds, and diabetic foot ulcers because of their softness and ease of water absorption, which minimizes tissue dehydration. Currently, the usage of hydrogels is more common because of their unique properties such as ease of administration and firmness with the shape of the wound. Hydrogels can retain maximum water due to which they are shown to be elastic and flexible. Both hydrogels and scaffolds are utilized for the uniform distribution of the growth nutrients. Covalent bonding between the growth factor and the hydrogel is one of these techniques. Granulocyte-macrophage colony-stimulating factor (GM-CSF) combined with hydrogel has reportedly been proven to be useful in treating burns and promoting tissue regeneration. The regeneration of a variety of wounded tissues has been studied extensively in pre-clinical studies employing hydrogels as drug delivery vehicles, with some promising results. In these experiments, growth factors were injected as an injectable solution or as hydrogels that had been implanted. In certain experiments, a hydrogel and growth factor mixture is positioned above a scaffold and implanted at the location of the injury. For instance, a hydrogel made of fibrin and hyaluronic acid that has been BMP-2 (bone morphogenetic protein-2) conjugated displays potent bone regeneration properties [77].

11.7.1 Heparin Hydrogel

Heparin hydrogel coated by a polylactide caprolactone scaffold aids in bone regeneration and formation [78].

11.7.2 Gelatin Hydrogel

A gelatin hydrogel with a tricalcium phosphate porous scaffold filled with fibrin gel mixed with vascular endothelial growth factor for bone defects and a poly-l-lactic acid (PLLA) scaffold loaded with fibroblast growth factor for bone regeneration. Researchers developed novel methods to create a covalent connection between the growth factors and hydrogels to prevent the rupture of growth factors from hydrogels. This led to the development of hydrogels with a novel feature of prolonged growth factor release from a heparin-binding growth factor hydrogel at the targeted site. Scientists have developed a fibrin hydrogel nanomaterial with a covalently bonded peptide that interacts with the growth factor (neurotrophin-3), a method that has been used to successfully treat spinal cord injuries [79].

11.7.3 Marketed Preparations Having Nanocompounds Used in Wound Healing

Various commercially available dressings contain AgNPs. Acticoat, a wound dressing comprising AgNPs with an average size of 15 nm, serves as an example of this. The majority of test volunteers experienced Acticoat's established benefits of pain relief, wound healing, and infection reduction at the wound site. For the treatment of burns, this coating is still being researched. Recent clinical trials found that using Anticoat along with creams containing silver sulphadiazine and chlorhexidine digluconate may be effective in preventing infections in burns [80, 81].

11.8 Conclusion

Inflammation, proliferation, and remodeling all take place throughout the complex three-stage process of wound healing. A variety of topical treatments with moist environments and antibacterial activity have been developed by researchers to promote a speedy recovery with minimal scarring. But because of bacterium biofilms and multidrug-resistant germs, treating wounds is still difficult. To overcome this issue, nanoparticles due to their vibrant advantages such as high surface-to-volume ratio implanted and used in a wide range of medicinal applications, including wound therapy.

Nanotechnology, often known as nanomedicine, is a rapidly growing subject in the medical field that provides significant therapeutic advancements for a variety of ailments, including wound healing. The primary goal of this review is to illustrate the diverse ways in which nanomedicine might be used to speed up the healing of wounds. To that end, we have extensively described how nanoparticles interact with wounds to promote the healing process.

Wound dressings with metal nanoparticle coatings show good antibacterial activity and are crucial to the healing of wounds. Gelatin, hydrogel, and other wound dressing materials coupled with peptide and polymeric nanostructures showed enhanced results for cell proliferation, epithelialization, collagen fiber deposition, tissue regeneration, and wound closure. The combination of nanoparticles and biopolymers accelerates tissue regeneration and wound healing.

References

1. Naskar, A., and Kim, K. S. (2020). Recent advances in nanomaterial-based wound-healing therapeutics, *Pharmaceutics*, **12**, 499.
2. Sandhiya, S., Dkhar, S. A., and Surendiran, A. (2009). Emerging trends of nanomedicine–an overview, *Fundam. Clin. Pharmacol.*, **23**, 263–269.
3. Li, J., Chen, J., and Kirsner, R. (2007). Pathophysiology of acute wound healing, *Clin. Dermatol.*, **25**, 9–18.
4. Schreml, S., Szeimies, R. M., Prantl, L., Landthaler, M., and Babilas, P. (2010). Wound healing in the 21st century, *J. Am. Acad. Dermatol.*, **63**, 866–881.
5. Negut, I., Grumezescu, V., and Grumezescu, A. M. (2018). Treatment strategies for infected wounds, *Molecules*, **23**, 2392.
6. Mihai, M. M., Holban, A. M., Giurcăneanu, C., Popa, L. G., Buzea, M., Filipov, M., and Popa, M. I. (2014). Identification and phenotypic characterization of the most frequent bacterial etiologies in chronic skin ulcers, *Rom. J. Morphol. Embryol.*, **55**, 1401–1408.

7. Mihai, M. M., Preda, M., Lungu, I., Gestal, M. C., Popa, M. I., and Holban, A. M. (2018). Nanocoatings for chronic wound repair—modulation of microbial colonization and biofilm formation, *Int. J. Mol. Sci.*, **19**, 1179.
8. Hamdan, S., Pastar, I., Drakulich, S., Dikici, E., Tomic-Canic, M., Deo, S., and Daunert, S. (2017). Nanotechnology-driven therapeutic interventions in wound healing: potential uses and applications, *ACS Cent. Sci.*, **3**, 163–175.
9. Lee, D. S., Sinno, S., and Khachemoune, A. (2011). Honey and wound healing, *Am. J. Clin. Dermatol.*, **12**, 181–190.
10. Oryan, A., Alemzadeh, E., and Moshiri, A. (2016). Biological properties and therapeutic activities of honey in wound healing: a narrative review and meta-analysis, *J. Tissue Viability*, **25**, 98–118.
11. Lusby, P. E., Coombes, A., and Wilkinson, J. M. (2002). Honey: a potent agent for wound healing, *J. Wound Care*, **29**, 295–300.
12. Al-Waili, N., Salom, K., and Al-Ghamdi, A. A. (2011). Honey for wound healing, ulcers, and burns; data supporting its use in clinical practice, *Sci. World J.*, **11**, 766–787.
13. Scepankova, H., Combarros-Fuertes, P., Fresno, J. M., Tornadijo, M. E., Dias, M. S., Pinto, C. A., and Estevinho, L. M. (2021). Role of honey in advanced wound care, *Molecules*, **26**, 4784.
14. Meo, S. A., Al-Asiri, S. A., Mahesar, A. L., and Ansari, M. J. (2017). Role of honey in modern medicine, *Saudi J. Biol. Sci.*, **24**, 975–978.
15. Gainza, G., Villullas, S., Pedraz, J. L., Hernandez, R. M., and Igartua, M. (2015). Advances in drug delivery systems (DDSs) to release growth factors for wound healing and skin regeneration, *Nanomed. Nanotechnol. Biol. Med.*, **11**, 1551–1573.
16. Majtan, J. (2014). Honey: an immunomodulator in wound healing, *Wound Repair Regeneration*, **22**, 187–192.
17. Molan, P. C. (1999). The role of honey in the management of wounds, *J. Wound Care*, **8**, 415–418.
18. Miller, M. C., and Nanchahal, J. (2005). Advances in the modulation of cutaneous wound healing and scarring, *BioDrugs*, **19**, 363–381.
19. Arafa, M. G., El-Kased, R. F., and Elmazar, M. M. (2018). Thermo-responsive gels containing gold nanoparticles as smart antibacterial and wound healing agents, *Sci. Rep.*, **8**, 1–16.
20. Mihai, M. M., Giurcăneanu, C., Popa, L. G., Nitipir, C., and Popa, M. I. (2015). Controversies and challenges of chronic wound infection diagnosis and treatment, *Mod. Med.*, **22**, 375–381.

21. Contardi, M., Heredia-Guerrero, J. A., Perotto, G., Valentini, P., Pompa, P. P., Spanò, R., and Bayer, I. S. (2017). Transparent ciprofloxacin-povidone antibiotic films and nanofiber mats as potential skin and wound care dressings, *Eur. J. Pharm. Sci.*, **104**, 133–144.

22. Losi, P., Briganti, E., Magera, A., Spiller, D., Ristori, C., Battolla, B., and Soldani, G. (2010). Tissue response to poly (ether) urethane-polydimethylsiloxane-fibrin composite scaffolds for controlled delivery of pro-angiogenic growth factors, *Biomaterials*, **31**, 5336–5344.

23. Upton, D., Solowiej, K., Hender, C., and Woo, K. Y. (2012). Stress and pain associated with dressing change in patients with chronic wounds, *J. Wound Care*, **21**, 53–61.

24. Han, G., and Ceilley, R. (2017). Chronic wound healing: a review of current management and treatments, *Adv. Ther.*, **34**, 599–610.

25. Martin, P. (1997). Wound healing: aiming for perfect skin regeneration, *Science*, **276**, 75–81.

26. Braund, R., Hook, S., and Medlicott, N. J. (2007). The role of topical growth factors in chronic wounds, *Curr. Drug Deliv.*, **4**, 195–204.

27. Eming, S. A., Krieg, T., and Davidson, J. M. (2007). Inflammation in wound repair: molecular and cellular mechanisms, *J. Invest. Dermatol.*, **127**, 514–525.

28. Velnar, T., Bailey, T., and Smrkolj, V. (2009). The wound healing process: an overview of the cellular and molecular mechanisms, *J. Int. Med. Res.*, **37**, 1528–1542.

29. Gong, C., Wu, Q., Wang, Y., Zhang, D., Luo, F., Zhao, X., and Qian, Z. (2013). A biodegradable hydrogel system containing curcumin encapsulated in micelles for cutaneous wound healing, *Biomaterials*, 34, 6377–6387.

30. Nguyen, T. T. T., Ghosh, C., Hwang, S. G., Tran, L. D., and Park, J. S. (2013). Characteristics of curcumin-loaded poly (lactic acid) nanofibers for wound healing, *J. Mater. Sci.*, 48, 7125–7133.

31. Schröfel, A., Kratošová, G., Šafařík, I., Šafaříková, M., Raška, I., and Shor, L. M. (2014). Applications of biosynthesized metallic nanoparticles—a review, *Acta Biomater.*, **10**, 4023–4042.

32. Loomba, L., and Scarabelli, T. (2013). Metallic nanoparticles and their medicinal potential. Part II: aluminosilicates, nanobiomagnets, quantum dots and cochleates, *Ther. Deliv.*, **4**, 1179–1196.

33. Kuppusamy, P., Yusoff, M. M., Maniam, G. P., and Govindan, N. (2016). Biosynthesis of metallic nanoparticles using plant derivatives and

their new avenues in pharmacological applications—an updated report, *Saudi Pharm. J.*, **24**, 473–484.

34. Gade, A., Ingle, A., Whiteley, C., and Rai, M. (2010). Mycogenic metal nanoparticles: progress and applications, *Biotechnol. Lett.*, **32**, 593–600.
35. Mody, V. V., Siwale, R., Singh, A., and Mody, H. R. (2010). Introduction to metallic nanoparticles, *J. Pharm. Bioallied Sci.*, **2**, 282.
36. Patil, S., and Chandrasekaran, R. (2020). Biogenic nanoparticles: a comprehensive perspective in synthesis, characterization, application and its challenges, *J. Genet. Eng. Biotechnol.*, **18**, 1–23.
37. Paladini, F., and Pollini, M. (2019). Antimicrobial silver nanoparticles for wound healing application: progress and future trends, *Materials*, **12**, 2540.
38. Konop, M., Damps, T., Misicka, A., and Rudnicka, L. (2016). Certain aspects of silver and silver nanoparticles in wound care: a minireview, *J. Nanomater.*, **10**, 2016.
39. Wei, L., Lu, J., Xu, H., Patel, A., Chen, Z. S., and Chen, G. (2015). Silver nanoparticles: synthesis, properties, and therapeutic applications, *Drug Discov.*, 20, 595–601.
40. Lau, P., Bidin, N., Islam, S., Shukri, W. N. B. W. M., Zakaria, N., Musa, N., and Krishnan, G. (2017). Influence of gold nanoparticles on wound healing treatment in rat model: photobiomodulation therapy, *Lasers Surg. Med.*, **49**, 380–386.
41. Shamaila, S., Zafar, N., Riaz, S., Sharif, R., Nazir, J., and Naseem, S. (2016). Gold nanoparticles: an efficient antimicrobial agent against enteric bacterial human pathogen, *Nanomaterials*, 6, 71.
42. Fayaz, A. M., Girilal, M., Mahdy, S. A., Somsundar, S. S., Venkatesan, R., and Kalaichelvan, P. T. (2011). Vancomycin bound biogenic gold nanoparticles: a different perspective for development of anti VRSA agents, *Process Biochem.*, **46**, 636–641.
43. Gu, H., Ho, P. L., Tong, E., Wang, L., and Xu, B. (2003). Presenting vancomycin on nanoparticles to enhance antimicrobial activities, *Nano Lett.*, **3**, 1261–1263.
44. Arafa, M. G., El-Kased, R. F., and Elmazar, M. M. (2018). Thermo-responsive gels containing gold nanoparticles as smart antibacterial and wound healing agents, *Sci. Rep.*, **8**, 1–16.
45. Shervani, Z., Taisuke, Y., Ifuku, S., Saimoto, H., and Morimoto, M. (2012). Preparation of gold nanoparticles loaded chitin nanofiber composite, *J. Sci. Res.*, **1**, 71–78.

46. Ponnanikajamideen, M., Rajeshkumar, S., Vanaja, M., and Annadurai, G. (2019). *In vivo* type 2 diabetes and wound-healing effects of antioxidant gold nanoparticles synthesized using the insulin plant *Chamaecostus cuspidatus* in albino rats, *Can. J. Diabetes*, **43**, 82–89.

47. Chhabra, H., Deshpande, R., Kanitkar, M., Jaiswal, A., Kale, V. P., and Bellare, J. R. (2016). A nano zinc oxide doped electrospun scaffold improves wound healing in a rodent model, *RSC Adv.*, **6**(2), 1428–1439.

48. Abdullah, B. J., Atasoy, N., and Omer, A. K. (2019). Evaluate the effects of platelet rich plasma (PRP) and zinc oxide ointment on skin wound healing, *Ann. Med. Surg.*, **37**, 30–37.

49. Ågren, M. S., Chvapil, M., and Franzén, L. (1991). Enhancement of re-epithelialization with topical zinc oxide in porcine partial-thickness wounds, *J. Surg. Res.*, **50**, 101–105.

50. Balaure, P. C., Holban, A. M., Grumezescu, A. M., Mogoşanu, G. D., Bălşeanu, T. A., Stan, M. S., and Mogoantă, L. (2019). *In vitro* and *in vivo* studies of novel fabricated bioactive dressings based on collagen and zinc oxide 3D scaffolds, *Int. J. Pharm.*, **557**, 199–207.

51. Foox, M., and Zilberman, M. (2015). Drug delivery from gelatin-based systems, *Expert Opin. Drug Deliv.*, **12**, 1547–1563.

52. Raja, I. S., and Fathima, N. N. (2018). Gelatin–cerium oxide nano-composite for enhanced excisional wound healing, *ACS Appl. Bio Mater.*, **1**, 487–495.

53. Guo, N., Zhang, L., Wang, J., Wang, S., Zou, Y., and Wang, X. (2020). Novel fabrication of morphology tailored nanostructures with Gelatin/Chitosan Co-polymeric bio-composited hydrogel system to accelerate bone fracture healing and hard tissue nursing care management, *Process Biochem.*, **90**, 177–183.

54. Pourshahrestani, S., Zeimaran, E., Kadri, N. A., Mutlu, N., and Boccaccini, A. R. (2020). Polymeric hydrogel systems as emerging biomaterial platforms to enable hemostasis and wound healing. *Adv. Healthc. Mater.*, **9**, 2000905.

55. Le Thi, P., Lee, Y., Tran, D. L., Thi, T. T. H., Kang, J. I., Park, K. M., and Park, K. D. (2020). In situ forming and reactive oxygen species-scavenging gelatin hydrogels for enhancing wound healing efficacy, *Acta Biomater.*, **103**, 142–152.

56. Bilgic, H., Demiriz, M., Ozler, M., Ide, T., Dogan, N., Gumus, S., and Hasirci, N. E. S. R. Ý. N. (2013). Gelatin based scaffolds and effect of EGF dose on wound healing, *J. Biomater. Tissue Eng.*, **3**, 205–211.

57. Malathi, S., Balashanmugam, P., Devasena, T., and Kalkura, S. N. (2021). Enhanced antibacterial activity and wound healing by a novel collagen blended ZnO nanoparticles embedded niosome nanocomposites. *J. Drug Deliv. Sci. Technol.*, **63**, 102498.

58. Wang, K., Pan, S., Qi, Z., Xia, P., Xu, H., Kong, W., and Fu, C. (2020). Recent advances in chitosan-based metal nanocomposites for wound healing applications, *Adv. Mater. Sci.*, 2020, Article ID 3827912 | https://doi.org/10.1155/2020/3827912.

59. Ali, A., and Ahmed, S. (2018). A review on chitosan and its nanocomposites in drug delivery. *Int. J. Bio. macromol.*, 109, 273–286.

60. Chen, H., Lan, G., Ran, L., Xiao, Y., Yu, K., Lu, B., and Lu, F. (2018). A novel wound dressing based on a Konjac glucomannan/silver nanoparticle composite sponge effectively kills bacteria and accelerates wound healing, *Carbohdr. Polym.*, **183**, 70–80.

61. Hajji, S., Ktari, N., Ben Salah, R., Boufi, S., Debeaufort, F., and Nasri, M. (2022). Development of nanocomposite films based on chitosan and gelatin loaded with chitosan-tripolyphosphate nanoparticles: antioxidant potentials and applications in wound healing, *J. Polym. Environ.*, **30**, 833–854.

62. Mihai, M. M., Dima, M. B., Dima, B., and Holban, A. M. (2019). Nanomaterials for wound healing and infection control, *Materials*, **12**, 2176.

63. Gao, Y., Wang, X., Zhang, Y., Li, J., Zhang, H., and Li, J. (2022). Novel fabrication of bi-metal oxide hybrid nanocomposites for synergetic enhancement of *in vivo* healing and wound care after caesarean section surgery, *Int. Wound J.*, **19**(7), 1705–1716. doi: 10.1111/iwj.13771.

64. Pérez, J. A. C., Sosa-Hernández, J. E., Hussain, S. M., Bilal, M., Parra-Saldivar, R., and Iqbal, H. M. (2019). Bioinspired biomaterials and enzyme-based biosensors for point-of-care applications with reference to cancer and bioimaging, *Biocatal. Agric. Biotechnol.*, **17**, 168–176.

65. Sun, T., Zhan, B., Zhang, W., Qin, D., Xia, G., Zhang, H., ... and Lee, W. H. (2018). Carboxymethyl chitosan nanoparticles loaded with bioactive peptide OH-CATH30 benefit nonscar wound healing, *Int. J. Nanomed.*, **13**, 5771.

66. Moniri, M., Boroumand Moghaddam, A., Azizi, S., Abdul Rahim, R., Bin Ariff, A., Zuhainis Saad, W., and Mohamad, R. (2017). Production and status of bacterial cellulose in biomedical engineering, *J. Nanomater.*, **7**, 257.

67. Lohani, A., and Verma, A. (2017). Vesicles: potential nano carriers for the delivery of skin cosmetics, *J. Cosmet. Laser. Ther.*, **19**, 485–493.

68. Seabra, A. B., Rai, M., and Durán, N. (2014). Nano carriers for nitric oxide delivery and its potential applications in plant physiological process: a mini review, *J. Plant Biochem. Biotechnol.*, **23**, 1–10.

69. Gutierrez Cisneros, C., Bloemen, V., and Mignon, A. (2021). Synthetic, natural, and semisynthetic polymer carriers for controlled nitric oxide release in dermal applications: a review, *Polymers*, **13**, 760.

70. Mihai, M. M., Dima, M. B., Dima, B., and Holban, A. M. (2019). Nanomaterials for wound healing and infection control, *Materials*, **12**, 2176.

71. Nguyen, M. H., Vu, N. B. D., Nguyen, T. H. N., Le, H. S., Le, H. T., Tran, T. T., and Park, H. J. (2019). *In vivo* comparison of wound healing and scar treatment effect between curcumin–oligochitosan nanoparticle complex and oligochitosan-coated curcumin-loaded-liposome, *J. Microencapsul.*, **36**, 156–168.

72. Moradi, A., Kheirollahkhani, Y., Fatahi, P., Abdollahifar, M. A., Amini, A., Naserzadeh, P., and Bayat, M. (2019). An improvement in acute wound healing in mice by the combined application of photobiomodulation and curcumin-loaded iron particles, *Lasers Med. Sci.*, **34**, 779–791.

73. Paolini, A., Leoni, L., Giannicchi, I., Abbaszadeh, Z., D'Oria, V., Mura, F., and Masotti, A. (2018). MicroRNAs delivery into human cells grown on 3D-printed PLA scaffolds coated with a novel fluorescent PAMAM dendrimer for biomedical applications, *Sci. Rep.*, **8**, 1–11.

74. Vedhanayagam, M., Unni Nair, B., and Sreeram, K. J. (2018). Collagen-ZnO scaffolds for wound healing applications: role of dendrimer functionalization and nanoparticle morphology, *ACS Appl. Bio Mater.*, **1**, 1942–1958.

75. Haik, J., Kornhaber, R., Blal, B., and Harats, M. (2017). The feasibility of a handheld electrospinning device for the application of nanofibrous wound dressings, *Adv. Wound Care*, **6**, 166–174.

76. Huang, D., Zuo, Y., Zou, Q., Wang, Y., Gao, S., Wang, X., ... and Li, Y. (2012). Reinforced nanohydroxyapatite/polyamide66 scaffolds by chitosan coating for bone tissue engineering, *J. Biomed. Mater. Res.*, **100**, 51–57.

77. Li, Y., Xu, T., Tu, Z., Dai, W., Xue, Y., Tang, C., and Lin, C. (2020). Bioactive antibacterial silica-based nanocomposites hydrogel scaffolds with high angiogenesis for promoting diabetic wound healing and skin repair, *Theranostics*, **10**, 4929.

78. Andreopoulos, F. M., and Persaud, I. (2006). Delivery of basic fibroblast growth factor (bFGF) from photoresponsive hydrogel scaffolds, *Biomaterials*, **27**, 2468–2476.

79. Zheng, M., Wang, X., Yue, O., Hou, M., Zhang, H., Beyer, S., and Guo, J. (2021). Skin-inspired gelatin-based flexible bio-electronic hydrogel for wound healing promotion and motion sensing, *Biomaterials*, **276**, 121026.

80. Kleintjes, W. G., Schoeman, D., and Collier, L. (2015). A pilot study of Cutimed® Sorbact® versus ACTICOAT versus Silverlon® for the treatment of burn wounds in a South African adult burn unit: general review, *Wound Healing Southern Africa*, **8**, 22–29.

81. Rigo, C., Ferroni, L., Tocco, I., Roman, M., Munivrana, I., Gardin, C., and Zavan, B. (2013). Active silver nanoparticles for wound healing, *Int. J. Mol. Sci.*, **14**, 4817–4840.

Multiple-Choice Questions

1. Phases of cutaneous wound healing include
   a. Hemostasis
   b. Inflammation
   c. Proliferation and remodeling
   d. All of the above
2. Nanotechnology is specifically used in the treatment of
   a. Diabetic wounds
   b. Chronic wounds
   c. Both a and b
   d. None of the above
3. Advantages of nanoplatforms are
   a. Adaptability
   b. Turnability
   c. Controlled and sustained release of active ingredient
   d. All of the above
4. What is the diameter of a nanoparticle?
   a. 1–50 nm
   b. 1–90 nm

c. 1–100 nm
d. 0.1–50 nm

5. Nanotechnology is the science of
   a. Building microbial devices and components
   b. Building small devices or components
   c. Building large devices or components
   d. None of the above
6. Main approaches of nanotechnology are
   a. Top-down technique
   b. Top-up technique
   c. Bottom-up technique
   d. Both a and c
7. Nanotechnology is also called as
   a. Microphysics
   b. Microbiology
   c. Small technology
   d. Atomic engineering
8. The term "nanotechnology" was coined by
   a. Norio Taniguchi
   b. Richard Feynman
   c. Eric Drexler
   d. SumioTijima
9. Father of nanotechnology
   a. Alexender Fleming
   b. Richard Feynman
   c. Norio Taniguchi
   d. Eric Drexler
10. Which of the following nanomaterial are not used in wound healing?
    a. Silver
    b. Gold
    c. Zinc
    d. Diamond

11. Nanotechnology is used in the treatment of
    a. Cancer
    b. Neurological disorders
    c. HIV/AIDS
    d. All of the above
12. Disadvantages of nanotechnology are
    a. Economic disruption
    b. Threats to security and privacy
    c. Both a and b
    d. None of the above
13. Properties of silver nanoparticle
    a. Antibacterial
    b. Antifungal
    c. Antiviral
    d. All of the above
14. In which year was nanotechnology first used in medicine?
    a. 1998
    b. 1999
    c. 1980
    d. 1975
15. The name of the first nanomedicine
    a. Doxil
    b. Abraxane
    c. Paclitaxel
    d. Irinotecan
16. Properties of nanofibers
    a. High porosity
    b. Controllable morphology
    c. Thermal stability
    d. All of the above
17. How do liposome help in wound healing?
    a. Protect from infection
    b. Create moist environment

c. Cover the wound
d. Both b and c

18. Which of this compound is used in wound healing in nanotechnology?
    a. Hydrogels
    b. Diamonds
    c. Rubber
    d. None of the above
19. Which of the following is incorrect about hydrogels used in nanotechnology?
    a. Forms physical barrier
    b. Provides moisture
    c. Remove excess exudates
    d. Form layers
20. NC gels are also known as?
    a. Nanocomposite hydrogels
    b. Nanocompost hydrogels
    c. Nanocolloid hydrogel
    d. Nanocare hydrogels
21. Properties of hydrogels
    a. Hydrophilicity
    b. Hydrophobicity
    c. Lipiphilicity
    d. Lipophobicity
22. Benefits of metal nanoparticles
    a. Ease of use
    b. Thermoliable
    c. More frequent dressing changes
    d. Prevent parasitic infection
23. Product containing nanoparticles
    a. Silver
    b. Gold
    c. Metal
    d. All of the above

24. Nonmetal used for healing wounds with its medicinal preparation
    a. Iodine
    b. Sodium
    c. Both a and b
    d. None of the above

25. In which year was nanotechnology first introduced?
    a. 1988
    b. 1980
    c. 1947
    d. 1959

Answer Key

1.	d	**2.**	c	**3.**	d	**4.**	c	**5.**	b	**6.**	d	**7.**	c
8.	a	**9.**	b	**10.**	d	**11.**	d	**12.**	c	**13.**	d	**14.**	b
15.	a	**16.**	d	**17.**	d	**18.**	a	**19.**	d	**20.**	a	**21.**	a
22.	c	**23.**	d	**24.**	a	**25.**	d						

Long-Answer-Type Questions

1. Explain in detail the role of nanoparticles in wound healing.
2. Explain in detail pathogenesis.
3. Explain in detail the nanoparticles used in wound healing.
4. Explain in detail the role of polymeric particles.
5. Explain in detail metallic particles.
6. Explain in detail different polymeric forms.
7. Explain in detail the role of nitric oxide.

Short-Answer-Type Questions

1. Describe in detail wound healing.
2. Describe the pathogenesis of the wound.
3. Explain in detail the metallic particles of action of silver.

4. Explain in detail the particles of action of gold.
5. Explain in detail polymeric nanostructures.
6. Explain in detail nanostructures.
7. Explain in detail gelatin.
8. Explain in detail the role of coatings and scaffolds.
9. Explain in detail nanocarriers.
10. Explain in detail the role of chitosan in nanodrug delivery.

Chapter 12

Nanodrug Delivery Systems for Cosmetics

Sonia Dhiman, Ashi Mannan, Devanshi Mehta, and Thakur Gurjeet Singh

Chitkara College of Pharmacy,
Chitkara University, Punjab, India

soniadhmn6@gmail.com

Nanotechnology is a budding field that has led to breakthroughs in novel drug delivery system-based cosmetic formulations and it is relatively a new, extremely promising, and well-researched area. It has been demonstrated that nanotechnology-based cosmetics overcome the shortcomings linked with conventional products while also adding more valuable properties to a formulation. Conventional delivery techniques have been substantially supplanted by nanoemulsions, liposomes, niosomes, microemulsions, nanostructured lipid carriers, solid lipid nanoparticles, and nanospheres. Nanocosmetics and nanocosmeceuticals for dental purposes, hair, nails, skin, as well as lips have been the subject of extensive research. Additionally, the incorporation of nanoparticles increases the efficacy of formulation and customer gratification. As a result, nanocosmeceuticals are replacing many conventional cosmeceuticals. Nonetheless, nanotoxicological

Nanotechnology and Drug Delivery: Principles and Applications
Edited by Rakesh K. Sindhu

ISBN 978-981-4968-83-6 (Hardcover), 978-1-003-43040-7 (eBook)
www.jennystanford.com

investigations on nanocosmeceuticals have shown several obstacles. This chapter provides a summary of the nanotechnology-based methodologies employed in the delivery of cosmetics and cosmeceuticals, as well as the techniques used to characterize them. It describes their benefits in addition to any potential health and environmental hazards. It is an essential resource for materials scientists and pharmaceutical scientists who wish to gain a deeper knowledge of how nanotechnology is being applied to the development of the next generation of cosmetics. Finally, the purpose of this chapter is to give a brief introduction to nanocosmetics and nanocosmeceuticals and discuss how they are used in the cosmetical industry, in order to help consumers and regulators understand the benefits as well as the toxicity associated with their extended use, thereby promoting its prudent usage.

12.1 Introduction

The use of cosmetics by humans dates back a long time, and both men and women place a great value on these goods, which are mostly used for improving the appearance of the skin. These products are usually applied externally and are made up of natural or synthetic derivatives [1]. Cosmetics are defined by the United States Food and Drug Administration (USFDA) as a formulation "intended to be applied to the human body for cleansing, beautifying, promoting attractive-ness, or altering the appearance without affecting the body's structure or functions." This expansive definition encompasses any substance suggested for use as a component of a cosmetic product, with the clear exclusion of soap [2]. However, the term "cosmeceutical" is not defined in this act. According to European Union Cosmetics Directive (EUCD) cosmetics are "any substance or preparation intended to be placed in contact with the various external parts of the human body (epidermis, hair system, nails, lips, and external genital organs) or with the teeth and the mucous membranes of the oral cavity with a view exclusively or mainly of cleaning them, perfuming them, changing their appearance and/or correcting body odors and/or protecting them or keeping them in good condition" [3]. As per the Drugs and Cosmetics Act 1940 and Rules 1945 cosmetic is defined as "any article intended to be rubbed, poured, sprinkled or sprayed on, or introduced into, or otherwise applied to the human body or any part thereof for cleansing, beautifying, promoting attractiveness, or altering the appearance, and includes any article intended for use as a component of cosmetic" [4]. Regardless of the above-mentioned definitions, many countries' cosmetic definitions are substantially broader. In certain developed countries, cosmetic is considered merely beauty materials [5]. Cosmeceuticals are cosmetics that contain therapeutically active substances that have special healing properties when applied to the skin using traditional cosmetics. Dermatological disorders such as aging effects, xeroderma, melasma, rhytids, blemishes, hair shaft fracture, and other disorders are treated with these products, which have demonstrable skin and hair regenerative effects. They promise an improvement in look by bridging the gap between medications and cosmetics [6, 7]. Currently, the market for personalized care is expanding quickly, and one of the personal care industry's fastest-growing segments is cosmeceuticals [8]. Since this is the fastest-growing industry, more research, exploration, and application of nanocosmeceuticals are required. Nanocosmeceuticals' positive and negative aspects are compared in Fig. 12.1.

Nanotechnology and nanodelivery systems are cutting-edge scientific disciplines involving the design, characterization, fabrication, and use of nanoscale materials, devices, and systems (1–100 nm). Nanotechnology, which is widely recognized as a game-changer, is the subject of intensive research in the cosmetics and cosmeceuticals industries [9, 10]. The inclusion of nanotechnology has led to improvements in cosmetic science, which have raised global consumer demand [11]. Nanomaterials are rapidly gaining popularity in this industry since they offer more advantages than conventional cosmetics. In addition, various nanomaterial combination holds the greatest contribution to the expansion of the global pharmaceutical and cosmetics arena. According to estimates, the global market for nanomaterials was worth USD 8.5 billion in 2019 and is expected to increase by up to 13.1% annually from 2020 to 2027 [12]. Even though gold and silver nanoparticles have been used in cosmetics for a while, the number of applications has grown recently.

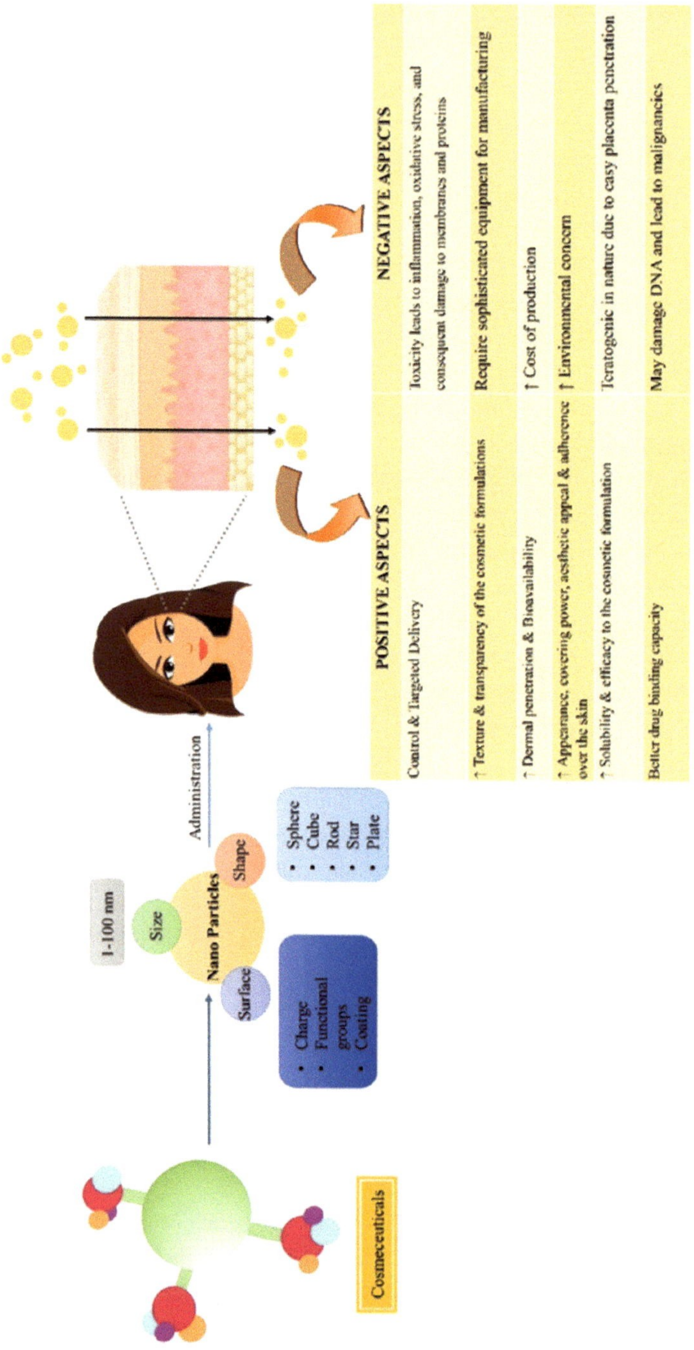

Figure 12.1 Nanocosmeceuticals' positive and negative aspects.

12.2 The Benefits and Limitations of Nanodrug Delivery Systems for Cosmetics

Cosmetic manufacturers use nano-sized components to improve a variety of characteristics, including enhanced sun protection factor (SPF)-based sun protection, tinted color texture, deeper skin permeability, prolonged stay effect, and delayed skin aging effects. Controlling active ingredient delivery, target-specific, and increasing drug-loading potential are ways to lengthen the duration of action. All of these reasons contribute to their rising consumer acceptance, necessitating scientific investigations to resolve safe usage issues. Anti-aging medications have frequently been made using nanocosmeceuticals. The products used for skincare, hair, and nails, among other things, are effectively promoted with the claim that they promote hair growth, protect hair shaft fracture, and improve the hydrating potential of skin and hair, hence enhancing the efficacy of cosmetic goods [13, 14]. In terms of stability, scalability, toxicity, expense, and so on, they have various disadvantages. Moreover, nanomaterials' toxicological and safety profiles are nowadays a matter of controversy. Nanoparticles interact better with their microenvironment because they are small, have a lot of surface area, and have a positive charge on their surface. The dosage of an active substance has a bigger impact on its bioavailability than its physicochemical properties [15]. In the case of beauty products, one of the primary issues associated with the creation of nanoformulations is that they may increase the concentration of active compounds entering the circulation, hence influencing toxicity.

12.3 Novel Nanocarriers for Cosmetic Drug Delivery Systems

12.3.1 Liposomes

Liposomes are most frequently used in cosmetic products which have a vesicular structure comprising a hydrophilic core surrounded by-layer of lipids. The fundamental lipid ingredient of liposomes are generally phospholipids, which are considered to have lesser harmful consequences [16]. Liposomes encapsulate the medicine and release its active elements in a regulated manner to prevent metabolic breakdown [17]. Liposomes may transport both hydrophobic and hydrophilic substances and has a unilamellar/multilamellar structure. Its particle size is > 20 nm [18]. In order to increase the physical and chemical stability of liposomes when distributed in water, antioxidants including carotenoids, CoQ10, and lycopene as well as active ingredients like vitamins A, E, and K have been included [19]. The essential component of liposomes is phosphatidylcholine, which is used in skincare and hair products, such as moisturizing creams, shampoos, and conditioners, because of its certain properties such as emollient and hair-smoothening potential. Numerous cosmeceuticals employ liposomes because they retain the active ingredient and are biocompatible as well as non-toxic [20]. Vegetable phospholipids are extensively utilized in cosmetics and dermatology as they contain a high concentration of esterified fatty acids. Due to this property, they are commonly employed for cosmetics meant for dermatological applications. Following the application of linoleic acid, the skin's barrier function improves rapidly and water loss diminishes. Due to their surface activity, vegetable and soy phospholipids are used to generate liposomes. These phospholipids are responsible for linoleic acid delivery into the skin [21, 22]. From the clinical studies [23] data, it has been observed that liposomes aid in the lessening of rhytid and have other beneficial benefits, such as lowering acne and enhancing skin smoothness. Liposomes are being used in cosmetic formulations such as antiperspirants, deodorants, body sprays, lipsticks, skin lotions, sunscreen, anti-aging creams, anti-alopecia agents, and skin-brightening creams.

12.3.2 Niosomes

Niosomes, a multilamellar or unilamellar structure are generated from the bilayer organization of surfactant macromolecules [24, 25]. The diameter ranges from 10 to 3000 nm [26]. Niosomes are prepared using nonionic surfactants like Tweens, Spans, Brijs, sorbitan ester, alkyl amides, polyoxyethylene alkyl ether, crown ester, and steroid-linked surfactants [27]. Niosomes transport hydrophilic as well as lipophilic drugs. Niosomes are a revolutionary medication delivery mechanism [28] for drugs that have poor permeation. They encapsulate the drug, which prolongs the drug's duration in systemic circulation and enhances its tissue penetration. Niosomes eliminate the disadvantages of liposomes, including instability, high cost, and oxidation susceptibility [29]. They are used in cosmetic and dermatological products because of their capacity to reversibly diminish the horny layer's barrier resistance, enabling the active component to penetrate the living tissues more swiftly. Numerous factors influence noisome formation, including surfactant nature and type, the characteristic of the drug, the composition of the lipid membrane, as well as parameters that affect the shape and size of niosomes [30]. Proniosomes are niosomes made up of nonionic surfactant vesicles that are immediately hydrated to generate niosome dispersions. Moreover, they are also employed to enhance medication delivery [31, 32].

Through the study and development of synthetic liposomes, L'Oréal prepared the production of niosomes in 1970. In 1987, L'Oréal patented niosomes and marketed them under the trade name Lancome. Numerous marketed niosomes cosmetic formulations are antirhytid creams, moisturizing and skin whitening creams, and anti-alopecia shampoos and conditioners.

12.3.3 Solid Lipid Nanoparticles

At the beginning of the 1990s, solid lipid nanoparticles (SLN) were introduced as an effective substitute for standard lipoidal carriers. Solid lipid nanoparticles range in size from 50 to 1000 nm [33]. They consist of a single layer of shells surrounding an oily or lipoidal center. A matrix drug is a form of drug delivery system in which the drug is homogenously dispersed or dissolved in the solid core which is made up of solid lipids or combinations of solid lipids. The hydrophobic chains of phospholipids are incorporated into the lipid matrix. They have a composition of complex glyceride mixtures, waxes, lipids, and triglycerides [34]. Active compounds that are lipophilic, hydrophilic, and poorly water-soluble can be coupled with physiological and biocompatible lipids to generate SLNs. By preparing SLN using biocompatible chemicals, toxicity concerns are minimized [35]. The two most common techniques for preparing SLNs are homogenization under high pressure and precipitation. It is possible to achieve prolonged release of active pharmaceutical ingredients (API) using this technology.

SLN with a drug-enriched core exhibits sustained release, whereas SLN with a drug-enriched shell demonstrates burst release [36, 37]. They have proved to be prominent in nanocosmetics because they are constituted of lipids (biodegradable) with minimal toxic effects. Due to their nanoscale size, they easily penetrate the skin's outer layer, hence enhancing the skin permeation of drugs [38].

Because SLNs are resistant to UV rays and function as physical sunscreens on their own, they can provide enhanced photo-protection with fewer negative effects when paired with molecular sunscreen [38]. To enhance UV protection, solid lipid nanoparticles are being produced as carriers for 3,4,5-trimethoxybenzoylchitin and vitamin E sunscreen [38]. SLNs have an occlusive feature that can be exploited to enhance skin moisture [39]. SLNs are also employed in perfume compositions since they delay the perfume's release over a longer length of time and are perfect for day creams [40, 41]. They have greater coalescence stability than liposomes due to their solid form and the restricted movement of incorporated API preventing their leakage from the drug delivery system.

12.3.4 Nanostructured Lipid Carriers

Nanostructured lipid carriers (NLCs) are nanocarriers that belong to second-generation nanoparticles consisting of lipid carriers, surfactants with nanostructures. They were developed to address the shortcomings of SLN [42, 43]. On the basis of formulation composition and production parameters, NLCs are divided into three types: imperfect, amorphous, and multiple emulsion type [44]. The usual diameter of NLCs falls between 10 and 1000 nm.

In recent years, there has been significant scientific and commercial interest in NLC due to the lower likelihood of systemic side effects. NLC has a greater drug-loading capability for entrapped bioactive chemicals than SLN due to its twisted shape. NLC formulation addresses other SLN issues, such as particle concentration and drug ejection during storage. They consist of biodegradable and physiological lipids with a low level of toxicity [45]. The modified drug delivery profile of NLC is characterized by a specialized pattern of drug release in which a sudden burst eventually leading to constant-rate continuous drug flow is achieved. Their occlusive qualities promote skin hydration, and their small size enables faster drug penetration across the stratum corneum. There is increased UV protection with fewer adverse effects, as well as steady drug integration during storage. In October 2005, the first products containing lipid nanoparticles, NanoRepair Q10® cream and NanoRepair Q10® serum, were released to the cosmetics market by Dr. Rimpler GmbH, Germany, giving greater skin penetration [46].

12.3.5 Nanoemulsions

Nanoemulsions are liquid dispersions that are kinetically or thermodynamically stable and comprise an oil phase, a water phase, and a surfactant. Depending on the manner of preparation, their structure can be altered to create a range of goods. On the basis of their composition, oil in water, water in oil, and bicontinuous nanoemulsions are the three varieties of nanoemulsions. They range in size from 50 to 200 nm. This is a dispersed phase consisting of nanodroplets with minimal oil/water interfacial tension [47]. They possess a hydrophobic core which is surrounded by a phospholipid monomolecular layer making them more appropriate to transport hydrophobic substances.

With nanoemulsions, flocculation, coalescence, sedimentation, and creaming are not issues, as they are with macromolecules. Nanoemulsions exhibit low viscosity, strong kinetic stability, a wide interfacial area, and a high solubilization capacity [48]. They have been commonly employed in cosmeceuticals (sunscreens, deodorants, lotions, nail enamels, shampoos, hair serums, and conditioners) as delivery vehicles [49]. Nanoemulsions are utilized in the formulation of cosmetics to offer quick penetration into stratum corneum, to transfer API, and to hydrate the skin. Gold nanoparticles are tiny gold particles with a diameter between 1 and 100 nm, and are known as colloidal gold when dispersed in water. The size range of gold nanoparticles or nanogold lies between 5 and 400 nm. The interaction between particles as well as the aggregation of nanogold particles are crucial for defining their characteristics [50]. They include nanospheres, nanoshells, nanoclusters, nanorods, nanostars, nanocubes, branching nanotriangles, and nanotriangles. Nanogold particles' resonance frequency is significantly affected by their shape, size, ambient conditions, and dielectric characteristics. Due to aggregation, the hue of nanogold ranges from red to violet to nearly black [51]. Natural inert gold nanoparticles are highly stable, biocompatible, and noncytotoxic. Nanogold is nonbleaching following membrane staining and is available conjugated and unconjugated [52]. Additionally, it is available in conjugated and unconjugated forms. Since they have nano-sized sphere particles, wide surface area, and crystallinity, they contain high drug-loading capacity and can easily penetrate skin cells [53].

Because of nanogold particles' potent antifungal as well as antibacterial activity, they are considered a promising candidate in cosmetics. Cosmetic companies like L'Oréal and L'Core Paris are using gold nanoparticles to make more effective creams and lotions. Increased blood circulation, anti-inflammatory qualities, antibacterial capabilities, improved skin firmness and elasticity, slowing the aging process, and revitalizing skin metabolism are some of the key benefits of nanogold in beauty care [54].

12.3.6 Nanospheres

Nanospheres are solid particles that have a spherical structure with a core-shell configuration. Their diameter lies below 200 nm. The medicine is shielded against chemical and enzymatic destruction by being entrapped, dissolved, connected, or encapsulated in nanospheres. The medication is physically and evenly disseminated in the polymer matrix system. In nature, nanospheres can be either crystalline or amorphous [55]. Because it can transform drugs with poor bioavailability, penetrability, and low solubility into effective pharmaceutical as well as cosmetic products, this technology has a lot of promise. Nanospheres can contain enzymes, DNA, and medicines in their cores [56].

The two types of nanospheres are biodegradable as well as nonbiodegradable in nature. Gelatin, starch (modified), and albumin nanospheres are all biodegradable, with polylactic acid being the sole acceptable polymer. Nanospheres have been explored in dermatological products and cosmetics for transferring API deeper into the stratum corneum layer accurately and efficiently. These minute pieces are helpful in preventing actinic aging. Nanospheres are increasingly being used in cosmetics, particularly in dermatological formulations including anti-acne, moisturizing, and antirhytid creams.

12.3.7 Dendrimers

Dendrimers are multivalent nanoparticles with bulbous, micellar nanostructures that are extensively branched and unimolecular. A dendrimer is usually made up of a core onto which one or more series of arborescent engrafted branches are grafted, and it exhibits a spherical three-dimensional morphology [57]. The presence of numerous series branches depicts the dendrimer's generation. They are tiny, with dimensions ranging from 2 to 20 nm [58]. Its additional characteristics, such as polyvalence, monodispersity, and stability, make them an attractive drug delivery carrier. For targeting reasons, terminal groups are changed to attach biologically active compounds. Drugs are both integrated into the interior and connected to the surface of dendrimers, allowing for regulated release from the inner core [59]. Dendrimers are a novel type of macromolecular architecture that is being employed in hair, skin, and nail care as nanotechnology-based cosmeceuticals. Dendrimers can be found in shampoos, sunscreens, hair styling gels, and anti-acne treatments, among other cosmetics.

12.3.8 Carbon Nanotubes

Carbon nanotubes (CNTs) are one of the most innovative nanotechnology innovations. They are made up of rolled graphene that has been hybridized with SP2. These are hollow cylindrical threads with graphene walls constructed as a hexagonal carbon lattice, rolled at specified and distinct "chiral" angles. Individual carbon nanotubes form "ropes" that are organically kept together by π-stacking. Their size ranges between 0.7 and 50 nm [60, 61]. CNTs are extremely small and light. Single-walled (SW), double-walled (DW), and multiwalled (MW) CNTs are the three varieties of carbon nanotubes. SW-CNTs comprise a 1–2 nm diameter graphene sheet (single rolled), DW-CNTs are composed of 2 concentric CNTs, and MW-CNTs comprise multiple layers of 2–50 nm diameter graphene tubes [62]. Laser ablation, arc discharge, flame synthesis, chemical vapor deposition, and silane solution are the most common CNT production processes.

12.3.9 Polymersomes

Polymersomes are artificial vesicles made up of block copolymer amphiphiles that self-assemble around a core aqueous cavity. They can be employed for both lipophilic and hydrophilic medicines because they have a hydrophilic inner core and a lipophilic bilayer, while the hydrophobic core generates a protein-friendly environment [63]. Polymerases are exceedingly versatile and biologically stable. Biodegradable or stimuli-responsive block copolymers can simply alter their drug encapsulation and release capabilities. The radius ranges from 50 nm to 5 micrometers or more [64]. Drugs, proteins, peptides, enzymes, DNA, and RNA fragments can all be encapsulated and protected by polymerases. In most cases, synthetic block copolymers have been employed to make polymersomes. Polymersomes with varied characteristics, responsiveness to stimuli, membrane thickness, and permeabilities can be generated since the composition and molecular weight of these polymers can be modified [65, 66]. They can target and control medication release thanks to the flexibility of the polymersome membrane. Because they have a thick and rigid bilayer, they are more stable than liposomes.

12.3.10 Cubosomes

Cubosomes are advanced nanoparticles that have a discrete structure with sub-micron-sized crystalline particles. Cubosomes are generated when aqueous lipid and surfactant solutions are combined in a precise ratio with water and a microstructure [40].

They are a bicontinuous cubic liquid phase in which two distinct regions of water are separated by surfactant-controlled bilayers and wrapped into a three-dimensional, periodic, and minimum surface, resulting in a densely packed structure [41].

Cubosomes have a honeycomb-like (cavernous) structure and have a slightly round appearance. Their diameter is between 10 and 500 nm, and they can incorporate all natural compounds (like lipophobic, lipophilic, and amphiphilic). They offer bioactive compounds having sustained and prolonged release with site-specificity [44, 45]. Cubosomes offer an appealing option for cosmetic products. Thus several cosmetics manufacturers are researching them.

The nanocarriers for cosmetics drug delivery systems are shown in Fig. 12.2.

12.4 Major Nanocosmeceuticals

The fastest-growing section of the personal care market is cosmetic pharmaceuticals. In nail, hair, lip, and skin care, a vast array of nanocosmeceuticals is used.

12.4.1 Skin Care

Cosmeceuticals for skin care products are used in the treatment of lichenification (skin texture). They augment the protection of the skin by increasing collagen production and ameliorating the production of reactive oxygen species (free radicals). Also, they possess the property to rejuvenate the skin by preserving the keratin. Nanoparticles of zinc oxide (ZnO) and titanium dioxide (TiO_2) are efficient in sun protective lotions for skin protecting by reaching stratum basale, rendering all products less oily, odorous, and transparent. Because they produce a thin film of humectants and retain moisture for an extended length of time, SLNs, nanoemulsions, liposomes, and niosomes are often employed in moisturizing formulations. Nanocosmeceutical anti-aging solutions that contain liposomes, nanocapsules, nanospheres as well as nanosomes, demonstrate benefits like collagen restoration, enhancing skin texture, skin firming, and tightening.

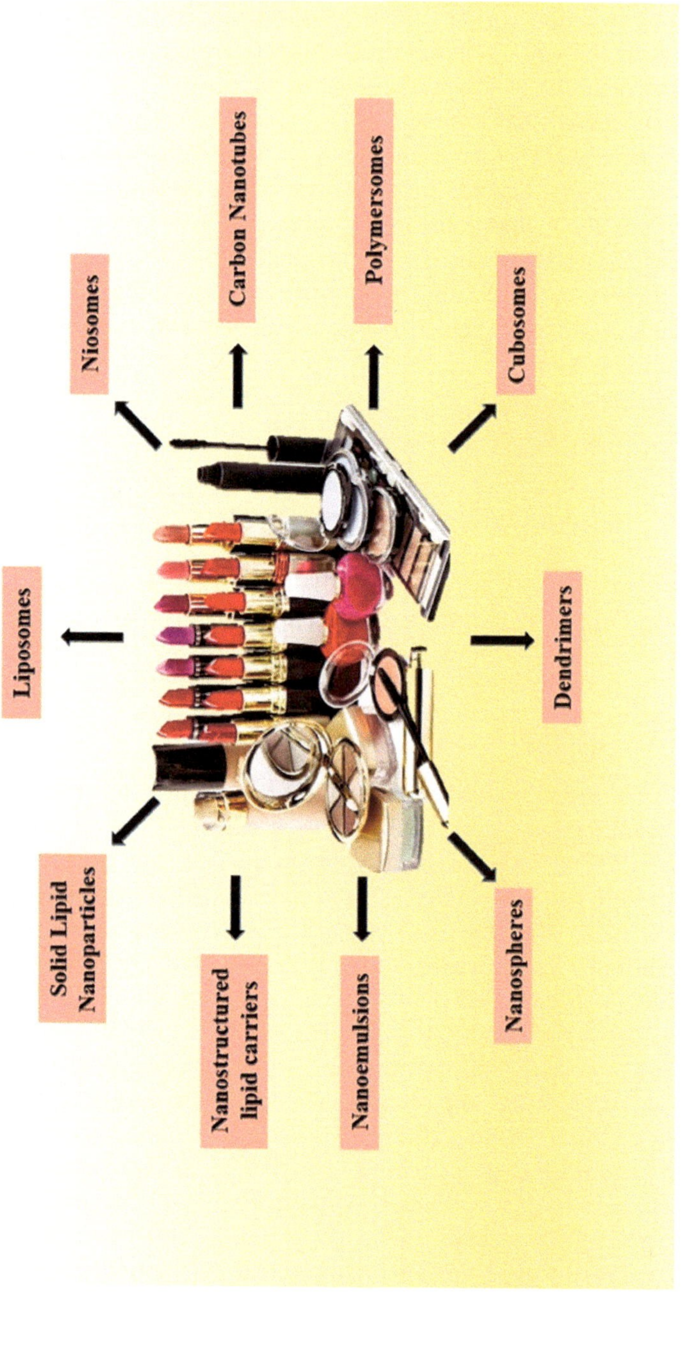

Figure 12.2 Nanocarriers for cosmetics drug delivery systems

12.4.2 Hair Care

Nanocosmeceutical goods for hair include shampoos, conditioning agents, hair growth boosters, coloring, and style treatments. Nanoparticles' inherent features and size make it possible to target hair follicles and shafts with an increased amount of active substance. By extending resident contact time with the scalp and hair follicles and generating a protective film, nanoparticles in shampoos trap moisture within the cuticles. The objective of conditioning nanocosmeceutical compounds is to add softness, sheen, silkiness, and gloss while also facilitating hair detangling. Novel carriers, including niosomes, microemulsions, nano-emulsions, nanospheres, and liposomes, play a crucial role in mending damaged cuticles, restoring texture and gloss, and making hair nongreasy, lustrous, and less brittle.

12.4.3 Lip Care

The nanocosmetics for lip care items include lipstick, balm, gloss, oil, and volumizer. A variety of nanoparticles can be used in lip gloss and lipstick to soften the lips by minimizing transepidermal water loss, as well as to prevent pigments from migrating from the lips and prolong the retention of lip color. Lip volumizer using liposomes augments lip volume, moisturizes and defines the lips, and fills in lip contour lines.

12.4.4 Nail Care

Nanocosmeceutical-based nail care solutions are superior to conventional ones. As a result of nanotechnology, nail polishes have advantages such as rapid drying, durability, chip resistance, and application simplicity. In order to improve the treatment of onychomycosis, medicated nail lacquer formulations like silica-coated silver nanoparticles have been created for efficient drug delivery of antifungals.

12.5 Characterization

12.5.1 Biological Evaluation of Nanocarriers

After nanocarriers have been well characterized, effectiveness and safety testing can be conducted [62]. Utilizing efficacy tests to evaluate its performance. Nanocarrier cellular toxicity is measured by cell viability and other safety studies [63, 64]. *In vitro* release and skin permeation/penetration assays are routinely employed as efficacy tests [9, 11, 13, 31]. Assays such as cell uptake [65, 66], antioxidant activity [67], moisturizing impact [62], and nanoencapsulated chemical content [68] are frequently utilized as efficacy assessments. Because *in vitro* release simulates the discharge of a chemical, it is commonly utilized. Typically, nanocarriers outperform conventional formulations (lacking nanocarriers), hence promoting the release of the nanoencapsulated material [69]. In addition, nanocarriers display a burst release followed by a continuous release [11, 13, 21, 31, 35]. This longer effect is advantageous because it minimizes the frequency of product reapplications. Moreover, the release characteristics of each nanocarrier vary to some degree [11, 21]. (for instance, see [21]) Consequently, it is conceivable, depending on the objective, to prepare NLC instead of SNL to enhance substance release. Alterations in nanocarrier constituents can also modulate biological effects. Quantitative differences in the nanocarrier composition affect the *in vitro* release and moisturizing impact [13]. The purpose of skin penetration/permeation investigations is to identify the position of a substance in the skin layers (penetration) and/or its presence in the receptor media (skin permeation) [5, 36]. In the same manner as *in vitro* release experiments influence skin distribution profiles, nanocarrier type influences skin distribution profiles. Nanoemulsions have a lower skin retention rate than NLC. Permeation may occur in nanoemulsions as well [6, 11]. They enable better skin penetration than conventional formulations, regardless of the kind of nanocarrier [8]. Permeation (detection in the bloodstream) is undesired in cosmetic products, whereas penetration/retention in the epidermis or dermis is desirable [8].

Table 12.1 Characterization parameters for nanocarriers

S.No	Parameter	Features
1	Physical-chemical	Particle size, particle morphology, surface area, pore diameter, agglomeration behavior, solubility, and other chemical properties such as molecular formula, chemical structure, final composition of nanomaterial, phase distinctiveness, and hydrophilic-lipophilic nature
2	Mathematical modeling	Simple, empirical algorithms to complex mathematical equations
3	Microscopic techniques	Particle-induced x-ray emission laser scanning confocal microscopy, radio labeling with positron emitter 45 V, high-resolution transmission electron microscopy
4	*In vitro* methods	Dermal absorption measurements on human/pig skin, phototoxicity testing via the 3T3NPRT, MM, and WEX, *in vitro* mammalian cell gene mutation test, genotoxicity/mutagenicity testing, Epskin or Epiderm, *in vitro* micronucleus test or *in vitro* mammalian chromosomes aberration test, skin corrosion testing via TER, embryotoxicity testing via three tests EST, skin irritation testing via Epiakin

It is also worth noting that nanoencapsulating vegetable components help them stay in the epidermis and dermis longer [5, 9, 35]. This study is significant because it assures the improved efficacy of vegetable elements loaded with nanocarriers, which is important given the growing popularity of natural substances in cosmetics [5]. Cell uptake is a study that confirms the location/ deposition of nanoencapsulated compounds on the skin in addition to skin permeation. Nanoencapsulation of vegetable components alters their skin distribution and enables skin retention, as revealed by confocal microscopy [38]. Additionally, increasing cellular absorption with nanocarriers with a positive electrical charge (CSLN) is an approach [68]. Cell viability, on the other hand, is, as previously said, a safety test. Nanosystems can be hazardous to cells and tissues, therefore verifying their safety is crucial. Nanocarriers with low cytotoxicity are deemed safe [11, 25, 26]. Other efficacy tests show that nanocarriers outperform. Nanoencapsulation increases the antioxidant activity of vegetable components [12, 26]. Nanocarriers also aid in skin moisturization [10, 34], with the moisturizing impact varying depending on the carrier makeup [10]. Entrapped compounds' photostability is increased by nanocarriers, which impacts their antioxidant activity. Because light degrades less of a material, more of it is accessible to act as an antioxidant [11, 24]. Characterization parameters for nanocarriers are shown in Table 12.1.

12.5.2 Biological Evaluation of Nanocosmetics

Nanocosmetics are evaluated using the same assays as nanocarriers, such as penetration/skin permeation, skin moisturization, and antioxidant activity. For semi-solid forms, other tests such as the sun protection factor (SPF) and ultraviolet A protection factor (UVA-PF) are utilized [31]. Substance buildup in skin layers and, if any, permeation are governed by skin penetration/permeation. Penetration and/or permeation will be desirable depending on the type of product. Antioxidants are better absorbed through the epidermis and dermis [69]. Furthermore, nanocosmetics components alter skin permeation/penetration, regardless of whether they are nanocarrier or semi-solid form substances [25]. Nanocosmetics have been demonstrated to retain and penetrate the skin better than traditional cosmetics [26]. SPF and UVA-PF efficacy tests are used to assess UVB and UVA protection, respectively [70]. In these tests, nanocosmetics outperformed conventional cosmetics. Cosmetics with varied quantitative compositions of nanocarriers have varying SPF and PF-UVA values [71]. Nanoencapsulation also increases UV protection (for example, see [16]). UV protection has also been achieved using nanocosmetics containing vegetable oil associations [12]. Moisturizing impact is routinely studied *in vitro* [19, 26] or in people [18, 20], and is a key component in moisturizing and anti-aging cosmetics [20]. Because of their adhesive capabilities, composition [18, 20], and semi-solid vehicle composition [17], cosmetics containing lipid nanocarriers have moisturizing effects. After irradiation, nanocosmetics retain antioxidant action. Once endogenous antioxidants are reduced by UV radiation exposure, these nanocosmetics can be employed as anti-aging cosmetics [26]. Another significant test is skin toxicity evaluation, which aims to detect any irritation induced by nanocosmetics [19]. Photo-stabilization is another benefit of nanocosmetics. Nanocosmetics can help nanoencapsulated substances last longer [23]. The biological efficiency of multifunctional nanocosmetics can also be improved [72]. Furthermore, a trend toward more complicated cosmetics that include nanocarriers, inorganic nanoparticles, and traditional cosmetic chemicals (without the use of nanotechnology) [73] has emerged.

12.6 Major Challenges of Using Nanomaterials for Cosmetic Applications

Nanoparticles have been discovered to cause a wide range of health and environmental problems in individuals and the environment. The toxicity of nanomaterials is determined by their attributes, which include their smaller size, chemical composition, surface structure, solubility, shape, and aggregation. Some of the causes of nanotoxicity are listed below:

12.6.1 Smaller Size of Nanoparticles

The microscopic size of nanoparticles distinguishes them. This can alter their physicochemical properties, allowing for enhanced absorption and interaction with biological tissues when compared to their bigger counterparts. Toxicity refers to the production of reactive oxygen species such as free radicals, which cause oxidative stress, inflammation, and damage to proteins, membranes, and DNA. These nanoparticles can easily enter the bloodstream via skin or inhalation and be delivered to multiple organs due to their small size. The large dose and long residence time of nanoparticles in important organs can cause malfunction. Carbon nanotubes have been found to kill kidney cells and stop them from growing further. Even at low dosages and without UV exposure, 20 nm titanium dioxide particles can totally damage super-coiled DNA, but 500 nm titanium dioxide particles have just a limited ability to produce DNA strand breaking. Mice treated with 2–5 nm TiO_2 nanoparticles demonstrated a significant but moderate inflammatory response, according to another study [74].

12.6.2 Shape of Nanoparticles

Nanoparticles come in a range of sizes, including spheres, tubes, sheets, and other shapes, which may contribute to the health hazards they represent. A study discovered that exposing the abdominal cavities of mice to long carbon nanotubes caused abdominal wall inflammation [75].

12.6.3 Surface Area of Nanoparticles

As the particle's size reduces, its surface area increases, enhancing its reactivity. Nanomaterials are extremely reactive due to their high surface area-to-mass ratio, which provides more surface area per weight for chemical reactions to occur. Due to their heightened reactivity, some nanoscale particles may be potentially explosive and/or photoactive, according to studies. If finely dispersed in air and come into touch with a sufficiently potent ignition source, several nanomaterials, such as nanoscale titanium dioxide and silicon dioxide, may explode [76].

12.6.4 Penetration of Nanoparticles via Skin

According to scientific studies, nanoparticles can permeate the skin, especially when the skin is flexed. Broken skin allows particles as small as 7000 nm to penetrate directly. Acne, eczema, and wounds may increase the absorption of nanoparticles into the bloodstream, which may lead to additional issues. A preliminary investigation found that psoriasis-affected skin was more permeable to nanoparticles than healthy skin. Recently, base carriers have been changed to promote skin penetration by integrating physical and chemical penetration enhancers and by producing novel vesicular systems, such as ethosomes and transferosomes, with enhanced skin penetrability. Additionally, bending and massaging the skin can aid nanoparticle penetration. According to one study [37–39], when skin is flexed, particles as small as 1000 nm can be absorbed through unbroken skin and reach living cells.

12.6.5 Cellular Toxicity of Zinc Oxide and Titanium Dioxide Nanoparticles

In a study, Minghong Wu and colleagues from Shanghai University found that zinc oxide (ZnO) nanoparticles found in sunscreens can injure or destroy stem cells in the brains of mice. To examine the possible neurotoxicity of ZnO nanoparticles, Wu et al. cultured mouse neural stem cells (NSCs) and treated them with zinc oxide nanoparticles ranging in size from 10 to 200 nm. After 24 h, the cell viability test demonstrated that ZnO nanoparticles exhibited harmful effects on NSCs that were dose-dependent but not size-dependent. Using confocal microscopy, transmission electron microscopy, and flow cytometry, a large number of NSCs exhibited apparent apoptotic characteristics. This toxicity of zinc oxide nanoparticles was found to be induced by zinc ions dissolved in the culture media or within the cells. The NN Research Group's Arnaud Magrez discovered that titanium dioxide-based nanofilaments were cytotoxic, which was affected by their shape and increased by the presence of surface defects created by chemical treatment. Internalization of nanofilaments and morphological alterations of cells have been observed [40–41, 77].

12.6.6 Route and Extent of Exposure

Human health concerns caused by nanoparticles depend on the route and degree of exposure to these substances. Nanomaterials generally enter the body through three routes.

12.6.6.1 Inhalation

According to the National Institute of Occupational Health and Safety, this is the most common method of nanoparticle exposure. If adequate safety devices are not employed, workers may inhale nanoparticles while manufacturing them, and consumers may inhale nanomaterials while using products using nanomaterials, such as spray versions of sunscreens containing nanoscale titanium dioxide. Officials from the National Institutes of Health report that while the vast majority of inhaled particles reach the pulmonary tract, animal studies suggest that certain inhaled nanomaterials may travel via the nasal nerves to the brain and get access to the blood, neurological system, and other organs.

12.6.6.2 Ingestion

Nanomaterials can be swallowed via hand-to-mouth transfer or purposeful intake. The bulk of nanoparticles quickly depart the body after intake; but, a tiny proportion may be retained and move to organs.

12.6.6.3 Through skin

Studies have demonstrated that some nanoparticles can permeate pig skin within 24 h of exposure. Studies analysed by the US Government Accountability Office (GAO) have raised concerns about the potential for sunscreen nanoparticles to penetrate the damaged skin [42–46].

12.6.7 Environmental Risks of Nanoparticles

The release of nanomaterials into water, air, and soil during the production, use, and disposal of these materials also endangers the environment. If these nanoparticles are antibacterial and discharged in sufficient amounts, they could potentially interfere with beneficial bacteria in sewage and wastewater treatment plants and contaminate water intended for reuse, according to several of the research evaluated by the US GAO. For instance, investigations have demonstrated that TiO_2 nanoparticles are harmful to the primary body systems of rainbow trout. In a study conducted by the University of Toledo, researchers revealed that nano-titanium dioxide used in personal care products inhibited the biological roles of bacteria after less than an hour of exposure. These findings suggest that these particles, which end up in municipal sewage treatment plants, could eradicate bacteria with crucial functions in ecosystems while also aiding in wastewater treatment. Carbon fullerenes have been reported to cause brain damage in largemouth bass, a species used as a model for defining ecotoxicological consequences by regulatory bodies. It has also been discovered that fullerenes are bactericidal and destroy water fleas. According to the Center for Biological and Environmental Nanotechnology at Rice University, nanoparticles have a propensity to bind to environmental contaminants, such as cadmium and petrochemicals. This property makes nanoparticles a potential pathway for the long-distance and extensive transfer of contaminants in groundwater. Several studies indicate that nanoparticles have the potential for biomagnification. An interdisciplinary team of UC Santa Barbara researchers produced a groundbreaking discovery about the biomagnification of nanoparticles in a basic microbial food chain.

The use of nanoparticles in cosmetics offers both advantages and problems, as with any other practice. Since nanoparticles have unique features compared to bulk materials, they may be able to modify biological traits. Consequently, research on nanoparticle toxicity is required. There is currently no consensus about the effect of particle size, shape, charge, particle interactions with biological cells, and linkages with toxicity and safety concerns. Due to their unique features, nanoparticles are employed in a wide variety of applications. On the other hand, it is hypothesized that these features are the basis for nanoparticle-induced toxicity, which results from the complex interaction between nanoparticle uniqueness (e.g., size, shape, surface chemistry, and charge), administered dose, and host immunity. Changes in these qualities may influence interactions between nanoparticles and biomolecules, proteins, cell lines, and tissues. It is essential to examine the intracellular activity and function of nanoparticles in order to produce effective and safe aesthetic nanoparticles.

It has been discovered that nanoparticles are highly reactive, resulting in the generation of a higher number of ROSs. Nanoparticles are capable of penetrating many barriers in the human body and affecting multiple systems, including the blood, respiratory system, and skin. These reactive oxygen species have an effect on macromolecules such as proteins, DNA, and cell membranes. Nanoparticles may be harmful to human cells and tissues, leading to the death of cells. Widely utilized TiO_2 nanoparticles have an effect on cell DNA because they generate ROS, which enhances the oxidative stress of fibroblast cells. The effect of photoactivated TiO_2 nanoparticles on skin fibroblast cells and nucleic acids. Titanium dioxide and zinc oxide nanoparticles absorb UV radiation and generate skin-damaging free radicals. This may lead to cellular damage and skin cancer. In addition to their size, the chemical composition of nanoparticles has an effect on the human system. The lungs of rats injected with nanoparticles exhibited certain inflammatory symptoms, and lung tumors were observed as a result. The danger posed by nanoparticles might vary based on the nature of the hazard and the extent of exposure. Brain impairment was observed in male progeny of pregnant mice exposed to TiO_2 nanoparticles. Traces of TiO_2 have long-lasting impacts on the brain. When considering cosmetics, the mode of exposure, topical application, is incapable of causing the type of exposure (inhalation) required to induce such harm. It was found when the method of application was changed to aerosols. The primary problem with cosmetics is that they can penetrate the skin and enter the bloodstream. Nanoparticles can transport cosmetics' active ingredients to the deeper layers of the skin. These compounds may cause irritation in humans. In addition to the beneficial impacts of nanomaterials on cells, their unfavorable consequences have also been explored. Aluminum oxide and iron oxide were evaluated for their toxicity *in vitro*. The ability of the free radicals created by aluminum oxide nanoparticles to induce concentration-dependent stem cell toxicity and inflammation, which may lead to illnesses such as atherosclerosis, was investigated. In addition, they compromised the blood-brain barrier and were directly neurotoxic to brain blood vessel cells.

The benefits of utilizing nanoparticles are frequently illustrated. Uncertainty surrounds the risks, health risks, and environmental problems linked with nanoparticle exposure. When nanoparticles are absorbed through the skin, respiratory tract, brain, and other organs, they can cause harm (via blood). It has been demonstrated that certain nanoparticles have detrimental effects on the brain. Current knowledge regarding the safety of nanoparticles is inadequate. There is a need for studies focusing on synthesis processes, characteristics, *in vitro* and *in vivo* safety assessments, and dose determinations.

Components of cosmetic products must be safe for use, and the items themselves must be labeled as such. The FDA is responsible for authorizing products for sale. Utilized cosmetics should be pure and effective, with no additives. In this context, the FDA has issued a distinct set of safety guidelines for the use of nanoparticles in cosmetics, titled "Guidance for Industry: Safety of Nanomaterials in Cosmetic Products." This document gives an overview of the safety risks posed by the use of nanoparticles in cosmetics and proposes to aid interested companies in identifying and evaluating significant safety measures [69–77].

12.7 Conclusions and Future Direction

Nanotechnology is currently recognized as a new and promising field, and it is utilized and valued in sectors such as cosmetics, cosmeceuticals, dermatology, biomedical applications, etc. Cosmetics and cosmeceuticals are more popular as a result of recent innovations and novel drug delivery techniques, which contribute to their growing market share. In addition, the incorporation of nanotechnology into cosmetics has expanded global acceptance. However, the toxicity linked with its penetrability is a serious worry that is often disregarded, resulting in negative health effects. Currently, innovative nanocarriers such as liposomes, ethosomes, cubosomes, NLC, SLNs, nanoemulsions, and niosomes are used to generate enhanced cosmetics and cosmeceuticals. Using several methods, nanosystems carry and administer these formulations over the skin, giving a variety of benefits such as UV protection, moisturization, wrinkle reduction, etc. Despite the fact that these nanomaterial-based products are gaining significant market value, there is a great dispute regarding their human safety and toxicity, necessitating further investigation. Therefore, cosmetic regulation should offer a detailed list of references and substances that produce unexpected environmental consequences for all users of cosmetic products, including consumers and professionals, to ensure the safety of cosmetic product use. Before these products are commercialized, toxicological or carcinogenicity studies should be conducted on cosmetics, including nanocosmetics and nanocosmeceuticals (and their constituents). Nanocosmeceuticals should be created so that they improve the health of customers. In addition, clinical trials similar to those undertaken for pharmaceuticals should be conducted to ensure the human safety of cosmeceutical formulations. Furthermore, the production, storage, import, and marketing of cosmeceuticals and nanoparticles included within them should be subject to stringent laws. To develop standard guidelines and regulations for the use of nanosystems in cosmetics and to help fill in current data gaps, researchers and global regulatory bodies must work together on a worldwide scale. Government agencies and non-governmental organizations should work together to develop and distribute effective consumer education materials. To educate people on the safe use of cosmetics including nanocosmetics and nanocosmeceuticals, they should develop customized programs, including written and video materials, multimedia, and seminars. In conclusion, there is a need for international regulatory harmonization in order to build a stronger regulatory framework for safety, efficacy, and marketing, which would eventually benefit the cosmetic industry while safeguarding consumers from any dangers. Additionally, customer awareness can aid in the improvement of the problem by enabling educated product selection.

Manufacturers of cosmetics utilize nanoscale compounds to improve UV protection, skin penetration, long-lasting effects, color intensity, and finish quality, among other benefits. Micellar nanoparticles are the new era of cosmetics being increasingly commercialized and attracting interest in both domestic and international markets. The ability of the nanoemulsion technology to generate small micellar nanoparticles with a large surface area enables the efficient delivery of bioactive components to the skin. Makeup removers, facial cleansers, anti-aging lotions, sunscreens, and other water-based cosmetic formulations all contain nanoemulsions of oil in water. The objective of this review is to investigate critically the properties, advantages, and production mechanisms of micellar nanoparticles in nanoemulsion systems. Consequently, this paper presents and examines the special advantages of a nanoemulsion system in the creation of micellar nanoparticles for cosmetics formulation, which are crucial aspects for the future development of micellar-based cosmetic segments.

References

1. Jones G. Globalization and beauty: a historical and firm perspective. *Entrep Multinatl* 2013; 41: 57–76.
2. Roberts R. Cosmetics marketing & industry trends: a 2020 ecommerce report on the state of online beauty. *Common Thread Collect* 2020.
3. Nozaki F. General aspects of cosmetics in relation to science and society: social, cultural, science, and marketing aspects. In: Sakamoto K, Lochhead RY, Maibach HI, Yamashita Y, eds, *Cosmetic Science and Technology: Theoretical Principles and Applications,* Elsevier 2017.
4. Tadros TF. Future developments in cosmetic formulations. *Int J Cosmetic Sci* 1992; 14(3): 93–111.
5. Farris PK, ed, *Cosmeceuticals and Cosmetic Practice.* Chichester, UK: Wiley 2013. p. 295.
6. Li BS, Cary JH, Maibach HI. Science behind cosmetics and skin care. In: Cornier J, Keck CM, Van de Voorde M, eds, *Nanocosmetics,* Cham: Springer International Publishing 2019. pp. 3–15.
7. Chen J, Dong X, Zhao J, Tang G. *In vivo* acute toxicity of titanium dioxide nanoparticles to mice after intraperitioneal injection. *J Appl Toxicol* 2009; 29: 330–337.
8. Claude O, Brigitte R. Engineered nanoparticles current knowledge about OHS risks and prevention measures, chemical substances and biological agents, Studies and Research Projects, REPORT R-656. (Last accessed on 2010). Available from: http://www.irsst.qc.ca/media/documents/PubIRSST/R-656.pdf.
9. Matthew C. Environmental health news, Nanoparticles from sunscreens damage microbes, scientific american. [Last accessed on 2009]. Available from: http://www.scientificamerican.com/article.cfm?id=nanoparticles-insunscreen&page=2.
10. Glaser DA. Anti-aging products and cosmeceuticals. *Facial Plast Surg Clin North Am* 2004; 12(3): 363–372.
11. Hu ZM, Liao Y, Chen et al. A novel preparation method for silicone oil nanoemulsions and its application for coating hair with silicone. *Int J Nanomed* 2012; 7: 5719–5724.
12. Bethany H. Zapping nanoparticles into nail polish: Laser ablation method makes cosmetic and biomedical coatings in a flash. *Chem Eng News* 2017; 95(12): 9.

13. Pereira L, Dias N, Carvalho J, Fernandes S, Santos C, Lima N. Synthesis, characterization and antifungal activity of chemically and fungal-produced silver nanoparticles against T richophytonrubrum. *J Appl Microbiol* 2014 Dec; 117(6): 1601–1613.
14. Singh P, Nanda A. Nanotechnology in cosmetics: a boon or bane? *Toxicol Environ Chem* 2012 Sep 1; 94(8): 1467–1479.
15. Bernauer U, Bodin L, Chaudhry Q, Coenraads PJ, Dusinska M, Gaffet E, Panteri E, Rogiers V, Rousselle C, Stepnik M, Vanhaecke T. SCCS Guidance on the Safety Assessment of Nanomaterials in Cosmetics- SCCS/1611/1. 2019.
16. Rosen J, Landriscina A, Friedman AJ. Nanotechnology-based cosmetics for hair care. *Cosmetics* 2015 Sep; 2(3): 211–224.
17. Kushwaha N, Minocha N, Kumar N. Use of nanotechnology in cosmeceuticals: a review. *Int J Pharm Sci Invent* 2020; 9: 43–51.
18. Smijs TG, Pavel S. Titanium dioxide and zinc oxide nanoparticles in sunscreens: focus on their safety and effectiveness. *Nanotechnol Sci Appl* 2011; 4: 95.
19. Cornier J, Keck CM, Van de Voorde M, eds, *Nanocosmetics: From Ideas to Products*, Springer; 2019 Jun 14.
20. Santos AC, Morais F, Simões A, Pereira I, Sequeira JA, Pereira-Silva M, Veiga F, Ribeiro A. Nanotechnology for the development of new cosmetic formulations. *Expert Opin Drug Deliv* 2019 Apr 3; 16(4): 313–330.
21. Ammar HO, Ghorab MM, Mostafa DM, Ibrahim ES. Folic acid loaded lipid nanocarriers with promoted skin antiaging and antioxidant efficacy. *J Drug Deliv Sci Technol* 2016 Feb 1; 31: 72–82.
22. Vickers NJ. Animal communication: when i'm calling you, will you answer too? *Curr Biol* 2017 Jul 24; 27(14): R713–R715.
23. Bose S, Michniak-Kohn B. Preparation and characterization of lipid based nanosystems for topical delivery of quercetin. *Eur J Pharm Sci* 2013; 48: 442–452.
24. Salunkhe SS, Bhatia NM, Pokharkar VB, et al. Topical delivery of Idebenone using nanostructured lipid carriers: evaluations of sunprotection and anti-oxidant effects. *J Pharm Invest* 2013; 43: 287–303.
25. Puglia C, Bonina F, Rizza P, et al. Lipid nanoparticles as carrier for octyl-methoxycinnamate: *in vitro* percutaneous absorption and photostability studies. *J Pharm Sci* 2012; 101: 301–311.

26. Puglia C, Damiani E, Offerta A, et al. Evaluation of nanostructured lipid carriers (NLC) and nanoemulsions as carriers for UV-filters: characterization, *in vitro* penetration and photostability studies. *Eur J Pharm Sci* 2014; 51: 211–217.

27. Mitri K, Shegokar R, Gohla S, et al. Lipid nanocarriers for dermal delivery of lutein: preparation, characterization, stability and performance. *Int J Pharm* 2011; 414: 267–275.

28. FDA. Final guidance for industry—safety of nanomaterials in cosmetic products. online: https://www.fda.gov/media/83957/download2014 (accessed on 14 April 2020).

29. European Union Observatory for Nanomaterials (EUON). online: https://euon.echa.europa.eu/ (accessed on 26 April 2020).

30. Nafisi S, Maibach, HI. *Nanotechnology in Cosmetics, in Cosmetic Science and Technology*, Sakamoto K, Lochhead RY, Maibach HI, Yamashita Y, eds, Elsevier: Amsterdam, The Netherlands, 2017; pp. 337–369.

31. Sankhyan A, Pawar PK. Metformin loaded non-ionic surfactant vesicles: optimization of formulation, effect of process variables and characterization. *Daru* 2013; 21(1), 7.

32. Pastrana H, Avila A, Tsai, CSJ Nanomaterials in cosmetic products: the challenges with regard to current legal frameworks and consumer exposure. *Nano Ethics* 2018; 12, 123–137.

33. Fytianos G, Rahdar A, Kyzas, GZ Nanomaterials in cosmetics: recent updates. *Nanomaterials* 2020; 10, 979.

34. Dhapte-Pawar V, Kadam S, Saptarsi S, Kenjale, PP Nano-cosmeceuticals: facets and aspects. *Futur. Sci. OA* 2020; 6, FSO613.

35. Loo CH, Basri M, Ismail R, et al. Effect of compositions in nano-structured lipid carriers (NLC) on skin hydration and occlusion. *Int J Nanomed* 2013; 8: 13–22.

36. Tichota DM, Silva AC, Sousa Lobo JM, et al. Design, characterization, and clinical evaluation of argan oil nanostructured lipid carriers to improve skin hydration. *Int J Nanomed* 2014; 9: 3855–3864.

37. Barua S, Kim H, Hong SC, et al. Moisturizing effect of serineloaded solid lipid nanoparticles and polysaccharide-rich extract of root Phragmitescommunis incorporated in hydrogel bases. *Arch Pharm Res* 2017; 40: 250–257.

38. Shetty PK, Venuvanka V, Jagani HV, et al. Development and evaluation of sunscreen creams containing morin-encapsulated nanoparticles for enhanced UV radiation protection and antioxidant activity. *Int J Nanomed* 2015; 10: 6477–6491.

39. Loo CH, Basri M, Ismail R, et al. Effect of compositions in nano-structured lipid carriers (NLC) on skin hydration and occlusion. *Int J Nanomed* 2018: 1–19.

40. De AzevedoRibeiro RC, Barreto SMAG, Ostrosky EA, et al. Production and characterization of cosmetic nanoemulsions containing Opuntiaficus-indica (L.) mill extract as moisturizing agent. *Molecules* 2015; 20: 2492–2509.

41. Lacatusu I, Arsenie LV, Badea G, et al. New cosmetic formulations with broad photoprotective and antioxidative activities designed by amaranth and pumpkin seed oils nanocarriers. *Ind Crops Prod* 2018; 123: 424–433.

42. Niculae G, Lacatusu I, Badea N, et al. Rice bran and raspberry seed oil-based nanocarriers with self-antioxidative properties as safe photoprotective formulations. *Photochem Photobiol Sci* 2014; 13: 703–716.

43. Niculae G, Badea N, Meghea A, et al. Coencapsulation of butylmethoxydibenzoylmethane and octocrylene into lipid nanocarriers: UV performance, photostability and *in vitro* release. *Photochem Photobiol* 2013; 89: 1085–1094.

44. Kwon MC, Choi WY, Seo YC, et al. Enhancement of the skin-protective activities of Centellaasiatica L. urban by a nano-encapsulation process. *J Biotechnol* 2012; 157: 100–106.

45. Badea G, Lăcătuşu I, Badea N, et al. Use of various vegetable oils in designing photoprotective nanostructured formulations for UV protection and antioxidant activity. *Ind Crops Prod* 2015; 67: 18–24.

46. Contri RV, Kulkamp-Guerreiro IC, da Silva SJ, et al. Nanoencapsulation of rose-hip oil prevents oil oxidation and allows obtainment of gel and film topical formulations. *AAPS PharmSciTech* 2016; 17: 863–871.

47. Ayumi NS, Sahudin S, Hussain Z, et al. Polymeric nanoparticles for topical delivery of alpha and beta arbutin: preparation and characterization. *Drug Deliv Transl Res* 2019; 9: 482–496.

48. Netto M, Pharm G, Jose J. Development, characterization, and evaluation of sunscreen cream containing solid lipid nanoparticles of silymarin. *J Cosmetic Dermatol* 2018; 17: 1073–1083.

49. Souza C, de Freitas LAP, Maia Campos PMBG. Topical formulation containing beeswax-based nanoparticles improved *in vivo* skin barrier function. *AAPS PharmSciTech* 2017; 18: 2505–2516.

50. Baccarin T, Lemos-Senna E. Potential application of nanoemulsions for skin delivery of pomegranate peel polyphenols. *AAPS PharmSciTech* 2017; 18: 3307–3314.

51. Kaul S, Gulati N, Verma D, Mukherjee S, Nagaich U. Role of nanotechnology in cosmeceuticals: a review of recent advances. *J Pharm* 2018; 2018: 1–19.

52. Sonneville-Aubrun O, Yukuyama MN, Pizzino, A. Application of nanoemulsions in cosmetics. In Jafari SM, McClements DJ, eds, *Nanoemulsions*, Academic Press: Cambridge, MA, USA, 2018; pp. 435–475.

53. Carrouel F, Viennot S, Ottolenghi L, Gaillard C, Bourgeois, D. Nanoparticles as anti-microbial, anti-inflammatory, and remineralizing agents in oral care cosmetics: a review of the current situation. *Nanomaterials* 2020; 10, 140.

54. Revia RA, Wagner BA, Zhang, M. A portable electrospinner for nanofiber synthesis and its application for cosmetic treatment of alopecia. *Nanomaterials* 2019; 9, 1317.

55. Singh S, Pandey SK, Vishwakarma, N. Functional nanomaterials for the cosmetics industry. *Handbook Funct Nanomater Ind Appl* 2020; 717–730, https://doi.org/10.1016/B978-0-12-816787-8.00022-3.

56. Raj S, Jose S, Sumod US, Sabitha, M. Nanotechnology in cosmetics: opportunities and challenges. *J Pharm Bioallied Sci* 2012; 4: 186–193.

57. Kaul S, Gulati N, Verma D, Mukherjee S, Nagaich, U. Role of nanotechnology in cosmeceuticals: a review of recent advances. *J Pharm* 2018; 3420204.

58. Santos AC, Morais F, Simões A, Pereira I, Sequeira JAD, Pereira-Silva M, Veiga F, Ribeiro, A. Nanotechnology for the development of new cosmetic formulations. *Expert Opin Drug Deliv* 2019; 16: 313–330.

59. Dhawan S, Sharma P, Nanda, S. Cosmetic nanoformulations and their intended use. In *Nanocosmetics*; Elsevier: Amsterdam, The Netherlands, 2020.

60. Souto EB, Fernandes AR, Martins-Gomes C, Coutinho TE, Durazzo A, Lucarini M, Souto SB, Silva AM, Santini, A. Nanomaterials for skin delivery of cosmeceuticals and pharmaceuticals. *Appl Sci* 2020; 10: 1594.

61. Ghasemiyeh P, Mohammadi-Samani, S. Potential of nanoparticles as permeation enhancers and targeted delivery options for skin: advantages and disadvantages. *Drug Des Devel Ther* 2020; 14: 3271–3289.

62. Joshi H, Hegde AR, Shetty PK, et al. Sunscreen creams containing naringenin nanoparticles: formulation development and *in vitro* and *in vivo* evaluations. *Photodermatol Photoimmun Photomed* 2017; 34: 69–81.

63. L'enabrunet, Delinay L, Ernestm H, Pedroj JA, Markr W. Comparative photoactivity and antibacterial properties of C60 fullerenes and titanium dioxide nanoparticles. *Environ Sci Technol* 2009; 43: 4355–4360.

64. Abla MJ, Banga AK. Formulation of tocopherolnanocarriers and *in vitro* delivery into human skin. *Int J Cosmet Sci* 2014; 36: 239–246.

65. Külkamp-Guerreiro IC, Terroso TF, Assumpção ER, et al. Development and stability of innovative semisolid formulations containing nanoencapsulatedlipoic acid for topical use. *J Nanosci Nanotechnol* 2012; 12: 7723–7732.

66. Oberdörster G, Oberdörster E, Oberdörster J. Nanotoxicology: an emerging discipline evolving from studies of ultrafine particles. *Environ Health Perspect* 2005; 113: 823–839.

67. Tarl WP, Jeffrey EG, Lynlee LL, Rokhaya F, Margaret B. Nanoparticles and microparticles for skin drug delivery. *Adv Drug Deliv Rev* 2011; 63: 470–491.

68. Magrez A, Kasas S, Salicio V, Pasquier N, Seo JW, Celio M, et al. Cellular toxicity of carbon-based nanomaterials. *Nano Lett* 2006; 6: 1121–1125.

69. Donalson K, Beswick P, Gilmour P. Free radical activity associated with the surface of particles: a unifying factor in determining biological activity? *Toxicol Lett* 1996; 88: 293–298.

70. Grassian VH, O'Shaughnessy PT, Adamcakova-Dodd A, Pettibone JM, Thorne PS. Inhalation Exposure study of titanium dioxide nanoparticles with a primary particle size of 2 to 5 nm. *Environ Health Perspect* 2007; 115: 397–402.

71. Chopra H, Dey PS, Das D, Bhattacharya T, Shah M, Mubin S, Maishu SP, Akter R, Rahman MH, Karthika C, Murad W, Qusty N, Qusti S, Alshammari EM, Batiha GE, Altalbawy FMA, Albooq MIM, Alamri BM. Curcumin nanoparticles as promising therapeutic agents for drug targets. *Molecules* 2021; 26(16): 4998.

72. Rouse J, Yang J, Ryman-Rasmussen J, Barron A, Monteiro-Riviere N. Effects of mechanical flexion on the penetration of fullerene amino acid derivatized peptide nanoparticles through skin. *Nano Lett* 2007; 7: 155–160.

73. Ryman-Rasmussen J, Riviere J, Monteiro-Riviere N. Penetration of intact skin by quantum dots with diverse physicochemical properties. *Toxicol Sci* 2006; 9: 159–165.

74. Kaewamatawong T, Kawamura N, Okajima M, Sawada M, Morita T, Shimada A. Acute pulmonary toxicity caused by exposure to colloidal silica: particle size dependent pathological changes in mice. *Toxicol Pathol* 2005; 33: 743–749.

75. Schulte P, Geraci C, Zumwalde R, Hoover M, Kuempel E. Occupational risk management of engineered nanoparticles. *J Occup Environ Hyg* 2008; 5: 239–249.

76. Chen-yu G, Chun-fen Y, Qi-lu L, et al. Development of a Quercetinloaded nanostructured lipid carrier formulation for topical delivery. *Int J Pharm* 2012; 430: 292–298.

77. Wu W, Samet JM, Peden DB, Bromberg PA. Phosphorylation of p65 Is required for zinc oxide nanoparticle–induced interleukin 8 expression in human bronchial epithelial cells. *Environ Health Perspect* 2010; 118: 982–987.

Multiple-Choice Questions

1. Under which US authority do cosmetics fall?
   a. United States Drug Act
   b. Food and Drug Administration
   c. United States Cosmetics Administration
   d. United States Food and Drug Administration (USFDA)
2. Liposomes help in the transport of
   a. Hydrophilic drugs
   b. Hydrophobic drugs
   c. Cationic drugs
   d. Both hydrophilic and hydrophobic drugs
3. Niosomes are used for drugs that have
   a. Molecular weight less than 400 Da
   b. Poor permeation rates
   c. Hydrophilic or hydrophobic characteristics
   d. Both b and c

4. Preparation of solid lipid nanoparticles is mainly done through
   a. Hot melt extrusion method
   b. Emulsion method
   c. Homogenization under high pressure and precipitation
   d. Solvent evaporation method
5. Out of the following which is not a NLC category?
   a. Perfect type
   b. Imperfect type
   c. Amorphous type
   d. Multiple type
6. Nanostructured lipid carriers are better than solid lipid nanoparticles in terms of
   a. Size and shape
   b. Confirmation
   c. Drug-loading capacity
   d. Stability
7. Which of the following does not belong to the classification of nanoemulsion?
   a. Oil in water
   b. Water in oil
   c. Multiple emulsion
   d. Bicontinous nanoemulsion
8. Drug entrapped within nanospheres is shielded against
   a. Enzymes
   b. Chemicals
   c. Microenvironment
   d. Both a and b
9. If a dendrimer has 3 series, it would be called
   a. 3 dendrimers
   b. 3rd generation dendrimer
   c. 3rd dendrimer
   d. None of the above

10. Carbon nanotubes may not be structurally
    a. Single-walled carbon nanotubes
    b. Double-walled carbon nanotubes
    c. Triple walled carbon nanotubes
    d. Multiwalled carbon nanotubes
11. In most cases, which type of polymers could be employed in the production of polymersomes?
    a. Copolymers
    b. Synthetic block copolymers
    c. Natural copolymers
    d. None of the above
12. Structurally cubosomes have two water layers separated by
    a. Lipophilic layer
    b. Hydrophilic bilayer
    c. Surfactant-controlled bilayer
    d. Surfactant layer
13. What is the API in sunscreens that prevent the sunrays from going deep into the skin layers?
    a. Zinc oxide
    b. Zinc dioxide
    c. Titanium dioxide
    d. Both a and c
    e. Both b and c
14. In nail nanocosmeceuticals, which metal provides antifungal properties?
    a. Silver
    b. Gold
    c. Copper
    d. Zinc
15. Which one has the highest retention rate?
    a. Nanolipid carriers
    b. Nanoemulsion
    c. Liposomes
    d. Cubosomes

16. What are the characterization parameters for nanocarriers?
    a. Physicochemical
    b. Invitro drug release
    c. Mathematical modeling
    d. Microscopic evaluation
    e. All of the above
17. What is the major advantage of nanotechnology?
    a. Biostabilization
    b. Loading capacity
    c. Increased surface area
    d. Optimization
18. Which sections of nano production are covered under the Drugs and Cosmetics Act, 1940?
    a. Import
    b. Production
    c. Storage
    d. Marketing
    e. All of the above
19. Titanium dioxide has a damaging action on the
    a. DNA
    b. Mitochondria
    c. Fibroblasts
    d. Both a and b
    e. Both a and c
20. What guidelines have been laid down by the FDA for nanocosmeceuticals?
    a. Drug and Cosmetics Act 1945
    b. Guidance for Industry: Safety of Nanomaterials in Cosmetic Products
    c. Guidelines for the Safety of Nanocosmeceuticals
    d. There is no such guideline

Answer Key

1.	d.	**2.**	d.	**3.**	d.	**4.**	c.	**5.**	a.	**6.**	c.	**7.**	c.
8.	d.	**9.**	b.	**10.**	c.	**11.**	b.	**12.**	c.	**13.**	d.	**14.**	a.
15.	a.	**16.**	e.	**17.**	a.	**18.**	e.	**19.**	e.	**20.**	b.		

Short-Answer-Type Questions

1. What are the benefits and limitations of nanodrug delivery systems for cosmetics?
2. Elaborate nanostructured lipid carriers (NLC) with examples.
3. What is the use of gold nanoparticles in cosmetics? Give a few examples.
4. What are dendrimers?
5. What are the different types of carbon nanotubes (CNT)?
6. Why are polymersomes better than liposomes?
7. How are solid lipid nanoparticles beneficial for nano-cosmeceuticals?

Long-Answer-Type Questions

1. Elaborate on various novel nanocarriers for cosmetic drug delivery systems.
2. Explain various characterizations of nanocarriers used in cosmetics.
3. Highlight the major challenges of using nanomaterials for cosmetic applications.
4. Discuss major nanocosmeceuticals.
5. Describe the applications of nanocarriers in cosmetic products.

Chapter 13

Novel Drug Delivery System for Rectal and Vaginal Targets

Shaima K. A.,[a] Astha Mishra,[b] M. Arockia Babu, Sarita Jangra,[c] and Rakesh K. Sindhu[d]

[a]*Shambhunath Institute of Pharmacy,*
Utthan Campus, Jhalwa, Paryagraj, Uttar Pradesh, India
[b]*Optometry department, Chitkara School of Health Sciences,*
Chitkara University, Punjab, India
[c]*Department of Pharmacy Practice,*
Chitkara College of Pharmacy, Chitkara University, Rajpura, Punjab, India
[d]*School of Pharmacy, Sharda University,*
Greater Noida, Uttar Pradesh, India

rakeshsindhu16@gmail.com

The drugs can be absorbed both locally and systemically through the vaginal and rectal route, which is a possible location for drug administration. More control over the distribution of drug molecules for local and systemic actions has been made possibly by the development of novel rectal drug delivery, including hollow-type suppositories, thermo-responsive and mucoadhesive liquid suppositories, and nanoparticulate systems. The use of mucoadhesive or bioadhesive polymers, pH or temperature-sensitive polymers, liposomes, nanoparticles, vaginal inserts, multiple emulsions, and hydrogels have all been developed to overcome the limitations of conventional dosage forms

Nanotechnology and Drug Delivery: Principles and Applications
Edited by Rakesh K. Sindhu

ISBN 978-981-4968-83-6 (Hardcover), 978-1-003-43040-7 (eBook)
www.jennystanford.com

administered through the vaginal route. These approaches enabled controlled and prolonged drug release. The potential of rectal and vaginal drug delivery systems may be unlocked through ongoing study and development in this area of drug delivery. The present chapter is a comprehensive review of novel approaches to rectal and vaginal drug delivery.

13.1 Introduction

Drug delivery is defined as the method of administering a drug to the human body to achieve its therapeutic effect. There are two types of drug delivery systems, conventional/traditional and novel drug delivery systems (NDDS). Researchers invented NDDS to reduce undesired effects and maximize therapeutic benefits by maintaining the concentration of a drug in the therapeutic window. Novel drug delivery systems are defined as a new approach that combines innovative development, formulations, new technologies, and new methodologies for delivering pharmaceutical compounds into the body as needed to safely achieve their desired therapeutic effects. It may include scientific site targeting within the body, improving drug potency, and controlled drug release with prolonged therapeutic effect. It involved the development of a novel, better and safer drug with a long half-life and therapeutic indices.

The most practical way to administer medication is orally. However, there are situations when this isn't possible from a clinical or pharmaceutical standpoint. In these situations, the rectal or vaginal route may be a viable alternative, as it can be utilized to deliver medications with both local and systemic effects. The rectal and vaginal routes were utilized to deliver medications with both systemic and local effects on the human body.

The research on NDDS has been under way for a long time, but it has intensified in the past couple of years. The development of several types of NDDS in the past few decades includes microparticles, nanoparticles, niosomes, and liposomes with the motive of delivering drugs to the targeted tissue to cure certain diseases.

Contraceptive suppositories made of crocodile excrement, honey, and sodium carbonate were one of the most intriguing compositions mentioned in ancient writings. Another historic source for vaginal prescription is the Papyrus Ebers (approximately 1550 BC), explaining acacia tips and honey-soaked lint-based contraceptive tampons. Gum arabic was traditionally obtained from the acacia bush. After a tampon was inserted, the gum generated lactic acid, acidifying the vagina [1–3]. Lactic acid is now a widely used and well-known spermicidal ingredient in contemporary contraceptive creams as well as gels [4, 5]. It is important to note that by the 15th century, drugs that can infiltrate the systemic circulation after being administered vaginally had been already discovered. The vaginal use of arsenic or other toxic drugs to cause suicide or abortion was a frequent, if heinous, practice [6].

The vaginal canal serves a variety of activities, including sexual functions, but it also plays a role in active immunologic and anatomically mediated processes that are critical for maintaining a microenvironment that is appropriate for "normal" bacteria [7, 8]. Many studies have shown that the vaginal environment contains various immune-related cells and receptors that aid the microbial environment. Community state types (CSTs) refer to the five major forms of vaginal microbes. The predominant species throughout four of them is *Lactobacillus* spp. (CST-I, -II, -III, -V); CST-IV, on the other hand, is made up of a combination of facultative anaerobes such as *Gardnerella*, *Autopodium*, and *Prevotella*. Depending on the ethnic background, the incidence of various CSTs varies.

The quantity of blood arteries in the vaginal region is a distinct advantage, particularly when it comes to systemic formulations. There are various advantages to vaginal administration over oral administration. These include dose decrease, less frequent dosing, fewer adverse effects, and no hepatic first-pass impact. However, several obstacles must be overcome, such as peristaltic movement of the vaginal wall or dilution of the vaginal fluid [9–16].

The most prevalent vaginal abnormalities include mucoid ectopy, aerobic vaginitis, candidiasis, bacterial vaginosis, cervicitis atrophic vaginitis, and desquamative inflammatory vaginitis. The most common vaginal infection in women between the ages of

15 and 44 is bacterial vaginosis (BV), according to statistics from the Centers for Disease Control and Prevention. In 2004, the frequency of BV in women in the United States was estimated to be around 21.2 million in the United States [17–20]. The second most common vaginal infection is candidiasis. Vulvar or vaginal malignancies are examples of other vaginal disorders. They are generally regarded as being rare; in 2017, vaginal cancer was diagnosed in 0.7 of every 100,000 women, and 2.6 per 100,000 women were diagnosed with vulvar cancer. The fact that the circumstances in the vaginal canal are extremely unstable must be taken into account while designing a vaginal formulation. Sexual activity, menstrual cycle, comorbid conditions, and patient age all have significant effects on acidity, vaginal fluid flow, and epithelial thickness [21–24].

Various types of natural or synthetic polymers are used in most vaginal medication delivery methods. Their primary responsibility is to ensure that the drug remains in contact at the site of action for as long as feasible, as well as to deliver a controlled drug release on a consistent and predictable basis. A wide range of vaginal medication delivery devices are now in use or being researched. Examples of these include patches, films, rings, suppositories, tablets, capsules, gels, creams, foams, pellets, microparticles, and nanoparticles. According to certain research changes in the normal composition and functions of vaginal flora are involved in the development of numerous vaginal disorders. Currently, vaginal formulations are used to administer drugs with a localized action, including antibiotics [25–29], spermicides [30, 31], and antimycotics [32], as well as to introduce pharmaceuticals into the systemic circulation [33–35], primarily for hormone therapy or contraception [36, 37]. Microbicides delivered vaginally to prevent HIV [38, 39], human papillomavirus (HPV) [40–42], or herpes simplex virus (HSV) [43–45] transmission are also attracting a lot of attention. Every year, more than 10 million people are affected by disorders of the female reproductive tract (FRT). Itching, burning, soreness, irregular bleeding, discharge, discomfort, and dyspareunia are common non-specific symptoms, and they cause significant distress in patients. Most of the above, however, have been linked to vaginal dermatoses, and allergic and irritating reactions.

Clinically, the rectal route is already being used to deliver several medicines for both local and systemic disorders. Constipation, hemorrhoids, anal fissures, inflammation, and hyperkalemia can all be treated locally. Pain, fever, nausea and vomiting, migraines, allergies, and drowsiness are all treated with rectal formulations for systemic medication distribution [46]. These rectal formulations are primarily used for short-term therapy and are based on traditional dosage forms like suppositories and enemas. Rectal dose forms can be produced at a lower cost than parenteral dosage forms and can be delivered by patients themselves without the assistance of a medical professional (e.g., intramuscular and intravenous injections). This is especially beneficial for rural populations and poor countries when it comes to certain pharmaceuticals that cannot be provided through other means. Patients, on the other hand, do not like the rectal route of administration due to cultural concerns and/or the risk of discomfort and leaking [47].

Standard treatment options are extensive and primarily consist of systemically injected antimicrobial medicines, while topical therapies may also be provided. Women who received intravaginal antimicrobial drugs were happier with their treatment than those who received oral antimicrobial agents in some clinical trials comparing oral and topical antimicrobial medicines [48, 49]. In addition, gastrointestinal problems and candida infection are caused by various oral antimicrobial medications. Furthermore, poor oral therapy adherence might lead to treatment failure, which can lead to recurrence or drug resistance. Intravaginal therapies, on the other hand, have several benefits, including the ability to bypass first metabolism, the convenience of administration, and fewer adverse effects. Studies have revealed that the vaginal route for drug administration is underutilized, and as a result, major attempts have been undertaken to improve this potential delivery method [50, 51] for both local and systemic effects. In fact, in recent years, researchers have looked into systemic vaginal absorption of a variety of therapeutic compounds (proteins, small interfering

RNAs, peptides, vaccines, oligonucleotides, antigens, and hormones) [52].

To date, a variety of topical dosage forms for vaginal drug delivery have been proposed, including lotions, aerosols, gels, creams, suppositories, ovules, and tablets, but their effectiveness is severely limited by poor permeability across the vaginal wall and rapid removal from the vaginal canal, which is further influenced by the presence of hormones. As a result, to compensate for the quick removal of the drug carrier, numerous and frequent local doses are required, resulting in an increase in drug side effects and a decrease in patient compliance. For these reasons, vaginal medication administration remains a difficulty, and the development of innovative effective local treatments that can remain in place and release active agents for an extended length of time is gaining traction [53–84].

The goal of this chapter is to provide the physiological and pharmacological factors that influence vaginal and rectal medication distribution, as well as a thorough examination of current advancements in vaginal and rectal medication delivery systems, identifying the most widely researched study areas, as well as assessing future trends and potential obstacles in rectal and vaginal medication delivery research.

13.2 Polymer-Based Vaginal Formulations

To have a localized impact or reach the systemic circulation when given a drug intravaginally, it must get past physiological and anatomical barriers. The drug form must also possess unique properties. For instance, it is necessary to adopt appropriate drug release parameters, have a longer transit time at the site of action, and guarantee mucosal adherence. Mucoadhesive preparations depending on the appropriate polymers are particularly intriguing and appear to have the most potential for vaginal medicine administration. This category includes both the pharmaceutical forms, such as tablets, creams, suppositories, and films, and also the new therapeutics forms, such as rings, nanoparticles, and films [85]. Classification of the vaginal dose forms is depicted in Fig. 13.1.

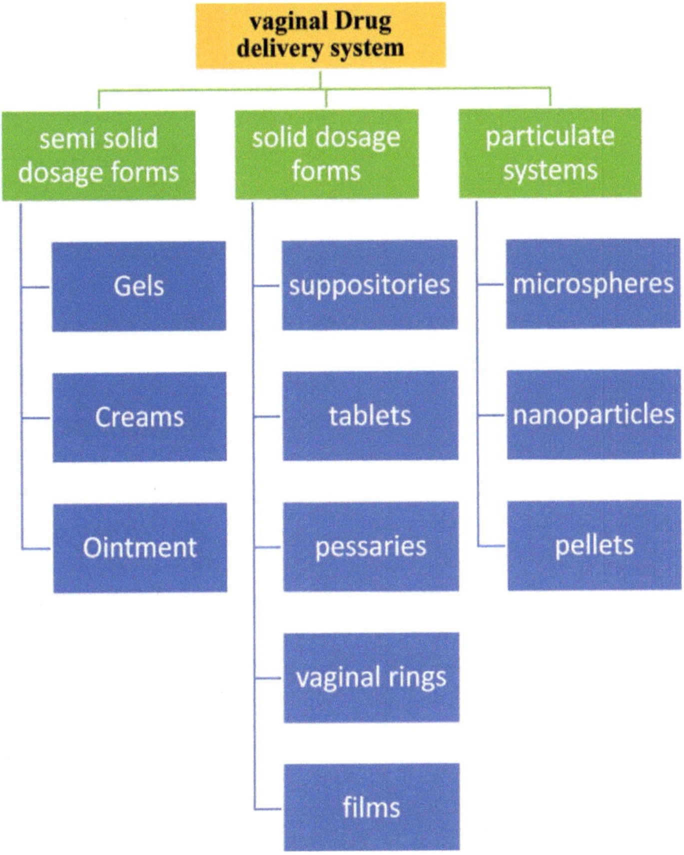

Figure 13.1 Classification of the vaginal dose forms.

13.2.1 Semisolid Formulations

Gels, creams, and ointments are semisolid formulations for vaginal usage [86, 87]. These systems have several advantages, including high acceptability, ease of usage, and reasonable production costs. Semisolid systems, on the other hand, are seen as troublesome due to the leakage, discomfort following application, messiness, and a short post-administration residence period, all of which could cause a lower efficacy. In order to boost the clinical effect experienced with vaginal semisolid products, frequent administration is occasionally required, which may be regarded as inconvenient [87, 89]. Another method involves using mucoadhesive polymers to improve interactions with the mucosal membrane and lengthen the time spent in the vaginal canal. According to certain studies, using eco-friendly polymers to increase the formulation viscosity after administration is a viable option. When the product comes into touch with vaginal conditions, it transforms from liquid to semisolid. Acceptability by patients is a significant factor in the administration and effectiveness of vaginal products. Patients prefer semisolid dosage forms over vaginal rings and vaginal suppositories because they are more convenient to apply [88, 90].

It is worth noting, however, that patient acceptability is a complicated topic that can be influenced by a variety of cultural, social, and other factors [91]. One of the areas of vaginal drug administration that have recently received the most attention is the development of devices with antiviral agents put into them as prospective HIV and sexually transmitted diseases (STD) preventive drugs. Dosing frequency was found to be the most important element influencing patients' preferences and choices in these goods [92]. Semisolids' limited retention time is mentioned as the major disadvantage in this regard [93].

13.2.1.1 Gels

Although gels are used in many scientific and non-scientific fields, it can be challenging to define a gel and other approaches to explain these systems exist as well. Gels are defined by Almdal et al. [94] as "solid, solid-like, soft materials comprised of two or more elements." One of the elements is liquid, and it is much more plentiful than the other one. Gels have unusual rheological features. It is also important to note that this definition excludes heterogeneous materials.

According to Rogovina et al. [94], a flexible solid made up of two or more components is known as a gel. The other is a three-dimensional network, while the first is a liquid. The type of gel depends on the kind of bonds that are present in the network. Strong covalent connections hold chemical gels together, whereas hydrogen bonds hold physical gels together. Low molecular weight gelators can also be utilized as the network-forming component [95, 96]. Hydrogels are water-based liquid components, while organogels are non-aqueous liquid components.

The majority of vaginal medicine administration gels are weak physical hydrogels created utilizing gelling agents derived from polymers.

The majority of the gel-based dosage forms under investigation are used to administer antimicrobial drugs to treat vaginal illnesses such as fungal [97, 98] and bacterial [99, 100] infections. On the other hand, a lot of research is focused on how to distribute contraceptive medications effectively and how to prevent HIV transmission [101]. Clinical trials on the efficacy and safety of several gel formulations, notably containing tenofovir and dapivirine, have been performed [102]. Mucoadhesive and thermosensitive systems should be highlighted when looking at the areas of pharmaceutical technology and drug carrier optimization that have received the greatest attention.

13.2.1.2 Mucoadhesive drug delivery systems

Mucoadhesion is caused by interactions between formulation components and the mucus layer that lines the surface of the vaginal mucous membrane. Hydrophilic glycoproteins having a high glycosylation level are the most important components of mucus. Mucin subunits are joined by disulfide bridges to create massive three-dimensional gel forms [103]. Electrostatic interactions, hydrogen bonds, or van der Waals interactions are the most common way that mucoadhesive composition elements engage with mucin. As a result, the presence of a large variety of functional groups, such as carboxyl or hydroxyl, amine groups, and sulfate, is the most crucial property of mucoadhesive polymers. Additional qualities include the presence of negative and positive charges in the molecules, attractive surface properties that allow the formulation to be applied to the mucous membrane, and chain flexibility that allows the interpenetration of the polymer and mucin lattices [104].

Chitosan, a cationic linear polysaccharide produced from chitin deacetylation and recognized for antibacterial [105] and wound-healing characteristics, is one of the most widely used bioadhesive polymers. Two kinds of chitosan with different molecular weights were investigated by Bonferoni et al. [106] as carriers for mucoadhesive gels intended to release lactic acid under regulated conditions. Given the variations in the release of active elements in various mediums, it was hypothesized that lactic acid was released as a result of diffusion and ionic displacement.

Ciprofloxacin hydrochloride and acyclovir were employed as active components. The utilized chitosan derivatives' ability to inhibit proteolytic enzymes, including carboxypeptidase A and leucine amino-peptidase, was investigated. It is believed that inhibiting these enzymes will increase the transport of hydrophilic and macromolecular materials across the mucosal membrane. Despite having good penetration results in comparison to controls, there were no statistically significant differences when compared to chitosan hydrochloride. Senyiit et al. [107] used miconazole and econazole nitrates to examine chitosan-based gels. In this study, the effects of polymer molecular weight in the release of active compounds, vaginal preservation, and mucoadhesive qualities were examined. All of the formulations in the study were also tested for antibacterial characteristics. It was found that the formulation with the best vaginal medicine distribution properties was one built with a medium molecular weight polymer.

Comparative research on several polymer creams designed for the complete administration of the antimuscarinic medication oxybutynin, which is used to treat an overactive bladder, was carried out by Demiröz et al. Hydroxypropyl methylcellulose (hydroxyl propyl methyl cellulose [HPMC] K100M), poloxamer 407, and chitosan were used as thickening agents. The highest cohesion and mucoadhesion were seen in the HPMC K100M condition. Furthermore, all semisolid formulations were evaluated *in vivo* against a tablet that is typically sold. The gel made of HPMC was found to be a useful alternative to the oral formulation.

Using covalent thioglycolic acid and cysteine treatments, Cevher et al. [109] looked at chitosan and polycarbophil hydrogels. The product served as carriers for clomiphene citrate, a drug that may be used to treat infection with human papillomavirus (HPV). Polycarbophil and its thiol derivatives were shown to extend drug release up to 72 h, whereas chitosan and its derivatives only lasted 12 h, which was less than ideal for the study's goal. Furthermore, it was found that both the type of polymer and the quantity of conjugating agent utilized had a significant impact on the mechanical characteristics of the suggested systems.

Hydroxypropyl methylcellulose is another often-used mucoadhesive polymer (HPMC). Bilensoy et al. [110] synthesized hydrogels with both Carbopol 934 and HPMC as a bioadhesive agent and thermosensitive poloxamer 407 as a thermosensitive polymer. Clotrimazole, a water-insoluble antifungal drug, was used as the active ingredient. Clotrimazole's solubility was improved using an inclusion complex with cyclodextrin. Clotrimazole complexation was proven to prolong the drug's release from hydrogels. Additionally, it was noted that Carbopol-based gels were incompatible because of precipitation. It is a positive breakthrough for vaginal drug administration that gels prepared from HPMC were stable and delivered the active component for a considerable amount of time.

A study by Aka-Any-Grah et al. concentrated on developing vaginal hydrogels that could tolerate being diluted with vaginal secretions and were both thermosensitive and mucoadhesive. As thermosensitive components, Pluronic®F127 was used in the formulations under research, or Pluronic®F127 and F68 together. HPMC, a mucoadhesive agent, was utilized. According to the outcomes of an ex vivo animal model, the dilution had no impact on the mucoadhesive properties of hydrogels created using a mixture of Pluronic's. However, even after dilution, both gels maintained a gelling temperature of around 30–35°C [111–113].

13.2.1.3 Thermosensitive dosage forms

Thermosensitive gels are more accurately referred to as stimuli-responsive systems because they thicken in response to physiological conditions. The stimuli-responsive system used in vaginal medicine administration that has received the most research persists as liquid at ambient temperature and transmutes into gels at body temperature. These therapies benefit from easy vaginal administration and effective interaction with the creases and gaps of the vaginal mucous membrane.

Thermogelation produces a more viscous medium that prolongs the active component release while also enhancing retention at the administration site. The most often utilized poloxamer, poloxamer 407, is one of the most regularly used thermosensitive polymers. Typically, it is seen as helpful as an excipient in dosage forms intended for use with various routes of administration because it is non-toxic. It also exhibits beneficial thermosensitive characteristics that allow the construction of liquid systems that solidify into gels at physiological temperatures.

The formulation used as a result is therefore more resistant to the vaginal clearance mechanisms. It is worth noting that the temperature of gelation and the properties of the gel are influenced by the system's composition. Poloxamer-based methods for vaginal drug delivery have substantial drawbacks due to their poor mucoadhesive characteristics. Additional bioadhesive excipients are used to extend the medication's stay at the administration site. Liu et al. looked at the effect of adding carrageenan to an in situ vaginal gel based on poloxamer 407.

The study's goal was to develop a sustained-release formulation for the delivery of acyclovir, a common antiviral drug used as a genital herpes treatment. Due to its effectiveness in preventing HIV infections, carrageenan was recognized as a good excipient for the vaginal medication delivery system. The addition of the macromolecular component had no effect on the gelation temperature, according to rheological experiments. Carrageenan was found to slow down the *in vitro* release of acyclovir, which was also linked to a slower rate of poloxamer 407 breakdown and gel erosion. The concentration of carrageenan had an impact on the effect that was seen [114–120].

A mouse model was used to explore the residence time *in vivo*. Compared to a standard poloxamer-based gel, the carrageenan-enhanced system had a much longer residence period in the trials.

Rossi et al. investigated systems of chitosan lactate and poloxamer 407 as well as mixes of glycerophosphate and chitosan lactate. Amoxicillin trihydrate was introduced into the systems under investigation. The objective of the study was to develop thermosensitive vehicles for vaginal mucositis that gelled at physiological temperatures. It was discovered that additional macromolecules could bring the poloxamer gelation temperature up to a physiological level [121–123].

The length of the gelation of the poloxamer/chitosan lactate combination was prolonged after being diluted with simulated vaginal fluid. There was no such impact detected in the chitosan derivatives mixture. However, compared to the poloxamer-based system, the latter had worse elastic characteristics and improved bioadhesion. For vaginal administration, Zhou et al. examined thermosensitive in situ creating hydrogel with baicalein. The active component was combined with hydroxypropyl-cyclodextrin to form an inclusion complex. Benzalkonium chloride, hydroxypropyl methylcellulose (HPMC), sodium alginate, poloxamer 188, and poloxamer 407 were used to make the hydrogel vehicle.

The generated formulation gelled at a temperature appropriate for in situ vaginal gel, and medication release followed the Peppas equation, indicating an erosion-based process. In an *in vivo* study using an animal model, the evaluated systems also showed adequate efficacy. Another study by Deshkarand Palve [114] described the in situ creation of a thermosensitive gel with an integrated cyclodextrin complex based on poloxamer [123–125].

Voriconazole, an antifungal drug with poor water solubility, was used in the study as the active ingredient. Spray drying was used to obtain the drug and hydroxypropyl-beta-cyclodextrin inclusion complex in the first phase. Following that, an in situ gelling formulation was created using poloxamers 407 and 188, as well as numerous other polymers as mucoadhesive agents. The ideal gelation temperature for vaginal compositions is between 30° and 35° Celsius. Poloxamer 188 was added to boost gelation temperature, whereas mucoadhesive agents have had the reverse effect.

Hypromellose, a mucoadhesive polymer, was present in the formulation with the most favorable properties for vaginal medication delivery 0.4% of it. The modified product displayed good bioadhesive properties and a gelation temperature of 31.7 ± 0.1 °C. Additionally, it was discovered that using an inclusion complex-based gel rather than a conventional one allowed for better voriconazole uptake by tissues in *in vivo* tests.

Rençber et al. conducted a similar investigation for generating clotrimazole-loaded gels, a common antifungal drug used to treat vaginal candidiasis. At roughly 34°C, the modified poloxamer 407, poloxamer 188, and Hypromellose mixture began to turn into gel. The examined system also showed appropriate mucoadhesive characteristics and persisted at the administration site for 24 h [126–130].

13.2.2 Suppositories, Tablets, and Pessaries

For many years, traditional solid vaginal dose forms, such as globules or suppositories, have been widely used. Unfortunately, they have a number of flaws, including a proclivity for discomfort and difficult application. Due to inadequate retention of the active medicinal ingredients caused by vaginal self-cleansing or leakages, the patient may need to apply multiple dosages each day. All of the aforementioned drawbacks cause patients a great deal of inconvenience, which can lead to low adherence and a lack of therapeutic benefit.

As a result, technicians are finding it difficult to modify old formulations. The development of current vaginal tablets is based on the phenomena of mucoadhesion. Years of study have led to the development of mini-tablets, tablets, pessaries, and other formulations with extended vaginal residence, sustained API release, acceptable efficacy, and patient convenience due to the use of natural and synthetic polymers with high mucoadhesive qualities.

These compositions are used mostly to treat skin infections caused by bacteria, viruses, and fungi, and PrEP (pre-exposure prophylaxis of sexual transmission of HIV) as well as inflammations, atrophic vaginitis, and dry vagina. Medications for cancer therapy and probiotics have both been delivered via vaginal tablets. It is crucial to remember that the recommended drugs need to sustain a long vaginal retention time in order to be very effective.

Hydroxypropyl methylcellulose (HPMC) emerged as the most popular and effective polymer among all those examined. The sustained-release polymer (HPMC), a single excipient used in tablet production, has been shown by McConville et al. to deliver efficient doses of the HIV microbiocide tenofovir for up to 24 h. Perioli et al. created HPMC tablets that had good hydration properties by producing a homogenous, gelled phase as well as, most importantly, prolonged benzydamine release.

Carbopol inclusion in the formulation led to the creation of a spongy, stiff substance that was unable to guarantee the drug's linear release while having outstanding mucoadhesive capabilities. Other authors offer proof to back up the advantages of using HPMC in a polymer mix. After analyzing mixes of chitosan, HPMC, Eudragit RS, and guar gum, Notario-Pérez et al. believe that the joint properties of HPMC and chitosan are the most advantageous. Tenofovir was released from the resultant pills for 72 h, and they stayed attached to the vaginal mucosa for 96 h, indicating that they could be used to enhance HIV prophylaxis in women in underdeveloped countries [131–135].

Cevher et al. presented a very original solution. Itraconazole's solubility and antifungal activity were improved by the introduction of cyclodextrin-inclusive complexes but its toxicity increased, leading to a prolonged drug residence and effectiveness. Contrarily, when combined with Carbopol®934P, the use of HPMC, xanthan gum mucoadhesive polymers lengthened the formulation residence duration. Additionally, HPMC may be utilized as a mucoadhesive carrier for spray-dried microspheres containing clotrimazole and *Pediococcus pentosaceus* SB83, a lyophilized bacteria having antilisterial and pH-reducing activity [136].

In this preparation, the polymers sodium carboxymethylcellulose, Carbopol, and HPMC worked together to minimize burst effects when the drug came into touch with bodily fluids. This allowed for a controlled release of the medication clotrimazole. Chitosan has been found in the literature to be particularly well-suited for the creation of mucoadhesive vaginal tablets. A porcine mucin gel, vaginal mucosa, and mucin gel were used by Szymaska et al. to examine the efficacy of clotrimazole tablets produced with varying concentrations of chitosan in three distinct scenarios.

The outcomes indicated that chitosan possesses bioadhesive characteristics. Due to their stable, prolonged release of clotrimazole and prolonged stay on the vaginal tissue, formulations comprising 25% and 40% chitosan were selected as the finest applicants for further study. Chitosan's behavior could potentially change in various ways. In formulations including thiolated poly(acrylic acid)-cysteine and the nitrated of econazole and miconazole, Baloðlu et al. advised their use [137].

Synthetic polymer-containing tablets were mucoadhesive and had a high water uptake ratio. It is crucial to keep in mind that thiolating the polymer and guarding the thiol groups from oxidation with an aromatic ligand produced S-protected chitosan. In this case, a carbodiimide-mediated amide bond was used to link NAC-6-MNA to chitosan. Better mucoadhesive properties, a longer duration for metronidazole, an antiprotozoal and antibacterial medication, to be released from vaginal tablets, and improved antimicrobial activity were all benefits of S-protected chitosan [138].

In the future, pectins might be used in vaginal medication delivery systems. A Carbopol 934 and pectin (2:1) mixture, according to Baloðlu et al., could be utilized as a moisturizer in the dry vagina as well as a carrier for topical active medications. This mixture has the maximum swelling volume and mucoadhesive strength. It additionally demonstrated the least level of pH reduction. When treating vaginal infections, acid-buffering bioadhesive tablets must be used because vaginal pH is a factor to be taken into account. Mixed vaginal infections can have a pH rise as a symptom or as a cause.

To maintain pH at 4.4, a sign of a healthy vagina, tablets with sodium monocitrate are used as a buffer. Furthermore, genitourinary infections can be successfully treated with drugs like metronidazole and clotrimazole as well as *Lactobacillus acidophilus* spores. A healthy vagina contains L. acidophilus, which is in charge of the pH acidity. For this active agent combination, sodium carboxymethyl cellulose and polycarbophil displayed the optimal behavior [139].

Hyaluronic acid (HA) is a perfect choice for vaginal drug delivery due to its occurrence in the human body and biological functions. Its structure can be tweaked to achieve even greater results. Using 6-mercaptonicotinamide, Nowak et al. thiolated and preactivated it, increasing its mucoadhesive characteristics and stability [140].

This solution makes use of the mucoadhesion provided by the creation of disulfide bonds between thiol groups while also keeping the material stable. Furthermore, it has been demonstrated that HA can operate as a therapeutic agent rather than just a drug carrier. Hyaluronic acid vaginal pills of 5 mg were contrasted with vaginal tablets of 25 mg estradiol. Both groups were successful in treating atrophic vaginitis. Although estradiol is now favored, HA may be helpful in those for whom hormonal management is either undesirable or contraindicated [141].

Mini-tablets have received a lot of attention recently. This dose type is said to be a better version of traditional tablets. Hiorth et al. investigation of various polymers led to the invention of mini-tablets that concentrate on the vaginal route of administration. The study's objective was to determine the most efficient way to distribute hexyl amino levulinate (HAL), a potential topical treatment for cervical cancer that uses photodynamic therapy.

This is important because vaginal delivery systems need to consider how a hormone level, a woman's age, and/or sexual activity might affect a range of properties, including pH and viscosity. The mechanical characteristics, bioadhesive strength, and drug release independent of vaginal pH of hydroxypropyl methylcellulose (HPMC) and hydroxypropyl methylcellulose (HPMC) were sufficient. Without any mucoadhesive characteristics, microcrystalline cellulose, methylcellulose, and hydroxyethyl cellulose were able to release complete medication dosages in a matter of minutes.

Utilizing multiparticulate medication delivery strategies, 1–3 mm mini-tablets, medication diffuses more widely inside the vagina, dissolves more quickly, and is retained for longer. Even a few mini-tablets lost have less of an effect than with conventional forms. Mini-tablets are simple to use, painless, and evenly spread because they can be placed into capsules or applicators. These benefits may aid in patient compliance and the maintenance of a strong therapeutic result.

McConville et al. offered a straightforward yet original and practical solution to the issue of versatile preventive tools by creating many-sided pills to aid in the prevention of pregnancy and sexually transmitted disease. The best medication release patterns and *in vivo* action were achieved by using Kollidon®SR and Kollidon®VA. The trial used the anti-herpes simplex drug acyclovir, the anti-retroviral drug dapivirine, and the hormone levonorgestrel as a method of birth control. The authors developed tablets with three to four layers that offered an API release that was quick or steady.

The highly encouraging results suggest that multifunctional, multi-layered tablets might be brought into the pharmaceutical industry. FOR instance, prepared tablets delivered an immediate surge of active chemicals together with a continual release of dapivirine, which has dual usage as an antiviral and contraceptive. By using these formulations, it may be possible to decrease the number of given forms while also improving patient comfort, which would boost therapy compliance and results. The described multifunctional dose formulations could be particularly beneficial in poor nations in terms of reducing HIV infections and the high birth rate.

Osmotic pump pills (OPTs) are frequently considered in oral medicine delivery systems, although Rastogi et al. claim that they can also be administered vaginally [142]. In order to wrap vaginal tablets of the potential antiviral drug IQP-0528 with a bioadhesive polymer (cellulose acetate or cellulose acetate phthalate) and a typical mechanism involving liquid consumption and drug release through an orifice, the researchers used this method.

The study's findings showed that it is possible to make tablets that transport active substances to the vaginal area for 2–5 days. Additionally, osmotic pump pills might have a drug that releases in a burst that is pH-dependent. Utilizing this -phenomena, a formulation for HIV prevention that adjusts the pH as sperm enter the vaginal canal can be created, activating the formulation. As a result, opts may help patients adhere to and use PrEP more effectively. Despite their lack of popularity, pessaries may be equally effective as other vaginal dosing forms.

With the help of bioadhesive polymers like polycarbophil, HPMC, and sodium salt of hyaluronic acid, Semi-synthetic solid triglyceride pessaries were created by Ceschel et al. to keep preparations in the vaginal canal for several days without causing any harm. Clotrimazole [143–145], which is used to treat typical mycotic infections, is a good example of an imidazole antimycotic chemical that can be transported by the specified pessaries.

13.2.3 Vaginal Rings

NuvaRing® (Merck and Co., Kenilworth, NJ, USA), Progering® (Laboratorios Andrómaco SA, Pealolén, Chile), Annovera®

(Therapeutics MDInc, Boca Raton, FL, USA), Ornibel®/Ginoring® (Exeltis, Madrid, Spain), and EluRyngTM (Merck and Co., Kenilworth, NJ, USA) are some of (Amneal Pharmaceuticals, Bridgewater, NJ, USA) Ethylene vinyl acetate (EVA) copolymers make up NuvaRing®. It has a diameter of 54 mm and a thickness of 4 mm.

Every day, it generates 0.012 mg of etonogestrel and 0.015 mg of ethinyl oestradiol. It is applied three times during the course of a one-week period. Contrarily, Progering® was manufactured of silicone elastomer. For three months, IT offers 10 mg of progesterone every day. Formulations that combine antiviral and contraceptive activity are the topic of some clinical research studies. Their goal is to improve contraceptive effectiveness and reduce HIV transmission through sexual contact.

Thurman et al. performed research to contrast the benefits of vaginal rings and oral contraceptives. It was discovered that topical drug distribution through the vaginal ring enables the administration of lower drug doses without causing a first-pass effect on the liver.

Vaginal rings also lessen pain and lengthen menstruation, which is another advantage. Additionally, they are comfortable and in control when applying their own ideas. These rings should not be sensed during normal activities and have no effect on sexual behavior. They can, however, induce vaginal bleeding and irritation [146].

13.2.4 Microspheres

Over 20 years ago, polymeric microspheres were investigated as a vaginal drug delivery system. Hyaluronic acid esters were used to make microspheres by Rochina and colleagues to transport salmon calcitonin. For formulation, they employed the solvent extraction approach. They were able to make smooth-surfaced, spherical microspheres with a diameter of about 10 m. The extraction of the peptide from the microspheres produced between 80% and 90% of the peptide, indicating good incorporation efficacy. *In vivo* measurement of the isolated peptide revealed that the microsphere manufacturing process had no impact on the biological activity of calcitonin. Another study that investigated the potential for repairing the vaginal environment with microparticles comprising probiotics and prebiotics also used the polymer hyaluronic acid.

The findings of a study on the design of a new vaginal bio-adhesive delivery system for probiotics and prebiotic encapsulated on the basis of pectinate-hyaluronic acid microparticles were given by Pliszczak et al. in 2011. The emulsification/gelation process was used to create microparticles, with calcium ions serving as the cross-linking agent. First, it was determined how important preparation and processing limitations affected the size distribution of unloaded microparticles. The bioadhesive characteristics of the gels used to make the final microparticles were also investigated using rheological studies. The ideal operational conditions for creating bio-sticky microparticles with probiotics and prebiotics were then determined using an experimental design.

The use of encapsulation technology may improve the effects of *Lactobacillus* species while safeguarding them during drying and storage. The final microparticles, with a mean diameter of 137 m, granted the full release of probiotic strains after 16 h in a simulated vaginal fluid at 37°C. To avoid problems with oral delivery, Maestrelli et al. [136] developed chitosan-alginate microspheres for cefixime vaginal administration. They used calcium chloride as the cross-linkage agent and ionotropic gelation to generate microparticles. When the drug-to-polymer ratio was optimized, entrapment efficacy grew with drug loading concentration in the beginning solution and peaked at 30 mg/ml.

It is interesting to note that water uptake peaked at the same 30 mg/mi drug loading concentration while microsphere swelling properties grew as more drug dose was entrapped in them. As indicated by the relationship between water uptake and medication release rate, the ideal formulation of microspheres is synthesized with 30 mg/ml cefixime. All formulations ensured in situ persistence for more than 2 h, according to mucoadhesion testing. Through microbiological research, it was discovered that the rate of cefixime discharge from microspheres and the fall in Escherichia coli viability were related.

They came to the conclusion that the microspheres formulation tested could be used to treat urogenital infections locally. Spray drying is an additional technique for producing microspheres that has been used by numerous groups and for a variety of polymers. Zhang et al. studied pH-sensitive and spray-dried mucoadhesive microspheres [147], and tenofovir was administered via polymethacrylate salt (a model HIV microbicide). Using the methacrylic copolymers Eudragit®L-100 and S-100 could result in a unique, low-swellable mucoadhesive substance.

The enhanced formulation contains a 2.3% (w/w) drug loading and an average size of 4.73 m. These microspheres have been demonstrated to respond swiftly to pH changes, releasing over 90% of the medication within 60 min. These microspheres significantly outperform the 1% HEC gel formulation in terms of mucoadhesion. These microspheres do not harm vaginal or endocervical epithelial cells, according to the results of this investigation, which also demonstrate that they do not induce an immune response.

There is no evidence of cytotoxicity in normal vaginal flora. In addition, methacrylic acid copolymers were used for the microsphere synthesis by Gupta et al. Their research objective was to produce and assess vaginal pills that included microspheres of clotrimazole.

Mucoadhesive polymers such as sodium carboxymethyl cellulose, Carbopol®934, and hydroxypropyl cellulose were utilized as excipients in the tablets formulation to generate a long-lasting therapeutic action at the site of infection. The spray drying techniques Eudragit RS-100 and Eudragit RL-100 were used to create these clotrimazole microspheres. According to the findings, the created vaginal formulations have a regulated medication release. Making mucoadhesive microparticles by spray-congealing in addition to spray drying is an innovative technique.

Albertini et al. studied adhesive microparticles for the vaginal delivery of econazole nitrate. Adhesive microparticles for the vaginal administration of econazole nitrate were investigated by

Albertini et al. [138] and found to be efficient. They used a lipid-hydrophilic matrix to make microparticles that contained both a medication and a mucoadhesive material and were spray-congealed. This technique, which includes atomizing a drug dispersion in a liquid carrier, could be helpful for producing mucoadhesive microparticles because it does not require the use of solvents.

Sodium carboxymethyl cellulose, poloxamers, and chitosan were among the mucoadhesive polymers that were investigated in the hydrophilic-hydrophobic meltable matrix (Gelucire 53/10, Gattefosse, France). When econazole was microencapsulated in the Gelucire 53/10, the solubility of the drug rose by 15 times. Albertini et al. came to the conclusion that this was due to the carrier's amphiphilic structure (HLB = 10).

Upon dissolving in the fluid, the carrier produces micelles, with the hydrophobic portion carrying the medicine and the hydrophilic portion carrying the medicine and the hydrophilic portion serving as an interface between the drug outside and the simulated vaginal fluid within. Poloxamers had the same effect when added to the lipophilic carrier as when Gelucire 53/10 was used alone, but chitosan and sodium carboxymethylcellulose reduced API solubility.

This is most likely due to the interaction between polymer solubilization and the carrier impact on drug wettability and solubility enhancement [148, 149]. In addition, the microparticles' mucoadhesive characteristics were studied. Importantly, mucoadhesive properties can prolong the antifungal agent residence time at the vaginal mucosa tissue infection sites.

The cohesion test results were best for the particles that included poloxamers. The researchers came to the conclusion that the spray-congealing process might be regarded as a novel and solvent-free way of creating mucoadhesive microparticles for econazole nitrate vaginal dispersion.

13.2.5 Pellets

Granules that range in size from 300 to 1000 microns are called pellets. Because of their diminutive size, they should adhere to the vaginal mucosa surface after vaginal administration and be less affected by gravity than vaginal tablets. Pellets have been proposed as probiotic bacterium matrices or as carriers for active substances. Santiago et al. [150] looked at how the normal protective microflora of the vaginal microbiota will be impacted by the addition of the carrier material.

They employed lyophilized lactose-based pellets with probiotic bacteria as well as starch-based pellets. Gelatin capsules containing pellets were manufactured for vaginal administration. A control group that was not given any medication was added in order to monitor the pH and microbiota organic changes during the menstrual cycle. The vaginal and ectocervical mucosa did not experience any negative effects during the course of the trial. The researchers found that lyophilized lactose/skimmed milk and probiotic strains or other medications can be delivered vaginally using fast-dissolving starch pellets as a carrier substance.

Poelvoorde et al. [106] examined the vaginal characteristics of pellets made of either non-dissolving microcrystalline cellulose or dissolving starch. Patients received pellets that had been enclosed in either hydroxypropyl methylcellulose capsules or hard gelatin capsules (HPMC). *In vivo* evaluations of pellet behavior (vaginal distribution and retention) and patient tolerance (annoyance, discomfort). Capsules constructed of HPMC had better mucoadhesive qualities right away, but gelatin capsules degraded faster.

Pellets made of starch degraded considerably faster than pellets made of microcrystalline cellulose after being released from capsules. Hard gelatin capsules had a faster *in vitro* disintegration rate than HPMC capsules, but they behaved similarly *in vivo*, with two out of five remaining intact 6 h after injection. The authors discovered that gradual capsule breaking would control the rate of drug release. If pellets were provided with another kind of applicator that did not require placing pellets inside of capsules, the drawback would be eliminated.

Although the main constituent in the pellets, high-amylose starch, lacked mucoadhesive properties, this formulation diffused more freely throughout the vaginal mucosa and was better maintained as a result of the pellets' disintegration. In order to continue this work, Mehta et al. [151] compared the effects of starch pellets and a cream of ceto macrogols. They sought to show the changes in tracer substance deposition following vaginal administration.

The researchers used a gamma scintigraphy technique as well as a magnetic resonance imaging method. The study involved using sheep as well as a group of volunteer humans. Pellets, due to their quick breakdown, were proven to cover the vaginal epithelium to a level comparable to cream. Metha et al. carried out an additional investigation based on the manufacturing of fast-dissolving tablets containing pellets. They anticipated that because tablets disintegrate faster than capsules, pellets would spread more quickly within the vaginal cavity, resulting in extended retention.

The researchers used gamma scintigraphy and MRI to assess the distribution and retention pf pellets compressed into fast-dissolving tablets in sheep and women. The dissolution of the tablet began within 30 min of treatment in sheep, and within 2–4 h, the whole vagina was covered in dissolved pellets, with a constant spread lasting up to 48 h. In females, breakdown took 4 h, while prolonged retention lasted up to 24 h [152].

The dissolving tablets containing starch-based pellets have a good intravaginal distribution and a long retention duration, making them an appealing vaginal drug delivery platform. By including medications from several therapeutic classes in the starch-based pellets, these tablets could be used as carriers for intravaginal administration. Hiorth et al. [153] prepared various trials with bioadhesive pellets based on the research stated above.

The purpose of this group's study research was to develop quick-release bioadhesive pellets comprising hexyl ester 5-aminolevulinic acid, a predecessor of the photoactive chemical, for vaginal medicine delivery. Unlike the previously described disintegrating pellet-based technique, the purpose of the up-to-date work was to create bioadhesive pellets with a quick active component release. Extrusion/spheronization was employed to make the pellets, and Carbopol®934 was used to provide them with bioadhesive characteristics that extend their duration in the vaginal system. Researchers aimed to employ the photodynamic approach in order to determine the utility of polymers in the management of cervical cancer.

The presence of 8% Carbopol has a good effect on the mucoadhesive qualities of pellets, according to research. They had bioadhesive characteristics when it came to vaginal tissue. In the *in vitro* dissolution test, the investigated pellets were mechanically stable and released the drug in phosphate buffer at pH = 4.0 and 6.8 within 20 min. Furthermore, the examined dosage formulations had a 6- to 7-week stability time. The proposed delivery devices were effective in delivering hexyl ester 5-aminolevulinic acid to the vaginal cavity.

13.2.6 Nanoparticles

Polymeric nanoparticles (NPs) have been frequently reported as vaginal medication carriers, as well as for locally and systemically acting medications, in recent years. NPs are small, very stable particles with diameters less than 1000 nm [154]. They have the ability to encapsulate a large range of APIs and distribute them in a skillful, long-term, and exact manner. The most prevalent uses of NPs in vaginal drug delivery are effective microbicide distribution, targeted siRNA delivery, tumor management, delivery of hydrophobic compounds, HIV prevention, protection or management of sexually transmitted diseases, and antibiotic delivery [143–146].

Natural (e.g., hyaluronic acid, chitosan) or synthetic polymers can be used to create such dosage forms. The majority of scientists are interested in synthetic chemicals such as (meth)acrylate polymers, polyethylene glycol (PEG), poly(lactic-co-glycolic) acid (PLGA), polyethylene glycol (PEG), polyesters (polycaprolactone), and many more. Polymeric liposomes (LIPs) or cyclodextrins (CD) nanoparticles (NPs), Nano spheres (NS), and nano capsules (NC) are all examples of NPs for vaginal administration [155]. Some medication formulation issues, such as poor water/oil solubility, API degradation, toxicity, or unattractive organoleptic qualities, can be solved with NPs.

13.2.6.1 Poly(lactic-co-glycolic) acid

PLGA is the most recently described polymer in terms of NPs. Das Neves et al. attempted to manufacture NPs from PLGA that were loaded with dapivirine in order to supply an effective antiretroviral medication delivery. Using an emulsion-solvent evaporation method, they found elements with a mean diameter of 170 nm. When compared to the free medication, the formulation had an early burst impact lasting up to 4 h, followed by a 24 h continuous release with lower or equivalent toxicity.

13.2.6.2 Polyethylene glycol

PEG-neutral, hydrophilic, and mucoadhesion-minimizing polymers are crucial for mucus penetration, allowing NPs' chemicals to pass through the molluscum contagiosum virus (MCV). Maisel et al. validated these features of PEG in their study. They demonstrated its anti-mucoadhesive properties ex vivo on human human cervicovaginal mucus (CVM) before administering PEG-coated NPs to a mouse's cervicovaginal tract. They observed homogenous diffusion into the vaginal epithelium as a result [156].

Jraholmen et al. created PEGylated liposomes with a diameter of 181 nm that can enter MCV and contain interferon alpha-2b for the local treatment of human papillomavirus (HPV). They found no release *in vitro*; however, ex vivo testing demonstrated increased TNF-2b penetration when compared to the control group. Because there were no mucin contacts, PEGylated liposomes were able to reach the deeper epithelium [157].

Lechantour et al. proposed another method for treating HPV-induced cervical lesions. They examined the use of siRNA-loaded PEGylated lipoplexes for vaginal delivery. Resulting in a novel vaginal injection of fluorescent PEGylated lipoplexes, *in vivo* investigations in mice indicated full and persistent covering of the mucosal epithelium. When lipoplexes were coated with PEG, active siRNA was released into the cytoplasm of HPV-positive cells, resulting in a biological response and the suppression of mucin protein aggregation on lipoplexes [158].

PEG is also an excellent option for administering photo-sensitizers. Wang et al. successfully solvothermal prepared boron-dipyrromethene (BDP)-loaded PEG-based NPs. *In vitro* and *in vivo* studies demonstrated that NPs improved cellular uptake and mucus penetration when compared to BDP-loaded polymeric micelles. Because of their extraordinary photothermal activity, activating tumor apoptosis upon irradiation, high efficacy, and safety, the scientists concluded that NPs are a capable strategy in the management of severe cervical intraepithelial neoplasia [159].

13.2.6.3 (Meth)acrylate polymers

Numerous (meth)acrylate polymers are also appropriate for nanocarriers. Frank et al. created NPs using Eudragit®RS100 and Eudragit®S100 as a model of lipophilic material loaded with Nile red and integrated into chitosan gel that serves as an intravaginal medium. When compared to free medicines, NPs with a diameter of roughly 200 nm had better Nile red penetration, particularly in the case of nano capsules (Eudragit®RS100) [160].

13.2.6.4 Polyesters (polycaprolactone)

Frank et al. developed polycaprolactone (PCL) as a basic polymer for NPs. To treat HPV infections, the scientists used a mix of nanocarriers and mucoadhesive semisolids to increase adherence and penetration through the vaginal mucosa. Two formulations were developed for this purpose: chitosan-coated poly(e-caprolactone)-nanocapsules were inserted into hydroxyethyl cellulose gel and poly(e-caprolactone)-nanocapsules were introduced into chitosan hydrogel. According to their findings, the most promising dosage form in terms of mucoadhesion, drug retention, and permeability is chitosan-coated NCs in combination with a mucoadhesive gel [161].

Only NCs demonstrated a high level of fungus reduction efficiency as competed to NSs and the medication solution. In addition, histological research revealed substantial variations between tissues that were connected to the levels of inflammatory cytokines. NC-treated mice had lower cytokine levels, but NS- and solution-treated mice had higher cytokine levels and tissue swelling. This indicates that PCL-NCs have a strong potential for improving itraconazole treatment and reducing cytotoxicity [162].

13.2.6.5 Polymers of a natural origin

Natural polymers are also being studied as a foundation for nanocarriers. Chitosan is a well-known natural polymer. Jraholmen et al. created chitosan-coated LIPs loaded with clotrimazole for local vaginal infection treatment in pregnant females to reduce systemic absorption. Chitosan was coated on sonicated liposomes in three different concentrations: 0.1%, 0.3%, and 0.6%.

13.2.7 Vaginal Films

Vaginal films are solid dosage forms made largely of plasticizers and aqueous polymers that may or may not contain an active ingredient [12]. They are produced with a variety of polymers to achieve mucoadhesion and desired active release profiles. As a result, they can overcome some of the difficulties that come with vaginal medication administration, such as cervical secretion, pH, permeability, and so on. They are preferred to conventional semisolid preparations because of their patient-friendly application, higher stability, improved residence time, and cosmetic benefits.

They are normally flexible, soft, odorless, and colorless, and when they come into contact with vaginal fluids, they scatter or dissolve, allowing them to adhere and stay in vaginal mucosa for long periods [162]. Polyvinyl alcohol [163–169] and cellulose derivatives [170–172] are the most often utilized polymers for making vaginal films, with a combination of both [173–176] being the most prevalent. Other polymers have also been investigated [177, 178] with or without the previously listed typical alternatives.

After being discovered to have antiviral activity against the HIV and genital herpes virus [180], it was considered that cellulose acetate phthalate was an inert medicinal component having film-forming capabilities. It has since been formulated with hydroxypropyl cellulose to create a compound of microbicidal vaginal film while maintaining activity. Polyethylene glycol (PEG) and glycerine are the most often utilized plasticizers to obtain acceptable film properties, but others have been used as well.

The most popular process for creating vaginal films is solvent casting, which involves pouring polymers, active ingredients, plasticizers, and other excipients into a mold. The mixture is then cast into films and allowed to dry at ambient temperature or with gentle heating. The films are not immediately placed into single-film-sized molds.

Regev et al. created dapivirine vaginal film utilizing a quality-by-design (QbD) approach and the hot-melt extrusion (HME) process [181]. HME films were discovered to be thicker, have less water content, heavier, and degrade more quickly than solvent cast SC films. HME could be useful in achieving continuous manufacturing and easier scalability, even if it isn't considerably better than solvent casting.

The quickest drug release was observed in single-layer films, which were immediately followed by a burst of discharge, double-layer films, and finally NPs in films, which had to lowest release. This implies that, depending on the therapeutic requirement, several techniques can be employed to attain a range of drug release profiles. Another recent invention was a freeze-dried vaginal sheet made of a gelatine-based gel by Machado et al. [182–190]. The vaginal sheet, which was created using lactose as a representative powdered ingredient, displayed buffering capabilities when used with a vaginal fluid stimulant while maintaining desired organoleptic properties, such as texture (VFS). Garg et al. distinguish three types of films: quick dissolving (flash release or flash dispersal) films, non-disintegrating films that can be used to manage residence length when paired with fast disintegrating films, and medium disintegrating films.

Vaginal films have been studied for a variety of purposes, the most popular of which is microbicidal and for vaginal diseases. As a preventive instrument for STDs, microbicidal vaginal films can be used. Because of their patient-friendly administration, films have acquired acceptance and preference over standard vaginal formulations [191]. Antiviral, antibacterial, and antifungal active substances are available as vaginal films.

Noncytotoxic contraceptive films made of sodium polystyrene sulfonate (PSS) were created and studied by Garg et al. Researchers and consumers alike are interested in multipurpose preventive technologies (MPTs) that act as contraceptives while also protecting against STDs. Nonoxyl-9 (N-9) was one of the first multipurpose drugs to be commercialized, but the later investigations reports showed negative results. A vaginal multipurpose preventive film called MB66 contains monoclonal antibodies, which have been shown to be successful in preventing infections following vaginal application.

In order to provide defense against HIV 1 and HSV 1 AND 2, Politch et al. created a film that combines two human mABs, VRC01 and HSV 8. In a phase 1 clinical trial, it was determined to be both secure and efficient. Yoo et al. demonstrate another use of vaginal films for treating female sexual arousal problems through mucosal administration of nitric oxide (NO), S-nitroglutathione (GSNO) films from a rat model showed improved vaginal blood perfusion without cytotoxicity and a longer duration of effect for GSNO, a NO donor. Notario et al. created smart microbicide films that are pH delicate and may modify the drug release behavior from a constant release profile under normal vaginal settings (pH 4–5) to a fast release in vaginal pH situations after ejaculation (pH 7–8) [192].

13.3 Novel Rectal Drug Delivery Approaches

Drug delivery via the rectum is a useful alternative route of administration to the oral route for patients who cannot swallow. Traditional rectal dosage forms have been historically used for localized treatments including the delivery of laxatives, treatment of hemorrhoids, and delivery of antipyretics. However, the recent trend shows an increase in the development of novel rectal delivery systems to deliver drugs directly into the systemic circulation by taking advantage of porto-systemic shunting. Novel rectal drug delivery systems including hollow-type suppositories, thermo-responsive and muco-adhesive liquid suppositories, and nanoparticulate systems incorporated into an appropriate vehicle have offered more control over the delivery of drug molecules for local or systemic actions. Continuous research and development in this field of drug delivery may unleash the hidden potential of rectal drug delivery systems [193]. Classification of rectal novel drug delivery system shown Fig. 13.2.

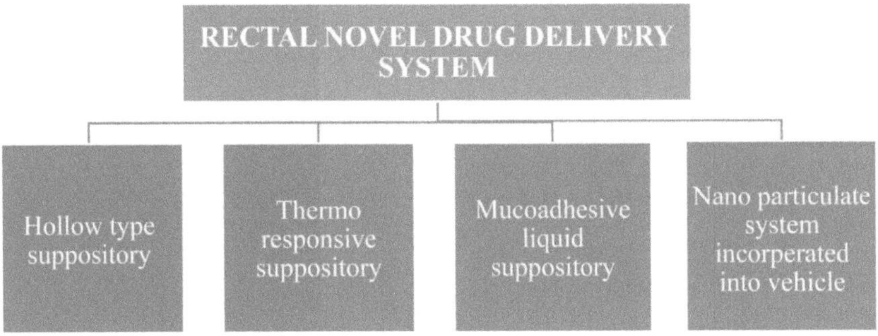

Figure 13.2 Rectal novel drug delivery system classification.

13.4 Thermosensitive Gelling System for Rectal Administration

The drawbacks of traditional solid suppositories can be resolved by developing a thermosensitive liquid suppository. Regrettably, only a few studies describe their therapeutic use. Recent trends, however, show that this model treatment system is progressing at a faster pace. The application of thermosensitive liquid suppositories for anticancer, analgesics, antiemetic, psychiatric, antihypertensive, anesthetic, antiallergic, antimalarial medicines, and insulin has recently been discovered [194–196].

13.4.1 Advantages

- Simple dosage form to administer
- Remains liquid at low temperature
- Acts as a mucoadhesive to rectal tissue without leakage after administration
- No damage to mucosal layers
- Reduces the sensation of foreign body
- Partial prevention of first-pass metabolism
- Rapid absorption of low molecular weight drugs
- Prevents overdosing
- Constant and static rectal environment
- Shielding enzymatically to unstable drugs

- Minimizing exposure of the gastric mucosa to irritant drugs
- Systemic as well as local effects [197–198]

13.4.2 Limitations

- ➢ The new field of research
- ➢ High production cost
- ➢ Preparation difficulties
- ➢ Difficulties in the selection of a temperature-sensitive polymer
- ➢ Rectal mucosa irritant drugs [199]

The elements that need to be considered for the development of the thermosensitive gelling system include the selection of temperature-sensitive polymer, gelation time, rheological properties, and composition of a thermosensitive liquid suppository [200]. Thermosensitive Liquid Suppositories composition and transport mechanism are shown in Table 13.1.

13.5 Mucoadhesive Liquid Suppository

In situ gelling suppositories are liquid suppositories at room temperature but convert to gel when exposed to body temperature. A liquid suppository of Nimesulide, a non-steroidal anti-inflammatory drug (NSAID) was created to increase patient compliance and systemic absorption in rheumatoid arthritis and other musculoskeletal conditions. To modulate the gel strength and impart mucoadhesive force to the suppository base, Poloxamers P188 and P407 temperature-sensitive gelatine property), HPMC, and Carbopol 934p were used by the cold method.

13.6 Nanoparticulate Rectal Drug Delivery Approaches

To increase the therapeutic outcomes of medication for both systemic and local therapy, incorporation of nanoparticles. Nanoparticulate methods have been used in rectal dosage forms.

Table 13.1 Thermosensitive liquid suppositories composition and transport mechanism

Drug/ category	Example	Composition	Mechanism	Ref.
Anaesthetic drugs	Lidocaine	P407: 5–25% P188: 1–5% HPMC: 0.5–1.0% Carbapol: 0.5–1.5%	Unknown	[201]
Antimalarial drug	Rectal chloroquine-p407 gel system	P407: 18–24% Carbopol: 0.3%,0.6%,0.9% PVP: 0.3%,0.6%,0.9% PCP: 0.3%,0.6%,0.9%	Fickian diffusion	[203]
Analgesic drugs	Ketorolac 10 mg	P407: 21% P188: 9% MC: 0.2%,0.6%,1.0% Sodium alginate: 0.2%,0.6%,1.0%	Fickian diffusion	[204]
Anticancer drugs	5-flurouracil 1%	P407: 10–20% Carbopol: 1.0% Pectin: 2.0%	Non-Fickian release	[205]
Antiemetic drugs	Ondansetron 0.8%	P407: 18% PVP: 0.8% Sodium alginate: 0.8% MC: 0.8%	Fickian diffusion	[206]
Antihyper-tensive drug	Candesartan	P407: 1.8% Chitosan: 0.2–0.8%	Unknown	[207]
Psychiatric drugs	Carbamazepine 10%	P407: 20% P188: 10%–20% MC: 1.0% Carbopol: 0.5%	Fickian diffusion	[208]
Insulin	Insulin 0.38%	P407: 15% P188: 20% Sodium Salicylate: 10–30% PCP: 0.2–0.6%	Unknown	[202]

The nanoparticulate rectal dosage forms are distinct from conservative rectal dosage forms in that they encapsulate or load the medicine into nanoparticles before dispersion in a formulation base. Nanoencapsulation would be used to preserve chemicals from degradation, increase the solubility of hydrophobic substances, and adjust drug release kinetics (e.g., prolonged-release or controlled release) [209].

13.6.1 Biological Benefits of Nanoparticulate Systems

- Extend encapsulated chemicals' residence time (even when diarrhea increases colonic motility).
- Improve cellular uptake.
- Facilitate easier gastrointestinal transport.
- Distribution of medication and medication release should be uniform.
- Encourage medication accumulation at the area of mucosal infection (e.g., inflamed tissues).

To successfully deploy nano drug delivery for rectal medication administration, two key aspects must be considered. The initial concern was the physicochemical properties (Size, composition, charge, and surface qualities) and the effective contact of nanoparticles with the colorectal and rectal mucosa. The base and nanoparticles interaction in the dosage form comes in second [210].

Nanoparticle interaction with the dosage form base comes in second. By permitting more contact between medication and the mucosal surface, mucosal penetration, cellular absorption, and drug release would all be improved. Nanoparticle stability in the pharmaceutical formulation should be taken into account during the manufacturing and storage stages. Rectal drug delivery success depends on mucosal adherence since it decreases the risk of nanoformulations being eliminated by leakage, mucus, or quick transit time (e.g., diarrhea) [211]. For rectal application, a variety of nanoparticulate technologies were explored.

13.6.2 Nanoparticulate Liquid Dosage Forms

Buffered solutions and aqueous liquids such as water are commonly used to make nanoparticles. Early investigations examine the importance of nanoparticulate systems for rectal medication treatment mainly for liquid dosage forms [212]. Proof of concept experiments is typically employed in aqueous solutions to reduce the interference of the formulation base with nanoparticles.

Nanoparticles with different sizes (500, 200, 100, and 40 nm) were examined. When healthy animals were used in the investigation and colitis was induced by 2,4,6-trinitrobenzene sulfonic acid (TNBS), it was possible for nanoparticles coated with PEG of all sizes to correctly diffuse across the tissue surface of the colon, suggesting enhanced medication administration. While keeping their mucus penetrating characteristics, hydrophilic surface chemistry produced by surface PEGylation of nanoparticles lessens their interaction with the digestive tract. There is only a little research on nanoparticle drug administration to the rectal mucosa in a liquid dosage form for systemic as well as local action.

The absorption of common nanoparticles and microparticles into the rectal mucosa of patients with and without IBD was studied by Schmidt et al. (2013). Poly(lactic-co-glycolic) acid nanoparticles (mean particle size of 3 m) and microparticles (mean particle size of 250 nm) were distributed in a saline solution containing 10% human albumin. The protein in the dispersal media stabilized the particles and lowered their surface charge via surface absorption. The microparticles were shown to have been deposited in the ulcerous lesion of patients with rectal Crohn's disease and ulcerative colitis, according to the results. Only traces of nanoparticles were found in the mucosal lining of IBD patients, indicating a clear size-dependent variation in particle accumulation. While microparticles accumulated and bioadhered to the inflamed mucosal membrane, there was no epithelial barrier penetration. Patients with IBD have been found to have nanoparticles translocate to their serosal compartment, which could result in systemic absorption. There were basically no nanoparticles or microparticles in the rectal mucosa of healthy control subjects. According to the researchers, local medicine delivery for intestinal disease in humans does not require nanoparticles. The difference in element size between animal and human studies is still unknown [213].

Osmolality and physiological pH have been widely considered for the development of rectal drug administration. Enemas can be tailored for systemic and/or local nanoparticle distribution, as demonstrated by Maisel et al. (2015). When compared to potassium-based enemas, enemas based on hypotonic sodium were discovered to be a viable liquid preparation base for enhancing the supply of PEGylated polystyrene nanoparticles on the colorectal epithelial surface. Enemas based on hypotonic sodium increased fluid absorption and homogenous dispersion of nanoparticles throughout the epithelial surface. By preventing nanoparticles from getting into close touch with the mucosal surface, hypertonic enemas caused fluid secretion and intestinal distention. Strongly hypertonic enemas can harm the intestinal epithelium when administered as a pre-treatment, allowing hypnotically delivered nanoparticles to penetrate the tissue. Overall, problems with nanoparticulate liquid dosage forms may be similar to those with conventional liquid dosage forms. Despite the fact that liquid dose forms spread more evenly in the rectum, they sometimes have low leakage and retention rates, which might result in inconsistent drug absorption [214].

The dosing frequency and clinical application will have a substantial impact on their effectiveness. Furthermore, preliminary study reports from liquid dosage forms demonstrated that nanoparticles may increase rectal drug delivery.

13.6.3 Nanoparticulate Solid Dosage Form

Rectal medication delivery utilizing solid dosage forms of nanoparticles has only been tested in a small number of trials. For the prospective treatment of severe seizures, Abdelbary (2009) et al. synthesized solid lipid nanoparticles (SLN) encapsulating the water-insoluble diazepam. The release patterns of the nanoparticles, the particle size, and the degree of entrapment efficiency would change if the surfactant, concentration, or kind of lipid matrix were altered. Sixty percent of the medication formulations had particles with diameters less than 500 nm, according to laser diffractometry and transmission electron microscopy [215].

Hard fat suppositories with nanoparticles were effectively incorporated (Witepsol W35 and Witepsol S58). SLN-containing suppositories had significantly longer drug release than free drug suppositories were demonstrated by *In vitro* tests. The SLN-containing suppository formulations delivered the drug faster than the free drug suppositories. The effectiveness of rectal formulations *in vivo* needs to be investigated further. Faster drug release into the physiological fluid may be possible with the diazepam-loaded SLNs' release profile, which is favorable for emergency medical treatments.

Mohamed et al. investigated the concept of drug-loaded nanoparticles with suppository substrates with varying solubility properties (2013). This work involved the incorporation of the hydrophilic medication metoclopramide into SLNs (particle sizes varying from 24.99 to 396.8 nm), which were then converted into suppositories by utilizing a lipophilic base. Most of the metoclopramide was released from SLNs by the suppositories with a coca butter base, which was probably due to the lower melting point and lack of hydrophilicity. As a result of the lipid coating on the nanoparticles, the formulation allowed for long-term drug release. In addition to showing extra sustained-release features *in vivo*, metoclopramide-loaded SLN suppositories showed the same gastric emptying percentage as the commercially available metoclopramide suppository (primperan), negating the necessity for multiple dosing [216].

Siczek et al. (2018) examined the use of cocoa butter suppositories to release silver from silver-coated glass beads for anti-inflammatory effects in IBD patients. Before being covered with silver, the borosilicate glass beads had a diameter of 1,000 mm. Silver was released quickly in *in vitro* drug release experiments employing silver-coated glass beads; more than half of the deposited metal was released in the first 30 min. About 30% of the silver was still on the glass beads after 24 h. The efficiency of the *in vivo* formulation as well as the rate of silver release from the suppository's silver-coated glass beads needs further research [217].

An X-ray CT examination of suppositories comprising silver-coated glass beads indicated a uniform circulation of the beads throughout the suppository volume with minimal sinking or agglomeration. Only a few research has employed nanoparticles in solid dose form for rectal drug administration; more research is required. Particularly *in vitro* and early *in vivo* studies demonstrate the drug formulation strategy's promise for drug release characteristics. To show that these nanoparticulate formulations are secure, bioavailable, and effective, proof of concept is still required.

13.6.4 Nanoparticulate Semisolid Dosage Forms

The thick viscosity of gels aids in rectum retention and increases drug absorption by increasing contact with the rectal mucosa. Gels have rectilinear transport capacity. The use of mucoadhesive polymers and/or thermosensitive polymers in the formulation base has resulted in a number of advancements in rectal medication delivery, much like with conventional semisolid dosage forms. The physicochemical qualities of the nanoparticles dictate the gel base and its composition, and they should ideally not interfere with drug release or nanoparticle contact with the rectal mucosa.

It has not been proven that mucoadhesive bases alone can transport nanoparticles into the rectum. For the transport of nanoparticles through the rectal mucosa, thermosensitive polymers in the drug composition base are becoming increasingly popular. These polymers develop a liquid dosage form that was easy to administer and disperse throughout the mucosa at room temperature before converting to a gel phase. Melo et al. investigated the colorectal retention and distribution of PLGA nanoparticles (poloxamer 407) embedded on a thermosensitive base (mean particle size 170–180 nm) [218].

In vitro experiments on drug release showed that dipivefrine-loaded nanoparticles in PBS released the drug more quickly and effectively than free drugs in a thermosensitive base did over the course of an 8 h period. Furthermore, testing on live mice demonstrated that the thermosensitive base dispersed nanoparticles in the colorectal region at a slower but larger rate. The nanoparticles were also retained in better condition in the colorectum. Din et al. (2017) established a novel irinotecan preparation for the treatment of rectal cancer. BY dispersing thermosensitive SLNs (mean particle size of 190 nm) in a solution of thermosensitive poloxamer, a double reverse thermosensitive nanocarrier system was created (DRTN) [219].

There has been little investigation into the use of thermosensitive and mucoadhesive polymers as the formulation base for rectal nanoparticle injection. In order to increase the bioavailability of tizanidine, Moawad et al. (2017) added nanotransferosome (mean particle size of 150 nm) to a formulation base that also contained mucoadhesive polymer hydroxypropyl methylcellulose and thermosensitive polymer. The fact that the rectal route avoids hepatic first-pass metabolism certainly contributed to the increase in bioavailability. The nanoparticles' permeation-enhancing effect was also credited with boosting the nanotransfersome gel's bioavailability [220].

More study is required to determine how semisolid dosage forms interact with nanoparticles, including

(i) Formulation stability
(ii) Nanoparticle movement in the semisolid dosage form
(iii) Formulation retention in the rectum
(iv) Drug release from nanoparticles
(v) Nanoparticle uptake and/or adhesion in the rectal mucosa

13.6.5 Rectal Formulations in Clinical Trials

Rectal medications are already on the market, with more under clinical studies. Table 13.1 demonstrates clinically authorized rectal medication compositions for local and systemic absorption. The drugs in these preparations usually have a wide therapeutic window between therapeutic and dangerous concentrations. This allows for a safety margin that accounts for variability in rectal medication absorption. Rectal medications that have been approved are mostly utilized for the short-term treatment of diseases [217].

In patients with ulcerative proctosigmoiditis, which is common in IBD, mesalazine, or corticosteroids, locally active drugs are given for a longer period of time to induce remission. According to clinical trials, budesonide rectal foam and enema are effective in these circumstances, while lowering the potential of systemic steroid-related side effects. Most of the rectal preparations used in the clinical trial would mix with currently licensed drugs with classic rectal administration such as enemas, rectal gel, and suppositories. Most of these compounds are still in clinical studies and are used to cure local diseases including IBD, fecal microbiota transplant, hemorrhoids, constipation, bowel preparation, and so on [220].

Table 13.2 Rectal drugs under clinical trial (clinical trials.gov.in)

Drug	Dosage form	Indication
Mesalamine	Enema	Healthy
Ibuprofen	Suppository	Healthy
Quetiapine	Suppository	Dementia, delirium
Hydrocortisone	Suppository	Internal hemorrhoids
Meloxicam	Suppository	Ankylosing Spondylitis
Balsalazide	Suppository	Ulcerative Colitis
Belladonna + Opium	Suppository	Nephrolithiasis
Tenofovir	Enema	HIV prevention
ALTH12	Enema	Ulcerative colitis
Promelaxin	Enema	Chronic functional constipation
IQP-0528	Rectal Gel	HIV prevention
Tenofovir	Rectal Gel	HIV prevention
Dapivirine	Rectal Gel	HIV prevention
Lidocaine + diclofenac	Rectal Gel	Anal fissure
Maraviroc	Rectal gel	HIV/AIDS

Pain is treated with rare rectal formulations that target on systemic drug absorption. Clinical trial formulations, similar to approved rectal dosage forms, are typically used for short-term treatment. The most innovative clinical trials are predicted to use thermosensitive rectal gels. Both healthy persons and people with ulcerative colitis have been examined for things like safety, preference, distribution, and retention. We expected to see more success in clinical research for rectal drug formulation [218].

13.7 Conclusion

Unique manufacturing techniques have evolved recently, allowing the new potential to produce highly advanced platforms for drug administration through vaginal and rectal routes, followed by systemic and local effects. Despite the fact that the vaginal route's full potential appears to be underutilized, the benefits of the vagina as a prospective pharmaceutical management site have been identified and are already being used.

One of the most significant research topics in vaginal drug delivery allows the local action, which is a natural result of a variety of diseases and ailments that can arise in the vagina, such as fungal, bacterial, and viral infections. Vaginal drug delivery techniques, on the other hand, are used to induce systemic effects. Hormone administration in menopausal treatment and contraception are the most intensively researched directions. Furthermore, vaginal drug formulations are being studied as potential prophylactic medicines for sexually transmitted illnesses, such as HIV. However, numerous vaginal physiological aspects, particularly the considerable fluctuation of vaginal circumstances, such as the pH, volume, and content of fluids, make drug distribution difficult. These conditions vary within individuals, which may contribute to various treatment responses in the same person. Even though the oral route is the most accessible and desirable method of drug delivery, there have been various cases where this is not practicable, either clinically or pharmaceutically. In these situations, the rectal route may be a viable option for administering medications with both local and systemic effects. Despite its benefits, the rectal route for medication administration is still underutilized.

The lengthening of the vaginal residency time is one of the most important research directions for polymers used in vaginal medicine delivery. Smart and mucoadhesive polymers that increase viscosity when exposed to physiological conditions are frequently investigated for this purpose. It is crucial to remember that the desired product features can be obtained by chemically tailoring the polymer properties. In the case of any newly manufactured excipient, however, comprehensive research on potential toxicity and irritation to the vaginal mucosa is required. The majority of the current literature concentrates on dosage form studies and uses *in vitro* tests and ex vivo animal models to study the features of the studied systems, which is insufficient for proper safety evaluation. As a result, the toxicity of possible vaginal medication delivery systems should be considered more carefully in future product reviews. Other issues with vaginal products include their safety. The risk of primary component leakage to the sexual companion during coitus has been identified in the case of hormone-loaded systems.

Unintended systemic exposure to the active component as a result of medication absorption into the systemic circulation via topical intravaginal preparations is another crucial point. Despite the fact that this phenomenon has been mentioned previously as a possible therapeutic issue, the available literature suggests that the risk of serious side effects is low because just a small quantity of the active component can be absorbed and have an impact on the entire body.

A large number of ideas and ongoing projects, as evidenced by several scientific papers, are pushing the technology of polymer-based vaginal formulations to a new level in order to deal with issues such as poor bioadhesion, thinning with vaginal fluids, short residence time, inadequate dispersal in the vaginal cavity, or fast drug release. However, the appropriate safety testing techniques for vagina or rectal drug delivery that were included at the start of the project might be valuable in the development of future pharmaceutical products.

To fully utilize the potential of this route to treat systemic and local disorders, continued advances in vaginal and rectal medication formulation, as well as detailed investigations on the biological interactions of rectal and vaginal drug administration, are required.

References

1. Contraception—An ancient interest—contraceptive, women, methods, and practice. Available online: https://science.jrank.org/pages/1761/Contraception-An-ancient-interest.html (accessed on 12 February 2020).
2. Smith, L. The Kahun Gynaecological Papyrus: Ancient Egyptian medicine. *J. Fam. Plan. Reprod. Health Care* 2011, 37, 54–55.

3. Hasan, I., Zulkifli, M., Ansari, A. H., Sherwani, A. M. K., Shakir, M. History of ancient Egyptian obstetrics & gynecology: A review. *J. Microb. Biotechnol. Res.* 2011, 1, 35–39.
4. Britton, L. E., Alspaugh, A., Greene, M. Z., McLemore, M. R. CE: An evidence-based update on contraception. *Am. J. Nursing*. 2020, 120, 22–33.
5. New Non-hormonal contraceptive gel found to be effective. Available online: https://www.pharmacytimes.com/view/newnon-hormonal-contraceptive-found-to-be-effective (accessed on 24 May 2021).
6. Whorton, J. C. *The Arsenic Century: How Victorian Britain was Poisoned at Home, Work, and Play*, Oxford University Press: Oxford. 2010, pp. 140–142.
7. Soderberg, S. F. Vaginal disorders. *Vet. Clin. N. Am. Small Anim. Pract.* 1986, 16, 543–559.
8. Siddique, S. A. Vaginal anatomy and physiology. *J. Pelvic Med. Surg.* 2003, 9, 263–272.
9. Hussain, A., Ahsan, F. The vagina as a route for systemic drug delivery. *J. Control Release* 2005, 103, 301–313.
10. Barton, D. L., Shuster, L. T., Dockter, T., Atherton, P. J., Thielen, J., Birrell, S. N., Sood, R., Griffin, P., Terstriep, S. A., Mattar, B., et al. Systemic and local effects of vaginal dehydroepiandrosterone (DHEA): NCCTG N10C1 (Alliance). *Support. Care Cancer* 2017, 26, 1335–1343.
11. Caramella, C. M., Rossi, S., Ferrari, F., Bonferroni, M. C., Sandri, G. Mucoadhesive and thermogelling systems for vaginal drug delivery. *Adv. Drug Deliv. Rev.* 2015, 92, 39–52.
12. Vermani, K., Garg, S. The scope and potential of vaginal drug delivery. *Pharm. Sci. Technol. Today* 2000, 3, 359–364.
13. Machado, R. M., Palmeira-De-Oliveira, A., Gaspar, C., de Oliveira, J. M., Palmeira-De-Oliveira, R. Studies and methodologies on vaginal drug permeation. *Adv. Drug Deliv. Rev.* 2015, 92, 14–26.
14. Machado, A., das Neves, J. Tissue-based *in vitro* and ex vivo models for vaginal permeability studies. In *Concepts and Models for Drug Permeability Studies: Cell and Tissue-based In vitro Culture Models*, Elsevier: Amsterdam, The Netherlands, 2016, 273–308.
15. Morrow, R. J., Woolfson, A. D., Donnelly, L., Curran, R., Andrews, G., Katinger, D., Malcolm, R. K. Sustained release of proteins from a modified vaginal ring device. *Eur. J. Pharm. Biopharm.* 2011, 77, 3–10. Available online: http://www.ncbi.nlm.nih.gov/pubmed/21055465.

16. Srikrishna, S., Cardozo, L. The vagina as a route for drug delivery: A review. *Int. Urogynecol. J.* 2012, 24, 537–543. Available online: https://link.springer.com/article/10.1007/s00192-012-2009-3.
17. Sherrard, J., Wilson, J., Donders, G., Mendling, W., Jensen, J. S. 2018 European (IUSTI/WHO) International Union against sexually transmitted infections (IUSTI) World Health Organization (WHO) guideline on the management of vaginal discharge. *Int. J. STD AIDS* 2018, 29, 1258–1272. Available online: https://pubmed.ncbi.nlm.nih.gov/30049258/ (accessed on 20 May 2020).
18. CDC—Bacterial Vaginosis Statistics. Available online: https://www.cdc.gov/std/bv/stats.htm.
19. Vaginal and Vulvar Cancers Statistics. Available online: https://www.cdc.gov/cancer/vagvulv/statistics/index.htm.
20. Koumans, E. H., Sternberg, M., Bruce, C., McQuillan, G., Kendrick, J., Sutton, M., Markowitz, L. E. The prevalence of bacterial vaginosis in the United States, 2001–2004, associations with symptoms, sexual behaviors, and reproductive health. *Sex. Transm. Dis.* 2007, 34, 864–869. Available online: https://pubmed.ncbi.nlm.nih.gov/17621244/.
21. Katz, D. F., Yuan, A., Gao, Y. Vaginal drug distribution modeling. *Adv. Drug Deliv. Rev.* 2015, 92, 2–13.
22. Melis, G. B., Ibba, M. T., Steri, B., Kotsonis, P., Matta, V., Paoletti, A. M. Role of pH as a regulator of vaginal physiological environment. *Minerva Ginecol.* 2000, 52, 111–121. Available online: http://www.ncbi.nlm.nih.gov/pubmed/10900941 (accessed on 13 February 2020).
23. Mercer, B. M., Miodovnik, M., Thurnau, G. R., Goldenberg, R. L., Das, A. F., Ramsey, R. D., Rabello, A. Y., Meis, P. J., Moawad, A. H., Iams, J. D., et al. The preterm prediction study: Significance of vaginal infections. National Institute of Child Health and Human Development Maternal-Fetal Medicine Units Network. *Am. J. Obs. Gynecol.* 1995, 173, 1231–1235. Available online: http://www.ncbi.nlm.nih.gov/entrez/query.fcgi?cmd=Retrieve&db=PubMed&dopt=Citation&list_uids=7485327.
24. Stojanovic, N., Plécaš, D., Plešinac, S. Normal vaginal flora, disorders, and application of probiotics in pregnancy. *Arch. Gynecol. Obstet.* 2012, 286, 325–332.
25. Donders, G. Diagnosis and management of bacterial vaginosis and other types of abnormal vaginal bacterial flora: A review. *Obstet. Gynecol. Surv.* 2010, 65, 462–473. Available online: http://www.ncbi.nlm.nih.gov/pubmed/20723268 (accessed on 12 February 2020).

26. Macklaim, J. M., Clemente, J. C., Knight, R., Gloor, G. B., Reid, G. Changes in vaginal microbiota following antimicrobial and probiotic therapy. *Microb. Ecol. Health Dis.* 2015, 26, 27799.

27. Tanphaichitr, N., Srakaew, N., Alonzi, R., Kiattiburut, W., Kongmanas, K., Zhi, R., Li, W., Baker, M., Wang, G., Hickling, D. Potential use of antimicrobial peptides as vaginal spermicides/microbicides. *Pharmaceuticals* 2016, 9, 13. Available online: http://www.ncbi.nlm.nih.gov/pubmed/26978373 (accessed on 12 February 2020).

28. Johal, H. S., Garg, T., Rath, G., Goyal, A. K. Advanced topical drug delivery system for the management of vaginal candidiasis. *Drug Deliv.* 2016, 23, 550–563.

29. Palmeira-de-Oliveira, R., Palmeira-de-Oliveira, A., Martinez-de-Oliveira, J. New strategies for local treatment of vaginal infections. *Adv. Drug Deliv. Rev.* 2015, 92, 105–122.

30. Baptista, M., Tavares, R., Ramalho-Santos, J. Spermicidal, and microbicidal compounds: In search of an efficient multipurpose strategy. *Curr. Med. Chem.* 2014, 21, 3693–3700. Available online: http://www.ncbi.nlm.nih.gov/pubmed/25174922 (accessed on 12 February 2020).

31. Subramanian, B., Agarwal, T., Ghorai, S. K., Mandal, P., Chattopadhyay, S., Basak, P., Maiti, T. K., Guha, S. K. Biocompatible polyvinyl alcohol and RISUG®blend polymeric films with spermicidal potential. *Biomed. Mater.* 2019, 14, 035017.

32. Daniel, S., Rotem, R., Koren, G., Lunenfeld, E., Levy, A. Vaginal antimycotics and the risk for spontaneous abortions. *Am. J. Obstet. Gynecol.* 2018, 218, 601.e1–601.e7. Available online: http://www.ncbi.nlm.nih.gov/pubmed/29510088.

33. El-Hammadi, M., Arias, J. Nano-sized platforms for vaginal drug delivery. *Curr. Pharm. Des.* 2015, 21, 1633–1644.

34. Gupta, S., Gabrani, R., Ali, J., Dang, S. Exploring novel approaches to vaginal drug delivery. *Recent Pat. Drug Deliv. Formula.* 2011, 5, 82–94.

35. Bassi, P., Kaur, G. Innovations in bioadhesive vaginal drug delivery system. *Expert Opin. Ther. Pat.* 2012, 22, 1019–1032. Available online: http://www.ncbi.nlm.nih.gov/pubmed/22860765.

36. Naumova, I., Castelo-Branco, C. Current treatment options for postmenopausal vaginal atrophy. *Int. J. Women's Health* 2018, 10, 387–395. Available online: http://www.ncbi.nlm.nih.gov/pubmed/30104904.

37. Veres, S., Miller, L., Burington, B. A comparison between the vaginal ring and oral contraceptives. *Obstet. Gynecol.* 2004, 104, 555–563. Available online: http://www.ncbi.nlm.nih.gov/pubmed/15339769.
38. Gao, Y., Yuan, A., Chuchuen, O., Ham, A., Yang, K. H., Katz, D. F. Vaginal deployment and tenofovir delivery by microbicide gels. *Drug Deliv. Transl. Res.* 2015, 5, 279–294. Available online: http://www.ncbi.nlm.nih.gov/pubmed/25874971.
39. Ferguson, L. M., Rohan, L. C. The importance of the vaginal delivery route for antiretrovirals in HIV prevention. *Ther. Deliv.* 2011, 2, 1535–1550. Available online: http://www.ncbi.nlm.nih.gov/pubmed/22468220, *Pharmaceutics* 2021, 13, 884 36 of 49.
40. Madanchi, H., Shoushtari, M., Kashani, H., Sardari, S. Antimicrobial peptides of the vaginal innate immunity and their role in the fight against sexually transmitted diseases. *N. Microbes N. Infect.* 2020, 34, 100627.
41. Novetsky, A. P., Keller, M. J., Gradissimo, A., Chen, Z., Morgan, S. L., Xue, X., Strickler, H. D., Fernández-Romero, J. A., Burk, R., Einstein, M. H. *In vitro* inhibition of human papillomavirus following use of a carrageenan-containing vaginal gel. *Gynecol. Oncol.* 2016, 143, 313–318.
42. Rodríguez, A., Kleinbeck, K., Mizenina, O., Kizima, L., Levendosky, K., Jean-Pierre, N., Villegas, G., Ford, B. E., Cooney, M. L., Teleshova, N., et al. *In vitro* and *in vivo* evaluation of two carrageenan-based formulations to prevent HPV acquisition. *Antivir. Res.* 2014, 108, 88–93.
43. Baptista, M., Ramalho-Santos, J. Spermicides, microbicides, and antiviral agents: Recent advances in the development of novel multi-functional compounds. *Mini Rev. Med. Chem.* 2009, 9, 1556–1567. Available online: http://www.eurekaselect.com/openurl/content.php?genre=article&issn=13895575&volume=9&issue=13&spage=1556.
44. First Multipurpose Gel Designed to Prevent HIV, HSV, and HPV Simultaneously in Women and Men Advances in Clinical Trials. Population Council. Available online: https://www.popcouncil.org/news/first-multipurpose-gel-designed-to-prevent-hiv-hsvand-hpv-simultaneously-i.
45. Price, C. F., Tyssen, D., Sonza, S., Davie, A., Evans, S., Lewis, G. R., Xia, S., Spelman, T., Hodsman, P., Moench, T. R., et al. SPL7013gel (vivagel®) retains potent HIV-1 and HSV-2 inhibitory activity following vaginal administration in humans. *PLoS ONE* 2011, 6, 24095.

46. Turner, C., Aye Mya Thein, N., Turner, P., Nosten, F., and White, N. J. Rectal pH in well and unwell infants. *J. Trop. Pediatr.* 2012, 58(4), 311–313. DOI: 10.1093/trope/fmr088.

47. Jannin, V., Lemagnen, G., Gueroult, P., Larrouture, D., and Tuleu, C. The rectal route in the 21st Century to treat children. *Adv. Drug Deliv. Rev.* 2014, 73, 34–49. DOI: 10.1016/j.addr.2014.05.012.

48. Ferris, D. G., Litaker, M. S., Woodward, L., Mathis, D., Hendrich, J. Treatment of bacterial vaginosis: A comparison of oral metronidazole, metronidazole vaginal gel, and clindamycin vaginal cream. *J. Fam. Pract.* 1995, 41, 443–449.

49. Paavonen, J., Mangioni, C., Martin, M. A., Wajszczuk, C. P. Vaginal clindamycin and oral metronidazole for bacterial vaginosis: A randomized trial. *Obstet. Gynecol.* 2000, 96, 256–260.

50. Alexander, N. J., Baker, E., Kaptein, M., Karck, U., Miller, L., Zampaglione, E. Why consider vaginal drug administration? *Fertil. Steril.* 2004, 82, 1–12.

51. Srikrishna, S., Cardozo, L. The vagina as a route for drug delivery: A review. *Int. Urogynecol. J. Pelvic Floor Dysfunct.* 2012, 24, 537–543.

52. Gupta, S., Gabrani, R., Ali, J., Dang, S. Exploring novel approaches to vaginal drug delivery. *Recent Pat. Drug Deliv. Formul.* 2011, 5, 82–94.

53. Vermani, K., Garg, S. The scope and potential of vaginal drug delivery. *Pharm. Sci. Technol. Today* 2000, 3, 359–364.

54. Barnhart, K. T., Izquierdo, A., Pretorius, E. S., Shera, D. M., Shabbout, M., Shaunik, A. Baseline dimensions of the human vagina. *Hum. Reprod.* 2006, 21, 1618–1622. Available online: http://www.ncbi.nlm.nih.gov/pubmed/16478763 (accessed on 13 February 2020).

55. Graziottin, A., Gambini, D. Anatomy and physiology of genital organs—women. In *Handbook of Clinical Neurology*, Elsevier: Amsterdam, The Netherlands, 2015, pp. 39–60.

56. Hickey, M., Pillai, G., Higham, J., Sullivan, M., Horncastle, D., Doherty, D., Stamp, G. Changes in endometrial blood vessels in the endometrium of women with hormone replacement therapy-related irregular bleeding. *Hum. Reprod.* 2003, 18, 1100–1106. Available online: http://www.ncbi.nlm.nih.gov/pubmed/12721191 (accessed on 13 February 2020).

57. Cunha, G. R. The dual origin of vaginal epithelium. *Am. J. Anat.* 1975, 143, 387–392.

58. Nilsson, K., Risberg, B., Heimer, G. The vaginal epithelium in the postmenopause—cytology, histology and pH as methods of

assessment. *Maturitas* 1995, 21, 51–56. Available online: http://www.ncbi.nlm.nih.gov/pubmed/7731384 (accessed on 13 February 2020).

59. Boutin, E. L., Cunha, G. R. Estrogen-induced epithelial proliferation and cornification are uncoupled in sinus vaginal epithelium associated with uterine stroma. *Differentiation* 1998, 62, 171–178.
60. Farage, M., Maibach, H. Lifetime changes in the vulva and vagina. *Arch. Gynecol. Obstet.* 2006, 273, 195–202.
61. Mårdh, P. A. The vaginal ecosystem. *Am. J. Obstet. Gynecol.* 1991, 165, 1163–1168.
62. Valore, E. V., Park, C. H., Igreti, S. L., Ganz, T. Antimicrobial components of vaginal fluid. *Am. J. Obstet. Gynecol.* 2002, 187, 561–568. Available online: http://www.ncbi.nlm.nih.gov/pubmed/12237628 (accessed on 13 February 2020).
63. Owen, D. H., Katz, D. F. A vaginal fluid simulant. *Contraception* 1999, 59, 91–95.
64. Chen, K. C., Forsyth, P. S., Buchanan, T. M., Holmes, K. K. Amine content of vaginal fluid from untreated and treated patients with nonspecific vaginitis. *J. Clin. Investig.* 1979, 63, 828–835. Available online: http://www.ncbi.nlm.nih.gov/pubmed/447831 (accessed on 13 February 2020).
65. Rajan, N., Cao, Q., Anderson, B. E., Pruden, D. L., Sensibar, J., Duncan, J. L., Schaeffer, A. J. Roles of glycoproteins and oligosaccharides found in human vaginal fluid in bacterial adherence. *Infect. Immun.* 1999, 67, 5027–5032. Available online: http://www.ncbi.nlm.nih.gov/pubmed/10496874 (accessed on 20 February 2020).
66. Sobel, J. D., Faro, S., Force, R. W., Foxman, B., Ledger, W., Nyirjesy, P. R., Reed, B. D., Summers, P. R. Vulvovaginal candidiasis: Epidemiologic, diagnostic, and therapeutic considerations. *Am. J. Obstet. Gynecol.* 1998, 178, 203–211.
67. Heine, P., McGregor, J. A. Trichomonas vaginalis: A reemerging pathogen. *Clin. Obstet. Gynecol.* 1993, 36, 137–144. Available online: http://www.ncbi.nlm.nih.gov/pubmed/8435938 (accessed on 20 February 2020).
68. Pascual, L. M., Daniele, M. B., Pájaro, C., Barberis, L. *Lactobacillus* species isolated from the vagina: Identification, hydrogen peroxide production and nonoxynol-9 resistance. *Contraception* 2006, 73, 78–81.
69. Linhares, I. M., Summers, P. R., Larsen, B., Giraldo, P. C., Witkin, S. S. Contemporary perspectives on vaginal pH and lactobacilli.

Am. J. Obstet. Gynecol. 2011, 204, 120.e1–120.e5. Available online: http://www.ncbi.nlm.nih.gov/pubmed/20832044 (accessed on 13 February 2020).

70. Caillouette, J. C., Sharp, J., Zimmerman, G. J., Roy, S. Vaginal pH as a marker for bacterial pathogens and menopausal status. *Am. J. Obstet. Gynecol.* 1997, 176, 1270–1277.

71. Andrews, G. P., Laverty, T. P., Jones, D. S. Mucoadhesive polymeric platforms for controlled drug delivery. *Eur. J. Pharm. Biopharm.* 2009, 71, 505–518. Available online: http://www.ncbi.nlm.nih.gov/pubmed/18984051 (accessed on 13 February 2020).

72. Kale, V. Vaginal mucosa—A promising site for drug therapy. *Br. J. Pharm. Res.* 2013, 3, 983–1000.

73. Sigurdsson, H. H., Kirch, J., Lehr, C.-M. Mucus as a barrier to lipophilic drugs. *Int. J. Pharm.* 2013, 453, 56–64. Available online: https://linkinghub.elsevier.com/retrieve/pii/S0378517313004572 (accessed on 13 February 2020).

74. Smart, J. D., Kellaway, I. W., Worthington, H. E. C. An *in vitro* investigation of mucosa-adhesive materials for use in controlled drug delivery. *Pharm. Pharmacol.* 2011, 36, 295–299.

75. Roy, S., Pal, K., Anis, A., Pramanik, K., Prabhakar, B. Polymers in mucoadhesive drug-delivery systems: A brief note. *Monomers Polym.* 2009, 12, 483–495.

76. Sriamornsak, P., Wattanakorn, N., Takeuchi, H. Study on the mucoadhesion mechanism of pectin by atomic force microscopy and mucin-particle method. *Carbohydr. Polym.* 2010, 79, 54–59.

77. Hartman, C. G. The permeability of the vaginal mucosa. *Ann. N. Y. Acad. Sci.* 1959, 83, 318–327. Available online: http://www.ncbi.nlm.nih.gov/pubmed/14400131 (accessed on 13 February 2020).

78. Das Neves, J., Bahia, M. F. Gels as vaginal drug delivery systems. *Int. J. Pharm.* 2006, 318, 1–14.

79. Van der Bijl, P., van Eyk, A. D. Comparative *in vitro* permeability of human vaginal, small intestinal and colonic mucosa. *Int. J. Pharm.* 2003, 261, 147–152. Available online: http://www.ncbi.nlm.nih.gov/pubmed/12878403 (accessed on 13 February 2020).

80. Der Bijl, P., van Eyk, A. D., Thompson, I. O. C., Stander, I. A. Diffusion rates of vasopressin through human vaginal and buccal mucosa. *Eur. J. Oral. Sci.* 1998, 106, 958–962. Available online: http://www.ncbi.nlm.nih.gov/pubmed/9786326 (accessed on 13 February 2020).

81. Van Eyk, A. D., Van der Bijl, P. Comparative permeability of various chemical markers through human vaginal and buccal mucosa as well as porcine buccal and mouth floor mucosa. *Arch. Oral Biol.* 2004, 49, 387–392. Available online: http://www.ncbi.nlm.nih. gov/pubmed/15041486 (accessed on 13 February 2020).

82. Waugh, A., Grant A. *Ross and Wilson: Anatomy and Physiology in Health and Illness.* (9th edn). Churchill Livingstone 2004, pp: 304–305.

83. Lakshmi Prasanna, J., Deepthi, B., Rama Rao, N. Rectal drug delivery: A promising route for enhancing drug absorption. *Asian J. Res. Pharm. Sci.* 2012, 2, 143–149.

84. Baviskar, P, Bedse, A, Sadique, S, Kunde, V, Jaiswal, S. Drug delivery on rectal absorption: suppositories. *Int. J. Pharm. Sci. Rev. Res.* 2013, 21, 70–76.

85. Harris, J. M. Poly (Ethylene Glycol) Chemistry: Biotechnical and Biomedical Applications, Springer: Berlin/Heidelberg, Germany, 2013, 1–385.

86. Machado, R. M., Palmeira-De-Oliveira, A., Martinez-De-Oliveira, J., Palmeira-De-Oliveira, R. Vaginal semisolid products: Technological performance considering physiologic parameters. *Eur. J. Pharm. Sci.* 2017, 109, 556–568.

87. Palmeira-De-Oliveira, R., Duarte, P., Palmeira-De-Oliveira, A., das Neves, J., Amaral, M. H., Breitenfeld, L., Martinez-De-Oliveira, J. Women's experiences, preferences and perceptions regarding vaginal products: Results from a cross-sectional web-based survey in Portugal. *Eur. J. Contracept. Reprod. Health Care* 2015, 20, 259–271.

88. Baloğlu, E., Bernkop-Schnürch, A., Karavana, S. Y., Þenyiðit, Z. A. Strategies to prolong the intravaginal residence time of drug delivery systems. *J. Pharm. Pharm. Sci.* 2009, 12, 312–336.

89. Palmeira-de-Oliveira, R., Duarte, P., Palmeira-de-Oliveira, A., das Neves, J., Amaral, M., Breitenfeld, L., Martinez-de-Oliveira, J. What do Portuguese women prefer regarding vaginal products? Results from a cross-sectional web-based survey. *Pharmaceutics* 2014, 6, 543–556.

90. Nappi, R. E., Liekens, G., Brandenburg, U. Attitudes, perceptions and knowledge about the vagina: The International Vagina Dialogue Survey. *Contraception* 2006, 73, 493–500.

91. Van Den Berg, J. J., Rosen, R. K., Bregman, D. E., Thompson, L. A., Jensen, K. M., Kiser, P. F., Katz, D. F., Buckheit, K., Buckheit, R. W., Jr., Morrow, K. M. Set it and forget it. Women's perceptions and opinions of long-acting topical vaginal gels. *AIDS Behav.* 2014, 18, 862–870.

92. Garg, S., Vermani, K., Garg, A., Anderson, R. A., Rencher, W. B., Zaneveld, L. J. D. Development and characterization of bioadhesive vaginal films of sodium polystyrene sulfonate (PSS), a novel contraceptive antimicrobial agent. *Pharm. Res.* 2005, 22, 584–595.

93. Almdal, K., Dyre, J., Hvidt, S., Kramer, O. Towards a phenomenological definition of the term "gel". *Polym. Gels Netw.* 1993, 1, 5–17.

94. Rogovina, L. Z., Vasil'Ev, V. G., Braudo, E. E. Definition of the concept of polymer gel. *Sci. Ser. C* 2008, 50, 85–92.

95. Yang, X., Zhang, G., Zhang, D. Stimuli responsive gels based on low molecular weight gelators. *J. Mater. Chem.* 2012, 22, 38–50.

96. Salah, S., Awad, G. E., Makhlouf, A. I. Improved vaginal retention and enhanced antifungal activity of miconazole microsponges gel: Formulation development and *in vivo* therapeutic efficacy in rats. *Eur. J. Pharm. Sci.* 2018, 114, 255–266.

97. Menard, J. P. Antibacterial treatment of bacterial vaginosis: Current and emerging therapies. *Int. J. Women's Health* 2011, 3, 295–305.

98. Friend, D. R. Advances in vaginal drug delivery. *Drug Deliv. Transl. Res.* 2011, 1, 183–184.

99. Rossi, S., Ferrari, F., Bonferoni, M. C., Sandri, G., Faccendini, A., Puccio, A., Caramella, C. Comparison of poloxamer-and chitosan-based thermally sensitive gels for the treatment of vaginal mucositis. *Drug Dev. Ind. Pharm.* 2013, 40, 352–360.

100. Yu, M., Vajdy, M. Mucosal HIV transmission and vaccination strategies through oral compared with vaginal and rectal routes. *Expert Opin. Biol. Ther.* 2010, 10, 1181–1195.

101. Home—ClinicalTrials.gov. Available online: https://clinicaltrials.gov/ (accessed on 28 January 2021).

102. De Araújo Pereira, R. R., Bruschi, M. L. Vaginal mucoadhesive drug delivery systems. *Drug Dev. Ind. Pharm.* 2012, 38, 643–652.

103. Khutoryanskiy, V. V. Advances in mucoadhesion and mucoadhesive polymers. *Macromol. Biosci.* 2011, 11, 748–764.

104. Kong, M., Chen, X. G., Xing, K., Park, H. J. Antimicrobial properties of chitosan and mode of action: A state of the art review. *Int. J. Food Microbiol.* 2010, 144, 51–63.

105. Bonferoni, M. C., Giunchedi, P., Scalia, S., Rossi, S., Sandri, G., Caramella, C. Chitosan gels for the vaginal delivery of lactic acid: Relevance of formulation parameters to mucoadhesion and release mechanisms. *AAPS PharmSciTech* 2006, 7, E141–E147.

106. Bonferoni, M. C., Sandri, G., Rossi, S., Ferrari, F., Gibin, S., Caramella, C. Chitosan citrate as multifunctional polymer for vaginal delivery. Evaluation of penetration enhancement and peptidase inhibition properties. *Eur. J. Pharm. Sci.* 2008, 33, 166–176.

107. Şenyiğit, Z. A., Karavana, S. Y., Eraç, B., Gürsel, Ö., Limoncu, M. H., Baloğlu, E. Evaluation of chitosan based vaginal bioadhesive gel formulations for antifungal drugs. *Acta Pharm.* 2014, 64, 139–156.

108. Demiröz, F. N. T., Acartürk, F., Erdoðan, D. Development of long-acting bioadhesive vaginal gels of oxybutynin: Formulation, *in vitro* and *in vivo* evaluations. *Int. J. Pharm.* 2013, 457, 25–39.

109. Cevher, E., Sensoy, D., Taha, M. A. M., Araman, A. Effect of thiolated polymers to textural and mucoadhesive properties of vaginal gel Formulations prepared with polycarbophil and chitosan. *AAPS PharmSciTech* 2008, 9, 953–965.

110. Bilensoy, E., Rouf, M. A., Vural, I., Šen, M., Hincal, A. A. Mucoadhesive, thermosensitive, prolonged-release vaginal gel for clotrimazole: β-cyclodextrin complex. *AAPS PharmSciTech* 2006, 7, E54–E60.

111. Aka-Any-Grah, A., Bouchemal, K., Koffi, A., Agnely, F., Zhang, M., Djabourov, M., Ponchel, G. Formulation of mucoadhesive vaginal hydrogels insensitive to dilution with vaginal fluids. *Eur. J. Pharm. Biopharm.* 2010, 76, 296–303.

112. Liu, Y., Zhu, Y., Wei, G., Lu, W. Effect of carrageenan on poloxamer-based in situ gel for vaginal use: Improved *in vitro* and *in vivo* sustained-release properties. *Eur. J. Pharm. Sci.* 2009, 37, 306–312.

113. Zhou, Q., Zhong, L., Wei, X., Dou, W., Chou, G., Wang, Z. Baicalein and hydroxypropyl-γ-cyclodextrin complex in poloxamer thermal sensitive hydrogel for vaginal administration. *Int. J. Pharm.* 2013, 454, 125–134.

114. Deshkar, S. S., Palve, V. K. Formulation and development of thermo-sensitive cyclodextrin-based in situ gel of voriconazole for vaginal delivery. *J. Drug Deliv. Sci. Technol.* 2019, 49, 277–285.

115. Rençber, S., Karavana, S. Y., Þenyiðit, Z. A., Eraç, B., Limoncu, M. H., Baloðlu, E. Mucoadhesive in situ gel formulation for vaginal delivery of clotrimazole: Formulation, preparation, and *in vitro*/*in vivo* evaluation. *Pharm. Dev. Technol.* 2016, 22, 551–561.

116. Cevher, E., Açma, A., Sinani, G., Aksu, B., Zloh, M., Mülazımoğlu, L. Bioadhesive tablets containing cyclodextrin complex of itraconazole for the treatment of vaginal candidiasis. *Int. J. Biol. Macromol.* 2014, 69, 124–136.

117. Gupta, N. V., Natasha, S., Getyala, A., Bhat, R. S. Bioadhesive vaginal tablets containing spray dried microspheres loaded with clotrimazole for treatment of vaginal Candidiasis. *Acta Pharm.* 2013, 63, 359–372.

118. Szymańska, E., Winnicka, K., Amelian, A., Cwalina, U. Vaginal chitosan tablets with clotrimazole-design and evaluation of mucoadhesive properties using porcine vaginal mucosa, mucin and gelatine. *Chem. Pharm. Bull.* 2014, 62, 160–167.

119. Baloğlu, E., Şenyığıt, Z. A., Karavana, S. Y., Vetter, A., Metın, D. Y., Polat, S. H., Guneri, T., Bernkop-Schnürch, A. *In vitro* evaluation of mucoadhesive vaginal tablets of antifungal drugs prepared with thiolated polymer and development of a new dissolution technique for vaginal formulations. *Chem. Pharm. Bull.* 2011, 59, 952–958.

120. Alam, M. A., Ahmad, F. J., Khan, Z. I., Khar, R. K., Ali, M. Development and evaluation of acid-buffering bioadhesive vaginal tablet for mixed vaginal infections. *AAPS PharmSciTech* 2007, 8, 229–236.

121. Ceschel, G. C., Maffei, P., Borgia, S. L., Ronchi, C., Rossi, S. Development of a mucoadhesive dosage form for vaginal administration. *Drug Dev. Ind. Pharm.* 2001, 27, 541–547.

122. McConville, C., Friend, D. R., Clark, M. R., Malcolm, K. Preformulation and development of a once-daily sustained-release tenofovir vaginal tablet tablet containing a single excipient. *J. Pharm. Sci.* 2013, 102, 1859–1868.

123. Notario-Pérez, F., Cazorla-Luna, R., Martín-Illana, A., Ruiz-Caro, R., Tamayo, A., Rubio, J., Veiga, M.-D. Optimization of tenofovir release from mucoadhesive vaginal tablets by polymer combination to prevent sexual transmission of HIV. *Carbohydr. Polym.* 2018, 179, 305–316.

124. McConville, C., Major, I., Devlin, B., Brimer, A. Development of a multi-layered vaginal tablet containing dapivirine, levonorgestrel and acyclovir for use as a multipurpose prevention technology. *Eur. J. Pharm. Biopharm.* 2016, 104, 171–179.

125. Rastogi, R., Teller, R. S., Mesquita, P. M. M., Herold, B. C., Kiser, P. F. Osmotic pump tablets for delivery of antiretrovirals to the vaginal mucosa. *Antivir. Res.* 2013, 100, 255–258.

126. Perioli, L., Ambrogi, V., Pagano, C., Massetti, E., Rossi, C. New solid mucoadhesive systems for benzydamine vaginal administration. *Colloids Surf. B Biointerfaces* 2011, 84, 413–420.

127. Ekin, M., Yaşar, L., Savan, K., Temur, M., Uhri, M., Gencer, I., Kıvanç, E. The comparison of hyaluronic acid vaginal tablets with estradiol

vaginal tablets in the treatment of atrophic vaginitis: A randomized controlled trial. *Arch. Gynecol. Obstet.* 2010, 283, 539–543.

128. Baloğlu, E., Özyazici, M., Hizarcioğlu, S. Y., Karavana, H. A. An *in vitro* investigation for vaginal bioadhesive formulations: Bioadhesive properties and swelling states of polymer mixtures. *Il Farmaco* 2003, 58, 391–396.

129. Hiorth, M., Nilsen, S., Tho, I. Bioadhesive mini-tablets for vaginal drug delivery. *Pharmaceutics* 2014, 6, 494–511. Available online: https://pubmed.ncbi.nlm.nih.gov/25166286/ (accessed on 21 March 2021).

130. Baffoe, C. S., Nguyen, N., Boyd, P., Wang, W., Morris, M., McConville, C. Disulfiram-loaded immediate and extended-release vaginal tablets for the localised treatment of cervical cancer. *J. Pharm. Pharmacol.* 2015, 67, 189–198.

131. Borges, S., Costa, P., Silva, J., Teixeira, P. Effects of processing and storage on pediococcuspentosaceus SB83 in vaginal formulations: Lyophilized powder and tablets. *Biomed. Res. Int.* 2013, 680767.

132. Nowak, J., Laffleur, F., Bernkop-Schnürch, A. Preactivated hyaluronic acid: A potential mucoadhesive polymer for vaginal delivery. *Int. J. Pharm.* 2015, 478, 383–389.

133. Thurman, A., Clark, M., Hurlburt, J., Doncel, G. Intravaginal rings as delivery systems for microbicides and multipurpose prevention technologies. *Int. J. Women's Health* 2013, 5, 695–708. Available online:/pmc/articles/PMC3808127/ (accessed on 24 April 2021).

134. Rochira, M., Miglietta, M. R., Richardson, J. L., Ferrari, L., Beccaro, M., Benedetti, L. Novel vaginal delivery systems for calcitonin. II. Preparation and characterization of HYAFF® microspheres containing calcitonin. *Int. J. Pharm.* 1996, 144, 19–26.

135. Pliszczak, D., Bourgeois, S., Bordes, C., Valour, J.-P., Mazoyer, M.-A., Orecchioni, A., Nakache, E., Lanteri, P. Improvement of an encapsulation process for the preparation of pro- and prebiotics-loaded bioadhesive microparticles by using experimental design. *Eur. J. Pharm. Sci.* 2011, 44, 83–92.

136. Maestrelli, F., Jug, M., Cirri, M., Kosalec, I., Mura, P. Characterization and microbiological evaluation of chitosan-alginate microspheres for cefixime vaginal administration. *Carbohydr. Polym.* 2018, 192, 176–183.

137. Zhang, T., Zhang, C., Agrahari, V., Murowchick, J. B., Oyler, N. A., Youan, B. B. C. Spray drying tenofovir loaded mucoadhesive and pH-sensitive

microspheres intended for HIV prevention. *Antivir. Res.* 2013, 97, 334–346.

138. Albertini, B., Passerini, N., Di Sabatino, M., Vitali, B., Brigidi, P., Rodriguez, L. Polymer-lipid based mucoadhesive microspheres prepared by spray-congealing for the vaginal delivery of econazole nitrate. *Eur. J. Pharm. Sci.* 2009, 36, 591–601.
139. Santiago, G. L., Verstraelen, H., Poelvoorde, N., De Corte, S., Claeys, G., Trog, M., De Backer, E., Saerens, B., Vervaet, C., De Boeck, F., et al. A pilot study evaluating the safety of vaginal administration of a multi-particulate pellet formulation. *Eur. J. Pharm. Biopharm.* 2009, 73, 399–403.
140. Mehta, S., De Beer, T., Remon, J. P., Vervaet, C. Effect of disintegrants on the properties of multiparticulate tablets comprising starch pellets and excipient granules. *Int. J. Pharm.* 2012, 422, 310–317.
141. Hiorth, M., Liereng, L., Reinertsen, R., Tho, I. Formulation of bio-adhesive hexylaminolevulinate pellets intended for photodynamic therapy in the treatment of cervical cancer. *Int. J. Pharm.* 2013, 441, 544–554.
142. Pinto Reis, C., Neufeld, R. J., Ribeiro, A. J., Veiga, F., Nanoencapsulation, I. Methods for preparation of drug-loaded polymeric nanoparticles. *Nanomed. Nanotechnol. Biol. Med.* 2006, 2, 8–21.
143. Das Neves, J., Sarmento, B. Precise engineering of dapivirine-loaded nanoparticles for the development of anti-HIV vaginal microbicides. *Acta Biomater.* 2015, 18, 77–87.
144. Gu, J., Yang, S., Ho, E. A. Biodegradable film for the targeted delivery of siRNA-loaded nanoparticles to vaginal immune cells. *Mol. Pharm.* 2015, 12, 2889–2903.
145. Yang, M., Yu, T., Wang, Y. Y., Lai, S. K., Zeng, Q., Miao, B., Hanes, J. Vaginal delivery of paclitaxel via nanoparticles with non-mucoadhesive surfaces suppresses cervical tumor growth. *Adv. Healthc. Mater.* 2014, 3, 1044–1052.
146. Melo, C. M., Cardoso, J. F., Perassoli, F. B., Neto, A. S. D. O., Pinto, L. M., Marques, M. B. D. F., Mussel, W. D. N., Magalhães, J., Moura, S. A. D. L., Araújo, M. G. D. F., et al. Amphotericin B-loaded Eudragit RL100 nanoparticles coated with hyaluronic acid for the treatment of vulvovaginal candidiasis. *Carbohydr. Polym.* 2020, 230, 115608.
147. Cunha-Reis, C., Machado, A., Barreiros, L., Araújo, F., Nunes, R., Seabra, V., Ferreira, D., Segundo, M., Sarmento, B., das Neves, J. Nanoparticles-in-film for the combined vaginal delivery of anti-HIV microbicide drugs. *J. Control. Release* 2016, 243, 43–53.

148. Jøraholmen, M. W., Basnet, P., Acharya, G., Škalko-Basnet, N. PEGylated liposomes for topical vaginal therapy improve delivery of interferon alpha. *Eur. J. Pharm. Biopharm.* 2017, 113, 132–139.

149. Santos, S. S., Lorenzoni, A., Pegoraro, N. S., Denardi, L. B., Alves, S. H., Schaffazick, S. R., Cruz, L. Formulation and *in vitro* evaluation of coconut oil-core cationic nanocapsules intended for vaginal delivery of clotrimazole. *Colloids Surf. B Biointerfaces* 2014, 116, 270–276.

150. Varan, C., Wickström, H., Sandler, N., Aktaş, Y., Bilensoy, E. Inkjet printing of antiviral PCL nanoparticles and anticancer cyclodextrin inclusion complexes on bioadhesive film for cervical administration. *Int. J. Pharm.* 2017, 531, 701–713.

151. Machado, A., Cunha-Reis, C., Araújo, F., Nunes, R., Seabra, V., Ferreira, D., das Neves, J., Sarmento, B. Development and *in vivo* safety assessment of tenofovir-loaded nanoparticles-in-film as a novel vaginal microbicide delivery system. *Acta Biomater.* 2016, 44, 332–340.

152. Sims, L. B., Curtis, L. T., Frieboes, H. B., Steinbach-Rankins, J. M. Enhanced uptake and transport of PLGA-modified nanoparticles in cervical cancer. *J. Nanobiotechnol.* 2016, 14, 1–12.

153. Maisel, K., Reddy, M., Xu, Q., Chattopadhyay, S., Cone, R., Ensign, L. M., Hanes, J. Nanoparticles coated with high molecular weight PEG penetrate mucus and provide uniform vaginal and colorectal distribution *in vivo*. *Nanomedicine* 2016, 11, 1337–1343.

154. Lechanteur, A., Furst, T., Evrard, B., Delvenne, P., Piel, G., Hubert, P. Promoting vaginal distribution of E7 and MCL-1 siRNA-silencing nanoparticles for cervical cancer treatment. *Mol. Pharm.* 2017, 14, 1706–1717.

155. Wang, X., Fu, L., Lin, W., Zhang, W., Pei, Q., Zheng, X., Liu, S., Zhang, T., Xie, Z. Vaginal delivery of mucus-penetrating organic nanoparticles for photothermal therapy against cervical intraepithelial neoplasia in mice. *J. Mater. Chem. B* 2019, 7, 4528–4537.

156. Frank, L. A., Chaves, P. S., D'Amore, C. M., Contri, R. V., Frank, A. G., Beck, R., Pohlmann, A. R., Buffon, A., Guterres, S. S. The use of chitosan as cationic coating or gel vehicle for polymeric nanocapsules: Increasing penetration and adhesion of imiquimod in vaginal tissue. *Eur. J. Pharm. Biopharm.* 2017, 114, 202–212.

157. Lucena, P. A., Nascimento, T. L., Gaeti, M. P. N., De Ávila, R. I., Mendes, L. P., Vieira, M. S., Fabrini, D., Amaral, A. C., Lima, E. M. *In vivo* vaginal fungal load reduction after treatment with itraconazole-loaded

polycaprolactone-nanoparticles. *J. Biomed. Nanotechnol.* 2018, 14, 1347–1358.

158. Marciello, M., Rossi, S., Caramella, C., Remuñán-López, C. Freeze-dried cylinders carrying chitosan nanoparticles for vaginal peptide delivery. *Carbohydr. Polym.* 2017, 170, 43–51.

159. Rossi, S., Vigani, B., Puccio, A., Bonferoni, M. C., Sandri, G., Ferrari, F. Chitosan ascorbate nanoparticles for the vaginal delivery of antibiotic drugs in atrophic vaginitis. *Mar. Drugs* 2017, 15, 319.

160. Lalan, M. S., Patel, V. N., Misra, A. Polymers in vaginal drug delivery: Recent advancements. In *Applications of Polymers in Drug Delivery*, Elsevier: Amsterdam, The Netherlands, 2021, pp. 281–303.

161. Yoo, J.-W., Dharmala, K., Lee, C. H. The physicodynamic properties of mucoadhesive polymeric films developed as female-controlled drug delivery system. *Int. J. Pharm.* 2006, 309, 139–145.

162. Machado, R. M., Palmeira-De-Oliveira, A., de Oliveira, J. M., Palmeira-De-Oliveira, R. Vaginal films for drug delivery. *J. Pharm. Sci.* 2013, 102, 2069–2081.

163. Rohan, L. C., Sassi, A. B. Vaginal drug delivery systems for HIV prevention. *AAPS J.* 2009, 11, 78–87.

164. Akil, A., Devlin, B., Cost, M., Rohan, L. C. Increased dapivirine tissue accumulation through vaginal film codelivery of dapivirine and tenofovir. *Mol. Pharm.* 2014, 11, 1533–1541.

165. Traore, Y. L., Fumakia, M., Gu, J., A Ho, E. Dynamic mechanical behaviour of nanoparticle loaded biodegradable PVA films for vaginal drug delivery. *J. Biomater. Appl.* 2018, 32, 1119–1126.

166. Cautela, M. P., Moshe, H., Sosnik, A., Sarmento, B., Das Neves, J. Composite films for vaginal delivery of tenofovir disoproxil fumarate and emtricitabine. *J. Pharm. Biopharm.* 2019, 138, 3–10.

167. Vartak, R., Patki, M., Menon, S., Jablonski, J., Mediouni, S., Fu, Y., Valente, S. T., Billack, B., Patel, K. β-cyclodextrin polymer/Soluplus® encapsulated Ebselen ternary complex (EβpolySol) as a potential therapy for vaginal candidiasis and pre-exposure prophylactic for HIV. *Int. J. Pharm.* 2020, 589, 119863.

168. Politch, J. A., Cu-Uvin, S., Moench, T. R., Tashima, K. T., Marathe, J. G., Guthrie, K. M., Cabral, H., Nyhuis, T., Brennan, M., Zeitlin, L., et al. Safety, acceptability, and pharmacokinetics of a monoclonal antibody-based vaginal multipurpose prevention film (MB66): A Phase I randomized trial. *PLoS Med.* 2021, 18, e1003495.

169. Ham, A. S., Rohan, L. C., Boczar, A., Yang, L., Buckheit, K. W., Buckheit, R. W. Vaginal film drug delivery of the pyrimidinedione IQP-0528 for the prevention of HIV infection. *Pharm. Res.* 2012, 29, 1897–1907.

170. Neurath, A. R., Strick, N., Li, Y.-Y. Water dispersible microbicidal cellulose acetate phthalate film. *BMC Infect. Dis.* 2003, 3, 27.

171. Kumar, L., Reddy, M. S., Shirodkar, R. K., Pai, G. K., Krishna, V. T., Verma, R. Preparation and characterisation of fluconazole vaginal films for the treatment of vaginal candidiasis. *Indian J. Pharm. Sci.* 2013, 75, 585–590.

172. Gahlot, N., Maheshwari, R. K. Formulation and development of vaginal films of poorly water-soluble drug, metronidazole, using mixed solvency concept and their evaluations. *J. Drug Deliv. Ther.* 2018, 8, 41–48.

173. Zhang, W., Parniak, M. A., Sarafianos, S. G., Cost, M. R., Rohan, L. C. Development of a vaginal delivery film containing EFdA, a novel anti-HIV nucleoside reverse transcriptase inhibitor. *Int. J. Pharm.* 2014, 461, 203–213.

174. Gong, T., Zhang, W., Parniak, M. A., Graebing, P. W., Moncla, B., Gupta, P., Empey, K. M., Rohan, L. C. Preformulation and vaginal film formulation development of microbicide drug candidate CSIC for HIV prevention. *J. Pharm. Innov.* 2017, 12, 142–154.

175. Zhang, W., Hu, M., Shi, Y., Gong, T., Dezzutti, C. S., Moncla, B., Sarafianos, S. G., Parniak, M. A., Rohan, L. C. Vaginal microbicide film combinations of two reverse transcriptase inhibitors, EFdA and CSIC, for the prevention of HIV-1 sexual transmission. *Pharm. Res.* 2015, 32, 2960–2972.

176. Akil, A., Parniak, M. A., Dezzuitti, C. S., Moncla, B. J., Cost, M. R., Li, M., Rohan, L. C. Development and characterization of a vaginal film containing dapivirine, a non-nucleoside reverse transcriptase inhibitor (NNRTI), for prevention of HIV-1 sexual transmission. *Drug Deliv. Transl. Res.* 2011, 1, 209–222.

177. Yoo, J.-W., Acharya, G., Lee, C. H. *In vivo* evaluation of vaginal films for mucosal delivery of nitric oxide. *Biomaterials* 2009, 30, 3978–3985.

178. Notario-Pérez, F., Martín-Illana, A., Cazorla-Luna, R., Ruiz-Caro, R., Bedoya, L.-M., Peña, J., Veiga, M.-D. Development of mucoadhesive vaginal films based on HPMC and zein as novel formulations to prevent sexual transmission of HIV. *Int. J. Pharm.* 2019, 570, 118643.

179. Gyotoku, T., Aurelian, L., Neurath, A. R. Cellulose acetate phthalate (CAP): An "inactive" pharmaceutical excipient with antiviral activity in the mouse model of genital herpesvirus infection. *Antivir. Chem. Chemother.* 1999, 10, 327–332.

180. Lu, H., Zhao, Q., Wallace, G., Liu, S., He, Y., Shattock, R., Neurath, A. R., Jiang, B. S. Cellulose acetate 1,2-benzenedicarboxylate inhibits infection by cell-free and cell-associated primary HIV-1 isolates. *AIDS Res. Hum. Retrovir.* 2006, 22, 411–418.

181. Regev, G., Patel, S. K., Moncla, B. J., Twist, J., Devlin, B., Rohan, L. C. Novel application of hot melt extrusion for the manufacturing of vaginal films containing microbicide candidate dapivirine. *AAPS PharmSciTech* 2019, 20, 239.

182. Machado, R. S. M., Tomás, M., Palmeira-De-Oliveira, A., de Oliveira, J. M., Palmeira-De-Oliveira, R. The vaginal sheet: An innovative form of vaginal film for the treatment of vaginal infections. *Drug Dev. Ind. Pharm.* 2020, 46, 135–145.

183. Garg, S., Goldman, D., Krumme, M., Rohan, L. C., Smoot, S., Friend, D. R. Advances in development, scale-up and manufacturing of microbicide gels, films, and tablets. *Antivir. Res.* 2010, 88, S19–S29.

184. Notario-Pérez, F., Cazorla-Luna, R., Martín-Illana, A., Galante, J., Ruiz-Caro, R., das Neves, J., Veiga, M.-D. Design, fabrication and characterisation of drug-loaded vaginal films: State-of-the-art. *J. Control. Release* 2020, 327, 477–499.

185. Garg, S., Tambwekar, K. R., Vermani, K., Kandarapu, R., Garg, A., Waller, D. P., Zaneveld, L. J. Development pharmaceutics of microbicide formulations. Part II: Formulation, evaluation, and challenges. *AIDS Patient Care STDs* 2003, 17, 377–399.

186. Drumond, N., van Riet-Nales, D. A., Karapinar-Çarkit, F., Stegemann, S. Patients' appropriateness, acceptability, usability and preferences for pharmaceutical preparations: Results from a literature review on clinical evidence. *Int. J. Pharm.* 2017, 521, 294–305.

187. Ghosal, K., Ranjan, A., Bhowmik, B. B. A novel vaginal drug delivery system: Anti-HIV bioadhesive film containing abacavir. *J. Mater. Sci. Mater. Med.* 2014, 25, 1679–1689.

188. Bassi, P., Kaur, G. Bioadhesive vaginal drug delivery of nystatin using a derivatized polymer: Development and characterization. *Eur. J. Pharm. Biopharm.* 2015, 96, 173–184.

189. Mishra, R., Soni, K., Mehta, T. Mucoadhesive vaginal film of fluconazole using cross-linked chitosan and pectin: *In vitro* and *in vivo* study. *J. Therm. Anal. Calorim.* 2017, 130, 1683–1695.

190. Dolci, L. S., Albertini, B., Di Filippo, M. F., Bonvicini, F., Passerini, N., Panzavolta, S. Development and *in vitro* evaluation of mucoadhesive gelatin films for the vaginal delivery of econazole. *Int. J. Pharm.* 2020, 591, 119979.

191. Frankman, O., Raabe, N., A Ingemansson, C. Clinical evaluation of C-film, a vaginal contraceptive. *J. Int. Med. Res.* 1975, 3, 292–296.

192. Hynes, J. S., Sales, J. M., Sheth, A. N., Lathrop, E., Haddad, L. B. Interest in multipurpose prevention technologies to prevent HIV/STIs and unintended pregnancy among young women in the United States. *Contraception* 2018, 97, 277–284.

193. Schreier, J., Sales, J., Sheth, A., Lathrop, E., Haddad, L. Interest in multipurpose prevention technologies for protection against unintended pregnancy, human immunodeficiency virus and other sexually transmitted infections among women in the United States. *Am. J. Obstet. Gynecol.* 2017, 217, 731.

194. Fernandes, T., Baxi, K., Sawarkar, S., Sarmento, B., das Neves, J. Vaginal multipurpose prevention technologies: Promising approaches for enhancing women's sexual and reproductive health. *Expert Opin. Drug Deliv.* 2020, 17, 379–393.

195. Repka, M., Repka, S., Mcginity, J. Bioadhesive hot-melt extruded film for topical and mucosal adhesion applications and drug delivery and process for preparation there of. U.S. Patent US6375963B1, 23 April 2002.

196. Leon, T., Gabel, P. Dissolvable vaginal deodorizing films and methods of vaginal deodorizing utilizing pliable dissolvable film. WO2004103232A1, 2 December 2004.

197. Maniar, M., Parandoosh, S. Ph-responsive film for intravaginal delivery of a beneficial agent. US20060018951A1, 4 April 2005.

198. Yang, J. T., Gao, H. M. *Lactobacillus* drug film. CN101199555A, 15 December 2006.

199. Staab, R. J. Methods for delivery of medication using a dissolvable device. US20130136784A1, 16 October 2009.

200. Notario-Pérez, F., Galante, J., Martín-Illana, A., Cazorla-Luna, R., Sarmento, B., Ruiz-Caro, R., das Neves, J., Veiga, M. D. Development of pH-sensitive vaginal films based on methacrylate copolymers for topical HIV-1 pre-exposure prophylaxis. *Acta Biomater.* 2021, 121, 316–327.

201. Dhamane, S., Kulkarni, A., Vaishali, P., Modase, M. Formulation and evaluation of rectal delivery system for the treatment of hemorrhoids. *Pharm. Reason.* 2018, 1, 42–50.

202. Yun, M., Choi, H., Jung, J., Kim, C. Development of a thermo-reversible insulin liquid suppository with bioavailability enhancement. *Int. J. Pharm.* 1999, 189, 137–145.

203. Abbas, Z., Aditya, N., Swamy, N. G. N. Fabrication and *in vitro* evaluation of mucoadhesive, thermoreversible, in situ gelling liquid sup-pository of chloroquine phosphate. *Indian J. Nov. Drug Deliv.* 2013, 5, 60–70.

204. Ramadan, E. M., Borg, T. M., Elkayal, M. O. Formulation and evaluation of novel mucoadhesive ketorolac tromethamine liquid suppository. *AJPP* 2009, 3, 124–132.

205. Kassab, H. J., Khalil, Y. I. 5-Fluorouracil mucoadhesive liquid formulation and evaluation. *World J. Pharm. Res.* 2014, 3, 119–135.

206. Ban, E., Kim, C.-K. Design and evaluation of ondansetron liquid suppository for the treatment of emesis. *Arch. Pharm. Res.* 2013, 36, 586–592.

207. Benedetti, M. S., Whomsley, R., Poggesi, I., Cawello, W., Mathy, F.-X., Delporte, M.-L., Papeleu, P., Watelet, J.-B. Drug metabolism and pharmacokinetics. *Drug Metab. Rev.* 2009, 41, 344–390.

208. El-Kamel, A., El-Khatib, M. Thermally reversible in situ gelling carbamazepine liquid suppository. *Drug Deliv.* 2006, 13, 143–148.

209. Purohit, T. J., Hanning, S. M., Wu, Z. Advances in rectal drug delivery systems. *Pharm. Dev. Technol.* 2018, 23(10), 942–952. https://doi.org/10.1080/10837450.2018.1484766.

210. Hua S., Marks E., Schneider J. J., Keely S. Advances in oral nano-delivery systems for colon targeted drug delivery in inflammatory bowel disease: selective targeting to diseased versus healthy tissue. *Nanomedicine* 2015, 11(5), 1117–1132. 10.1016/j.nano.2015.02.018.

211. Zhang S., Langer R., Traverso G. Nanoparticulate drug delivery systems targeting inflammation for treatment of inflammatory bowel disease. *Nano Today*. 2017, 16, 82–96. 10.1016/j.nantod.2017.08.006.

212. Mesquita L., Galante J., Nunes R., Sarmento B., das Neves J. Pharmaceutical vehicles for vaginal and rectal administration of anti-HIV microbicide nanosystems. *Pharmaceutics* 2019, 11(3), 145. 10.3390/pharmaceutics11030145.

213. Maisel K., Chattopadhyay S., Moench T., Hendrix C., Cone R., Ensign L. M., et al. Enema ion compositions for enhancing colorectal drug delivery. *J. Control Release* 2015, 209, 280–287. 10.1016/j.jconrel.2015.04.040.

214. Abdelbary G., Fahmy R. H. Diazepam-loaded solid lipid nanoparticles: design and characterization. *AAPS PharmSciTech.* 2009, 10(1), 211–219. 10.1208/s12249-009-9197-2.

215. Mohamed R. A., Abass H. A., Attia M. A., Heikal O. A. Formulation and evaluation of metoclopramide solid lipid nanoparticles for rectal suppository. *J. Pharm. Pharmacol.* 2013, 65(11), 1607–1621. 10.1111/jphp.12136.

216. Sercombe L., Veerati T., Moheimani F., Wu S. Y., Sood A. K., Hua S. Advances and challenges of liposome assisted drug delivery. *Front. Pharmacol.* 6, 2015, 286. 10.3389/fphar.2015.00286.

217. Melo M., Nunes R., Sarmento B., das Neves J. Colorectal distribution and retention of polymeric nanoparticles following incorporation into a thermosensitive enema. *Biomater. Sci.* 2019, 7, 3801–3811. 10.1039/C9BM00759H.

218. Din F. U., Mustapha O., Kim D. W., Rashid R., Park J. H., Choi J. Y., et al. Novel dual-reverse thermosensitive solid lipid nanoparticle-loaded hydrogel for rectal administration of flurbiprofen with improved bioavailability and reduced initial burst effect. *Eur. J. Pharm. Biopharm.* 2015, 94, 64–72. 10.1016/j.ejpb.2015.04.019.

219. Din F. U., Mustapha O., Kim D. W., Rashid R., Park J. H., Choi J. Y., et al. Novel dual-reverse thermosensitive solid lipid nanoparticle-loaded hydrogel for rectal administration of flurbiprofen with improved bioavailability and reduced initial burst effect. *Eur. J. Pharm. Biopharm.* 2015, 94, 64–72. 10.1016/j.ejpb.2015.04.019.

220. Gross V., Bar-Meir S., Lavy A., Mickisch O., Tulassay Z., Pronai L., et al. Budesonide foam versus budesonide enema in active ulcerative proctitis and proctosigmoiditis. *Aliment. Pharmacol. Therapeut.* 2006, 1523(2), 303–312.

Multiple-Choice Questions

1. The spermicidal ingredient in contemporary contraceptive gels and creams

    a. Lactic acid
    b. Acetic acid
    c. Hydrochloric acid
    d. All

2. An inner mucosal tissue layer of the vagina made up of stratified squamous epithelium
   a. Stratified squamous epithelium
   b. Non-stratified squamous epithelium
   c. Both a and b
   d. None
3. The vaginal microbial environment consists of
   a. CST-IV
   b. *Gardnerella*
   c. *Atopobium*
   d. All of them
4. The advantage of vaginal administration is
   a. Less frequent dosing
   b. Less adverse effects
   c. No hepatic first-pass impact
   d. All
5. Obstacles to be overcome before developing vaginal formulations
   a. Vaginal fluid dilution
   b. Peristaltic movement of the vaginal wall
   c. Both a and b
   d. None of these
6. The most prevalent vaginal abnormalities
   a. Atrophic vaginitis
   b. Desquamative inflammatory vaginitis
   c. Mucoid ectopy
   d. All of these
7. Functions of natural or synthetic polymers used in most vaginal formulations are
   a. The drug remains in contact with the site of action for as long as feasible
   b. Delivers a controlled drug release on a consistent and predictable basis

   c. Both a and b
   d. None of these

8. The rectal formulations are used to treat
   a. Constipation
   b. Hemorrhoids
   c. Anal fissures
   d. All

9. Compared to parenteral dosage forms, rectal dosage forms are
   a. Often less expensive to produce
   b. Self-administered by patients
   c. Do not require a medically trained person
   d. All of these

10. Patients do not like the rectal route of administration due to
    a. Cultural concerns
    b. Risk of discomfort
    c. Leaking
    d. All of these

11. Women who received intravaginal antimicrobial drugs were happier with their treatment than those who received oral antimicrobial agents.
    a. Yes
    b. No

12. The semisolid formulations for vaginal usage
    a. Gels
    b. Creams
    c. Ointments
    d. All of these

13. Advantages of semisolid formulations
    a. High acceptability
    b. Ease of use
    c. Reasonable production costs
    d. All of these

14. Which of the following factors strengthens the clinical impact of vaginal semisolid products?
    a. Frequent administration
    b. Using mucoadhesive polymers
    c. Both a and b
    d. None of these
15. A vaginal gel dosage form is a flexible solid made up of two or more components.
    a. Yes
    b. No
16. ____________ connections hold chemical gels together.
    a. Strong covalent
    b. Hydrogen bonds
    c. Both a and b
    d. None of these
17. Hydrogen bonds hold ________ together.
    a. Physical gels
    b. Chemical gels
    c. Both a and b
    d. None of these
18. Hydrogels are
    a. Water-based liquid components
    b. Non-aqueous liquid components
    c. Both a and b
    d. All of these
19. Organogels are
    a. Non-aqueous liquid components
    b. Water-based liquid components
    c. Both a and b
    d. None of these
20. Mucoadhesion is caused by interactions between formulation components and the mucus layer that lines the surface of the vaginal mucous membrane.
    a. Yes
    b. No

21. Mucins are
    a. Water-soluble glycoproteins
    b. High degree of glycosylation
    c. Most essential components of mucus
    d. All of these
22. ________ join the subunits of mucin, forming enormous three-dimensional gel formations.
    a. Disulfide bridges
    b. Nitrogen
    c. Phosphorus
    d. All of these
23. Mucoadhesive formulation components interact with mucin via
    a. Hydrogen bonds
    b. Van der Waals interactions
    c. Electrostatic interactions
    d. All of these
24. Chitosan is a
    a. A cationic linear polysaccharide
    b. Produced from chitin deacetylation
    c. Both a and b
    d. None of these
25. Chitosan is recognized for
    a. Antibacterial
    b. Wound-healing characteristics
    c. Bioadhesive polymers
    d. All
26. Smaller the polymer's molecular weight, the stronger the bioadhesive contacts.
    a. Yes
    b. No
27. Traditional solid vaginal dose forms
    a. Globules
    b. Suppositories

c. Both a and b
d. None of these

28. Hydroxypropyl methylcellulose (HPMC) is a
    a. Polymer
    b. Lipid
    c. Carbohydrate
    d. None of these

29. Pectins could be used in vaginal medicine delivery systems in the future.
    a. Yes
    b. No

30. Osmotic pump tablets (OPTs) can also be administered vaginally
    a. Yes
    b. No

31. Pessaries may be equally effective as other vaginal dosing forms.
    a. Yes
    b. No

32. Topical distribution of the medicine through the vaginal ring allows for lower drug doses while also avoiding a first-pass impact on the liver.
    a. Yes
    b. No

33. The benefit of vaginal rings is
    a. Reduce pain
    b. Should not be sensed during normal activities
    c. No effect on sexual behavior
    d. All of these

34. Polymeric microspheres were tested as a medication carrier for vaginal administration more than 20 years ago.
    a. Yes
    b. No

35. The process used to create microparticles
    a. Emulsification
    b. Gelation
    c. Both a and b
    d. None of these
36. The encapsulation technology has the potential to increase the effects of *Lactobacillus* sp. while also protecting them during the drying and storage process.
    a. Yes
    b. No
37. Chitosan-alginate microspheres are used for
    a. Cefixime vaginal administration
    b. Dopamine
    c. All of these
    d. None of these
38. The optimum formulation of microspheres is produced with 30 mg/mL cefixime, as determined by the connection between water uptake and drug release rate.
    a. Yes
    b. No
39. Pellets have been suggested as carriers for active compounds or as matrices for probiotic bacteria.
    a. Yes
    b. No
40. Polymeric nanoparticles (NPs) are
    a. Drug carriers for vaginal delivery
    b. Small and very stable particles
    c. Particles that have a diameter of less than 1000 nm
    d. All of these
41. Synthetic polymers are
    a. Poly(lactic-co-glycolic) acid (PLGA)
    b. Polyethylene glycol (PEG)
    c. (Meth)acrylate polymers and polyesters (polycaprolactone)
    d. All of these

42. Vaginal films are solid dosage forms made largely of aqueous polymers and plasticizers that may or may not contain an active ingredient
    a. True
    b. False
43. Vaginal films
    a. Are soft and flexible
    b. Are preferably colorless and odorless
    c. Scatter or dissolve when they come into contact with vaginal fluids, allowing them to adhere and stay in the vaginal mucosa for long periods.
    d. All of these
44. Traditional rectal drug forms including solid dosage forms include
    a. Capsules
    b. Suppositories
    c. Tablets
    d. All of these
45. Enemas are the most popular liquid dosage form for rectal drug delivery
    a. True
    b. False

Answer Key

1.	a	**2.**	a	**3.**	d	**4.**	d	**5.**	c	**6.**	d	**7.**	c
8.	d	**9.**	d	**10.**	d	**11.**	a	**12.**	d	**13.**	d	**14.**	c
15.	a	**16.**	a	**17.**	a	**18.**	a	**19.**	a	**20.**	a	**21.**	d
22.	a	**23.**	d	**24.**	c	**25.**	d	**26.**	a	**27.**	c	**28.**	a
29.	a	**30.**	a	**31.**	a	**32.**	a	**33.**	d	**34.**	a	**35.**	c
36.	a	**37.**	a	**38.**	a	**39.**	a	**40.**	d	**41.**	d	**42.**	a
43.	d	**44.**	d	**45.**	a								

Short-Answer-Type Questions

1. List physiological characteristics considered for vaginal drug development.
2. List the physiological characteristics considered for rectal drug development.
3. Explain the mucoadhesion process.
4. Write a short note on vaginal films.
5. Write a short note on microspheres.
6. Write a short note on pellets.

Long-Answer-Type Questions

1. Explain in detail the NDDS for vaginal formulations.
2. Explain in detail the NDDS for rectal formulations.

Chapter 14

Nanonutraceuticals and Their Applications

Kashish Wilson,[a] Anju Bala,[a] Megha,[a] Rakesh K. Sindhu,[b] Manish Kumar Jeengar,[c] Inderjeet Verma,[a] Rajan Swami,[d] and Chander Parkash Dora[d]

[a]*Maharishi Markandeshwar College of Pharmacy, MM (DU), Mullana, Ambala, Haryana, India*
[b]*School of Pharmacy, Sharda University, Greater Noida, Uttar Pradesh, India*
[c]*School of Pharmacy, Amrita Vishwa Vidyapeetham, Kochi, Kerala, India*
[d]*Chitkara College of Pharmacy, Chitkara University, Punjab, India*

chanddora@gmail.com

Plant-based sources have always been a focal point in the origination of newer therapeutic entities. For cancer therapy, numerous phytoconstituents are available, such as taxanes (paclitaxel, docetaxel), vinca alkaloids (vincristine), podophyllotoxins (etoposide), and camptothecin. Moreover, like synthetic molecules, these also possess challenges such as poor solubility, stability, and target-ability for delivery purposes. To overcome these issues, various technologies have been explored and commercialized. Nanotechnology-based delivery approach is one of the innovative platforms to improvise cancer therapeutics by enhancing the solubility of hydrophobic phytodrugs, increasing their stability, permeability, and targeting cancerous cells. This

Nanotechnology and Drug Delivery: Principles and Applications
Edited by Rakesh K. Sindhu

ISBN 978-981-4968-83-6 (Hardcover), 978-1-003-43040-7 (eBook)
www.jennystanford.com

chapter discusses and explores different formulation strategies involving nanotechnologies such as lipid nanoparticles (solid lipid, nanostructured lipid carriers, liposomes) and polymeric and lipid-polymer hybrid nanoparticles to deliver drugs based on plant resources.

14.1 Plant Bioactives Used in Cancer Therapy

Cancer is mainly treated surgically by removing the solid tumors and afterward, followed by treatment with radiation and chemotherapy, which result in numerous side effects [1]. Another major problem of traditional chemotherapeutic agents is drug resistance caused by various mechanisms [2]. These issues can be reduced by utilizing natural sources. It was found that more than 80% of anticancer drugs belong to natural origin. Out of the natural sources medicinal plants are considered as the safest chemopreventive agents [3]. Plant bioactives are phytochemicals capable of modulating metabolic functions, which results in improving health [4]. They are extensively studied as a potential source for treating various diseases. They show structural diversity as it has a greater number of chiral centers and varied rings as compared to synthetic drugs. This helps in the target selectivity and hence reduces the unwanted side effects [5].

Plant bioactives such as curcumin, resveratrol, genistein, psoralen, and epigenin contain polyphenols and are vastly studied for their use in cancer therapy [6]. Curcumin is extracted from *Curcuma longa* and exhibits its anticancer activity due to its immunomodulating action by controlling different signaling pathways and regulating levels of cyclooxygenase-2, cytokines, and reactive oxygen species. It has shown therapeutic benefits in various forms of cancer such as lung, pancreatic, gastric, prostate, and brain tumors [7]. Another phenolic compound used in cancer therapy is resveratrol extracted from fruits and vegetables mainly berries, pines, grapes, and peanuts. It has also shown activity in skin, pancreatic, colon, prostate, liver, and breast cancers [8]. Quercetin is a flavonoid compound majorly present in our daily diet. It acts by varying cell cycle progression, inhibiting cell proliferation, and angiogenesis, thus promoting apoptosis. This compound shows excellent results in treating a wide range of cancers [9]. Paclitaxel is obtained from *Taxus brevifolia* and acts by resisting microtubulin depolymerization and it blocks mitosis progression [10]. Etoposide is obtained from podophyllin and is primarily useful in treating lung cancer and ovarian cancer. It acts by inhibiting DNA topoisomerase II, which leads to the inhibition of DNA synthesis at the pre-mitotic stage [11]. Various *in vitro* studies related to plant bioactive on cancer cell lines are summarized in Table 14.1.

Plant bioactives show a synergistic effect in combination with other plant bioactives. The main intention to give drugs in combination is a reduction in dose and toxicity. In a study, resveratrol and etoposide were given in combination to treat liver carcinoma and colon cancer, which improved the antiproliferative effect [12]. Quercetin and curcumin increase the apoptotic effect in breast cancer when used in combination. However, these plant bioactive compounds have poor bioavailability, which can be improved by developing an appropriate formulation [13]. Other plant bioactive combinations were indirubin and vinblastine in cervical cancer treatment [14], curcumin and resveratrol in colon cancer treatment [15], and quercetin and resveratrol in prostate cancer treatment [16].

This similar kind of synergistic behavior has also been seen in the combination of plant bioactives and synthetic antineoplastic drugs for anticancer activities. Curcumin reverses the 5-Fluorouracil (5-FU) resistance by downregulation of NFk B signaling and increases the activity in gastric cancer [17]. *Rauwolfia vomitoria* extract reduced the tumor burden by up to 90% in ovarian carcinoma when combined with carboplatin [18]. Another combination that shows synergistic effects is quercetin with doxorubicin (useful in various forms of cancer, including breast cancer) [19], berberine with tamoxifen (also useful in breast cancer treatment) [20], and curcumin with cisplatin (useful in ovarian cancer) [21].

Table 14.1 Cytotoxic effects shown by different plant bioactives

Plant bioactive	Cancer	Dose	Outcome	Refs
Curcumin	Colorectal	6.25–50 μM	Induce DNA impairment and mitosis phase arrest	[22]
Curcumin	Breast	100 μM	Telomerase inhibitor	[23]
Quercetin	Colon	0.1–100 μM	Apoptosis inducer and cell growth inhibitor	[24]
Paclitaxel	Lung	50 nM	Cause cell death via caspase-independent routes	[25]
Resveratrol	Ovarian	160 mg/kg	Shows antineoplastic action by inhibiting glucose uptake	[26]
Procyanudine B3	Prostate	10–100 μM	Act by inhibiting p300-dependent acetylation of androgen receptor	[27]
Topotecan	Breast	IC_{50}:0.218 μM	Increased oxidative stress in MCF-7 cell lines	[28]
Fisetin	Lung	10–40 μM	Kinase 1 and 2 inhibitor	[29]
Piceatannol	Prostate	20 mg/kg	Decrease interleukin-6 signaling	[30]
Gallic acid	Ovarian	40 μM	Antiproliferation and vascular endothelial growth factor expression inhibition	[31]
Genistein	Colon	50 μM	Shows negative effect on epidermal growth factor	[32]

14.2 Various Challenges to Deliver Plant-Derived Molecules

Despite various studies having been carried out, cancer is the leading cause of death all over the world. Cancer treatment is available with various synthetic chemotherapeutic agents but toxicity issues such as nephrotoxicity and skin toxicity have been reported from various synthetic drugs such as doxorubicin and 5-fluorouracil. Thus, an alternative arrangement is adopted for producing safe and less expensive cancer treatment. Plant-based molecules in the form of nanocarriers are adopted for cancer as they have good potential as antitumor agents. Moreover, they are safe and environment-friendly. Generally, they are a variety of plant-derived molecules available, such as vincristine, vinblastine, taxol, curcumin, and other agents. The basic challenges for these agents are poor aqueous solubility and their adverse effects [33]. Irrespective of enormous therapies for cancer by various plant-derived molecules, there have been various challenges in providing favorable outcomes in clinical studies [34, 35]. The major issues encountered with various polyphenolic plant-derived agents are less water solubility, reduced stability, and poor bioavailability. The extraction of these plant-derived molecules requires specific solvents, which may increase the cost of extraction processes [36]. There are plant-derived polyphenolic compounds when taken orally, they show very inferior bioavailability [37]. Further, the metabolism of these natural compounds occurs in the small intestine as well as the liver, which leads to reduced targeting in the main tissue in the bloodstream [38]. Thus, various Phase II enzymes convert these polyphenolic compounds into various methylated derivatives in which their ability for therapeutic action is still not known. Apparently, the mobile dose for the production of pharmacological activity is very less in experimental design because the amount of aglycone part of polyphenolic compound concentration is reduced compared with its mobile dose. Thus, to showcase the active role of plant resources in cancer therapy, nanotechnology is used for the production of plant resources [39]. To overcome the challenges of the clinical application of polyphenolic resources of plants, targeted delivery is secured by the formation of nanosized carriers for natural resources. In this way, these carriers help to transfer these natural resources to the site of tissue such as malignant to achieve maximum anticancer properties along with minimum production of toxicity in the bloodstream [40]. In order to produce a targeting effect in stipulated cells, plant resources nanoformulation need to be prepared on the basis of unique alteration in their size and shape. The targeting to the tumor cells is primarily active and passive.

In active targeting, various natural actives-loaded nanocarriers selectively target the site of the tumorous cells concerned, which leads to the avoidance of several adverse effects that were otherwise shown in conventional formulations. Passive targeting also plays a similar role in targeting tumor cells by nanoformulation of plant resources through the enhanced permeation and retention

(EPR) phenomenon of nanotechnology. In cases of other selective routes, there would be chances of unstable maturation of solid tumors, and natural resources might come in the state of higher permeability as well as retention passage which leads to the formation of nanoformulation as the best mode of treatment of solid tumors [41].

The other challenges faced by nanoformulation for adopting the process of targeting are formulation issues, passage in the body, simultaneous relation with the living system, and minimal reduction in toxicity so that a complete plant active loaded in nanoformulations can be formulated. The prime concern of formulation is the ability of nanoparticles to act as an antigenic agent on their own. The bioavailability and safety concern is related to the size and shape of the nanoformulation. Thus, nanoformulations of the size range of 20–30 nm are adopted as they are easily cleared by the excretory system, and size less than 200 nm is engulfed via the process of phagocytosis [42]. Furthermore, the stability of a nanosystem is also affected by other parameters such as surface charge, and lipophilic character along with various interactions with functional groups of the various other biomacromolecules. These nanoformulations have shown excellent results in cases of safe hemolysis such as thrombocytopenia and lysis of erythrocytes [43]. The formulated nanoformulation might react with plasma protein; thus it will tend to act as a particle of foreign nature. This phenomenon leads to simultaneous galvanization of contingent passage that can cause supersensitive reactions and anaplasia trauma along with various immune reactions such as neural chemotaxis [44].

All these toxicological problems associated with the formulation of plant-based nanoformulation lead to safety challenges. The systems discussed above many are prone to toxicities issues. In order to obtain an ideal plant-based nanoformulation, minor adjustments must be done in various segments such as size, surface charge, lipophilicity, permeability, retention, and allergic reaction, and various immune responses must be handled and discussed so that the plant-based nanoformulation can be designed.

14.3 Applications of Nanotechnology

Various nanoformulations have been developed and are in different phases to cater to the need of clinical requirements [45]. The encapsulation of plant-derived molecules is done easily through nanoformulation due to nanosized, big surface and volume ratio and biophysical characteristics. This will help to improve the pharmacotherapeutics activity of encapsulated plant molecules to a large extent [46]. Sustained drug release along with stability of *in vivo* and immense systemic circulation can be achieved through plant-based molecules charging in the nanocarriers. The other significant advantages of plant derived molecules loaded nanocarriers are versatility, biocompatibility, biodegradability and targetability.

Further, nanotechnology tends to enhance the bioavailability of drugs by modulating the biophysical characteristics like inferior solubility in water along with reduced stable nature with chemicals [47]. Additionally, the loaded drug can be protected through encapsulation, which safeguards the drug from the savage biological surroundings in the passage of systemic circulation, which tends to enhance the bioavailability. Thus, nanocarriers are utilized to deliver drugs with poor solubility and/or stability.

In cancer therapy, the biggest challenge is the limitation of drug permeation in the target tumor cells, which can be overcome by the formulation of plant-based molecule nanomedicine, which tends to improve drug permeation to designated tumor cells [48].

Other applications of nanotechnology are the improvement of drug therapeutic characteristics and reduced ill-effects of drugs because a precise dose is adopted for the procurement of sustained release in tumor cells in which the clearance rate can be minimized.

Furthermore, the toxicity issues of drugs can be resolved by the formulation of nanocarriers as they can modulate and achieve extreme intracellular agglomeration of respective drugs inside the tumor cells which results in high effectiveness in cancer therapy [49].

Drug pharmacokinetic as well as pharmacodynamic activity can be enhanced because the formation of nanocarriers tends to protect plant-based anticancer agents from the excretory processes. Finally, the formulation of these plant-based nano-carriers can reduce the tumor through the formulation of anticancer agents.

Currently, nanotechnology has great capability in cancer treatment in combination with various engineering biologics that enable the development of new techniques, which can be proved through clinical trials in these fields [50].

14.4 Different Types of Formulation

14.4.1 Lipid-Based Formulations

Although polymer-based nanoformulations are one of the best alternatives for sustained-release systems in a clinical setup, toxicity issues and lack of scale-up moderation of polymers have led formulation scientists to work on other substitutes. Moreover, lipids-based systems offer various advantages over polymer systems, such as reduced toxicity, enhanced drug loading capability, biocompatible, biodegradable, and extremely high bioavailability along with sustained release as a well-defined drug delivery system to the main administration site [51]. The various lipid drug delivery systems are discussed in the following subsections.

14.4.1.1 Liposomes

Generally, liposomes are composed of bilayer phospholipids vesicles which are in tapered proportions containing phospholipids and cholesterol for their structural formation in their central core region [52]. This structural formation helps in gathering the main hydrophilic drug inside the core region, whereas bilayers include all hydrophobic proportions in the drug. The most important characteristic of liposomes is to increase the pharmacokinetics of the drug and to help in reducing toxicity with increased effective therapy [53]. The main method of synthesis of liposome is extrusion or sonication in lipid and polymer is mixed in molar proportion to form nanoformulation by the process of extrusion. There is a variety of liposome plant-based nanoformulations of drugs such as quercetin, diospyrin, and nuxvomica, which are studied, formulated, and analyzed shown in Table 14.2. Liposomal formulation of nuxvomica elicited anti-inflammatory, anticancer, and analgesic activity [54]. The responsible alkaloids isolated from the seeds of nuxvomica were brucine and strychnine. Both alkaloids have the profound ability to work in colon cancer by reducing cell multiplication and growth. Inhibition in the maturation of DLD1 xenografted tumor in nude mice was observed when the liposomal formulation of strychnine and brucine was used [55]. Brucine and strychnine can produce inhibitory effects against HepG2 cell multiplication. Various other formulations of liposomal plant-derived molecules have been formulated such as pegylated liposome containing resveratrol and 5-fluorouracil tends to increase the uptake of caspase-3 that leads to apoptosis in the treatment of squamous carcinoma [56]. There are other liposome forms, such as co-loaded liposomal form of Epigallocatechin-3-gallate and paclitaxel, that showed good entrapment ability along with induced apoptosis in the treatment of lung cancer [57]. Further, liposomal encapsulation of curcumin and resveratrol also have shown anticancer and antioxidant activity [58].

14.4.1.2 Solid lipid nanoparticles

Basically, these particles are nanosphere-type carriers that contain a solid and lipid junction (50–1000 nm) which is composed of waxes and triglycerides. Their melting point is more than the body temperature [59]. Generally, these are carrier systems that comprise solid lipids, and various methods employed for manufacturing the same are ultrafiltration, ultrasonication, and surfactant flocculation [60]. Several plant-based solid lipid nanoparticles have been reported for their anticancer outcomes in Table 14.2. Drugs like curcumin and paclitaxel in the form of folate lipid nanoparticle lead to a sustained release of combined drugs in the therapy of osteocarcinoma [61]. A study of lipid nanocapsule of quercetin with Epigallocatechin-3-gallate was eventually performed to enhance the stability, solubility, and further therapeutic activity was enhanced. Further, encapsulation in the form of suspension which is colloidal in nature tends to diminish the oxidation factor of quercetin, and in this way the stability of Epigallocatechin-3-gallate is achieved leading to the formation of a stable suspension [62]. The novel formulations that contain a combination of plant-based molecules and synthetic drugs produce sustained release and minimization of toxicity issues in the treatment of cancer. Solid lipid nanoparticles were also made of curcumin with encapsulation with drugs like aspirin and sulforaphane, which tends to impart enhanced controlled release, and this formulation's low dose helps to decrease cell viability as well as reduced apoptosis in the cell lines [60]. Micellar nanocapsules in the form of Epigallocatechin-3-gallate and Herceptin help good targeting at the tumor and reduce its growth in the breast cancer treatment [63].

14.4.1.3 Double emulsion

This type of formulation is biphasic (oil and aqueous phase) and thermodynamically stable and composed of a dispersed phase distributed in the form of minute globules (0.1–100 μm) in a continuous medium with the help of an emulsifying agent, whereas a nanoemulsion includes the nano size of these minute globules, which helps in achieving controlled release along good penetration the selected plant-based molecules [64]. High-pressure homogenization was utilized to develop these types of formulations [65]. Double emulsion was adopted by Merlin et al. to prepare polylactic glycolic acid nanoparticles of ferulic acid, which showed enhanced action of anticancer property through ferulic acid nanoparticles in terms of simple ferulic acid. The formulation nanoparticles of ferulic acid acts on cell lines of cancer and promote apoptosis that shows the high efficiency of plant-based molecule in the form of a novel drug delivery system [66]. There are varieties of double-based emulsions of plant-based molecules, such as quercetin and docetaxel, which are reported and analyzed for the antioxidant and anticancer properties mentioned in Table 14.2.

Table 14.2 Various lipid plant-based nanoformulation for cancer therapy

Type of nanoformulation	Name of phytoconstituent	Carrier used	Remarks	Refs
Liposome	Quercetin	Phosphatidylethanolamine	Increased medicinal potency and antioxidant activity	[41]
	Nuxvomica	Hydrogenated soybean	High Drug entrapment and increased formulation stability	[54]
	Diospyrin	Dipalmitoyl phosphatidylcholine	Anticancer and increase activity against tumor	[67]
	Curcumin	Dimyristoyl phosphatidylcholine	Excellent drug targeting and cytotoxic effect	[68]
	Resveratrol	Phosphatidylcholine	Cell proliferation inhibition in breast cancer	[69]
	Vincristine and Vinblastine	Triethyl ammonium sucrose octasulfate	Drug targeting and stability enhanced	[70]
Solid lipid nanoparticles	Capsaicin	Stearic acid	Controlled release and enhanced anticancer activity	[71]
	Pomegranate extract	Stearic acid	Enhanced activity	[72]
	Curcumin	Phosphatidylcholine	Enhance stability of formulation	[73]
	Quercetin	Compritol	Enhanced anticancer activity	[74]
Double emulsion	Quercetin	Polylactic glycolic acid	Permeation of drug is improved	[75]
	Docetaxel	Polylactic acid and Polyethylene glycolic acid	Increased the retention time of formed drug	[76]

14.4.2 Polymer-Based Formulation

Despite significant advancements in medical technology, cancer treatment remains difficult due to the low cure rate. To overcome these challenges, nano-size-based formulations have been designed for their controlled delivery. Along with the other approaches, polymeric nanoparticles have also become a choice of delivery platform to carry the nutraceuticals to the target site, especially to elicit their anticancer potential due to the EPR phenomenon [77]. Moreover, to cater to toxicity issues associated with the nano size of formulations [78], various polymers viz. natural or synthetic have been synthesized and evaluated for different cancers [79, 80]. Natural polymeric nanoparticles offer a once-in-a-lifetime potential to make significant advancements in cancer treatment while limiting the negative effects of conventional chemotherapies on patients [81]. Natural substances can interfere with the carcinogenetic process at several stages, including initiation, development, and promotion. It could be utilized further to avoid multidrug resistance developed in conventional combinatorial therapy [82]. Natural chemicals administered through nanoparticles have improved absorption and reduced the toxicity associated with high treatment dosages [83]. Due to the poor solubility of nutraceuticals and thus poor bioavailability, response, or activity is shown in the sub-therapeutic domain. To cater to this, a high dose is needed, which leads to high toxicity associated with dose dependency [84]. So, nanotechnology was utilized and different types viz. micelle, polymerosomes, dendrimers, hybrid of polymeric nanoparticles were formulated and evaluated for their anticancer potential (Fig. 14.1). These nanoparticles can be prepared via emulsification, nano-precipitation, electrospraying, and microfluidic technologies. Moreover, nanoparticles can be functionalized/targeted with different type of ligands viz. small molecules, aptamers and peptides to improve the site specificity, circulation time and overall therapeutic efficacy [85].

Various natural polymers like biomaterials (e.g., chitosan, albumin, dextran, hyaluronic acid) were utilized for the preparation of nanoparticles for the treatment of different cancers [86].

Various advantages like biocompatibility, biodegradability, and non-immunogenicity make these polymers an ideal carrier for loading anticancer nutraceuticals [87]. Various polymers (e.g. Polylactic acid, polyglycolic acid and poly (D,L-lactic-co-glycolic acid)) containing lactic acid and glycolic acid like monomers are widely utilized in encapsulating nutraceuticals. Other polymers (hydrophilic type) like hyaluronic acid (HA) and chitosan are also used for anticancer therapy, where HA is widely utilized as targeted formulation by targeting HA receptors expressed in various cancerous sites. Similarly, nucleic acid-based polymers are also utilized to deliver doxorubicin and curcumin as an anticancer therapy [88]. Moreover, in some situations, the combination of polymers is utilized to formulate a robust delivery system to show a tuned release profile.

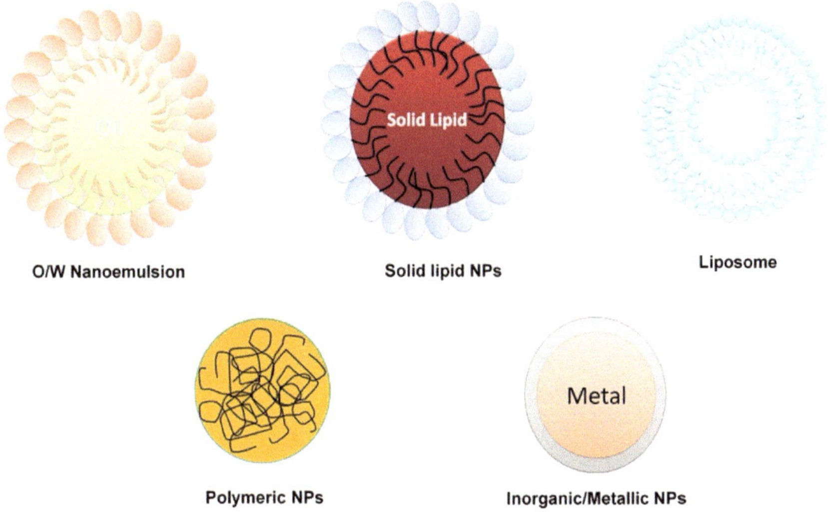

Figure 14.1 Various nanoformulations used for delivering Nutraceuticals.

14.4.2.1 Chitosan

Deacetylation of chitin produces chitosan, a linear cationic amino polysaccharide, which is made up of 1,4 glycosidic linkages that connect N-acetyl-D-glucosamine and -D-glucosamine. It elicits higher biocompatibility, mucoadhesive, antimicrobial, and nontoxic properties than other polymers [88]. However, except at low or acidic pH, chitosan is weakly soluble, limiting its applicability. This challenge can be limited by using synthetic analogs of the parent molecule to control other biological activities. The nanoformulation was prepared with chitosan to target the cancer stem-like cells (CSLCs). This could be explained by the increased internalization of the nanocarrier due to its size (20), which thus leads to more release/diffusion into the cytoplasm, gradually moving into the nucleus and showing its cytotoxicity [89]. Moreover, chitosan can be modified/functionalized to utilize in different novel delivery systems such as microspheres, nanoparticles, hydrogels, and micelles for the treatment of cancer [90]. In one example, chitosan ascorbate nanoparticles were formulated by falsification/ionotropic gelation method and evaluated for the treatment of cervical cancer (evaluated the cell viability in HeLa cell lines) [91]. In another example, siRNA-loaded chitosan nanoparticles were formulated to treat non-small lung cancer by targeting of epidermal growth factor receptor, and it was found that the targeted formulation inhibited tumor growth more effectively than the nontargeted stem-like cancer cells formulation (NSCLC) [92].

Moreover, folic acid-decorated chitosan nanoparticles of curcumin were formulated and successfully evaluated for folate receptor-expressed breast cancer cell lines. Modification of amine groups of chitosan with folic acid significantly modifies the property of parent characteristics of chitosan and turns nanoparticles into a target carrier [93]. Vivek et al. also evaluated the toxicity of curcumin-loaded chitosan NPs and found them more effective in breast cancer cells (MCF-7 cells), wherein they showed more efficacy than free curcumin, while the blank NPs solicited no toxicity in noncancerous L929 cells [94]. Furthermore, glycyrrhetinic acid (GA)-modified chitosan NPs were prepared to target glycyrrhetinic acid receptors of hepatic cells (QGY-7703 cells) for liver cancer treatments [95, 96].

14.4.2.2 Poly (lactic-co-glycolic acid) (PLGA)

Poly (lactic-co-glycolic acid) (PLGA) has been widely employed as a medication carrier approved by the US FDA and European

Medicine Agency in clinical medicine among a variety of biodegradable polymers [97]. It has a promising degrading property that makes it appropriate for hydrophilic or hydrophobic drug sustained release. They can also easily conjugate with specific target molecules, allowing them to change their surface features and increase interactions in order to reach certain tissues or cells. Due to the biodegradability and low toxicity of its monomers, PLGA is widely used in the development of nanomedicine. Currently, it is the most extensively used synthetic polymer in the manufacture of drug-loaded nanoparticles for cancer therapy [98]. It was used in the enhancement of solubility, bioavailability, and therapeutic efficacy of β-sitosterol against breast cancer cells [99]. It was also proved with the example of rutin, when PLGA nanoparticle-loaded drug improved the antioxidant potential and overall efficacy of the treatment of hepatic carcinoma [100].

14.4.2.3 Albumin

Albumin is the most often employed protein-based natural component for cancer medication delivery. In one example, albumin nanoparticles of piceatannol were formulated using a cross-linking agent (glutaraldehyde) and evaluated the toxicity for colon cancer cell lines (CaCo-2 and HT-29 cells). These nanoparticles have shown higher uptake through endocytosis and elucidate improved colon cancer therapeutics. Results of a study showed that albumin nanoparticles suppressed tumor growth in the murine model much more effectively [101].

Jithan et al. created albumin nanoparticles of curcumin to improve the therapeutics of breast cancer. Their experimental study reported that albumin NPs improved the solubility and provides sustained release. These NPs have also shown greater anticancer activity than free curcumin in treating breast carcinoma cells (MDA-MB-231) [102].

14.4.2.4 Gelatin

Gelatin can be used to treat a variety of malignancies as a medication carrier. Karthikeyan et al. formulated gelatin-based resveratrol-loaded nanoparticles and evaluated its therapeutics in lung carcinoma cells, wherein *in vitro* release study elucidated sustained release pattern after the immediate release profile of the drug. Moreover, the drug was quickly absorbed when loaded in nanoformulation and showed higher anticancer activity in Swiss albino mice [103].

14.4.3 Metallic and Other Formulations

Metal nanoparticles are formulations having a size range between 1–100 nm with the advantage of surface charge, dynamic structure, and large surface area. Moreover, owing to nanostructure and surface charge, it can easily interact with the biomolecules thus resulting in better targeting [104]. Positively charged nanoparticles elucidate a higher internalization rate than negatively charged or neutral particles because the interaction with the negative charge exists on the cell membrane [105]. Metal nanoparticles also have different biomedical applications and are also used for diagnostic purposes for imaging cancer cells [106].

A number of metal nanoparticles have been synthesized from different metals such as silver, gold, copper, and platinum that exert anticancerous effects [107]. Gold nanoparticles are an effective carrier system as they are chemically inert and biocompatible. Studies have revealed the use of gold nanoparticles in treating different kinds of cancers, namely colorectal, renal, cervical, leukemia, and bone marrow cancer [108]. Another metal is silver, which was used in ancient times to treat various infectious diseases and also in World War I [109]. Later on, its use in cancer therapy was explored. Many studies have shown the use of silver nanoparticles in breast, prostate, lung, skin, hepatic, cervical, nasopharyngeal, and colorectal cancer. Silver nanoparticles can be developed into different sizes and shapes by utilizing different reducing agents [110]. Similarly, copper nanoparticles are also extensively used as a carrier for delivering anticancer drugs. Moreover, their experimental procedures are simple and economical and can be obtained in high yield [111].

These metallic nanoparticles are also utilized to deliver plant bioactives in cancer therapy. Numerous studies have been conducted by utilizing different metallic formulations of plant bioactive in which gold, silver, and copper metals are used. These formulations show effective results in treating cancer by actively targeting the cancer cells or reducing side effects. Silver nanoparticles of Adenium obesum (Desert Rose) were biosynthesized and acted by generating reactive oxygen species that further induced apoptosis and autophagy. TEM images revealed the size of the particles is between 10 and 30 nm and most of them are spherical. Anticancer activity was investigated on MCF-7 (breast cancer) cell lines. IC50 value was determined to be 217 μg/ml [112]. Copper oxide nanoparticles of black bean extract were synthesized using the green synthesis technique. An *in vitro* anticancer study was performed on the HeLa cell line. The results indicated that copper oxide nanoparticles induce reactive oxygen species depending on dose and reduce cervical cancer [122]. Table 14.3 presents the list of metallic formulations of different plant bioactives.

14.5 Conclusion

This chapter focused on gathering information about nanodelivery systems utilized for carrying nutraceuticals. It is evident, especially in the COVID-19 era, that the whole world is inclined toward the more usage of natural constituents to improve the preventive measures taken against various pathological conditions such as inflammation, cancer, diabetes, and poor immunity-associated disorders. However, due to various limitations like solubility, permeability and stability associated with nutraceuticals, it is difficult to commercialize them in nanoforms. Here, we were able to successfully review the various delivery systems based on nanotechnology such as polymeric, lipidic, and metallic nanoparticles to improve the bioavailability, efficacy, and safety of nutraceuticals. Moreover, various formulations of nutraceuticals based on these novel technologies are available in the market and several others are under study.

Table 14.3 List of metal nanoparticles used for delivering plant bioactives in cancer therapy

Plant bioactive	Metal	Cancer type	Cell line	Size	Shape	Mechanism	Refs.
Curcumin	Gold	Colon Breast	HCT-116 MCF-7	26 nm	Spherical	Improved antiproliferative and apoptotic induction on both cell lines as compared to free curcumin, improved stability	[113]
Resveratrol	Gold	Breast	MCF-7	22.28 ± 2.98 nm	Spherical	Reduced progression of breast cancer by influencing cyclooxygenase-2, nuclear transcription factor-κB, Phosphoinositide 3 kinase	[114]
Quercetin	Gold	Breast	MCF-7, MDA-MB-231	5.2 nm	Spherical	Angiogenesis, migration, invasiveness, and tumor growth	[115]
Paclitaxel	Gold	Breast	MDA-MB-231	61.86 ± 3.01 nm	Spherical	Induced apoptosis with generation of reactive oxygen species that alter mitochondrial membrane potential; deliver the drug to photoacoustic imaging cancer cells	[116]
Moringa oleifera	Silver	Cervical	HeLa	40 nm	Pentagonal and spherical	Act by inducing apoptosis through reactive oxygen species (ROS) generation cervical cancer cell lines	[117]
Camptothecin	Silver	Cervical	HeLa	20 nm	Spherical	Induce cell death by changing permeability of mitochondrial membrane that leads to activation of caspase 9, 6 and 3 and increases ROS formation	[118]
Azadirachta indica	Copper oxide	Cervical	HeLa	12 nm	Spherical	Apoptosis, Increased cell proliferation	[119]
Punica granatum	Silver	Lung	A549	30 nm	Spherical	Execute apoptosis through activation of caspase	[120]
Quercetin	Zinc oxide	Breast	MCF-7	40 nm	Spherical	Induced apoptotic cell death via increasing oxidative stress and mitochondrial damage	[121]

References

1. DeSantis CE, Lin CC, Mariotto AB, Siegel RL, Stein KD, Kramer JL, et al. Cancer treatment and survivorship statistics, 2014. *CA: A Cancer Journal for Clinicians* 2014; 64: 252–71.
2. Housman G, Byler S, Heerboth S, Lapinska K, Longacre M, Snyder N, et al. Drug resistance in cancer: An overview. *Cancers* 2014; 6: 1769–1792.
3. Bishayee A, Sethi G. Bioactive natural products in cancer prevention and therapy: Progress and promise. *Seminars in Cancer Biology* 2016; 40-41: 1–3.
4. Correia RT, Borges KC, Medeiros MF, Genovese MI. Bioactive compounds and phenolic-linked functionality of powdered tropical fruit residues. *Food Science and Technology International* 2012; 18: 539–47.
5. Wang H, Oo Khor T, Shu L, Su Z-Y, Fuentes F, Lee J-H, et al. Plants vs. cancer: A review on natural phytochemicals in preventing and treating cancers and their druggability. *Anti-Cancer Agents in Medicinal Chemistry (Formerly Current Medicinal Chemistry-Anti-Cancer Agents)* 2012; 12: 1281–305.
6. Asensi M, Ortega A, Mena S, Feddi F, Estrela JM. Natural polyphenols in cancer therapy. *Critical Reviews in Clinical Laboratory Sciences* 2011; 48: 197–216.
7. Zoi V, Galani V, Lianos GD, Voulgaris S, Kyritsis AP, Alexiou GA. The role of curcumin in cancer treatment. *Biomedicines* 2021; 9: 1086.
8. Ko J-H, Sethi G, Um J-Y, Shanmugam MK, Arfuso F, Kumar AP, et al. The role of resveratrol in cancer therapy. *International Journal of Molecular Sciences* 2017; 18: 2589.
9. Tang S-M, Deng X-T, Zhou J, Li Q-P, Ge X-X, Miao L. Pharmacological basis and new insights of quercetin action in respect to its anti-cancer effects. *Biomedicine & Pharmacotherapy* 2020; 121: 109604.
10. Zhu L, Chen L. Progress in research on paclitaxel and tumor immunotherapy. *Cellular & Molecular Biology Letters* 2019; 24: 1–11.
11. Najar IA, Johri RK. Pharmaceutical and pharmacological approaches for bioavailability enhancement of etoposide. *Journal of Biosciences* 2014; 39: 139–44.
12. Amiri F, Zarnani A-H, Zand H, Koohdani F, Jeddi-Tehrani M, Vafa M. Synergistic anti-proliferative effect of resveratrol and etoposide on

human hepatocellular and colon cancer cell lines. *European Journal of Pharmacology* 2013; 718: 34–40.

13. Mansourizadeh F, Alberti D, Bitonto V, Tripepi M, Sepehri H, Khoee S, et al. Efficient synergistic combination effect of Quercetin with Curcumin on breast cancer cell apoptosis through their loading into Apo ferritin cavity. *Colloids and Surfaces B: Biointerfaces* 2020; 191: 110982.
14. Mohan L, Raghav D, Ashraf SM, Sebastian J, Rathinasamy K. Indirubin, a bis-indole alkaloid binds to tubulin and exhibits antimitotic activity against HeLa cells in synergism with vinblastine. *Biomedicine & Pharmacotherapy* 2018; 105: 506–17.
15. Majumdar AP, Banerjee S, Nautiyal J, Patel BB, Patel V, Du J, et al. Curcumin synergizes with resveratrol to inhibit colon cancer. *Nutrition and Cancer* 2009; 61: 544–53.
16. Singh CK, Chhabra G, Ndiaye MA, Siddiqui IA, Panackal JE, Mintie CA, et al. Quercetin–resveratrol combination for prostate cancer management in TRAMP mice. *Cancers* 2020; 12: 2141.
17. Kang Y, Hu W, Bai E, Zheng H, Liu Z, Wu J, et al. Curcumin sensitizes human gastric cancer cells to 5-fluorouracil through inhibition of the NFκB survival-signaling pathway. *Onco Targets and Therapy* 2016; 9: 7373.
18. Yu J, Ma Y, Drisko J, Chen Q. Antitumor activities of Rauwolfia vomitoria extract and potentiation of carboplatin effects against ovarian cancer. *Current Therapeutic Research* 2013; 75: 8–14.
19. Zanini C, Giribaldi G, Mandili G, Carta F, Crescenzio N, Bisaro B, et al. Inhibition of heat shock proteins (HSP) expression by quercetin and differential doxorubicin sensitization in neuroblastoma and Ewing's sarcoma cell lines. *Journal of Neurochemistry* 2007; 103: 1344–54.
20. Wen C, Wu L, Fu L, Zhang X, Zhou H. Berberine enhances the anti-tumor activity of tamoxifen in drug-sensitive MCF-7 and drug-resistant MCF-7/TAM cells. *Molecular Medicine Reports* 2016; 14: 2250–6.
21. Montopoli M, Ragazzi E, Froldi G, Caparrotta L. Cell-cycle inhibition and apoptosis induced by curcumin and cisplatin or oxaliplatin in human ovarian carcinoma cells. *Cell Proliferation* 2009; 42: 195–206.
22. Lu J-J, Cai Y-J, Ding J. Curcumin induces DNA damage and caffeine-insensitive cell cycle arrest in colorectal carcinoma HCT116 cells. *Molecular and Cellular Biochemistry* 2011; 354: 247–52.

23. Ramachandran C, Fonseca HB, Jhabvala P, Escalon EA, Melnick SJ. Curcumin inhibits telomerase activity through human telomerase reverse transcritpase in MCF-7 breast cancer cell line. *Cancer Letters* 2002; 184: 1–6.

24. Linsalata M, Orlando A, Messa C, Refolo MG, Russo F. Quercetin inhibits human DLD-1 colon cancer cell growth and polyamine biosynthesis. *Anticancer Research* 2010; 30: 3501–7.

25. Huisman C, Ferreira CG, Bröker LE, Rodriguez JA, Smit EF, Postmus PE, et al. Paclitaxel triggers cell death primarily via caspase-independent routes in the non-small cell lung cancer cell line NCI-H460. *Clinical Cancer Research* 2002; 8: 596–606.

26. Tan L, Wang W, He G, Kuick RD, Gossner G, Kueck AS, et al. Resveratrol inhibits ovarian tumor growth in an *in vivo* mouse model. *Cancer* 2016; 122: 722–9.

27. Choi K-C, Park S, Lim BJ, Sung A-R, Lee Y-H, Shiota M, et al. Procyanidin B3, an inhibitor of histone acetyltransferase, enhances the action of antagonist for prostate cancer cells via inhibition of p300-dependent acetylation of androgen receptor. *Biochemical Journal* 2011; 433: 235–44.

28. Timur M, Akbas SH, Ozben T. The effect of Topotecan on oxidative stress in MCF-7 human breast cancer cell line. *Acta Biochimica Polonica* 2005; 52: 897–902.

29. Liao Y-C, Shih Y-W, Chao C-H, Lee X-Y, Chiang T-A. Involvement of the ERK signaling pathway in fisetin reduces invasion and migration in the human lung cancer cell line A549. *Journal of Agricultural and Food Chemistry* 2009; 57: 8933–41.

30. Kwon GT, Jung JI, Song HR, Woo EY, Jun J-G, Kim J-K, et al. Piceatannol inhibits migration and invasion of prostate cancer cells: Possible mediation by decreased interleukin-6 signaling. *The Journal of Nutritional Biochemistry* 2012; 23: 228–38.

31. He Z, Li B, Rankin GO, Rojanasakul Y, Chen YC. Selecting bioactive phenolic compounds as potential agents to inhibit proliferation and VEGF expression in human ovarian cancer cells. *Oncology Letters* 2015; 9: 1444–50.

32. Qi W, Weber CR, Wasland K, Savkovic SD. Genistein inhibits proliferation of colon cancer cells by attenuating a negative effect of epidermal growth factor on tumor suppressor FOXO3 activity. *BMC Cancer* 2011; 11: 1–9.

33. Cragg G, Kingston D, Newman D. *Anticancer Agents from Natural Products*, ed 2. Boca Raton, CRC. Taylor & Francis, 2012.

34. Jeetah R, Bhaw-Luximon A, Jhurry D. Nanopharmaceutics: Phyto-chemical-based controlled or sustained drug-delivery systems for cancer treatment. *Journal of Biomedical Nanotechnology* 2014; 10: 1810–40.

35. Leonarduzzi G, Testa G, Sottero B, Gamba P, Poli G. Design and development of nanovehicle-based delivery systems for preventive or therapeutic supplementation with flavonoids. *Current Medicinal Chemistry* 2010; 17: 74–95.

36. Adhami VM, Mukhtar H. Human cancer chemoprevention: hurdles and challenges. In: Pezzuto, J., Suh, N. (eds) *Natural Products in Cancer Prevention and Therapy. Topics in Current Chemistry*, Springer, Berlin, Heidelberg. 2012; 329: 203–20.

37. Khan N, Adhami VM, Siddiqui IA, Bharali DJ, Mousa SA, Mukhtar H. Oral administration of naturally occurring chitosan based nanoformulated green tea polyphenol EGCG effectively inhibits prostate cancer cell growth in a xenograft model. AACR; In: *Proceedings of the 103rd Annual Meeting of the American Association for Cancer Research*; 2012 Mar 31–Apr 4; Chicago, IL. Philadelphia (PA): Cancer Res 2012; 72(8 Suppl): Abstract nr 5438.

38. Majumdar D, Jung KH, Zhang H, Nannapaneni S, Wang X, Amin AR, et al. Luteolin nanoparticle in chemoprevention: *In vitro* and *in vivo* anticancer activity. *Cancer Prevention Research (Philadelphia, Pa)* 2014; 7: 65–73.

39. Rodriguez-Mateos A, Vauzour D, Krueger CG, Shanmuganayagam D, Reed J, Calani L, et al. Bioavailability, bioactivity and impact on health of dietary flavonoids and related compounds: An update. *Archives of Toxicology* 2014; 88: 1803–53.

40. Rahman M, Beg S, Ahmed A, Swain S. Emergence of functionalized nanomedicines in cancer chemotherapy: Recent advancements, current challenges and toxicity considerations. *Recent Patents on Nanomedicine* 2013; 3: 128–39.

41. Ghosh D, Ghosh S, Sarkar S, Ghosh A, Das N, Saha KD, et al. Quercetin in vesicular delivery systems: Evaluation in combating arsenic-induced acute liver toxicity associated gene expression in rat model. *Chemico-Biological Interactions* 2010; 186: 61–71.

42. Moghimi SM, Hunter AC, Murray JC. Long-circulating and target-specific nanoparticles: Theory to practice. *Pharmacological Reviews* 2001; 53: 283–318.

43. Dobrovolskaia MA, McNeil SE. Immunological properties of engineered nanomaterials. *Nature Nanotechnology*: 2007; 2: 469–78.

44. Dobrovolskaia MA, Aggarwal P, Hall JB, McNeil SE. Preclinical studies to understand nanoparticle interaction with the immune system and its potential effects on nanoparticle biodistribution. *Molecular Pharmaceutics* 2008; 5: 487–95.

45. Bertrand N, Wu J, Xu X, Kamaly N, Farokhzad OC. Cancer nanotechnology: The impact of passive and active targeting in the era of modern cancer biology. *Advanced Drug Delivery Reviews* 2014; 66: 2–25.

46. Sun T, Zhang YS, Pang B, Hyun DC, Yang M, Xia Y. Engineered nanoparticles for drug delivery in cancer therapy. *Angewandte Chemie.* 2014; 53: 12320–64.

47. Peer D, Karp JM, Hong S, Farokhzad OC, Margalit R, Langer R. Nanocarriers as an emerging platform for cancer therapy. Balogh LP (ed) *Nano-Enabled Medical Applications*, Jenny Stanford Publishing. 2020: 61–91.

48. Brigger I, Dubernet C, Couvreur P. Nanoparticles in cancer therapy and diagnosis. *Advanced Drug Delivery Reviews* 2012; 64: 24–36.

49. Markman JL, Rekechenetskiy A, Holler E, Ljubimova JY. Nanomedicine therapeutic approaches to overcome cancer drug resistance. *Advanced Drug Delivery Reviews* 2013; 65: 1866–79.

50. Estanqueiro M, Amaral MH, Conceição J, Lobo JMS. Nanotechnological carriers for cancer chemotherapy: The state of the art. *Colloids and surfaces B: Biointerfaces* 2015; 126: 631–48.

51. Muller RH, Keck CM. Challenges and solutions for the delivery of biotech drugs—a review of drug nanocrystal technology and lipid nanoparticles. *Journal of Biotechnology* 2004; 113: 151–70.

52. Akbarzadeh A, Rezaei-Sadabady R, Davaran S, Joo SW, Zarghami N, Hanifehpour Y, et al. Liposome: Classification, preparation, and applications. *Nanoscale Research Letters* 2013; 8: 1–9.

53. Anselmo AC, Mitragotri S. Nanoparticles in the clinic. *Bioengineering & Translational Medicine* 2016; 1: 10–29.

54. Chen J, Lin A, Chen Z, Wang W, Zhang T, Cai H, et al. Ammonium sulfate gradient loading of brucine into liposomes: Effect of phospholipid composition on entrapment efficiency and physicochemical properties *in vitro*. *Drug Development and Industrial Pharmacy* 2010; 36: 245–53.

55. Ruiz-Torres V, Encinar JA, Herranz-López M, Pérez-Sánchez A, Galiano V, Barrajón-Catalán E, et al. An updated review on marine anticancer compounds: The use of virtual screening for the discovery of small-molecule cancer drugs. *Molecules* 2017; 22: 1037.

56. Mohan A, Narayanan S, Sethuraman S, Krishnan UM. Novel resveratrol and 5-fluorouracil coencapsulated in PEGylated nanoliposomes improve chemotherapeutic efficacy of combination against head and neck squamous cell carcinoma. *BioMed Research International* 2014; 2014: 1–14.

57. Ramadass SK, Anantharaman NV, Subramanian S, Sivasubramanian S, Madhan B. Paclitaxel/epigallocatechin gallate coloaded liposome: A synergistic delivery to control the invasiveness of MDA-MB-231 breast cancer cells. *Colloids and Surfaces B: Biointerfaces* 2015; 125: 65–72.

58. Narayanan NK, Nargi D, Randolph C, Narayanan BA. Liposome encapsulation of curcumin and resveratrol in combination reduces prostate cancer incidence in PTEN knockout mice. *International Journal of Cancer* 2009; 125: 1–8.

59. Wissing SA, Müller RH. The influence of solid lipid nanoparticles on skin hydration and viscoelasticity—*in vivo* study. *European Journal of Pharmaceutics and Biopharmaceutics* 2003; 56: 67–72.

60. Grandhi BK, Thakkar A, Wang J, Prabhu S. A novel combinatorial nanotechnology-based oral chemopreventive regimen demonstrates significant suppression of pancreatic cancer neoplastic lesions. *Cancer Prevention Research* 2013; 6: 1015–25.

61. Baek J-S, Cho C-W. A multifunctional lipid nanoparticle for co-delivery of paclitaxel and curcumin for targeted delivery and enhanced cytotoxicity in multidrug resistant breast cancer cells. *Oncotarget* 2017; 8: 30369.

62. Barras A, Mezzetti A, Richard A, Lazzaroni S, Roux S, Melnyk P, et al. Formulation and characterization of polyphenol-loaded lipid nanocapsules. *International Journal of Pharmaceutics* 2009; 379: 270–7.

63. Chung JE, Tan S, Gao SJ, Yongvongsoontorn N, Kim SH, Lee JH, et al. Self-assembled micellar nanocomplexes comprising green tea catechin derivatives and protein drugs for cancer therapy. *Nature Nanotechnology* 2014; 9: 907–12.

64. Bayón-Cordero L, Alkorta I, Arana L. Application of solid lipid nanoparticles to improve the efficiency of anticancer drugs. *Nanomaterials* 2019; 9: 474.

65. Sharma M. Applications of nanotechnology based dosage forms for delivery of herbal drugs. *Research and Reviews: Journal of Pharmaceutics and Nanotechnology* 2014; 2: 23–30.

66. Merlin JJ, Prasad NR, Shibli S. Ferulic acid loaded poly-d,l-lactide-co-glycolide nanoparticles: Systematic study of particle size, drug encapsulation efficiency and anticancer effect in non-small cell lung carcinoma cell line *in vitro*. *Biomedicine & Preventive Nutrition* 2012; 2: 69–76.

67. Hazra B, Kumar B, Biswas S, Pandey B, Mishra K. Enhancement of the tumour inhibitory activity, *in vivo*, of diospyrin, a plant-derived quinonoid, through liposomal encapsulation. *Toxicology Letters* 2005; 157: 109–17.

68. Thangapazham RL, Puri A, Tele S, Blumenthal R, Maheshwari RK. Evaluation of a nanotechnology-based carrier for delivery of curcumin in prostate cancer cells. *International Journal of Oncology* 2008; 32: 1119–23.

69. Meng J, Guo F, Xu H, Liang W, Wang C, Yang X-D. Combination therapy using co-encapsulated resveratrol and paclitaxel in liposomes for drug resistance reversal in breast cancer cells *in vivo*. *Scientific Reports* 2016; 6: 1–11.

70. Noble CO, Guo Z, Hayes ME, Marks JD, Park JW, Benz CC, et al. Characterization of highly stable liposomal and immunoliposomal formulations of vincristine and vinblastine. *Cancer Chemotherapy and Pharmacology* 2009; 64: 741–51.

71. Kunjiappan S, Sankaranarayanan M, Kumar BK, Pavadai P, Babkiewicz E, Maszczyk P, et al. Capsaicin-loaded solid lipid nanoparticles: Design, biodistribution, in silico modeling and *in vitro* cytotoxicity evaluation. *Nanotechnology* 2020; 32: 095101.

72. Badawi NM, Teaima MH, El-Say KM, Attia DA, El-Nabarawi MA, Elmazar MM. Pomegranate extract-loaded solid lipid nanoparticles: Design, optimization, and *in vitro* cytotoxicity study. *International Journal of Nanomedicine* 2018; 13: 1313.

73. Battaglia L, Gallarate M. Lipid nanoparticles: State of the art, new preparation methods and challenges in drug delivery. *Expert Opinion on Drug Delivery* 2012; 9: 497–508.

74. Niazvand F, Orazizadeh M, Khorsandi L, Abbaspour M, Mansouri E, Khodadadi A. Effects of quercetin-loaded nanoparticles on MCF-7 human breast cancer cells. *Medicina* 2019; 55: 114.

75. Malik P, Shankar R, Malik V, Sharma N, Mukherjee TK. Green chemistry based benign routes for nanoparticle synthesis. *Journal of Nanoparticles* 2014; 2014: 1–14.

76. Kumar S, Dilbaghi N, Saharan R, Bhanjana G. Nanotechnology as emerging tool for enhancing solubility of poorly water-soluble drugs. *Bionanoscience* 2012; 2: 227–50.

77. Kapoor DN, Bhatia A, Kaur R, Sharma R, Kaur G, Dhawan S. PLGA: A unique polymer for drug delivery. *Therapeutic Delivery* 2015; 6: 41–58.
78. Khan I, Saeed K, Khan I. Nanoparticles: Properties, applications and toxicities. *Arabian Journal of Chemistry* 2019; 12: 908–31.
79. Tan H-L, Teow S-Y, Pushpamalar J. Application of metal nanoparticle–hydrogel composites in tissue regeneration. *Bioengineering* 2019; 6: 17.
80. Yew YP, Shameli K, Mohamad SEB, Nagao Y, Teow S-Y, Lee KX, et al. Potential anticancer activity of protocatechuic acid loaded in montmorillonite/Fe_3O_4 nanocomposites stabilized by seaweed *Kappaphycus alvarezii*. *International Journal of Pharmaceutics* 2019; 572: 118743.
81. Cuenca AG, Jiang H, Hochwald SN, Delano M, Cance WG, Grobmyer SR. Emerging implications of nanotechnology on cancer diagnostics and therapeutics. *Cancer* 2006; 107: 459–66.
82. Nie S, Xing Y, Kim GJ, Simons JW. Nanotechnology applications in cancer. *Annual Review of Biomedical Engineering* 2007; 9: 257–88.
83. Ferrari M. Cancer nanotechnology: Opportunities and challenges. *Nature Reviews Cancer* 2005; 5: 161–71.
84. Issa AY, Volate SR, Wargovich MJ. The role of phytochemicals in inhibition of cancer and inflammation: New directions and perspectives. *Journal of Food Composition and Analysis* 2006; 19: 405–19.
85. Wong KH, Lu A, Chen X, Yang Z. Natural ingredient-based polymeric nanoparticles for cancer treatment. *Molecules* 2020; 25: 3620.
86. Sohail R, Abbas SR. Evaluation of amygdalin-loaded alginate-chitosan nanoparticles as biocompatible drug delivery carriers for anticancerous efficacy. *International Journal of Biological Macromolecules* 2020; 153: 36–45.
87. Darge HF, Andrgie AT, Tsai H-C, Lai J-Y. Polysaccharide and polypeptide based injectable thermo-sensitive hydrogels for local biomedical applications. *International Journal of Biological Macromolecules* 2019; 133: 545–63.
88. Thummarati P, Suksiriworapong J, Sakchaisri K, Junyaprasert VB. Effect of chemical linkers of curcumin conjugated hyaluronic acid on nanoparticle properties and *in vitro* performances in various cancer cells. *Journal of Drug Delivery Science and Technology* 2021; 61: 102323.

89. Benhabiles M, Salah R, Lounici H, Drouiche N, Goosen M, Mameri N. Antibacterial activity of chitin, chitosan and its oligomers prepared from shrimp shell waste. *Food Hydrocolloids* 2012; 29: 48–56.

90. Argüelles-Monal WM, Lizardi-Mendoza J, Fernández-Quiroz D, Recillas-Mota MT, Montiel-Herrera M. Chitosan derivatives: Introducing new functionalities with a controlled molecular architecture for innovative materials. *Polymers* 2018; 10: 342.

91. Sekar V, Rajendran K, Vallinayagam S, Deepak V, Mahadevan S. Synthesis and characterization of chitosan ascorbate nanoparticles for therapeutic inhibition for cervical cancer and their in silico modeling. *Journal of Industrial and Engineering Chemistry* 2018; 62: 239–49.

92. Nascimento AV, Singh A, Bousbaa H, Ferreira D, Sarmento B, Amiji MM. Mad2 checkpoint gene silencing using epidermal growth factor receptor-targeted chitosan nanoparticles in non-small cell lung cancer model. *Molecular Pharmaceutics* 2014; 11: 3515–27.

93. Wu Z, Lu J, Wang X, Hu B, Ye H, Fan J, et al. Optimization for production of exopolysaccharides with antitumor activity *in vitro* from *Paecilomyces hepiali*. *Carbohydrate Polymers* 2014; 99: 226–34.

94. Vivek R, Babu VN, Thangam R, Subramanian K, Kannan S. pH-responsive drug delivery of chitosan nanoparticles as Tamoxifen carriers for effective anti-tumor activity in breast cancer cells. *Colloids and Surfaces B: Biointerfaces* 2013; 111: 117–23.

95. Sheng-Jun M, Yue-Qi B, Hui J, Da-Peng W, Ru H, Shi-Xiang H. Preparation, characterization and uptake by primary cultured rat hepatocytes of liposomes surface-modified with glycyrrhetinic acid. *Die Pharmazie-An International Journal of Pharmaceutical Sciences* 2007; 62: 614–9.

96. Tian Q, Zhang C-N, Wang X-H, Wang W, Huang W, Cha R-T, et al. Glycyrrhetinic acid-modified chitosan/poly (ethylene glycol) nanoparticles for liver-targeted delivery. *Biomaterials* 2010; 31: 4748–56.

97. Chaubal M. Polylactides/glycolides-excipients for injectable drug delivery and beyond. *Drug Delivery Technology* 2002; 2: 34–6.

98. Loureiro JA, Pereira MC. PLGA based drug carrier and pharmaceutical applications: the most recent advances. *Pharmaceutics* 2020; 12: 1–5.

99. Andima M, Costabile G, Isert L, Ndakala AJ, Derese S, Merkel OM. Evaluation of β-Sitosterol loaded PLGA and PEG-PLA nanoparticles

for effective treatment of breast cancer: Preparation, physicochemical characterization, and antitumor activity. *Pharmaceutics* 2018; 10: 232.

100. Pandey P, Rahman M, Bhatt PC, Beg S, Paul B, Hafeez A, et al. Implication of nano-antioxidant therapy for treatment of hepatocellular carcinoma using PLGA nanoparticles of rutin. *Nanomedicine* 2018; 13: 849–70.

101. Aljabali AAA, Bakshi HA, Hakkim FL, Haggag YA, Al-Batanyeh KM, Al Zoubi MS, et al. Albumin nano-encapsulation of piceatannol enhances its anticancer potential in colon cancer via downregulation of nuclear p65 and HIF-1α. *Cancers* 2020; 12: 113.

102. Jithan A, Madhavi K, Madhavi M, Prabhakar K. Preparation and characterization of albumin nanoparticles encapsulating curcumin intended for the treatment of breast cancer. *International Journal of Pharmaceutical Investigation* 2011; 1: 119.

103. Karthikeyan S, Prasad NR, Ganamani A, Balamurugan E. Anticancer activity of resveratrol-loaded gelatin nanoparticles on NCI-H460 non-small cell lung cancer cells. *Biomedicine & Preventive Nutrition* 2013; 3: 64–73.

104. Rai M, Ingle AP, Birla S, Yadav A, Santos CAD. Strategic role of selected noble metal nanoparticles in medicine. *Critical Reviews in Microbiology* 2016; 42: 696–719.

105. Jurj A, Braicu C, Pop L-A, Tomuleasa C, Gherman CD, Berindan-Neagoe I. The new era of nanotechnology, an alternative to change cancer treatment. *Drug Design, Development and Therapy* 2017; 11: 2871.

106. Sharma A, Goyal AK, Rath G. Recent advances in metal nanoparticles in cancer therapy. *Journal of Drug Targeting* 2018; 26: 617–32.

107. Yang N, Gong F, Zhou Y, Hao Y, Dong Z, Lei H, et al. A general In-Situ reduction method to prepare core-shell liquid-metal/metal nanoparticles for photothermally enhanced catalytic cancer therapy. *Biomaterials* 2021; 277: 121125.

108. Raghunandan D, Ravishankar B, Sharanbasava G, Mahesh DB, Harsoor V, Yalagatti MS, et al. Anti-cancer studies of noble metal nanoparticles synthesized using different plant extracts. *Cancer Nanotechnology* 2011; 2: 57–65.

109. Bondarenko O, Juganson K, Ivask A, Kasemets K, Mortimer M, Kahru A. Toxicity of Ag, CuO and ZnO nanoparticles to selected environmentally relevant test organisms and mammalian cells *in vitro*: A critical review. *Archives of Toxicology* 2013; 87: 1181–200.

110. Khodashenas B, Ghorbani HR. Synthesis of silver nanoparticles with different shapes. *Arabian Journal of Chemistry* 2019; 12: 1823–38.

111. Halevas E, Pantazaki A. Copper nanoparticles as therapeutic anticancer agents. *Nanomedicine and Nanotechnology Journal* 2018; 2: 119–39.

112. Farah MA, Ali MA, Chen S-M, Li Y, Al-Hemaid FM, Abou-Tarboush FM, et al. Silver nanoparticles synthesized from *Adenium obesum* leaf extract induced DNA damage, apoptosis and autophagy via generation of reactive oxygen species. *Colloids and Surfaces B: Biointerfaces* 2016; 141: 158–69.

113. Elbialy NS, Abdelfatah EA, Khalil WA. Antitumor activity of curcumin-green synthesized gold nanoparticles: *In vitro* study. *BioNanoScience* 2019; 9: 813–20.

114. Park SY, Chae SY, Park JO, Lee KJ, Park G. Gold-conjugated resveratrol nanoparticles attenuate the invasion and MMP-9 and COX-2 expression in breast cancer cells. *Oncology Reports* 2016; 35: 3248–56.

115. Balakrishnan S, Bhat F, Raja Singh P, Mukherjee S, Elumalai P, Das S, et al. Gold nanoparticle–conjugated quercetin inhibits epithelial–mesenchymal transition, angiogenesis and invasiveness via EGFR/VEGFR-2-mediated pathway in breast cancer. *Cell Proliferation* 2016; 49: 678–97.

116. Manivasagan P, Bharathiraja S, Bui NQ, Lim IG, Oh J. Paclitaxel-loaded chitosan oligosaccharide-stabilized gold nanoparticles as novel agents for drug delivery and photoacoustic imaging of cancer cells. *International Journal of Pharmaceutics* 2016; 511: 367–79.

117. Vasanth K, Ilango K, MohanKumar R, Agrawal A, Dubey GP. Anticancer activity of Moringa oleifera mediated silver nanoparticles on human cervical carcinoma cells by apoptosis induction. *Colloids and Surfaces B: Biointerfaces* 2014; 117: 354–9.

118. Yuan Y-G, Zhang S, Hwang J-Y, Kong I-K. Silver nanoparticles potentiates cytotoxicity and apoptotic potential of camptothecin in human cervical cancer cells. *Oxidative Medicine and Cellular Longevity* 2018; 2018: 1–21.

119. Rehana D, Mahendiran D, Kumar RS, Rahiman AK. Evaluation of antioxidant and anticancer activity of copper oxide nanoparticles synthesized using medicinally important plant extracts. *Biomedicine & Pharmacotherapy* 2017; 89: 1067–77.

120. Padinjarathil H, Joseph MM, Unnikrishnan B, Preethi G, Shiji R, Archana M, et al. Galactomannan endowed biogenic silver nanoparticles exposed enhanced cancer cytotoxicity with excellent biocompatibility. *International Journal of Biological Macromolecules* 2018; 118: 1174–82.

121. Sadhukhan P, Kundu M, Chatterjee S, Ghosh N, Manna P, Das J, et al. Targeted delivery of quercetin via pH-responsive zinc oxide nanoparticles for breast cancer therapy. *Materials Science and Engineering: C* 2019; 100: 129–40.

122. Nagajyothi PC, Muthuraman P, Sreekanth TVM, Kim DH, Shim J. Green synthesis: In-vitro anticancer activity of copper oxide nanoparticles against human cervical carcinoma cells. *Arabian Journal of Chemistry*. 2017; 10: 215–225.

Multiple-Choice Questions

1. Quercetin is a ____________ compound.
   a. Flavonoid
   b. Lipid
   c. Carbohydrate
   d. None
2. A well-known example of taxanes is ____________.
   a. Paclitaxel
   b. Docetaxel
   c. Both a & b
   d. None of these
3. Nanotechnology improves the ___________ of nutraceuticals.
   a. Solubility
   b. Stability
   c. Permeability
   d. All of the above
4. Paclitaxel act as an anticancer agent with the mechanism of ____________.
   a. Resisting microtubulin depolymerization
   b. Inhibiting DNA Topoisomerase II
   c. Both a and b
   d. None

5. Etoposide acts as an anticancer agent with the mechanism of ____________.
   a. Resisting microtubulin depolymerization
   b. Inhibiting DNA Topoisomerase II
   c. Both a and b
   d. None
6. The major issue of polyphenolic bioactive is ____________.
   a. High Solubility
   b. Poor solubility
   c. Sustained release
   d. All of the above
7. Enhanced permeation and retention phenomenon is a type of ____________.
   a. Active transport
   b. Passive transport
   c. Both a and b
   d. None
8. Nanoparticles having size less than 200 nm are engulfed by ____________
   a. Pinocytosis
   b. Phagocytosis
   c. Both a and b
   d. None
9. Curcumin is extracted from ____________
   a. *Taxus brevifolia*
   b. *Curcumin longa*
   c. Both a and b
   d. None
10. Liposome can load ____________ type of nutraceuticals
    a. Hydrophilic
    b. Hydrophobic
    c. Both a and b
    d. None of the above
11. How can one make a drug-targeted delivery system?
    a. Ideal size of the carrier
    b. Specific site ligand

c. Both a and b
d. None of these

12. Nanoparticles can be prepared by ___________.
    a. Electrospraying
    b. Nanoprecipitation
    c. Microfluidization
    d. All of the above
13. Different types of ligands (aptamers and peptides) are used in ___________.
    a. Active targeting
    b. Passive targeting
    c. Both a and b
    d. None
14. Major component of liposomes are ___________.
    a. Phospholipid
    b. Cholesterol
    c. Both a and b
    d. None
15. Hyaluronic acid is an example of ___________ polymer.
    a. Hydrophilic
    b. Hydrophobic
    c. Both a and b
    d. None of the above
16. Glutaraldehyde is an example of___________.
    a. Surface active agent
    b. Cross-linking agent
    c. Both a and b
    d. None of these
17. Chitosan is an example of___________.
    a. Carbohydrate
    b. Protein
    c. Fatty acid
    d. Vitamin
18. Albumin is an example of___________.
    a. Carbohydrate
    b. Protein

c. Fatty acid
d. Vitamin

19. ____________ charged particles show higher internalization.

a. Positively
b. Negatively
c. Neutral
d. All of these

20. Which type of nanoparticles (NPs) are treated as an ideal candidates for the delivery of cancer?

a. Polymeric NPs
b. Solid lipid NPs
c. Metallic NPs
d. All of these

21. *Adenium obesum* is also known as______________.

a. Milk Thistle
b. Desert Rose
c. Both a and b
d. None

22. HeLa cells are an example of______________ cancer cell lines.

a. Cervical
b. Breast
c. Colon
d. Lung

23. MCF-7 cells are an example of_____________ cancer cell lines.

a. Cervical
b. Breast
c. Colon
d. Lung

24. Which monomers are used to synthesize PLGA?

a. Glycolic acid
b. Lactic acid
c. Both a and b
d. All of these

25. Glycyrrhetinic acid receptors are present on _________ cells
    a. Lung
    b. Kidney
    c. Breast
    d. Hepatic

Answer Key

1.	a	**2.**	c	**3.**	d	**4.**	b	**5.**	d	**6.**	b	**7.**	b
8.	b	**9.**	b	**10.**	c	**11.**	c	**12.**	d	**13.**	a	**14.**	c
15.	a	**16.**	b	**17.**	a	**18.**	b	**19.**	a	**20.**	a	**21.**	b
22.	a	**23.**	b	**24.**	c	**25.**	d						

Short-Answer-Type Questions

1. Elaborate on various applications of nanotechnology in delivering nutraceuticals.
2. Delineate the role of nanonutraceuticals in cancer research.
3. How can be physiochemical properties of hydrophobic nutraceuticals improved?
4. Elaborate various types of nutraceuticals.
5. Explain the advantage of lipidic formulations in overcoming the challenges of nutraceuticals.
6. Delineate the role of metallic nanoparticles in delivering nutraceuticals.
7. Write a note on polymeric nanonutraceuticals.

Long-Answer-Type Questions

1. Explain the different challenges to delivering bioactives, especially in cancer.
2. Elaborate on various nanoformulations developed for the delivery of nutraceuticals.
3. Delineate the role of nanotechnology in the treatment of cancer.

Index